KU-320-693

Handbook of Cancer Chemotherapy

Fifth Edition

Handbook of Cancer Chemotherapy

Fifth Edition

Edited by

Roland T. Skeel, M.D.
Chief of Hematology and Oncology
Richard D. Ruppert Health Center, Toledo, Ohio

LIPPINCOTT WILLIAMS & WILKINS
A **Wolters Kluwer** Company
Philadelphia · Baltimore · New York · London
Buenos Aires · Hong Kong · Sydney · Tokyo

Developmental Editor: Sara Lauber
Manufacturing Manager: Kevin Watt
Production Manager: Robert Pancotti
Production Editor: Brandy Mui
Cover Designer: Jeane Norton
Indexer: Lisa Mullenneaux
Compositor: Circle Graphics
Printer: RR Donnelley-Crawfordsville

© 1999, by Lippincott Williams & Wilkins. All rights reserved. This book is
protected by copyright. No part of it may be reproduced, stored in a retrieval
system, or transmitted, in any form or by any means—electronic, mechanical,
photocopy, recording, or otherwise—without the prior written consent of the
publisher, except for brief quotations embodied in critical articles and reviews.
For information write **Lippincott Williams & Wilkins, 227 East
Washington Square, Philadelphia, PA 19106-3780.**
     Materials appearing in this book prepared by individuals as part of
their official duties as U.S. Government employees are not covered by the
above-mentioned copyright.

Printed in the United States of America
9 8 7 6 5 4 3 2

Library of Congress Cataloging-in-Publication Data
Handbook of cancer chemotherapy/Roland T. Skeel, editor
          p. cm
     Includes bibliographical references and index.
     ISBN: 0-7817-1617-9 (paperback)
     1. Cancer—Chemotherapy—Handbooks, manuals, etc.   I. Skeel, Roland T.
     [DNLM: 1. Neoplasms—drug therapy—handbooks. QZ 39 H2355 1999.]
RC271.C5H36   1999
616.99′4061—dc21
DNLM/DLC
for Library of Congress   99-21311
                                                                    CIP

Care has been taken to confirm the accuracy of the information presented and
to describe generally accepted practices. However, the authors, editors, and
publisher are not responsible for errors or omissions or for any consequences
from application of the information in this book and make no warranty,
expressed or implied, with respect to the contents of the publication.
     The authors, editor, and publisher have exerted every effort to ensure that
drug selection and dosage set forth in this text are in accordance with current
recommendations and practice at the time of publication. However, in view of
ongoing research, changes in government regulations, and the constant flow of
information relating to drug therapy and drug reactions, the reader is urged to
check the package insert for each drug for any change in indications and dosage
and for added warnings and precautions. This is particularly important when the
recommended agent is a new or infrequently employed drug.
     Some drugs and medical devices presented in this publication have
Food and Drug Administration (FDA) clearance for limited use in restricted
research settings. It is the responsibility of the health care provider to
ascertain the FDA status of each drug or device planned for use in their
clinical practice.

Contents

Section I.
Basic Principles and Considerations of Rational Chemotherapy

Section II.
Chemotherapeutic and Biotherapeutic Agents and Their Use

Section III.
Chemotherapy of Human Cancer

Section IV.
Selected Aspects of Supportive
Care of Patients with Cancer

Appendices

Contributing Authors

Jane B. Alavi, M.D.
*Associate Professor, Department of Medicine Division of
Hematology and Oncology, University of Pennsylvania,
3400 Spruce Street, Philadelphia, Pennsylvania 19104*

Robert S. Benjamin, M.D.
*Department of Melanoma / Sarcoma Medical, Oncology,
M.D. Anderson Cancer Center, 1515 Holcombe Boulevard,
Box 77, Houston, Texas 77030*

Eduardo D. Bruera, M.D.
*Grey Nuns Community Hospital and Health Centre, Palliative
Care Program, 1100 Youville Drive West, Room 4324,
Edmonton, Alberta T6L 5X8, Canada*

Charles S. Cleeland, M.D.
*McCullough Professor of Cancer Research, Pain Research
Group, University of Texas, M.D. Anderson Cancer Center,
1100 Holcombe Boulevard, Box 221, Houston, Texas
77030-4095*

Ronald C. DeConti, M.D.
*Medical Director, Medical Oncology, H. Lee Moffitt Cancer
Center & Research Institute, 12902 Magnolia Drive,
Tampa, Florida 33612*

Kathy S.N. Franco-Bronson, M.D.
*Director of Residency Training, Head of Consultation-Liaison
Psychiatry, Department of Psychiatry and Psychology,
Cleveland Clinic Foundation, 9500 Euclid Avenue,
Room P-57, Cleveland, Ohio 44195-5001*

Walter H. Gajewski, M.D.
*Brown University School of Medicine, Women and Infants
Hospital, 101 Dudley Street, Providence, Rhode Island
02905-2499*

Patricia A. Ganz, M.D.
*Director Division of Cancer Prevention and Control Research,
Josson Comprehensive Cancer Center, Los Angeles,
California*

C.O. Granai, M.D.
*Brown University School of Medicine, Women and Infants
Hospital, 101 Dudley Street, Providence, Rhode Island
02905-2499*

John P. Greer
*Department of Medicine, Division of Hematology, Vanderbilt
University School of Medicine, 2220 Pierce Avenue, Room
551, MRB-2, Nashville, Tennessee 37232-6305*

Lynne Jahnke, M.D.
Division of Hematology and Oncology, Kaiser-Permanente Hospital, San Francisco, California

Chatchada Karanes, M.D.
Professor, Division of Hematology and Oncology, Barbara Ann Karmanos Cancer Institute, Wayne State University School of Medicine, Harper Hospital, 3990 John R Street, 4 Violet South, Detroit, Michigan 48201

Nurjehan A. Khan, M.D.
Medical Director, Blood Services, American Red Cross, Western Lake Erie Region, 3510 Executive Parkway, Toledo, Ohio 43606

Samir N. Khleif, M.D.
National Cancer Institute—Bethesda Naval Hospital, 8901 Wisconsin Avenue, Building 8, Room 5101, Bethesda, Maryland 20889-5101

Neil A. Lachant, M.D., F.A.C.P.
Professor of Medicine and Oncology, Barbara Ann Karmanos Cancer Institute, Wayne State University School of Medicine, Division of Hematology/Oncology, Harper Hospital, 3990 John R Street, 4 Brush South, Detroit, Michigan 48201

Robert D. Legare
Brown University School of Medicine, Women and Infants Hospital, 101 Dudley Street, Providence, Rhode Island 02905-2499

Rodger D. MacArthur, M.D.
Associate Professor, Division of Infectious Diseases, Wayne State University, 4201 St. Antoine; UHC 7D, Detroit, Michigan 48201

John C. Marsh, M.D.
Professor of Medicine (Emeritus), Departments of Internal Medicine and Pharmacology, Yale University School of Medicine, P.O. Box 208032, 333 Cedar Street, New Haven, Connecticut 06520-8032

Larry Nathanson, M.D., F.A.C.P.
Professor of Medicine (Emeritus), Department of Medicine, S.U.N.Y. Stony Brook School of Medicine, Oncology Consultants, 3 Gray Gardens East, Cambridge, Massachusetts 02138

Craig R. Nichols, M.D.
Division Chief, Department of Hematology and Medical Oncology, 3181 SW Sam Jackson Park Road, OP 28, Portland, Oregon 97201

Martin M. Oken, M.D.
Director, Virginia-Piper Cancer Institute, Abbott-Northwestern, 800 East 28th Street, Minneapolis, Minnesota 55407-3799

Carol S. Palackdharry, M.D., M.S.
Medical College of Ohio, P.O. Box 10008, Toledo, Ohio 43614

David R. Parkinson, M.D.
Novartis, Oncology Therapeutics, 59 Route #10, East Hanver, New Jersey 07936-1080

Walter D.Y. Quan, Jr, M.D.
Assistant Clinical Professor, Department of Medicine, Division of Hematology and Oncology, Case Western Reserve University, St. Luke's Medical Center, Cleveland, Ohio 44139

Scott B. Saxman, M.D.
Assistant Professor, Department of Medicine, Indiana University School of Medicine, 535 Barnhill Drive, Room RT 440, Indianapolis, Indiana 46202

David J. Schifeling, M.D., F.A.C.P.
Marshfield Clinic, Regional Cancer Center, 900 West Clairemont Avenue, Eau Claire, Wisconsin 54701

Joan H. Schiller, M.D.
Professor, Department of Medicine, Medical Oncology, University of Wisconsin Medical School, 600 Highland Avenue, Room K4/666, Madison, Wisconsin 53792-0001

Roland T. Skeel, M.D.
Chief of Hematology and Oncology, Department of Medicine, Medical College of Ohio, Richard D. Ruppert Health Center, 3120 Glendale Avenue, Toledo, Ohio 43614-5809

Mary R. Smith, M.D.
Professor, Associate Dean for Clinical Undergraduate and Graduate Medical Education, Medical College of Ohio, 3045 Arlington Avenue, Toledo, Ohio 43614-5805

Richard S. Stein, M.D.
Associate Professor, Department of Medicine, Division of Hematology, Vanderbilt University School of Medicine, 2220 Pierce Avenue, Room 551, MRB-2, Nashville, Tennessee 37232-6305

Janelle Tipton, M.S.N., R.N., O.C.N.
Medical College of Ohio, 3045 Arlington Avenue Room 4114, P.O. Box 10008, Toledo, Ohio 43614

Salvatore Veltri, M.D.
Medical College of Ohio, P.O. Box 10008, 3045 Arlington Avenue, Toledo, Ohio 43614

David H. Vesole, M.D., Ph.D., F.A.C.P.
*Associate Professor of Medicine, Clinical Director, Bone Marrow
    Transplant Program, Medical College of Wisconsin, 9200
    West Wisconsin Avenue, Milwaukee, Wisconsin 53226*

Jamie H. Von Roenn, M.D.
*Associate Professor of Medicine, Division of Hematology/Oncology,
    Northwestern University Medical School, 233 E. Erie, Suite
    700, Chicago, Illinois 60611*

Peter White, M.D.
*Medical College of Ohio, P.O. Box 10008, 3045 Arlington
    Avenue, Toledo, Ohio 43614*

Kristi S. Williams, M.D.
*Medical College of Ohio, P.O. Box 10008, 3045 Arlington
    Avenue, Toledo, Ohio 43614*

Preface

This edition of the *Handbook of Cancer Chemotherapy* has been revised to keep it the most useful chemotherapy handbook available. The chapter on high-dose chemotherapy with progenitor cell and cytokine support has been extensively expanded in recognition of the growing importance of peripheral blood stem cell transplant in community practices, particularly for breast cancer and lymphomas. Primary indications, usual dosage and schedule, and expected toxicities have been added for the large number of new drugs and biologic agents that oncologists have begun to use during the last five years. New data have also been added to the information on many of the older agents.

Each of the chapters dealing with specific cancer sites has been revised to reflect the best current medical practice and to point the way toward future advances. The section on basic principles of therapy and the section on supportive care have been streamlined to highlight those issues that are essential to the daily care of patients with cancer. Because cancer screening is important to reducing cancer deaths, American Cancer Society screening guidelines have been added to the appendix, as well as a short list of helpful internet addresses for cancer information.

The Handbook continues to be a practical pocket— or desk— reference with a wealth of information for oncology specialists, non-oncology physicians, house officers, oncology nurses, pharmacists, and medical students. It can even be read and understood by many patients and their families who want to be able to find practical information about their cancer and its treatment. Unlike many other books, the Handbook combines in one place the most current rationale and specific details necessary to safely administer chemotherapy for most adult cancers.

The hope for a more specific, radically improved medical treatment for cancer has been stimulated by the tremendous recent increase in information on the molecular basis of cancer, including the basic mechanisms of cell growth and death, and the alterations found in cancer. In the past few years, the potential for more specific and effective therapy of cancer by interference with oncogenes and oncogene products, or by manipulation of tumor suppressor genes or their products, has just begun to be realized. The recent availability of rituximab, a genetically engineered chimeric murine/human monoclonal antibody directed against the CD20 antigen found on the surface of normal B-cell lymphocytes, and trastuzumab, a recombinant humanized monoclonal antibody that targets the extracellular domain of the HER2 growth factor receptor (p185^{HER2}), will be only the first salvo in a barrage of new biologic agents based on the explosion of knowledge about the biologic basis for cancer cell development, growth, and metastasis.

Cure of cancer with chemotherapy or other systemic treatment has been a longterm aspiration for many people: those engaged in cancer research, physicians who are daily faced with anxious patients who have cancer, and others in the health professions. It also remains a fervent hope of patients and their families. Cure is possible for a small percentage of patients with some common tumors, particularly when there is only micrometastasis, and for some patients with more advanced tumors such as lymphomas. For most patients chemotherapy remains palliative at best. Although cures in advanced cancer are still uncommonly seen, continuing research into ways to enhance inherent biologic responses of the host to cancer, and to support patients undergoing the rigors of cancer treatment, has resulted in improved therapy in several cancers. Current trials that combine biologic therapies with each other and with chemotherapy offer a realistic expectation of accelerated progress in the control of cancer. We believe that with the additions and revisions in this edition, the Handbook will continue to be a valuable resource for physicians, nurses, students, and others as we move into the new millennium.

Roland T. Skeel, M.D.

I.

Basic Principles and Considerations of Rational Chemotherapy

Biologic and Pharmacologic Basis of Cancer Chemotherapy

Roland T. Skeel

I. **General mechanisms by which chemotherapeutic agents control cancer.** The purpose of treating cancer with chemotherapeutic agents is to prevent cancer cells from multiplying, invading, metastasizing, and ultimately killing the host (patient). Most agents currently in use appear to exert their effect primarily on cell multiplication and tumor growth. Because cell multiplication is a characteristic of many normal cells as well as cancer cells, most cancer chemotherapeutic agents also have toxic effects on normal cells, particularly those with a rapid rate of turnover, such as bone marrow and mucous membrane cells. The goal in selecting an effective drug, therefore, is to find an agent that has a marked growth-inhibitory or controlling effect on the cancer cell and a minimal toxic effect on the host. In the most effective chemotherapeutic regimens, the drugs are capable not only of inhibiting but also of completely eradicating all neoplastic cells while sufficiently preserving normal marrow and other target organs to permit a return to normal, or at least satisfactory, function.

Ideally, the pharmacologist or medicinal chemist would like to look at the cancer cell, discover how it differs from the normal host cell, and then design a chemotherapeutic agent to capitalize on that difference. In practice, often less rational means are used. The effectiveness of agents is discovered by treating either animal or human neoplasms, after which the pharmacologist attempts to discover why the agent works as well as it does. With few exceptions, the reasons chemotherapeutic and biologic agents are more effective against cancer cells than against normal cells are poorly understood. With the rapid expansion of information about cell biology and the factors within the neoplastic cell that control cell growth, the strictly empiric method of discovering effective new agents may be about to change. For example, antibodies against the protein product of the over-expressed HER-2/neu oncogene have been demonstrated to have definite (though limited) effectiveness in controlling metastatic breast cancer. This increased understanding of cancer cell biology promises to provide more specific and selective ways of controlling cancer cell growth in the next 10 years.

Inhibition of cell multiplication and tumor growth can take place at several levels within the cell.
1. Macromolecular synthesis and function
2. Cytoplasmic organization
3. Cell membrane synthesis function
4. Environment of cancer cell growth

3

A. **Standard agents.** Most agents currently in use or under investigation, with the exception of immunotherapeutic agents and other biologic response modifiers (BRMs), appear to have their primary effect on either macromolecular synthesis or function. This effect means that they interfere with the synthesis of either DNA, RNA, or proteins, or with the appropriate functioning of the preformed molecule. When interference in macromolecular synthesis or function in the neoplastic cell population is sufficiently great, a proportion of the cells die. Some cells die because of the direct effect of the chemotherapeutic agent. In other instances, the chemotherapy may trigger differentiation, senescence, or apoptosis, the cell's own mechanism of programmed death.

   Cell death may or may not take place at the time of exposure to the drug. Often, a cell must undergo several divisions before the lethal event that took place earlier finally results in the death of the cell. Because only a proportion of the cells die as a result of a given treatment, repeated doses of chemotherapy must be used to continue to reduce the cell number (Fig. 1-1). In an ideal system, each time the dose is repeated, the same proportion of cells—not the same absolute number—is killed. In the example shown in Fig. 1-1, 99.9% (3 logs) of the cancer cells are killed with each treatment, and there is a 10-fold (1 log) growth between treatments, for a net reduction of 2 logs with each treatment. Starting at 10^{10} cells (about 10 g, or 10 cm^3 leukemia cells), it would take five treatments to reach fewer than 10^0, or 1, cell. Such a model makes certain assumptions that rarely are strictly true in clinical practice.

   1. All cells in a tumor population are equally sensitive to a drug.
   2. Drug accessibility and cell sensitivity are independent of the location of the cells within the host and of local host factors, such as blood supply and surrounding fibrosis.
   3. Cell sensitivity does not change during the course of therapy.

   The lack of curability of most initially sensitive tumors is probably a reflection of the degree to which these assumptions do not hold true.

B. **Biologic response modifiers.** Within individual cells and cell populations are intricate interrelated mechanisms that promote or suppress cell growth, lead to cell differentiation, or set the cell on the path to inevitable death (apoptosis). These activities appear to be controlled in large part by normal and mutated promoter genes, tumor-suppressor genes, and their products. Included in these products are a host of cell growth factors. Some of these factors have been biosynthesized and are now used in standard

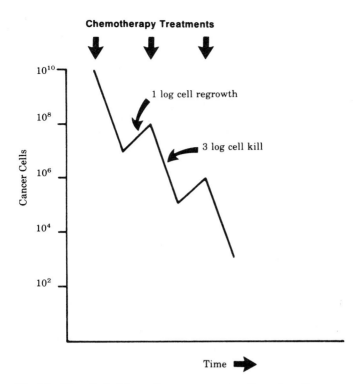

Fig. 1-1.   *The effect of chemotherapy on cancer cell numbers.* In an ideal system, chemotherapy kills a constant proportion of the remaining cancer cells with each dose. Between doses, cell regrowth occurs. When therapy is successful, cell killing is greater than cell growth.

and investigational therapy; they are discussed more fully in Chapter 2.

The recent expansion of our understanding of the biologic control of normal cells and tumor growth at the molecular level has only begun to offer improved therapy for cancer, though it has helped to explain differences in response among populations of patients. New discoveries in cancer cell biology have provided insights into apoptosis, cell cycling control, angiogenesis, metastasis, cell signal transduction, cell surface receptors, differentiation, and growth factor modulation. New drugs in clinical trials have been designed to block growth factor receptors, prevent oncogene activity, block the cell cycle, restore apoptosis, inhibit angiogenesis, restore lost function of tumor suppressor genes, or selectively kill tumors

containing abnormal genes. Further understanding
of each of these holds a great potential for providing
powerful and more selective means to control neoplastic cell growth and may lead to effective cancer
treatments in the next decade.

II. **Tumor cell kinetics and chemotherapy.** Cancer cells,
unlike other body cells, are characterized by a growth
process whereby their sensitivity to normal controlling
factors has been partially or completely lost. As a result of
this uncontrolled growth, it was once thought that cancer
cells grew or multiplied faster than normal cells and that
this growth rate was responsible for the sensitivity of
cancer cells to chemotherapy. Now it is known that most
cancer cells grow less rapidly than the more active, normal cells, such as bone marrow. Thus, although the growth
rate of many cancers is faster than that of normal surrounding tissues, growth rate alone cannot explain the
greater sensitivity of cancer cells to chemotherapy.

  A. **Tumor growth.** The growth of a tumor depends on
several interrelated factors.

    1. **Cell cycle time,** or the average time for a cell
that has just completed mitosis to grow, re-
divide, and again pass through mitosis, deter-
mines the maximum growth rate of a tumor but
probably does not determine drug sensitivity.
The relative proportion of cell cycle time taken
up by the DNA synthesis phase may relate
to drug sensitivity of some types (S-phase–
specific) of chemotherapeutic agents.

    2. **Growth fraction,** or the fraction of cells under-
going cell division, contains the portion of cells
that are sensitive to drugs whose major effect is
exerted on cells that are dividing actively. If the
growth fraction approaches 1 and the cell death
rate is low, the tumor doubling time approximates the cell cycle time.

    3. **Total number of cells in the population**
(determined at some arbitrary time at which
the growth measurement is started) is clinically
important because it is an index of how advanced is the cancer; it frequently correlates
with normal organ dysfunction. As the total
number of cells increases, so does the number of
resistant cells, which in turn leads to decreased
curability. Large tumors may also have greater
compromise of blood supply and oxygenation,
which can impair drug delivery to the tumor
cells as well as impaired sensitivity to both
chemotherapy and radiotherapy.

    4. **Intrinsic cell death rate** of tumors is difficult
to measure in patients, but probably makes a
major and positive contribution by slowing the
growth rate of many solid tumors.

  B. **Cell cycle.** The cell cycle of cancer cells is qualitatively the same as that of normal cells (Fig. 1-2).

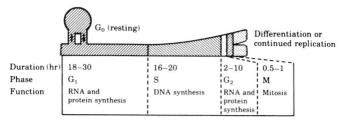

Duration (hr)	18–30	16–20	2–10	0.5–1
Phase	G_1	S	G_2	M
Function	RNA and protein synthesis	DNA synthesis	RNA and protein synthesis	Mitosis

Fig. 1-2. *Cell cycle time for human tissues* has a wide range (16–260 hours), with marked differences among normal and tumor tissues. Normal marrow and gastrointestinal-lining cells have cell cycle times of 24–48 hours. Representative durations and the kinetic or synthetic activity are indicated for each phase.

Each cell begins its growth during a postmitotic period, a phase called G_1, during which enzymes necessary for DNA production, other proteins, and RNA are produced. G_1 is followed by a period of DNA *synthesis* (S) in which essentially all DNA synthesis for a given cycle takes place. When DNA synthesis is complete, the cell enters a *premitotic period* (G_2), during which further protein and RNA synthesis occurs. This gap is followed immediately by *mitosis* (M), at the end of which actual physical division takes place, two daughter cells are formed, and each cell again enters G_1. G_1 phase is in equilibrium with a *resting state* called G_0. Cells in G_0 are relatively inactive with respect to macromolecular synthesis and are consequently insensitive to many chemotherapeutic agents, particularly those that affect macromolecular synthesis.

C.   **Phase and cell cycle specificity.** Most chemotherapeutic agents can be grouped according to whether they depend on cells being in cycle (i.e., not in G_0) and, if they depend on the cell being in cycle, whether their activity is greater when the cell is in a specific phase of the cycle. Most agents cannot be assigned to one category exclusively. Nonetheless, these classifications can be helpful for understanding drug activity.

1.   **Phase-specific drugs.** Agents that are most active against cells in a specific phase of the cell cycle are called *cell cycle phase–specific drugs.* A partial list of these drugs is shown in Table 1-1.

a.   **Implications of phase-specific drugs.** Phase specificity has important implications for cancer chemotherapy.

(1)   **Limitation to single-exposure cell kill.** With a phase-specific agent, there is a limit to the number of cells that can be killed with a single in-

Table 1-1. Cell cycle phase-specific chemotherapeutic agents

Phase of greatest activity	Class	Type	Characteristic agents
Gap 1 (G_1)	Natural product	Enzyme	Asparaginase
	Hormone	Corticosteroid	Prednisone
G_1/S junction	Antimetabolite	Purine analog	Cladribine
DNA synthesis (S)	Antimetabolite	Pyrimidine analog	Cytarabine, fluorouracil, gemcitabine
	Antimetabolite	Folic acid analog	Methotrexate
	Antimetabolite	Purine analog	Thioguanine, fludarabine
	Natural product	Topoisomerase I inhibitor	Topotecan
	Miscellaneous	Substituted urea	Hydroxyurea
Gap 2 (G_2)	Natural product	Antibiotic	Bleomycin
	Natural product	Topoisomerase II inhibitor	Etoposide
	Natural product	Microtubule polymerization and stabilization	Paclitaxel (Taxol)
Mitosis (M)	Natural product	Mitotic inhibitor	Vinblastine, vincristine, vindesine, vinorelbine

stantaneous (or very short) drug exposure because only those cells in the sensitive phase are killed. A higher dose kills no more cells.

(2) **Increasing cell kill by prolonged exposure.** To kill more cells requires either prolonged exposure to, or repeated doses of, the drug to allow more cells to enter the sensitive phase of the cycle. Theoretically, all cells could be killed if the blood level, or more importantly the intracellular concentration, of the drug remained sufficiently high while all cells in the target population passed through one complete cell cycle. This theory assumes that the drug does not prevent the passage of cells from one (insensitive) phase to another (sensitive) phase.

(3) **Recruitment.** A higher number of cells could be killed by a phase-specific drug if the proportion of cells in the sensitive phase could be increased (recruited).

b. **Cytarabine.** One of the best examples of a phase-specific agent is cytarabine (ara-C), which is an inhibitor of DNA synthesis and thus is active only in the S phase (at standard doses). When used in doses of 100–200 mg/m^2 daily (i.e., not "high-dose Ara-C") Ara-C is rapidly deaminated *in vivo* to an inactive compound, ara-U, and rapid injections result in very short, effective levels of ara-C. As a result, single doses of ara-C are nontoxic to the normal hematopoietic system and are generally ineffective for treating leukemia. If the drug is given as a daily rapid injection, some patients with leukemia respond well, but not nearly as well as when ara-C is given every 12 hours. The apparent reason for the greater effectiveness of the 12-hour schedule is that the S phase (DNA synthesis) of human acute nonlymphocytic leukemia cells lasts about 18 to 20 hours. If the drug is given every 24 hours, some cells that have not entered the S phase when the drug is first administered would not be sensitive to its effect. Therefore, these cells could pass all the way through the S phase before the next dose was administered and would completely escape any cytotoxic effect. However, when the drug is given every 12 hours, no cell that was "in cycle" would be able to escape exposure to ara-C because none would be able to get through one complete S phase without the drug being present.

If all cells were in active cycle, that is, if none were resting in a prolonged G_1 or G_0 phase, it would be theoretically possible to kill any cells in a population by a continuous or scheduled exposure equivalent to one complete cell cycle. Experiments with patients who have acute leukemia have shown that if tritiated thymidine is used to label cells as they enter DNA synthesis, it may be 7 to 10 days before the maximum number of leukemia cells have passed through the S phase. This factor means that, barring permutations caused by itself or other drugs, for ara-C to have a maximum effect on the leukemia, the repeated exposure must be continued for a 7-to-10 day period. Clinically, continuous infusion or administration of ara-C every 12 hours for 5 days or longer appears to be most effective for treating patients with newly diagnosed acute nonlymphocytic leukemia. However, even with such prolonged exposure, it appears that a few of the cells do not pass through the S phase.

2. **Cell cycle–specific drugs.** Agents that are effective while cells are actively in cycle but that are not dependent on the cell being in a particular phase are called *cell cycle–specific* (or *phase-nonspecific*) *drugs*. This group includes most of the alkylating agents, the antitumor antibiotics, and some miscellaneous agents, examples of which are shown in Table 1-2. Some agents in this group are not totally phase nonspecific; they may have greater activity in one phase than in another but not to the degree of the phase-specific agents. Many agents also appear to have some activity in cells that are not in cycle, although not as much as when the cells are rapidly dividing.

3. **Cell cycle–nonspecific drugs.** A third group of drugs appears to be effective whether cancer cells are in cycle or are resting. In this respect, these agents are similar to photon irradiation, that is, both types of therapy are effective irrespective of whether or not the cancer cell is in cycle. Drugs in this category are called *cell cycle–nonspecific drugs* and include mechlorethamine (nitrogen mustard) and the nitrosoureas (see Table 1-2).

D. **Changes in tumor cell kinetics and therapy implications.** As cancer cells grow from a few cells to a lethal tumor burden, certain changes occur in the growth rate of the population and affect the strate-

Table 1-2.   Cell cycle–specific and cell cycle–nonspecific chemotherapeutic agents

Class	Type	Characteristic agents
Cell cycle–specific		
Alkylating agent	Nitrogen mustard	Chlorambucil, cyclophosphamide melphalan
	Alkyl sulfonate	Busulfan
	Triazene	Dacarbazine
	Metal salt	Cisplatin, carboplatin
Natural product	Antibiotic	Dactinomycin, daunorubicin, doxorubicin, idarubicin
Cell cycle–nonspecific		
Alkylating agent	Nitrogen mustard	Mechlorethamine
	Nitrosourea	Carmustine, lomustine

gies of chemotherapy. These changes have been determined by observing the characteristics of experimental tumors in animals and neoplastic cells growing in tissue culture. Such model systems readily permit accurate cell number determinations to be made and growth rates to be determined. (Because tumor cells cannot be injected or implanted into humans and permitted to grow, studies of growth rates of intact tumors in humans must be limited largely to observing the growth rate of macroscopic tumors.)

1. **Stages of tumor growth.** Immediately after inoculating a tissue culture or an experimental animal with tumor cells, there is a *lag phase* during which there is little tumor growth; presumably, the cells in this phase are becoming accustomed to the new environment and are preparing to enter into cycle. The lag phase is followed by a period of rapid growth called *log phase,* during which there are repeated doublings of the cell number. In populations in which the growth fraction approaches 100% and the cell death rate is low, the population doubles within a period approximating the cell cycle time. As the cell number or tumor size becomes macroscopic, the doubling time of the tumor cell population becomes prolonged and levels off (plateau phase). Most clinically measurable human cancers are probably in the plateau phase, which may account, in part, for the slow doubling time observed in many human cancers (30 to 300 days). Because the

rate of change in the slope of the growth curve during the premeasurable period is unknown for most human cancers, extrapolation from two points when the mass is measurable to estimate the onset of the growth of the malignancy is subject to considerable error. The prolongation in tumor doubling time in the plateau phase may be due to a smaller growth fraction, a change in the cell cycle time, an increased intrinsic death rate (predominantly apoptosis which is a programmed and highly orchestrated cell death that occurs both naturally and under the influence of many types of chemotherapy), or a combination of these factors. Factors responsible for these changes include decreased nutrients or growth promotion factors, increased inhibitory metabolites or inhibitory growth factors, and inhibition of growth by other cell-cell interactions.

2. **Growth rate and effectiveness of chemotherapy.** Chemotherapeutic agents are most effective during the period of logarithmic growth. As might be expected, this result is particularly true for the antimetabolites, which are largely S-phase specific. As a result, when human tumors become macroscopic, the effectiveness of many chemotherapeutic agents is reduced because only part of the cell population is dividing actively. Theoretically, if the cell population could be reduced sufficiently by other means, such as surgery or radiotherapy, chemotherapy would be more effective because a higher fraction of the remaining cells would be in logarithmic growth. The validity of this theoretical premise is supported by the varying degrees of success of surgery plus chemotherapy, or radiotherapy plus chemotherapy in the treatment of breast cancer, colon cancer, Wilms' tumor, ovarian cancer, small cell anaplastic cell carcinoma of the lung, non–small cell carcinoma of the lung, head and neck cancers, and osteosarcomas.

III. **Combination chemotherapy.** Combinations of drugs are frequently more effective in producing responses and prolonging life than are the same drugs used sequentially. Combinations are likely to be more effective than single agents for several reasons.

A. **Reasons for effectiveness of combinations**

1. **Prevention of resistant clones.** If 1 in 10^5 cells is resistant to drug A and 1 in 10^5 cells is resistant to drug B, it is likely that treating a macroscopic tumor (which generally would have more than 10^9 cells) with either agent alone would result in several clones of cells that are resistant to that drug. If, after treatment with drug A, a resistant clone has grown to

macroscopic size (if the same mutant frequency persists for drug B), resistance to that agent will also emerge. If both drugs are used at the outset of therapy or in close sequence, however, the likelihood of a cell being resistant to both drugs (excluding for a moment the situation of pleiotropic drug resistance) is only 1 in 10^{10}. Thus, the combination confers considerable advantage against the emergence of resistant clones. Compounding the problem of preexisting resistant clones is the resistance that develops through spontaneous mutation in the absence of drug exposure. The use of multiple drugs with independent mechanisms of action or alternating non–cross-resistant combinations (as well as the use of surgery or radiotherapy to eliminate macroscopic tumor) theoretically minimizes the chances for outgrowth of resistant clones and increases the likelihood of remission or cure.

2. **Cytotoxicity to resting and dividing cells.** The combination of a drug that is cell cycle specific (phase-nonspecific) or cell cycle nonspecific with a drug that is cell cycle phase specific can kill cells that are dividing slowly as well as those that are dividing actively. The use of cell cycle–nonspecific drugs can also help recruit cells into a more actively dividing state, which results in their being more sensitive to the cell cycle phase–specific agents.

3. **Biochemical enhancement of effect**

   a. **Combinations of individually effective drugs** that affect different biochemical pathways or steps in a single pathway can enhance each other.

   b. **Combinations of an active agent with an inactive agent** can potentially result in beneficial effects by several mechanisms.

      (1) **An intracellular increase** in the drug or its active metabolites, by either increasing influx or decreasing efflux (e.g., calcium-channel inhibitors with multiple agents affected by multidrug resistance [MDR] due to P-glycoprotein overexpression).

      (2) **Reduced metabolic inactivation** of the drug (e.g., inhibition of cytidine deaminase inactivation of ara-C with tetrahydrouridine.

      (3) **Cooperative inhibition** of a single enzyme or reaction (e.g., leucovorin enhancement of fluorouracil inhibition of thymidylate synthetase).

      (4) **Enhancement of drug action** by inhibition of competing metabolites (e.g., N-phosphonacetyl-L-aspartic

acid [PALA] inhibition of *de novo* pyrimidine synthesis with resultant increased incorporation of 5-fluorouridine triphosphate [5FUTP] into RNA).

4. **Sanctuary access.** Combinations can be used to provide access to sanctuary sites for reasons such as drug solubility or affinity of specific tissues for a particular drug type.

5. **Rescue.** Combinations can be used in which one agent rescues the host from the toxic effects of another drug (e.g., leucovorin administration after high-dose methotrexate).

B. **Principles of agent selection.** When selecting appropriate agents for use in a combination, the following principles should be observed:

1. **Choose individually active drugs.** Do not use a combination in which one agent is inactive when used alone unless there is a clear, specific biochemical or pharmacologic reason to do so, for example, high-dose methotrexate followed by leucovorin rescue, or leucovorin followed by fluorouracil. *This principle is not applicable to the combined use of BRMs and chemotherapeutic agents* because the cooperativity of BRMs and chemotherapy may not depend on the independent cytotoxic effect of the BRMs.

2. **When possible, choose drugs in which the dose-limiting toxicities differ** qualitatively or in time of occurrence. Often, however, two or more agents that have marrow toxicity must be used, and the selection of a safe dose of each is critical. As a starting point, two drugs in combination can usually be given at two thirds of the dose used when the drugs are given alone. Whenever a new drug combination is tried, a careful evaluation of both expected and unanticipated toxicities must be carried out.

3. **Select agents for a combination for which there is a biochemical or pharmacologic rationale.** Preferably, this rationale has been tested in an animal tumor system and in the appropriate model system, and the combination has been found to be better than either agent alone.

4. **Be cautious when attempting to improve on a successful two-drug combination** by adding a third, fourth, and fifth drug simultaneously. Although this approach may be beneficial, two undesirable results may be seen:

   a. **An intolerable level of toxicity** that leads to excessive morbidity and mortality.

   b. **Unchanged or reduced antitumor effect** because of the necessity to reduce the dose of the most effective drugs to a level below which antitumor responses are not seen, despite the theoretical advantages of the combination. Therefore, the addition of each new agent to a combination must be considered carefully, the principles of combination therapy closely followed, and controlled clinical trials carried out to compare the efficacy of any new regimen with a more established (standard) treatment program.

C. **Clinical effectiveness of combinations.** Combinations of drugs have been clearly demonstrated to be better than single agents for treating many, but not all, human cancers. The survival benefit of combinations of drugs compared with that of the same drugs used sequentially has been marked in diseases such as acute lymphocytic and acute nonlymphocytic leukemia, Hodgkin's lymphoma, non-Hodgkin's lymphomas with more aggressive behavior (intermediate and high-grade), breast carcinoma, anaplastic small cell carcinoma of the lung, and testicular carcinoma. The benefit is less evident in cancers such as non–small cell carcinoma of the lung, non-Hodgkin's lymphomas with favorable prognoses, ovarian carcinoma, head and neck carcinomas, melanoma, and colorectal carcinomas, although reports exist for each of these tumors in which combinations are better in one respect or another than single agents.

IV. **Resistance to antineoplastic agents.** Resistance to antineoplastic chemotherapy is a combined characteristic of a specific drug, a specific tumor, and a specific host whereby the drug is ineffective in controlling the tumor without excessive toxicity. Resistance of a tumor to a drug is the reciprocal of selectivity of that drug for that tumor. The problem for the medical oncologist or pharmacologist is not simply to find an agent that is cytotoxic but to find one that selectively kills neoplastic cells while preserving the essential host cells and their function. Were it not for the problem of resistance of human cancer to antineoplastic agents or, conversely, the lack of selectivity of those agents, cancer chemotherapy would be similar to antibacterial chemotherapy in which complete eradication of infection is regularly observed. Such a utopian state of cancer chemotherapy has not yet been achieved for most human cancers. The problem of resistance and ways to overcome or even exploit it remains an area of major interest for the chemotherapist.

Resistance to antineoplastic chemotherapeutic agents may be either natural or acquired. *Natural resistance* refers to the initial unresponsiveness of a tumor to a given drug, and *acquired resistance* refers to the unresponsiveness that emerges after initially successful treatment. There are three basic categories of resistance to chemotherapy: kinetic, biochemical, and pharmacologic.

A. **Cell kinetics and resistance.** Resistance based on cell population kinetics relates to cycle and phase specificity, growth fractions and the implications of these factors for responsiveness to specific agents, and schedules of drug administration. A particular problem with many human tumors is that they are in a plateau growth phase with a small growth fraction. This factor renders many of the cells insensitive to the antimetabolites and relatively unresponsive to many of the other chemotherapeutic agents. Strategies to overcome resistance due to cell kinetics include the following:

1. Reducing tumor bulk with surgery or radiotherapy
2. Using combinations to include drugs that affect resting populations (with many G_0 cells)
3. Scheduling of drugs to prevent phase escape or to synchronize cell populations and increase cell kill

B. **Biochemical causes of resistance.** Resistance can occur for biochemical reasons, including the inability of a tumor to convert a drug to its active form, the ability of a tumor to inactivate a drug, or the location of a tumor at a site where substrates are present that bypass an otherwise lethal blockade. How cells become resistant is only partially understood. There can be decreased drug uptake, increased efflux, changes in the levels or structure of the intracellular target, reduced intracellular activation or increased inactivation of the drug, or increased rate of repair of damaged DNA. In one pre–B cell leukemia cell line, bcl-2 overexpression or decreased expression of the homolog *bax* renders cells resistant to several chemotherapeutic agents. Because bcl-2 blocks apoptosis, it has been proposed that its overexpression blocks chemotherapy-induced apoptosis. The interrelationship between mutations of p53, HER2/neu, and a host of other oncogenes and tumor suppressor genes, and resistance to the cytotoxic effects of radiotherapy, chemotherapeutic, hormonal, and biologic agents, when better understood, may further our understanding of resistance and provide new therapeutic strategies.

Multidrug resistance (MDR), also called *pleiotropic drug resistance,* is a phenomenon whereby treatment with one agent confers resistance not only to that drug and others of its class but also to several other unrelated agents. MDR is commonly mediated by an enhanced energy-dependent drug efflux mechanism that results in lower intracellular drug concentrations. With this type of MDR, overexpression of a membrane transport protein called *P-glycoprotein* (P-pleiotropic) is observed commonly. Other multidrug resistance proteins are the Multidrug-Resistance Protein (MRP) found in human lung cancer lines and the Lung-Resistance Protein (LRP). These proteins appear to have differing expression in different sets of neoplasms. Drugs that are effective in reversing resistance to P-glycoprotein do not reverse MRP.

Combination chemotherapy can overcome biochemical resistance by increasing the amount of active drug intracellularly as a result of biochemical interactions or effects on drug transport across the cell membrane. Calcium-channel blockers, antiarrhythmics, cyclosporin A analogs (e.g., PSC-833, a nonimmunosuppressive derivative of cyclosporin D), and other agents have been found to modulate the MDR effect *in vitro*, and some beneficial effects have been observed clinically.

The use of a second agent to rescue normal cells may also permit the use of high doses of the first agent, which can overcome the resistance caused by a low rate of conversion to the active metabolite or a high rate of inactivation. Another way to overcome resistance is to follow marrow-lethal doses of chemotherapy by posttherapy infusion of stem cells obtained from the peripheral blood or bone marrow. This experimental technique shows some promise for the treatment of lymphomas, chronic granulocytic leukemia, breast cancer, and a few other cancers. A more widely applicable technique may be to combine high-dose chemotherapy with blood cell growth factors, for example, granulocyte colony-stimulating factor (G-CSF) and granulocyte-macrophage colony-stimulating factor (GM-CSF) or oprelvekin (IL-11), to stimulate platelets. These and other marrow-protective and marrow-stimulating agents are being used increasingly and may enhance the effectiveness of chemotherapy in the treatment of several types of cancer. High-dose therapy is discussed more extensively in Chapter 6.

C. **Pharmacologic causes of resistance.** Apparent resistance to cancer chemotherapy can result from poor or erratic absorption, increased excretion or catabolism, and drug interactions, all leading to inadequate blood levels of the drug. Strictly speaking, this result is not true resistance; but to the degree that the insufficient blood levels are not appreciated by the clinician, resistance appears to be present. The variation from patient to patient at the highest tolerated dose has led to dose-modification schemes that permit dose escalation when the toxicities of the chemotherapy regimen are minimal or nonexistent as well as dose reduction when toxicities are great. This regulation is particularly important for some chemotherapeutic agents for which the dose-response curve is steep. Selection of the appropriate dose on the basis of predicted pharmacologic behavior is essential for some agents not only to avoid serious toxicity, but also to optimize effectiveness. This has been applied successfully to dose selection of carboplatin by predicting the time $\times$ concentration product (area under the curve or AUC) based on the individual patient's creatinine clearance.

True pharmacologic resistance is caused by the poor transport of agents into certain body tissues and tumor cells. For example, the central nervous system (CNS) is a site that many drugs do not reach well. Several drug characteristics favor transport into the CNS, including high lipid solubility and low molecular weight. For tumors that originate in the CNS or metastasize there, the drugs of choice should be those that achieve effective antitumor concentration in the brain tissue, and that are also effective against the tumor cell type being treated.

D. **Nonselectivity and resistance.** Nonselectivity is not a mechanism for resistance but rather an acknowledgment that for most cancers and most drugs, the reasons for resistance and selectivity are only partially understood. Given a limited understanding of the biochemical differences between normal and malignant cells, it is gratifying that chemotherapy is successful as frequently as it is. With the burgeoning of knowledge about the cancer cell, there is reason to hope that in 20 years we view current chemotherapy regimens as a crude beginning and will have found many more tumor target-directed agents that have a high potential for curing the human cancers that now defy treatment.

SELECTED READINGS

Baguley BC, Holdaway KM, Fray LM. Design of DNA intercalators to overcome topoisomerase II-mediated multi-drug resistance. *JNCI* 1990;82:398–402.

Baserga R. The cell cycle. *N Engl J Med* 1981;304:453–459.

Barinaga M. From bench top to bedside. *Science* 1997;278:1036–1039.

Clarkson B, Fried J, Strife A, Sakai Y, Ota K, Okita T. Studies of cellular proliferation in human leukemia. 3. Behavior of leukemic cells in three adults with acute leukemia given continuous infusions of 3H-thymidine for 8 or 10 days. *Cancer* 1970;25:1237–1260.

Dalton WS, Grogan TM, Meltzer PS, et al. Drug-resistance in multiple myeloma and non-Hodgkin's lymphoma: detection of P-glycoprotein and potential circumvention by addition of verapamil to chemotherapy. *J Clin Oncol* 1989;7:415–424.

Endicott JA, Ling U. The biochemistry of P-glycoprotein-mediated multidrug resistance. *Annu Rev Biochem* 1989;58:137–171.

Friedland ML. Combination chemotherapy. In: Perry MC, ed. *The Chemotherapy Source Book*. Baltimore: Williams & Wilkins, 1996; 63–78.

Goldie JH. Drug resistance. In: Perry MC, ed. *The Chemotherapy Source Book*. Baltimore: Williams & Wilkins, 1992:54–66.

Goldie JH, Coldman AJ. A mathematical model for relating drug sensitivity of tumors to their spontaneous mutation rate. *Cancer Treat Rep* 1979;63:1727–1733.

Kinzler KW, Vogelstein B. Cancer therapy meets p53. *N Engl J Med* 1994;331:49–50.

Schabel FM, Jr. The use of tumor growth kinetics in planning "curative" chemotherapy of advanced solid tumors. *Cancer Res* 1969; 29:2384–2398.

Sikic BI. Modulation of multidrug resistance: at the threshold. *J Clin Oncol* 1993;11:1629–1635.

Slingerland JM, Tannock IF. Cell proliferation and cell death. In: Tannock IF, Hill RP, eds. *The Basic Science of Oncology.* New York: McGraw-Hill, 1998;134–165.

Van Noorden CFJ, Meade-Tollin LC, Bosman FT. Metastasis. *American Scientist* 1998;86:130–141.

Yarbro JW. The scientific basis of cancer chemotherapy. In: Perry MC, ed., *The Chemotherapy Source Book.* Baltimore: Williams & Wilkins, 1996:3–18.

2

Principles of Therapy with Biologic Response Modifiers and Their Role in Cancer Management

David R. Parkinson

I. **Definition and approaches to biologic therapy.** The term *biologic therapy* describes a variety of agents and therapeutic approaches that continue to evolve from increased understanding of the biology of tumor cells and their relationship to the surrounding environment. Historically, this has involved immunologic approaches to treatment. The recognition the cells and antigens involved in antitumor mechanisms; the isolation and production in pharmacologic amounts of the proteins (cytokines) that regulate the differentiation, proliferation, and activity of immune cells; and the development of monoclonal antibody (MoAb) technology have all permitted clinical applications in humans based on promising concepts derived from preclinical studies in animal tumor models. More recently, treatment approaches based on preventing development of tumor-associated vasculature and approaches actually targeting this vasculature have emerged as promising new therapeutic strategies to affect the tumor environment.

II. **Biologic agents.** Biologic agents have generally consisted either of genetically engineered versions of naturally occurring proteins or therapeutic molecules based on these proteins. For example, a series of regulatory proteins termed *cytokines* have been studied for their use in cancer therapy. These proteins bind to specific cell surface receptors differentially expressed on cells of the hematopoietic and lymphoid systems and are responsible for controlling the growth, development, and functional activity of these cells. The range of biologic effects of these cytokines suggests wide possible therapeutic applications but has also complicated their clinical use when administered in pharmacologic quantities as drugs.

   A. **Cytokines as therapeutic agents.** Several of the central regulatory cytokines that have been isolated have undergone clinical trial, and some are now in general clinical use for oncologic and other indications. Others are still under study for their possible roles in cancer medicine.

      1. **Interleukin-1 (IL-1).** The two forms of IL-1 (IL-1α and IL-1β) are produced by a wide range of cells after stimulation. These cytokines, which bind to a common receptor, are among the most pleiotropic with regard to

their biologic properties. IL-1 plays an important role in inflammation, inducing fever and acute-phase reactant release; may play a role in tissue repair after injury; and has been implicated in tumor-associated cachexia. Furthermore, IL-1 has immunostimulatory properties that help to activate T lymphocytes and to induce the production of other cytokines. It both induces and is a cofactor for hematopoietic growth factors such as granulocyte and monocyte colony-stimulating factors. Experimentally, IL-1 is both a chemoprotector and a radioprotector, protecting animals against otherwise lethal myelosuppressive doses of cytotoxic agents. For these reasons, IL-1 has been studied in wound healing, as an adjuvant in vaccine trials, and for use in association with chemotherapy and irradiation; despite promising preclinical data, however, no role has been defined for IL-1 in clinical medicine.

2. **Interleukin-2.** IL-2 is a cytokine product of activated T cells that binds to a specific cell surface receptor on activated T lymphocytes; the protein stimulates T-cell proliferation but also activates natural killer (NK) cells. Because of its powerful immunostimulatory properties, IL-2 has been widely studied for its antitumor properties. In animals, IL-2 is active as a single agent in a dose- and schedule-dependent manner. For a given IL-2 treatment schedule, antitumor activity can be enhanced by the addition of other cytokines, such as interferon-α (IFN-α) and tumor necrosis factor-α (TNF-α), or by the concomitant use of activated antitumor lymphocytes or MoAbs directed against the tumor.

IL-2 has antitumor activity when used alone in high doses in patients with renal cell carcinoma and malignant melanoma. The greatest antitumor effects have been observed with high-dose IL-2 therapy. Single-agent, bolus IL-2 administered intravenously at a dose of 600,000 or 720,000 IU every 8 hours for up to 5 days has received U.S. Food and Drug Administration (FDA) approval for the treatment of patients with metastatic renal cell carcinoma and metastatic melanoma. Such intensive treatment can be administered only to patients carefully selected for cardiopulmonary status. This therapy is associated with significant toxicity and should be administered only by physicians experienced in its use.

3. **Interleukin-4.** IL-4 stimulates B cells and, together with IL-2, is a growth factor for cytotoxic T cells. This wide range of immunostimulatory

properties has led to clinical trials but not to a defined role in cancer therapy.

4. **Interleukin-6.** The IL-6 molecule possess widespread biologic effects. In addition to playing a central role in the induction of the acute-phase response, it is important in B-cell growth and differentiation and may serve as an autocrine growth factor in myeloma as well as a contributing factor to cancer-related cachexia; strategies to inhibit IL-6 production, such as the use of bisphosphonates, are therefore under study.

5. **Interleukin-12.** Another growth factor for early lymphoid progenitors, this cytokine is also important in T-cell activation and is being studied in clinical trials for its antitumor activity.

6. **Interferon-α.** Described initially for their antiviral properties, IFN-α and IFN-β, the type I IFNs, subserve a wide variety of biologic effects, some of which have proved useful in therapy for both malignant and nonmalignant diseases. IFN-α has been most widely studied. Its immunomodulatory effect includes activation of NK cells, modulation of antibody production by B lymphocytes, and induction on the tumor cell surface of major histocompatibility complex (MHC) antigens, making the tumor more susceptible to immune-mediated killing. However, the principal antitumor effects of this interferon are probably related to its direct antiproliferative effects.

    IFN-α is an active, FDA-approved agent in hairy-cell leukemia and in the early phase of chronic myelogenous leukemia. It also has activity in low-grade non-Hodgkin's lymphoma, multiple myeloma, and cutaneous T-cell lymphoma. Some solid tumors, principally melanoma and renal cell carcinoma, but also some squamous cell and basal cell carcinomas of the skin, have responded to interferon. Other clinical indications for the use of IFN-α include chronic infection with hepatitis C, condyloma acuminatum, and juvenile laryngeal carcinomatosis.

7. **Interferon-γ.** This interferon has weaker antiviral and a wider range of immunobiologic properties than IFN-α. It activates monocytes and macrophages, thereby upregulating Fc receptors, enhancing phagocytosis, and killing intracellular organisms. It increases the surface expression of MHC and tumor-associated antigens. IFN-γ has been disappointing as an antitumor agent when used alone, and it is now being studied in combination with other biologic agents. It is effective (and approved for clinical use) in chronic granulomatous disease,

in which its prophylactic use decreases the incidence and severity of infections.

8. **Tumor necrosis factor.** Originally named for their antitumor effects in animal models, TNF-α and TNF-β (*lymphotoxin*) are the products of activated macrophages, share a common receptor, and subserve a wide variety of biologic effects. They serve as growth factors for fibroblasts, have some antiviral activity, activate procoagulase activity on endothelial cells, and activate osteoclasts. Immunomodulatory effects include the induction of surface MHC antigens and interaction with other cytokines, such as IL-2, but TNF is directly cytotoxic to some cells, possibly through the induction of oxygen radicals. TNF may play a role in tumor cachexia. Acute intravenous administration of TNF leads to decreased systemic vascular resistance mediated through the induction of nitric oxide in endothelial cells. The TNF generated during gram-negative shock may be responsible for the lethality of these infections, and strategies for the treatment of this condition involve blocking the effects of TNF. As a single agent, TNF has been inactive systemically in cancer therapy in humans, perhaps because toxicity, principally hypotension, has limited the doses that can be administered systemically. It has been used more successfully in the treatment of recurrent extremity melanoma and soft tissue sarcomas when administered by isolated limb perfusion together with melphalan. This approach minimizes systemic toxicity and maximizes tumor exposure to the agent.

B. **Hematopoietic growth factors in cancer therapy**

1. **Erythropoietin.** Erythropoietin promotes the proliferation and differentiation of committed erythroid precursors. In addition to its nonmalignant indications, use of this factor results in decreased transfusion requirements during chemotherapy.

2. **Granulocyte colony-stimulating factor (G-CSF)** is a growth factor with proliferative activity for bone marrow progenitors committed to the neutrophil line. As discussed elsewhere in this volume, G-CSF is widely used in the setting of cytotoxic chemotherapy for solid tumors and leukemia to accelerate recovery of neutrophils and lessen the risk of bacterial infection.

3. **Granulocyte-macrophage colony-stimulating factor (GM-CSF).** To a greater degree than G-CSF, GM-CSF exhibits its predominant proliferative effects on multipotential stem cells. This protein also inhibits neutrophil mi-

gration, potentiates the functions of neutrophils and macrophages, and results in production of a spectrum of cytokines from these activated cells; therefore, it has been studied for its ability to reconstitute bone marrow and to activate macrophages. GM-CSF has also been approved for use after cytotoxic induction and maintenance chemotherapy for acute leukemia.

4. **Interleukin-3.** Also known as *multi-CSF,* IL-3 stimulates early multipotent marrow stem cells. Initial clinical trials using IL-3 after administration of cytotoxic chemotherapy were disappointing; however, IL-3–like proteins are being studied in similar clinical settings.

5. **Interleukin-11.** Another cytokine active on early hematopoietic cells, IL-11 has been demonstrated in controlled trials to accelerate the recovery of platelets after cytotoxic chemotherapy and has been approved for clinical use for that indication.

6. **Macrophage colony-stimulating factor.** Also known as colony-stimulating factor 1, this growth factor is relatively lineage specific, responsible for the proliferation and activation of monocytes. Clinical trials have not yet defined a role for this protein in clinical medicine.

7. **Thrombopoietin.** This hematopoietic growth factor enhances megakaryocyte development and is being studied in clinical trials for prevention and treatment of thrombocytopenia associated with cytotoxic chemotherapy, in similar settings to those in which IL-11 has been studied.

C. **Other growth factors and regulatory proteins**
   1. **Transforming growth factors (TGFs).** This group of regulatory molecules has profound effects on growth and differentiation. TGF-α is related to epidermal growth factor (EGF) and binds to the EGF receptor. TGF-β, a protein with a wide range of biologic effects, also enhances wound healing. It is being studied clinically for this use and for possible prevention or treatment of chemotherapy-associated mucositis as well as in a range of nonmalignant indications.

   2. **Other growth and differentiation factors.** It is becoming increasingly clear that a spectrum of proteins important in the control of growth, differentiation, and function exists for all organ systems. Further understanding of these proteins and their receptors will permit greater understanding of their roles in normal and disordered biology. Some of these proteins or their receptors may ultimately find a direct therapeutic role, or alternatively, they may

themselves represent targets for specific cancer therapeutics development.

D. Monoclonal antibodies. Antibodies that bind to tumor-associated cell surface antigens can result in the destruction of tumor cells through a number of possible mechanisms, including activation of complement and antibody-dependent cell-mediated cytotoxicity. Furthermore, these antibodies may be useful as means of targeting cytotoxic radioisotopes, toxins, or drugs to tumors, enhancing their delivery to tumors while minimizing systemic exposure. MoAb technology has made important contributions to cancer medicine by providing tools to allow the study of differentiation-associated antigens and the phenotypic characterization of both hematopoietic and solid tumors. Antigens expressed with relative specificity on tumor cell surfaces have been defined and have served as targets for diagnostic and therapeutic application of antibodies.

1. **Murine monoclonal antibodies.** The first MoAbs used *in vivo* diagnostically and therapeutically were murine. Studies have pointed out the ability of particular MoAbs to bind selectively to tumors but have also revealed the complexities involved in the clinical use of these agents. Relative distribution and densities of antigen on normal and malignant tissues, the affinity of the antibody for the antigen, and the behavior of the antigen after antibody binding all have effects on the success of this approach. The internal modulation of antigen from the cell surface after antibody binding is an impediment to treatment strategies using antibody alone, a necessity for immunotoxin or chemo-immune conjugates, and irrelevant to radioisotope therapeutic strategies.

   MoAbs are weak activators of the human immune system, and when used alone against T- or B-cell lymphoid malignancies, they have generally exhibited only transient antitumor activity. The antibodies against solid tumors have been largely inactive when studied in clinical trials. A problem with the repeated use of murine MoAb has been the development of human antimouse antibodies (HAMAs).

2. **Chimeric, human, and humanized monoclonal antibodies.** Although human antibodies have the theoretical advantage of less immunogenicity, longer half-lives, and greater immunologic activity, they have been difficult to generate in pharmacologic quantities. Solutions to this problem have included the generation of genetically engineered antibodies, which combine the antigen-binding properties of the murine antibodies with the advantages

of a human antibody backbone (chimeric antibody) or which have had mouse-specific sequences altered (humanized antibody) to decrease immunogenicity. Recently, large clinical trials have demonstrated the clinical utility of some of these antibody-based therapeutic agents. For example, rituximab (Rituxan) is a *primatized* (derived from a primate antibody) antibody reactive with the CD20 antigen on B cells; this agent has been approved for use in the treatment of chemotherapy-refractory follicular non-Hodgkin's lymphoma. More recently, trastuzumab (Herceptin), a humanized MoAb reactive with the Her-2/neu antigen overexpressed on some breast carcinoma cells, has been shown both to have single-agent clinical activity and in combination to add to the antitumor activity of paclitaxel or doxorubicin plus cyclophosphamide in the treatment of metastatic breast carcinoma.

3. **Antibody fragments.** Small antigen-binding proteins, either antibody fragments such as $F(ab')_2$, or single-chain antigen-binding proteins, may have shorter half-lives, greater access to tumor, and advantages as targeting agents.

E. **Antiangiogenesis agents.** A number of agents are being studied clinically for their ability to interfere with tumor new blood vessel formation. Several interfere with the production or binding of either basic fibroblast growth factor or vascular endothelial-derived growth factor (VEGF), two important angiogenic polypeptides. Numerous other agents have been demonstrated to have antiangiogenic activity, including IFN-α, analogs of the antibiotic fumagillin (e.g., TNP-1470), and thalidomide. Furthermore, several small molecule inhibitors of the VEGF receptor tyrosine kinase are under clinical development, a good example of how more conventional therapeutic development increasingly is merging into biologic therapy.

III. **Biologic strategies in cancer therapy**

A. **Single-agent therapy.** As noted already, some cytokines, principally IFN-α and IL-2, have been active as single agents in cancer therapy. In the case of IFN-α, the doses necessary for an antitumor effect range from the very low doses used in hairy-cell leukemia (as low as 2 to 5 MU/day of IFN-α_{2a} or IFN-α_{2b} given subcutaneously) to the higher doses necessary for melanoma (as it was used in adjuvant melanoma trials conducted by the Eastern Cooperative Oncology Group), which are associated with significant side effects. This problem is even more of an issue with IL-2, as noted already, of which the dose necessary for an antitumor effect may be associated with life-threatening toxicity. Current treatment strategies are designed to understand mechanisms of both antitumor effects and toxic effects in the expectation of developing less morbid, more effective therapy. One long-discussed but unproven tenet of biologic therapy is that because the optimal immunobiologic effects (optimal biologic dose) observed with an agent may be significantly less than the maximally tolerated dose (MTD), clinically useful effects may be observed at low, nontoxic doses. However, the validity of this concept can be tested only through clinical trials. At least with IL-2, the MTD appears to be associated with the greatest clinical activity in both melanoma and renal cell cancer.

B. Combination therapy. Because preclinical models suggest that combinations of biologic agents have greater therapeutic effects than single agents, clinical trials have studied the effects of immunostimulatory cytokines such as IL-2 administered together with MoAbs or with activated antitumor lymphocytes such as lymphokine activated killer (LAK) cells or cells generated from the tumor. Preclinical studies suggest that certain combinations of biologic and cytotoxic agents may be synergistic. TNF, for example, is both a radiosensitizer and an enhancer of the antitumor effects of topoisomerase inhibitors such as etoposide. IFN similarly enhances the antitumor activity of cisplatin and fluorouracil, and these combinations have been studied extensively in clinical trials; these approaches, however, have not resulted in any clear demonstration of enhanced chemotherapeutic effect.

C. Adoptive cellular therapy, gene therapy, and cancer vaccines. This treatment strategy involves the transfer of antitumor effective cells to the tumorbearing host. These cells have principally been either LAK cells generated by *in vitro* activation of peripheral blood lymphocytes with IL-2 or expanded populations of lymphocytes generated from the tumor. In some cases, these tumor-infiltrating lymphocytes (TILs) can be shown to exhibit specific cytotoxicity against the autologous tumor. Although this treatment approach is still experimental, it has allowed the isolation and characterization of human melanoma antigens recognized by T cells, including MAGE-1 and MAGE-3, MART-1, gp100, and tyrosinase. Cloned antigens have been used in the creation of vaccines involving peptides or vaccinia virus. Alternatively, gene transfer techniques with molecules such as GM-CSF have been used to increase the immunogenicity of autologous tumor cells for use in vaccination strategies. Numerous cancer vaccine strategies involving different antigens are in early development in attempts to induce active and specific antitumor immunity.

D. **Targeted therapy.** As noted already, tumor-associated surface structures, either tumor-associated antigens or receptors, can be used for targeted therapy with cytotoxic toxins, chemotherapeutic agents, or radionuclides.

   1. **Immunotoxin.** Conjugates of plant toxins, such as ricin, or bacterial toxins, such as *Pseudomonas* species exotoxin to MoAbs, have been used in therapeutic approaches, with responses noted in non-Hodgkin's lymphoma and chronic lymphocytic leukemia. Disadvantages of this strategy include the fact that target antigens must be internalized after antibody binding, antigen-negative cells can escape, and the plant toxin may be immunogenic.

   2. **Chimeric toxins.** Fusion genes composed of the cytotoxic portions of bacterial genes (e.g., diphtheria toxin or *Pseudomonas* species exotoxin) and targeting ligands (e.g., the cytokines IL-2 or TGF-α) can be used to produce cytotoxic chimeric proteins that target specifically cells expressing the respective high-affinity receptor. IL-2/diphtheria toxin fusion protein has been demonstrated to be active in the clinic against IL-2 receptor–expressing malignancies, particularly mycosis fungoides.

   3. **Radioimmunotherapy.** The selective targeting of radioisotopes to tumor presents many theoretical advantages over external-beam irradiation with regard to therapeutic index. In addition, owing to the bystander effect, even antigen-negative cells may be killed in this approach, and antibody need not be internalized for the therapy to be effective. Difficulties have included the necessity of developing more stable "linker" chemistry for the attachment of isotopes other than iodine, the poor radiation characteristics of the iodine isotopes used in the initial studies, and the limitation of dose escalation by myelosuppression using the initial radioimmune conjugates. Nevertheless, radioiodinated MoAbs against B-cell antigens have been used successfully in the treatment of chemotherapy-refractory non-Hodgkin's lymphoma, with high response rates reported in chemotherapy-refractory patients. Conjugates using isotopes such as yttrium-90 linked with MoAbs or small oligopeptide ligands, such as octreotide, are under development; together with dose fractionation and hematopoietic growth factors, these conjugates may permit delivery of therapeutic doses of radiation to solid tumors.

   4. **Chemoimmunotherapy.** This potential therapeutic strategy has been hindered by a lack

of good conjugation technology and appropriate chemotherapeutic agents. Doxorubicin-antibody constructs have been studied clinically, with little objective antitumor activity in solid tumors and with toxicity apparently related to specific antigen binding. Other constructs, including antitumor antibiotics of greater specific activity, such as calicheamicin, are under development.

E. **Reduction of chemotherapy or irradiation toxicity.** The hematopoietic growth factors have been studied extensively with regard to their ability to decrease the length of myelosuppression, the depth of the neutrophil nadir, the number of febrile events, and the incidence of mucositis after administration of cytotoxic drugs or radiation. There are several settings in which these factors have been used in association with myelosuppressive chemotherapy. The American Society of Clinical Oncology has produced a set of guidelines on the clinical use of G-CSF and GM-CSF, the two FDA-approved mycloid growth factors, which were published in the *Journal of Clinical Oncology* in November 1994. Use of these factors is recommended for the following indications:

1. The reduction of a likelihood of first-cycle neutropenia when this likelihood is otherwise 40% or higher (primary prophylaxis)

2. In further cycles of chemotherapy after occurrence of febrile neutropenia, when maintenance of dose intensity rather than dose reduction is appropriate (secondary prophylaxis)

3. After high-dose chemotherapy followed by peripheral blood stem cell or autologous bone marrow support

4. Rarely, in the treatment of established febrile neutropenia, generally only when the infection is life-threatening or is expected to require prolonged antibiotic or antifungal therapy

The recommended dosage of G-CSF (filgrastim) is 5 µg/kg/day and that of GM-CSF (sargramostim) is 250 µg/m²/day.

F. **Increasing the effectiveness of chemotherapy or irradiation.** Less clear than the toxicity reduction issue is whether the use of myeloid growth factors permits significant increases in dose intensity for chemotherapy through either dose escalation or a decrease in the interval between chemotherapy cycles. The agents are also being used in conjunction with bone marrow transplantation in attempts to decrease the morbidity and mortality associated with that procedure.

G. **Differentiation therapy.** Many of the myeloid growth and immune-stimulating factors described already also have differentiation-inducing properties. The hematopoietic factors, including IL-3 and

GM-CSF, are being studied in disorders of bone marrow differentiation, including myelodysplasia and aplastic anemia. Similarly, the interleukins may find application in certain patients with some inherited or acquired immunodeficiency states. A group of agents active in differentiation, the retinoids, are under study for both treatment and prevention of malignancy. Tretinoin (all *trans*-retinoic acid) is active in inducing remission of acute promyelocytic leukemia and has been approved for clinical use in this indication. Isotretinoin (13-*cis*-retinoic acid) has induced remissions of advanced squamous cell carcinomas of the skin and cervix and cutaneous T-cell lymphoma and has been demonstrated to prolong remission when used in the adjuvant setting in childhood neuroblastoma. Isotretinoin administered after primary treatment has also been shown to reduce the incidence of secondary malignancies in patients who have had squamous cell carcinoma of the head and neck. Preclinical studies suggest that these agents may be even more active when used together with some of the cytokines and growth factors discussed earlier.

IV. Toxicities of biologic therapy. In general, the predictable toxicities of biologic agents are dose and schedule related. Administration of the IFNs on a daily basis is associated with systemic symptoms, including fever, fatigue, and myalgia. Nonsteroidal antiinflammatory agents and acetaminophen are useful for alleviating these symptoms, although tachyphylaxis occurs with continued therapy, and these symptoms diminish over time.

A. Toxicities associated with IL-2 are dose dependent. The importance of careful patient selection for high-dose IL-2 therapy cannot be overemphasized because the high-dose IL-2 regimens are associated with significant cardiovascular complications, including hypotension and the development of a full-blown capillary leak syndrome. Clinical manifestations include decreased serum albumin, weight gain, and development of peripheral edema in the setting of fluid support for blood pressure. This fluid overload can be associated with pulmonary compromise. Other cardiac complications of high-dose IL-2 therapy include arrhythmias, principally supraventricular, and myocardial infarction. The latter complication is largely avoided by prescreening patient candidates for the presence of ischemic heart disease. Patients on IL-2 develop a characteristic erythematous rash that may progress to desquamation. IL-2 therapy can exacerbate preexisting psoriasis and, rarely, is associated with the development of a pemphigus-like syndrome. Patients on IL-2 characteristically have a decreased appetite and may develop nausea and occasional diarrhea. The development of hypothyroidism has been described in association with IL-2 therapy and rarely with IFN therapy. Development of neuropsychiatric changes, such as confusion, during IL-2 therapy is a reason to halt therapy. Like other IL-2 effects, these problems are reversible, but unlike the others, the neuropsychiatric changes may continue to progress after discontinuation of therapy. Although corticosteroids prevent or attenuate most IL-2–related side effects, presumably by preventing the release of such IL2–induced cytokines as TNF and IFN-γ, concern about the potential deleterious consequences on the antitumor effects of IL-2 precludes their use except in life-threatening situations.

   B.   **MoAb administration** has been associated with hypotension and shortness of breath. The risk of anaphylaxis, which is greater with repeated dosing, has led to routine administration of an intravenous test dose with anaphylactic precautions (including epinephrine, steroids, and antihistamines) on hand. The toxicities of the immunoconjugates are largely related to those of the linked cytotoxic moiety; for example, the use of ricin-conjugated immunotoxins has been associated with myalgias, elevated serum creatine phosphokinase levels, and occasional rhabdomyolysis, all features of ricin poisoning. Clinical experience with trastuzumab (Herceptin) has suggested that combination therapy with this drug plus doxorubicin and cyclophosphamide not only may result in greater antitumor activity but also may be associated with increased cardiotoxicity.

V.   **Current status of biologic agents in cancer therapy.** As noted in Table 2-1, biologic agents have found clinical applications in some cancer-related situations. Many more potential applications are under investigation, limited only by our understanding of the biologic characteristics of these agents and their effects on normal and malignant cells.

Table 2-1.   Current status of biologic agents in cancer therapy

Agent	Status
Interferon-α	Approved by the Food and Drug Administration (FDA) for hairy-cell leukemia, AIDS-related Kaposi's sarcoma, and chronic myelogenous leukemia
	Responses also seen in low-grade non-Hodgkin's lymphoma, cutaneous T-cell lymphomas
	Activity in nonmalignant indications, including condyloma acuminatum,

continued

Table 2-1.   (*Continued*)

Agent	Status
	chronic hepatitis B and C, juvenile laryngeal papillomatosis
Interferon-β	No approved indication in cancer therapy; has many properties similar to interferon-α; FDA-approved in therapy of multiple sclerosis
Interferon-γ	Active prophylactically in decreasing infections in chronic granulomatous disease (FDA approved); under investigation in cancer biotherapy for macrophage-stimulating and tumor antigen–upregulating properties
Interleukin-1	Despite abundant preclinical evidence regarding chemoprotective and radio-protective properties, no clinical role has been defined
Interleukin-2	Single-agent activity in metastatic renal cell carcinoma and malignant melanoma (FDA-approved indications)
Interleukin-4	Investigational: as an immunostimulatory agent
Interleukin-11	FDA-approved for use after cytotoxic chemotherapy; accelerates platelet recovery
Interleukin-12	Investigational; in clinical trials, potential T-cell–enhancing agent
Transforming growth factor-β (TGF-β)	Potential uses to decrease chemotherapy-associated mucositis or for myeloprotection; remains investigational
Granulocyte colony-stimulating factor (G-CSF)	Decreases length of myelosuppression after administration of cytotoxic agents; reduces length of neutropenia and incidence of febrile episodes during cytotoxic chemotherapy (FDA approved)
Granulocyte-macrophage colony-stimulating factor (GM-CSF)	Marrow-restorative properties similar to G-CSF (FDA approved); also being studied for monocyte proliferation and activating characteristics
	Investigational: under study for myelorestorative properties; also being studied in aplastic anemia and myelodysplasia
Interleukin-3	Investigational: under study for platelet-stimulating activities
Macrophage colony-stimulating factor (M-CSF; CSF-1)	Clearly defined preclinical proliferative and activating effects on monocytes; no clinical role established

continued

Table 2-1.   (*Continued*)

Agent	Status
Monoclonal antibodies (MoAb)	Anti-CD3 murine MoAb approved for treatment of allograft rejection; rituximab (Rituxan) (anti-CD2), approved for non-Hodgkin's lymphoma; traztuzumab (Herceptin) (anti-Her-2/neu) active alone and with chemotherapy in metastatic breast carcinoma
Immunotoxins	Investigational: demonstrate antitumor activity in refractory non-Hodgkin's lymphoma and chronic lymphocytic leukemia
Fusion toxins	Interleukin-2–diphtheria toxin conjugate has produced antitumor activity in mycosis fungoides; other cytokine-toxic conjugates under development
Radioimmuno-conjugates	Investigational: anti-B cell–iodine-131 conjugates have been active in refractory B-cell lymphomas
Antiangiogenesis factors	Investigational: interference with tumor new blood vessel formation (e.g., fumagillin analogs, thalidomide, angiostatin, endostatin)
Antineovasculature factors	Agents directed against epitopes selectively expressed on tumor neovasculature (e.g. $\alpha_v\beta_3$-integrin)

SELECTED READINGS

American Society of Clinical Oncology.Recommendations for the use of hematopoietic colony-stimulating factors: evidence-based, clinical practice guidelines. *J Clin Oncol* 1994;12:2471–2508.

Parkinson DR. Immune therapies for cancer. In: Brain MC, Carbone PP, eds. *Current therapy in hematology-oncology.* 5th ed. Philadelphia: Mosby, 1995:34–38.

Parkinson DR, Grimm EA. Cytokines: biology and applications in cancer medicine. In: Holland JF, Frie, E, Bast R, Kufe D, Morton D, Weichselbaum R, eds. *Cancer medicine.* 4th ed. Baltimore: Williams & Wilkins, 1996:1213–1226.

Sznol M, Parkinson DR. Clinical applications of IL-2. *Oncology* 1994;8:61–67.

Systematic Assessment of the Patient with Cancer and Long-term Medical Complications of Treatment

Roland T. Skeel and Patricia A. Ganz

I. **Establishing the diagnosis**
   A. **Pathologic diagnosis is critical.** Obviously, the diagnosis of cancer must be firmly established before chemotherapy or any other treatment is administered, but the critical nature of an accurate diagnosis warrants a reminder. As a rule, there must be cytologic or histologic evidence of neoplastic cells together with a clinical picture consistent with the diagnosis of the cancer under consideration. Most commonly, patients present to their physician with a complaint such as a cough, bleeding, pain, or a lump; through a logical sequence of evaluation, the presence of cancer is revealed on a cytologic or histologic specimen. Less frequently, lesions are discovered fortuitously during routine examination, systematic screening for cancer, or evaluation of an unrelated disorder. With some types of cancer, pathologists can establish the diagnosis based on small amounts of material obtained from needle biopsies, aspirations, or tissue scrapings. Other cancers require larger pieces of tissue for special staining, immunohistologic evaluation, flow cytometry, examination by electron microscopy, or more sophisticated studies, such as evaluation for gene rearrangement.

   It is often helpful to confer with the pathologist before obtaining a specimen to determine what kind and size of specimen is adequate to establish the complete diagnosis. When a tissue diagnosis of cancer is made by the pathologist, it is incumbent on the clinician to review the material with the pathologist. This practice is good medicine (and good learning); it also allows the clinician to tell the patient that he or she has actually seen the cancer. In addition, it prevents the physician from administering chemotherapy without a pathologic diagnosis. The pathologist often gives a better consultation—not just a tissue diagnosis—when the clinician shows a personal interest.
   B. **Pathologic and clinical diagnosis must be consistent.** Once the tissue diagnosis is established, the clinician must be certain that the pathologic diagnosis is consistent with the clinical findings. If the two are not consistent, a search must be made

for additional information, clinical or pathologic, that allows the clinician to make a unified diagnosis. A pathologic diagnosis, like a clinical diagnosis, is also an opinion with varying levels of certainty. The first part of the pathologic diagnosis—and usually the easier part—is an opinion about whether the tissue examined is neoplastic. Because most pathologists rarely render a diagnosis of cancer unless the degree of certainty is high, a positive diagnosis of cancer is generally reliable. Absence of definitively diagnosed cancer in a specimen does not mean that cancer is not present, however; it means only that it could not be diagnosed on the tissue obtained, and clinical circumstances must establish if additional tissue sampling is necessary. The second part of the pathologist's diagnosis is an opinion about the type of cancer. This determination is not necessary in all circumstances but is nearly always helpful in selecting the most appropriate therapy and making a determination of prognosis.

C. **Treatment without a pathologic diagnosis.** There are rare circumstances in which treatment is undertaken before a pathologic diagnosis is established. Such circumstances are clearly exceptions, however, and involve fewer than 1% of all patients with cancer. Therapy is begun without a pathologic diagnosis only when the following conditions are met:

1. When withholding prompt treatment or carrying out the procedures required to establish the diagnosis would greatly increase a patient's morbidity or risk of mortality, and

2. When the likelihood of a benign diagnosis is remote

Two examples of such circumstances are (a) a patient with a primary tumor of the midbrain and (b) a patient with superior vena cava syndrome with no accessible supraclavicular nodes and no endobronchial disease found on bronchoscopy in whom the risk of bleeding from mediastinoscopy is deemed greater than the risk of administering radiotherapy for a disease of uncertain nature.

II. **Staging.** Once the diagnosis of cancer is firmly established, it is important to determine the anatomic extent or stage of the disease. The steps taken for staging vary considerably among cancers because of the differing natural histories of the tumors.

A. **Staging system criteria.** For most cancers, a system of staging has been established based on the following factors:

1. Natural history and mode of spread of the cancer

2. Prognostic import for the staging parameters used

3. Value of the criteria used for decisions about therapy

B. **Staging and therapy decisions.** In the past, surgery and radiotherapy were used to treat patients with cancer in early stages, and chemotherapy was used when surgery and radiotherapy were no longer effective or when the disease was in an advanced stage at presentation. In such circumstances, chemotherapy was only palliative (except for gestational choriocarcinoma), and in the absence of exquisitely sensitive tumors or strikingly potent drugs, the likelihood of increasing the survival was low. As we have learned more about the genetic determinants of cancer growth, tumor cell kinetics, and the development of resistance, the value of early intervention with chemotherapy has been transposed from animal models to human cancers. To plan this intervention and evaluate its effectiveness, careful staging has become increasingly important. Only when the exact extent of disease has been established can the most rational plan of treatment for the individual patient be devised, whether it is surgery, radiotherapy, chemotherapy, or biologic therapy alone or in combination. Although no single staging system is universally used for all cancers, the system developed jointly by the American Joint Committee on Cancer (AJCC) and the TNM Committee of the International Union Against Cancer (UICC) is most widely used for staging solid tumors. It is based on the status of the primary tumor (T), regional lymph nodes (N), and distant metastasis (M). For some cancers, tumor grade (G) is also taken into account. The stage of the tumor is based on a condensation of the total possible TNM and G categories to create stage groupings, usually stages 0, I, II, III, and IV, which are relatively homogeneous with respect to prognosis. When relevant to the specific cancers whose chemotherapy is discussed in Part III of this *Handbook,* the staging system or systems most commonly used for that cancer are discussed.

III. **Performance status.** The performance status refers to the level of activity of which a patient is capable. It is an independent measure (independent from the anatomic extent or histologic characteristics of the cancer) of how much the cancer or comorbid conditions have affected the patient and a prognostic indicator of how well the patient is likely to respond to treatment.

A. **Types of performance status scales.** Two performance status scales are in wide use.

1. **The Karnofsky Performance Status Scale** (Table 3-1) has 10 levels of activity. It has the advantage of allowing discrimination over a wide scale but the disadvantages of being difficult to remember easily and perhaps of making discriminations that are not clinically useful.

2. **The Eastern Cooperative Oncology Group (ECOG) Performance Status Scale** (Table 3-2) has the advantages of being easy to remem-

Table 3-1. Karnofsky Performance Status Scale

Functional capability	Level of activity
Able to carry on normal activity; no special care needed	100%—Normal; no complaints, no evidence of disease 90%—Able to carry on normal activity; minor signs or symptoms of disease 80%—Normal activity with effort; some signs or symptoms of disease
Unable to work; able to live at home; cares for most personal needs; needs varying amount of assistance	70%—Cares for self; unable to carry on normal activity or to do active work 60%—Requires occasional assistance but is able to care for most of own needs 50%—Requires considerable assistance and frequent medical care
Unable to care for self; requires equivalent of institutional or hospital care	40%—Disabled; requires special medical care and assistance 30%—Severely disabled; hospitalization indicated, although death not imminent 20%—Very sick; hospitalization necessary; active supportive treatment necessary 10%—Moribund; fatal processes progressing rapidly 0%—Dead

ber and making discriminations that are clinically useful.

3. **Using the criteria of each scale,** patients who are fully active or have mild symptoms respond more frequently to treatment and survive longer than do patients who are less active or have severe symptoms. A clear designation of the performance status distribution of patients in therapeutic clinical trials is thus critical in determining comparability and generalizability of trials and effectiveness of the treatments used.

B. **Use of performance status for choosing treatment.** In the individualization of therapy, the performance status is often a useful parameter for helping the clinician decide whether the patient will benefit from treatment or will be made worse. For example, unless there is some reason to expect a dramatic response of a cancer to chemotherapy, treatment is

**Table 3-2.   Eastern Cooperative
Oncology Group Performance Status Scale**

Grade	Level of activity
0	Fully active; able to carry on all predisease performance without restriction (Karnofsky 90%–100%)
1	Restricted in physically strenuous activity but ambulatory and able to carry out work of a light or sedentary nature, e.g., light house work, office work (Karnofsky 70%–80%)
2	Ambulatory and capable of all self-care but unable to carry out any work activities; up and about more than 50% of waking hours (Karnofsky 50%–60%)
3	Capable of only limited self-care, confined to bed or chair more than 50% of waking hours (Karnofsky 30%–40%)
4	Completely disabled; cannot carry on any self-care; totally confined to bed or chair (Karnofsky 10%–20%)

often withheld from patients with an ECOG performance status of 4 because responses to therapy are infrequent and toxic effects of the treatment are likely to be great.

C. **Quality of life.** A related but partially independent measure of performance status can be determined based on patients' own perceptions of their quality of life (QOL). QOL evaluations have been shown to be independent predictors of tumor response and survival in some cancers, and they are important components in a comprehensive assessment of response to therapy. For some cancers, improvement in quality of life measures early in the course of treatment are the most reliable indicators of survival.

IV. **Response to therapy.** Response to therapy may be measured by (a) survival, (b) objective change in tumor size or in tumor product (e.g., immunoglobulin in myeloma), and (c) subjective change.

A. **Survival.** One goal of cancer therapy is to allow patients to live as long and with the same QOL as they would have if they did not have the cancer. If this goal is achieved, it can be said that the patient is cured of the cancer (though biologically the cancer may still be present). From a practical standpoint, we do not wait to see if patients live a normal life-span before saying that a given treatment is capable of achieving a cure, but we follow a cohort of patients to see if their survival within a given time span is different from a comparable cohort without the cancer. For the evaluation of response to *adjuvant therapy* (additional treatment after surgery or radiotherapy that is given to treat potential nonmeasurable, micrometastatic disease) or *neoadjuvant therapy* (chemotherapy or biologic therapy given as initial treatment before surgery or radiotherapy), survival analysis (rather than tumor response) must be used as the definitive objective measure of antineoplastic effect. With neoadjuvant therapy, tumor response and resectability are also partial determinants of effectiveness.

It is, of course, possible that a patient may be cured of the cancer but die early owing to complications associated with the treatment. Even with complications (unless they are acute ones such as bleeding or infection), survival of patients who have been cured of the cancer is likely to be longer than if the treatment had not been given, though shorter than if the patient never had the cancer.

If cure is not possible, the reduced goal is to allow the patient to live longer than if the therapy under consideration were not given. It is important for physicians to know if, and with what likelihood, any given treatment will result in a longer life. Such information helps the physician to choose whether to recommend treatment and the patient to decide whether to undertake the recommended treatment program.

B. Objective response. Although survival is important to the individual patient, it is not easy to predict how long a patient is going to live; thus, survival does not give an early measurement of treatment effectiveness. Tumor regression, on the other hand, frequently occurs early in the course of effective treatment and is therefore a readily used measurement of treatment benefit. Tumor regression can be determined by the reduced size of a tumor or the reduction of tumor products.

   1. Tumor size. When tumor size is measured, responses are usually classified as follows:

   a. Complete response is the disappearance of all evidence of the cancer for at least two measurement periods separated by at least 4 weeks.

   b. Partial response is a decrease of 50% or more in the sum of the products of the largest diameter and the diameter perpendicular to the largest (diameter product) of all measurable lesions with no appearance of any new lesions for at least 4 weeks. When there are more than three or four measurable lesions, representative lesions are usually measured, rather than all lesions.

   c. Stable disease is a decrease of less than 50% to an increase of less than 25% in the diameter product of any measurable lesions.

   d. Progression is an increase of more than 25% in the diameter product or the appearance of any new lesions.

e.   **Time to progression** is an additional indicator that is often used. It takes into account the fact that from the patient perspective, complete response, partial response, and stable disease may be meaningless distinctions, so long as the tumor is not causing symptoms or impairment of function. It also takes into account that some agents result in disease stability for a substantial period, despite failure to produce measurable disease shrinkage. Time to progression can also be used as an indicator of disease status when there was no measurable disease at the outset of therapy or when the therapeutic modalities were not comparable. For example, if one wanted to compare the results of surgery alone to those of chemotherapy alone, time to progression from the onset of treatment would allow a valid comparison of the effectiveness of the treatments, whereas the traditional tumor response criteria would not. Time to progression thus places each of the agents or modalities on an even basis.

f.   **If survival curves** of patient populations having different categories of response are compared, those patients with a complete response frequently survive longer than those with a lesser response. If a sizable number of complete responses occurs with a treatment regimen, the survival rate of patients treated with that regimen is likely to be significantly greater than that of patients who are untreated. When the number of complete responders in a population rises to about 50%, the possibility of cure for a small number of patients begins to appear. With increasing percentages of complete responders, the frequency of cures is likely to increase correspondingly.

Although patients who have partial response to a treatment usually survive longer than those who have stable disease or progression, it is often not easy to demonstrate that the overall survival of the treated population is better than that of a comparable untreated group. In part, this difficulty may be due to a phenomenon of small numbers. If only 15% to 20% of a population respond to therapy, the median survival rate may not change at all, and the numbers may not be high enough to demonstrate a significant difference in survival duration of the longest surviving 5% to 10% of patients (the "tail" of the curves) for treated and untreated populations. It is also possible that the patients who achieve a partial response to therapy are those who have less aggressive disease at the outset of treatment and thus will survive longer than the nonresponders regardless of therapy. These caveats notwithstanding, most clinicians and patients welcome a partial response as a sign that offers hope for longer survival and improved quality of life.

2. **Tumor products.** For many cancers, objective tumor size changes are difficult or impossible to document. For some of these neoplasms, tumor products (hormones, antigens, antibodies) may be measurable and may provide a good, objective way to evaluate tumor response. Two examples of such markers that closely reflect tumor cell mass are the abnormal immunoglobulins (M proteins) produced in multiple myeloma and the human chorionic gonadotropin (β-hCG) produced in choriocarcinoma and testicular cancer.

3. **Evaluable disease.** Other objective changes may occur but are not easily quantifiable. When these changes are not easily measurable, they may be termed *evaluable*. For example, neurologic changes secondary to primary brain tumors cannot be measured with a caliper, but they can be evaluated using neurologic testing. An arbitrary system of grading the degree of severity of the neurologic deficit can be devised to permit objective evaluation of tumor response.

4. **Performance status changes** may also be used as a measure of objective change, although in many respects the performance status is more representative of the subjective than the objective status of the disease.

C. **Subjective change and QOL considerations.** A subjective change is one that is perceived by the patient but not necessarily by the physician or others around the patient. Subjective improvement and an acceptable QOL are often of far greater importance to the patient than objective improvement: If the cancer shrinks but the patient feels worse than before treatment, he or she is not likely to believe that the treatment was worthwhile. It is not valid to look at subjective change in isolation, however, because temporary worsening in the perceived state of well-being may be necessary to achieve subsequent long-term improvement.

This point is particularly well illustrated by the combined-modality treatment in which chemotherapy is used to treat micrometastases after surgical removal of the macroscopic tumor. In such a circumstance, the patient is likely to feel entirely well after the primary surgical procedure, but the side effects of chemotherapy increase the symptoms and make the patient feel subjectively worse for the period of treatment. The winner's stakes are valuable, however, because if the chemotherapy treatment of the micrometastases is successful, the patient will be cured of the cancer and can be expected to have a normal or near-normal life expectancy rather than dying from recurrent disease. Most patients agree that the temporary subjective worsening is not only tolerable but well worth the price if cure of the cancer is a distinct possibility. This judgment depends on the severity and duration of symptoms, functional impairment, and perceptions of illness as well as on the expected benefit (increased likelihood of survival) anticipated as a result of the treatment.

When chemotherapy is given with a palliative intent, patients (and less often physicians) may be unwilling to tolerate significant side effects or subjective worsening. Fortunately, subjective improvement often accompanies objective improvement, so those patients in whom there is measurable improvement of the cancer also feel better. The degree of subjective worsening each patient is willing to tolerate varies, and the patient and physician together must discuss and evaluate whether the chemotherapy treatment program is worth continuing. Such discussions should include a clear presentation of the scientific facts that include objective survival and tumor response data together with whatever QOL information has been documented for the treatment proposed. Moreover, the expressed desires and the social, economic, psychological, and spiritual situation of the patient and his or her family must be sensitively considered.

V. **Toxicity**
    A. **Factors affecting toxicity.** One of the characteristics that distinguishes cancer chemotherapeutic agents from most other drugs is the frequency and severity of anticipated side effects at usual therapeutic doses. Because of the severity of the side effects, it is critical to monitor the patient carefully for adverse reactions so that therapy can be modified before the toxicity becomes life-threatening. Most toxicities vary according to the following factors:
        1. Specific agent
        2. Dose
        3. Schedule of administration
        4. Route of administration
        5. Predisposing factors in the patient, which may be known and predictive for toxicity or unknown and result in unexpected toxic effects
    B. **Clinical testing of new drugs for toxicity.** Before the introduction of any agent into wide clinical use,

the agent must undergo testing in carefully controlled clinical trials. The first set of clinical trials are called *Phase I trials.* They are carried out with the express purpose of determining toxicity in humans and establishing the maximum tolerated dose, although they are done only in patients who might benefit from the drug. Such trials are undertaken only after extensive tests in animals have been completed. Much human toxicity is predicted by animal studies, but because of significant species differences, initial doses used in human studies are several times lower than doses at which toxicity is first seen in animals. Phase I trials are carried out using several schedules, and the dose is escalated in successive groups of patients once the toxicity of the prior dose has been established.

At the completion of Phase I trials, there is usually a great deal of information about the spectrum and anticipated severity of acute drug effects (toxicity). However, because patients in Phase I trials often do not live long enough to undergo many months of treatment, chronic or cumulative effects may not be discovered. Discovery of these toxicities may occur only after widespread use of the drug in *Phase II trials* (to establish the spectrum of effectiveness of the drug) or *Phase III trials* (to compare the new drug or combination with standard therapy).

C. **Common acute toxicities.** Some toxicities are relatively common among cancer chemotherapeutic agents. Common acute toxicities include the following:
1. Myelosuppression with leukopenia, thrombocytopenia, and anemia
2. Nausea and vomiting
3. Mucous membrane ulceration
4. Alopecia

Aside from nausea and vomiting, these toxicities occur because of the cytotoxic effects of chemotherapy on rapidly dividing normal cells of the bone marrow and epithelium (e.g., mucous membranes, skin, hair follicles).

D. **Selective toxicities.** Other toxicities are less common and are specific to individual drugs or classes of drugs. Examples of drugs and their related toxicities include the following:
1. Vinca alkaloids: neurotoxicity
2. Ifosfamide and cyclophosphamide: hemorrhagic cystitis
3. Anthracyclines: cardiomyopathy
4. Bleomycin: pulmonary fibrosis
5. Asparaginase: anaphylaxis (allergic reaction)
6. Cisplatin: renal toxicity, neurotoxicity
7. Ifosfamide: central nervous system toxicity
8. Mitomycin: hemolytic-uremic syndrome
9. Procarbazine: food and drug interactions
10. Paclitaxel: neurotoxicity, acute hypersensitivity reactions

11.   Fludarabine, cladribine, pentostatin: prolonged suppression of cellular immunity with risk of opportunistic infection

E.   **Recognition and evaluation of toxicity.** Anyone who administers chemotherapeutic agents *must* be familiar with the expected and the unusual toxicities of the agent the patient is receiving, be prepared to avert severe toxicity when possible, and be able to manage toxic complications when they cannot be avoided. The specific toxicities of commonly used individual chemotherapeutic agents are detailed in Chapter 5.

For the purpose of reporting toxicity in a uniform manner, *criteria* are often established to grade the severity of the toxicity. For many years, a simplified set of criteria has been used by several National Cancer Institute (NCI)–supported clinical trials groups for the most common toxic manifestations. Although this document is helpful, it is in many respects incomplete. To address this issue, a new set of more comprehensive toxicity criteria have been developed and are now available on the Internet. A sample showing one section (Blood and Bone Marrow) from the new common toxicity criteria (3 pages of 33) is shown in Table 3-3. The complete common toxicity criteria, generic reporting forms, and a host of other helpful information can be obtained on the internet at **http://ctep.info.nih.gov/**. The complete set of criteria and generic reporting forms can be downloaded as needed. All new clinical trials approved by the NCI Cancer Therapy Evaluation Program (CTEP) will use these new toxicity criteria. Such standardization is important in the evaluation of the toxicity of cancer treatment. Small flipbooks with the Common Toxicity Criteria (CTC) can be obtained from the NCI Cancer Therapy Evaluation Program by sending an email request to **info@ctep.nci.nih.**

F.   **Acute toxicity management.** Prevention and treatment of myelosuppression and its consequences are discussed in Chapters 2, 6, 28, and 29. Management of nausea and vomiting, mucositis, and alopecia, as well as diarrhea, nutrition problems, and drug extravasation, are discussed in Chapter 27. Other acute toxicities are discussed with the individual drugs in Chapter 5. Long-term medical problems are a special issue and are highlighted in the section that follows.

VI.   **Late physical effects of cancer treatment**

A.   **Late organ toxicities** may be minimized by limiting doses when thresholds are known. In most instances, however, individual patient effects cannot be predicted. Treatment is primarily symptomatic.

1.   **Cardiac toxicity** (e.g., congestive cardiomyopathy) is most commonly associated with high total

Text continued on page 51

**Table 3-3. Representative section from the New Cancer
Therapy Evaluation Program (CTEP) Common Toxicity Criteria Version 2.0**

Category	0	1	2	3	4
			Blood and bone marrow		
Bone marrow cellularity	Normal for age	Mildly hypocellular or 25% reduction from normal cellularity for age	Moderately hypocellular or >25 to ≤50% reduction from normal cellularity for age or >2 but <4 wk to recovery of normal bone marrow cellularity	Severely hypocellular or >50 to ≤75% reduction in cellularity for age or 4–6 wk to recovery of normal bone marrow cellularity	Aplasia or >6 wk to recovery of normal bone marrow cellularity
Normal ranges Children (≤18 yr) Younger adults (19–59 yr) Older adults (≥60 yr)	90% Cellularity average 60%–70% Cellularity average 50% Cellularity average				

Note: Grade bone marrow cellularity for changes related only to treatment, not disease.

| CD4 count | WNL | < LLN–500/mm^3 | 200–< 500/mm^3 | 50–< 200/mm^3 | < 50/mm^3 |

continued

Table 3-3. (*Continued*)

Category	0	1	2	3	4
			Blood and bone marrow		
Haptoglobin	Normal	Decreased	—	Absent	—
Hemoglobin (Hgb)	WNL	< LLN–10.0 g/dl < LLN–100 g/L < LLN–6.2 mmol/L	8.0–< 10.0 g/dl 80–< 100 g/L 4.9–< 6.2 mmol/L	6.5–< 8.0 g/dl 65–80 g/L 4.0–< 4.9 mmol/L	< 6.5 g/dl < 65 g/L < 4.0 mmol/L

Note: The following criteria may be used for leukemia studies or bone marrow infiltrative/myelophthisic process if the protocol so specifies:

Category	0	1	2	3	4
For leukemia studies or bone marrow infiltrative or myelophthisic processes	WNL	10%–<25% Decrease from pretreatment	25%–<50% Decrease from pretreatment	50%–<75% Decrease from pretreatment	≥75% Decrease from pretreatment
Hemolysis (e.g., immune hemolytic anemia, drug-related hemolysis, other)	None	Only laboratory evidence of hemolysis (e.g., direct antiglobulin test [DAT, Coombs'] schistocytes)	Evidence of red blood cell destruction and ≥2 g decrease in hemoglobin; no transfusion	Requiring transfusion or medical intervention (e.g., steroids)	Catastrophic consequences of hemolysis (e.g., renal failure, hypotension, bronchospasm, emergency splenectomy)

Also consider haptoglobin, hemoglobin

	WNL	Grade 1	Grade 2	Grade 3	Grade 4
Leukocytes (total white blood cells)	WNL	< LLN–3.0 × 10⁹/L <LLN–3,000/mm³	≥2.0–<3.0 × 10⁹/L ≥2,000–<3,000/mm³	≥1.0–<2.0 × 10⁹/L ≥1,000–<2,000/mm³	< 1.0 × 10⁹/L < 1,000/mm³
For BMT studies:	WNL	≥2.0–<3.0 × 10⁹/L ≥2,000–<3,000/mm³	≥1.0–<2.0 × 10⁹/L ≥1,000–<2,000/mm³	≥0.5–<1.0 × 10⁹/L ≥500–<1,000/mm³	<0.5 × 10⁹/L <500/mm³
Note: The following criteria using age, race, and sex normal values may be used for pediatric studies if the protocol so specifies:		≥75–<100% LLN	≥50–<75% LLN	≥25–<50% LLN	<25% LLN
Lymphopenia	WNL	<LLN–1.0 × 10⁹/L <LLN–1,000/mm³	≥0.5–<1.0 × 10⁹/L ≥500–<1,000/mm³	<0.5 × 10⁹/L <500/mm³	—
Note: The following criteria using age, race, and sex normal values may be used for pediatric studies if the protocol so specifies.		≥75%–<100% LLN	≥50%–<75% LLN	≥25%–<50% LLN	<25% LLN
Neutrophils/granulocytes (ANC/AGC)	WNL	≥1.5–<2.0 × 10⁹/L ≥1,500–<2,000/mm³	≥1.0–<1.5 × 10⁹/L ≥1,000–<1,500/mm³	≥0.5–<1.0 × 10⁹/L ≥500–<1,000/mm³	<0.5×10⁹/L <500/mm³
For BMT:	WNL	≥1.0–<1.5 × 10⁹/L ≥1,000–<1,500/mm³	≥0.5–<1.0 × 10⁹/L ≥500–<1,000/mm³	≥0.1–<0.5 × 10⁹/L ≥100–<500/mm³	<0.1×10⁹/L <100/mm³
Note: The following criteria may be used for leukemia studies or bone marrow infiltrative or myelophthisic process if the protocol so specifies:					
For leukemia studies or bone marrow infiltrative or myelophthisic process	WNL	10%–<25% Decrease from baseline	25%–<50% Decrease from baseline	50%–<75% Decrease from baseline	≥75% Decrease from baseline

continued

Table 3-3. *(Continued)*

Category	0	1	2	3	4
			Blood and bone marrow		
Platelets	WNL	$<$LLN–$<$75.0 $\times$ 10⁹/L $<$LLN–75,000/mm³	≥50.0–$<$75.0 $\times$ 10⁹/L ≥50,000–$<$75,000/mm³	≥10.0–$<$ 50.0 $\times$ 10⁹/L ≥10,000–$<$50,000/mm³	$<$10.0 $\times$ 10⁹/L $<$10,000/mm³
For BMT:	WNL	≥50.0–$<$75.0 $\times$ 10⁹/L ≥50,000–$<$75,000/mm³	≥20.0 – $<$ 50.0 $\times$ 10⁹/L ≥20,000–$<$50,000/mm³	≥10.0–$<$20.0 $\times$ 10⁹/L ≥10,000–$<$20,000/mm³	$<$10.0 $\times$ 10⁹/L $<$10,000/mm³

Note: The following criteria may be used for leukemia studies or bone marrow infiltrative or myelophthisic process if the protocol so specifies:

Category	0	1	2	3	4
For leukemia studies or bone marrow infiltrative or myelophthisic process	WNL	10%–$<$25% Decrease from baseline	25%–$<$50% Decrease from baseline	50%–$<$75% Decrease from baseline	≥75% Decrease from baseline
Transfusion: Platelets	None	—	—	Yes	Platelet transfusions and other measures required to improve platelet increment; platelet transfusion refractoriness associated

with life-threatening bleeding (e.g., HLA or cross-matched platelet transfusions)

	None	One platelet transfusion in 24 h	Two platelet transfusions in 24 h	Three or more platelet transfusions in 24 h	Platelet transfusions and other measures required to improve platelet increment; platelet transfusion refractoriness associated with life-threatening bleeding (e.g., HLA or cross-matched platelet transfusions)
For BMT:	None	One platelet transfusion in 24 h	Two platelet transfusions in 24 h	Three or more platelet transfusions in 24 h	

Also consider platelets.

	None	—	—	Yes	—
Transfusion: packed red blood cells (pRBCs)	None	—	—	Yes	—

continued

Table 3-3. *(Continued)*

Category	0	1	2	3	4
			Blood and bone marrow		
For BMT:	None	≤2 U pRBCs (≤15 ml/kg) in 24 h, elective or planned	3 U pRBCs (>15–≤30 ml/kg) in 24 h, elective or planned	≥4 U pRBCs (>30 ml/kg) in 24 h	Hemorrhage or hemolysis associated with life-threatening anemia; medical intervention required to improve hemoglobin

Also consider hemoglobin.

Blood and bone marrow—other	None	Mild	Moderate	Severe	Life-threatening or disabling
(Specify: ———)					

LLN, Lower limit of normal; WNL, Within normal limits; DAT, Direct antiglobulin test; BMT, Bone marrow transplant; ANC, Absolute neutrophil count; AGC, Absolute granulocyte count; From Cancer Therapy Evaluation Program Homepage (**http://ctep.info.nih.gov**). Common Toxicity Criteria (CTC) Version 2.0.

doses of doxorubicin or daunorubicin. In addition, high-dose cyclophosphamide as used in transplantation regimens may contribute to congestive cardiomyopathies. When mediastinal irradiation is combined with these chemotherapeutic agents, cardiac toxicity may occur at lower doses. Although evaluation of ventricular ejection fraction with echocardiography or nuclear radiography studies has been useful for acutely monitoring the effects of these agents on the cardiac ejection fraction, studies have reported late onset of congestive heart failure during pregnancy or the initiation of vigorous exercise programs in adults who were previously treated for cancer as children or young adults. The cardiac reserve in these previously treated cancer patients may be marginal. It is probable that there are some changes that take place even at low doses, and it is only because of the great reserve in cardiac function that effects are not measurable until higher doses have been used. Mediastinal irradiation also may accelerate atherogenesis.

Because of the large number of women with breast cancer who are treated with doxorubicin as part of an adjuvant chemotherapy regimen, this group is of special concern and warrants ongoing clinical follow-up.

2. **Pulmonary toxicity** has been classically associated with high doses of bleomycin (>400 U). However, a number of other agents have been associated with pulmonary fibrosis (e.g., alkylating agents, methotrexate, nitrosoureas). Premature respiratory insufficiency, especially with exertion, may become evident with aging.

3. **Nephrotoxicity** is a potential toxicity of several agents (e.g., cisplatin, methotrexate, nitrosoureas). These agents can be associated with both acute and chronic toxicities. Rarely, some patients may require hemodialysis as a result of chronic toxicity.

4. **Neurotoxicity** has been particularly associated with the vinca alkaloids, cisplatin, epipodophyllotoxins, and paclitaxel. Peripheral neuropathy can cause considerable sensory and motor disability. Autonomic dysfunction may produce debilitating postural hypotension. Whole-brain irradiation, with or without chemotherapy, can be a cause of progressive dementia and dysfunction in some long-term survivors. This is particularly a problem for patients with primary brain tumors and for patients with small cell lung cancer who have received prophylactic therapy. Survivors of childhood leukemia have developed a variety of neuropsychological abnormalities related to central nervous system prophylaxis

that included whole-brain irradiation. Recently, it has been demonstrated that some patients who have received adjuvant chemotherapy for carcinoma of the breast also have measurable cognitive deficits such as difficulties with memory or concentration. This appears to be greater for women who have received high-dose chemotherapy plus tamoxifen (32% of women) but is measurably present (17%) in women who have received standard-dose chemotherapy plus tamoxifen.

5. **Hematologic and immunologic impairment** is usually acute and temporally related to the cancer treatment (e.g., chemotherapy or radiation therapy). In some instances, however, there can be persistent cytopenias, as with alkylating agents. Immunologic impairment is a long-term problem for patients with Hodgkin's disease, which may be due to the underlying disease as well as to the treatments that are used. Fludarabine, cladribine, and pentostatin cause profound suppression of CD4 and CD8 lymphocytes and render patients treated susceptible to opportunistic infections. Patients who have undergone splenectomy are also at risk of overwhelming bacterial infections. Complete immunologic reconstitution may take 2 years after marrow ablative therapy requiring stem cell reconstitution.

B. **Second malignancies**

1. **Acute myelogenous leukemia** may occur secondarily to combined modality treatment (e.g., radiation therapy and chemotherapy in Hodgkin's disease) or prolonged therapy with alkylating agents or nitrosoureas (e.g., for multiple myeloma). In general, this form of treatment-related acute leukemia arises in the setting of myelodysplasia and is refractory to intensive treatment. Treatment with the epipodophyllotoxins also has been associated with the development of acute nonlymphocytic leukemia. This may be the result of a specific gene rearrangement between chromosome 9 and chromosome 11 that creates a new cancer-causing oncogene: ALL-1/AF-9. The peak time of occurrence of secondary acute leukemia in patients with Hodgkin's disease is 5 to 7 years after treatment, with an actuarial risk of 6% to 12% by 15 years. Thus, a slowly developing anemia in a survivor of Hodgkin's disease should alert the clinician to the possibility of a secondary myelodysplasia or leukemia. Fortunately, secondary leukemias have not been reported in increased frequencies in women treated with standard adjuvant therapy for breast cancer (e.g., cyclophosphamide, metho-

trexate, and fluorouracil [CMF]), although treatments using higher-than-standard doses of cyclophosphamide (with doxorubicin) have been associated with increased risk of acute nonlymphocytic leukemia.

2. **Solid tumors and other malignancies** are seen with increased frequency in survivors who have been treated with chemotherapy or radiation therapy. Non-Hodgkin's lymphomas have been reported as a late complication in patients treated for Hodgkin's disease or multiple myeloma. Patients treated with long-term cyclophosphamide are at risk of bladder cancer. Patients who have received mantle irradiation for Hodgkin's disease have an increased risk of breast cancer, osteosarcoma, bronchogenic carcinoma, and mesothelioma. In these cases, the second neoplasm is usually in the irradiated field. In general, the risk of solid tumor begins to increase during the second decade of survival after Hodgkin's disease. As a result, young women who have received mantle irradiation for Hodgkin's disease should be screened more carefully for breast cancer by starting at an age earlier than what is advised in standard screening recommendations.

C. **Other sequelae**

1. **Endocrine problems** are a result of cancer treatment. Patients receiving radiation therapy to the head and neck region may develop subclinical or clinical hypothyroidism. This is a particular risk in patients receiving mantle irradiation for Hodgkin's disease. Biennial assessment of thyroid-stimulating hormone (TSH) should be undertaken in these patients. Thyroid replacement therapy should be given if the TSH level rises, to decrease the risk of thyroid cancer. Short stature may be a result of pituitary irradiation and growth hormone deficiency.

2. **Premature menopause** may occur in women who have received certain chemotherapeutic agents (e.g., alkylating agents, procarbazine) or abdominal and pelvic irradiation. The risk is age related, with women older than 30 years at the time of treatment having the greatest risk of treatment-induced amenorrhea and menopause. Early hormone replacement therapy should be considered in such women, if not otherwise contraindicated, to reduce the risk of accelerated osteoporosis and premature heart disease from estrogen deficiency.

3. **Gonadal failure or dysfunction** can lead to infertility in both male and female cancer survivors during their peak reproductive years. Azoospermia is common, but the condition

may improve over time after the completion of therapy. Retroperitoneal dissection in testicular cancer may produce infertility due to retrograde ejaculation. Psychological counseling should be provided to these patients to help them adjust to these long-term sequelae of therapy. Cryopreservation of sperm before treatment should be considered in men. For women, there are limited means available to preserve ova or protect against ovarian failure associated with treatment. Abdominal irradiation in young girls can lead to pregnancy loss due to decreased uterine capacity.

4. **The musculoskeletal system** can be affected by radiation therapy, especially in children and young adults. Radiation may injure the growth plates of long bones and lead to muscle atrophy. Short stature may be a result of direct injury to bone.

SELECTED READINGS

American Joint Committee on Cancer. *AJCC cancer staging manual.* 5th ed. Philadelphia: JB Lippincott Co, 1997.

Curtis RE, Boice J-D Jr, Stovall M, et al. Risk of leukemia after chemotherapy and radiation treatment for breast cancer. *N Engl J Med* 1992;326:1745–1751.

Goldhirsch A, Gelber PD, Simes RJ, Glasziou P, Coates AS. Costs and benefits of adjuvant therapy in breast cancer: a quality-adjusted survival analysis. *J Clin Oncol* 1989;7:36–44.

Kennealey GT, Mitchell MS. Factors that influence the therapeutic response. In: Becker FF, ed. *Cancer: a comprehensive treatise.* Vol. 5. New York: Plenum Publishing, 1977.

Loescher LJ, Welch-McCaffrey D, Leigh SA, Hoffman B, Meyskens FL Jr. Surviving adult cancers. Part 1: Physiologic effects. *Ann Intern Med* 1989;111:411–432.

Oken MM, Creech PH, Tormey DC, et al. Toxicity and response criteria of the Eastern Cooperative Oncology Group. *Am J Clin Oncol* 1982;5:649–655.

Pedersen-Bjergaard J, Sigsgaard TC, Nielsen D, et al. Acute monocytic or myelomonocytic leukemia with balanced chromosome translocations to band 11q23 after therapy with 4-epidoxorubicin and cisplatin or cyclophosphamide for breast cancer. *J Clin Oncol* 1992;10:1444–1451.

Perry MC. Toxicity: ten years later. *Semin Oncol* 1992;19: 453–457.

Pfeifer JD, Wick MR. The pathologic evaluation of neoplastic diseases. In: Holleb AI, Fink DJ, Murphy GP, eds. *Clinical oncology.* Atlanta: American Cancer Society, 1991:7–24.

Pui CH, Ribeiro RC, Hancock ML, et al. Acute myeloid leukemia in children treated with epipodophyllotoxins for acute lymphoblastic leukemia. *N Engl J Med* 1991;325:1682–1687.

Smith MA, Rubinstein L, Ungerleider RS. Therapy-related acute myeloid leukemia following treatment with epipodophyllotoxins: estimating the risks. *Med Pediatr Oncol* 1994;23:86–98.

van Dam FS, Schagen SB, Muller MJ, et al. Impairment of cognitive function in women receiving adjuvant treatment for high-risk breast cancer: high-dose versus standard-dose chemotherapy. *J Natl Cancer Inst* 1998;90:210–218.

van Leeuwen FE, Klokman JW, Hagenbeek A, et al. Second cancer risk following Hodgkin's disease: a 20-year follow-up study. *J Clin Oncol* 1994;12:312–325.

Selection of Treatment for the Patient with Cancer

Roland T. Skeel

I. **Setting treatment goals**
   A. **Medical perspective.** Before a physician decides on a course of treatment for a patient with cancer, the goal of treatment must be clearly defined. If the goal is to cure the patient of cancer, the strategy of therapy is likely to be different from the strategy chosen if the purpose is to prolong life or to relieve symptoms. To set the goal of therapy, the physician must be:
   - familiar with the natural history and behavior of the cancer to be treated;
   - knowledgeable about the principles and practice of therapy for each of the treatment modalities that may be effective in that cancer;
   - well grounded in the ethical principles of the treatment of patients with cancer;
   - familiar with the theory and use of antineoplastic agents;
   - informed about the particular therapy for the cancer in question; and
   - aware of the patient's individual circumstances, including stage of disease, performance status, social situation, and concurrent illnesses.

   Armed with this information and with the treatment goals in mind, the physician can plan a course of treatment and make a recommendation to the patient.

   Components of the treatment plan include the following:
   1. Should the cancer be treated at all, and if so, is the treatment to be designed for cure, prolongation of life, or palliation of symptoms?
   2. How aggressive should the therapy be to achieve the defined objective?
   3. Which modalities of therapy will be used and in what sequence?
   4. How will the treatment efficacy be determined?
   5. What are the criteria for deciding the duration of therapy?

   B. **Patient perspective.** Although most often the medical recommendation is accepted, some patients reject it as inappropriate for them for a variety of reasons. Some ask the physician for another recommendation, and others seek the opinion of a second physician. The physician must clearly present the reasons for the treatment recommendations and why they seem to be the best way to achieve the treatment objective. At the same time, it is important for the physician to allow the patient to share in setting treatment goals because it is the patient who must undergo the rigors of treatment and be willing to abide by its consequences. The physician has the obligation to make a treatment recommendation, but the patient always has the right to reject that advice without fear that the physician will be upset, dislike the patient, or refuse to continue to give the patient care.

II. **Choice of cancer treatment modality**

   A. **Surgery.** The oldest, most established, and still most effective way to cure most cancers is surgery. Surgery is selected as the treatment if the cancer is limited to one area and if it is anticipated that all cancer cells can be removed without unduly compromising vital structures. If it is believed that the patient can survive the operation and return to a worthwhile life, surgery is recommended. Surgery is not recommended if the risk of surgery is greater than the risk of the cancer, if metastasis always occurs despite complete removal of the primary tumor, or if the patient will be left so debilitated that although cured of cancer he or she feels that life is not worthwhile. If metastasis regularly (or always) occurs despite complete removal of the primary tumor, the benefits of removal of the gross tumor should be clearly defined before surgery is undertaken.

   Most commonly, surgery is reserved for treatment of the primary neoplasm, although at times it may be used effectively to remove isolated metastases (e.g., in lung, brain, liver) with curative intent. Surgery is also used palliatively, such as for decompression of the brain in patients with glioma or biliary bypass in patients with carcinoma of the pancreas. In nearly all nonhematologic cancers, a surgeon should be consulted to determine the role of surgery in the optimal treatment of the patient.

   B. **Radiotherapy.** Radiotherapy is used for the treatment of local or regional disease when surgery cannot completely remove the cancer or when it would unduly disrupt normal structures or functions. In the treatment of some cancers, radiotherapy is as effective as surgery for eradicating the tumor. In this circumstance, factors such as the anticipated side effects of the treatment, the expertise and experience of local oncologists, and the preference of the patient may influence the choice of treatment.

   One determinant of the appropriateness of radiotherapy is the inherent sensitivity of the cancer to ionizing radiation. Some kinds of cancer (e.g., the lymphomas and seminomas) are sensitive to radiotherapy. Other kinds (e.g., melanomas and sarcomas) tend to be less sensitive. Such considerations do not preclude the use of radiotherapy, however, and it is helpful to obtain the evaluation of the radiotherapist before initiating treatment so that treatment planning can take into consideration the possible contribution of this modality.

Although radiotherapy is frequently used as the primary or curative mode of therapy, it is also well suited to palliative management of problems, such as bony metastases, superior vena cava syndrome, and local nodal metastases. The use of radiotherapy in the management of spinal cord compression and superior vena cava syndrome is discussed in Chapter 30.

C. **Chemotherapy.** Chemotherapy has as its primary role the treatment of disease that is no longer confined to one site or region and has spread systemically. In the earliest days of chemotherapy, this interpretation directed its use to diseases that regularly presented in a disseminated form (e.g., leukemia) or after disease recurred following primary management with surgery or radiotherapy. It is now understood that widespread systemic micrometastases commonly occur early in cancer. These metastases are associated with certain predictive factors, such as the axillary node metastases of carcinoma of the breast and the large tumor size and poorly differentiated histologic features of sarcomas. Therefore, chemotherapy is now applied earlier to treat systemic disease. When this treatment is used for micrometastases, the response of an individual patient cannot be measured. Rather, the effectiveness of therapy must be determined by comparing the survival of high-risk patients who receive therapy with similar (control) patients who do not receive therapy for the micrometastases. Chemotherapy also has a role in the treatment of localized or regional disease. These specialized uses are discussed in Chapter 31.

D. **Biologic response modifiers.** It has long intrigued cancer biologists that cancer does not occur randomly but preferentially selects specific populations, the young, the elderly, the immunosuppressed (certain types of cancer only), and those with a strong family history of cancer. These observations have led cancer biologists to postulate that some kind of biologic control over the emergence of cancer exists, which some people have and others do not, at least at the time the cancer becomes established. One prime candidate for the mechanism of biologic control of cancer has been immunity. That immunity plays some role in controlling the development of cancer has been clearly demonstrated in animal models and a few, though not most, human neoplasms. Other biologic factors, including those controlled by oncogenes and tumor-suppressor genes and their protein products, are becoming better defined and are in all likelihood even more important than classical immunity in the development of cancer.

In an attempt to exploit and enhance the biologic control that is presumed to exist to some degree in everyone, a variety of agents called *biologic response modifiers* have been used in the treatment of cancer. Two classes of biologic response modifiers, the interferons and lymphokines (of which interleukin-2 is an example), have been studied intensively, and there is evidence of their substantial activity in some types of cancer. This area of intensive research promises to provide an important component of effective cancer therapy. Principles of biologic response modification are discussed in Chapter 2.

E. **Combined-modality therapy.** Neither surgery, radiotherapy, biotherapy, nor chemotherapy alone is appropriate for the treatment of all cancers. Frequently, patients present with cancer in which there is a bulky primary lesion, macroscopically evident regional disease, and presumed microscopic or submicroscopic systemic disease. For this reason, oncologists have turned to a multidisciplinary approach to the treatment of cancer, selecting two or more modalities of therapy for sequential or simultaneous use. This approach requires close cooperation among the surgical oncologist, radiation oncologist, and medical oncologist to provide the patient with the best overall treatment plan. Although combined-modality therapy is neither effective nor desirable for all kinds or stages of cancers, the regular practice of a multidisciplinary approach provides the best opportunity to exploit the advantages of each mode of treatment.

III. **Palliative care.** The medical oncologist is often seen as the coordinator of cancer treatment. In this role, the cancer is focused on, and the broader perspective of the oncologist as a coordinator of the patient's care—in partnership with the patient—may become obscured. Decisions about what therapy to use and how aggressively to treat the cancer are critically important to medically sound patient care. Decisions about when to stop active cancer treatment are also vitally important and may be among the most difficult responsibilities for the oncologist. Quality of life is often enhanced in patients responding to chemotherapy and other cancer treatments; it just as surely deteriorates more rapidly when the tumor does not respond to therapy and the patient experiences the toxicity of treatment along with the pain, fatigue, cachexia, and other symptoms of the cancer. For the 50% of patients with cancer who are not cured, the decision to stop antineoplastic therapy is just as important as the selection of chemotherapy regimens earlier in the disease. There comes a time when the best advice a physician can give is for the patient to forgo additional chemotherapy or any other active cancer treatment.

The introduction and rapid acceptance of hospice programs throughout the United States during the past 25 years reflect the need for this kind of care. Hospice programs have effectively addressed the special physical, psychological, social, and spiritual needs of patients approaching the end of life and have provided the unique skills required to maintain the best possible quality of life as long as possible. Yet too often physicians are reluctant to "give up" and are unable to recognize or to accept when the patient will be helped more by an acknowledgement that active cancer therapy will not improve survival or enhance quality of life.

Oncologists and others caring for patients with cancer who have been trained as acute care physicians can learn specific techniques to enhance the quality of life from those who are expert in palliative care. For example, one might compare the quality of death in hospitalized patients given "maintenance" intravenous hydration with that of hospice home care patients offered oral fluids and mouth care to assuage thirst. The former method may result in an overhydrated, edematous patient who dies with an uncomfortable-sounding "death rattle" that is disconcerting to family and staff; the latter usually results in a visibly more comfortable patient who is more likely to die with less edema and without as much apparent respiratory distress.

Legitimate questions also can be raised about medical costs toward the end of life that are incurred when physicians give "futile" and "marginal" care. Development of guidelines by physicians and hospitals that define futile care, along with thoughtful consideration of when the therapy offered patients has marginal value, may enable physicians to improve the quality of life for patients and at the same time hold down one component of the rising spiral of health care costs.

SELECTED READINGS

Emanuel EJ et al. Ethics of randomized clinical trials. *J Clin Oncol* 1998;16:365–366.

Lundberg GO. American health care system management objectives: the aura of inevitability becomes incarnate. *JAMA* 1993;269: 2254–2255.

Skeel RT. Quality of life dimensions that are most important to cancer patients. *Oncology* 1993;7:55–61.

Skeel RT. Measurement of outcomes in supportive oncology. In: Ann Berger et al., (ed.) Principles and Practice of Supportive Oncology. Philadelphia: Lippincott–Raven, 1998; 875–888.

Taylor LM, Feldstein ML, Skeel RT, Pandga KJ, Ng P, and Carboue PP. Fundamental dilemmas of the randomized clinical trial process: results of a survey of the 1737 Eastern Cooperative Oncology Group Investigators. *J Clin Oncol* 1994;12:1776–1805.

Chemotherapeutic and Biotherapeutic Agents and Their Use

Antineoplastic Drugs and Biologic Response Modifiers: Classification, Use, and Toxicity of Clinically Useful Agents

Roland T. Skeel

I. **Classes of drugs.** Chemotherapeutic agents are customarily divided into several classes. For two of the classes, the *alkylating agents* and the *antimetabolites,* the names indicate the mechanism of cytotoxic action of the drugs in their class. For the *hormonal agents,* the name designates the physiologic behavior of the drug, and for the *natural products,* the name reflects the source of the agents. The *biologic response modifiers,* agents that mimic, stimulate, enhance, inhibit, or otherwise alter the host responses to the cancer, are discussed extensively in Chapter 2. Drugs that do not fit easily into other categories are grouped together as *miscellaneous agents.* Data for individual agents are given in Section III of this chapter.

Within each class are several types of agents (Table 5-1). As with the criteria for separating into class, the types are also grouped according to the mechanism of action, biochemical structure or derivation, or physiologic action. In some instances, these groupings into classes and types are arbitrary, and some drugs seem to fit into either more than one category or none. However, the classification of chemotherapeutic agents in this fashion is helpful in several respects. For example, because the antimetabolites interfere with purine and pyrimidine metabolism and the formation of DNA and RNA, they are all at least cell cycle specific and in some instances primarily cell cycle phase specific. The nitrosourea group of alkylating agents, on the other hand, contains drugs that are predominantly or entirely cell cycle nonspecific. Such knowledge can be helpful in planning therapy for tumors when sufficient kinetic information permits a rational selection of agents and when drugs are selected for use in combination.

The classification scheme also may help to predict cross-resistance between drugs. Tumors that are resistant to one of the nitrogen-mustard types of alkylating agents thus would be likely to be resistant to another of that same type, but not necessarily to one of the other types of alkylating agents, such as the nitrosoureas or the metal salts (e.g., cisplatin). The classification system does not help in predicting multidrug resistance, which may have several phenotypes.

Table 5-1.   Useful chemotherapeutic agents

Class and Type	Agents
Alkylating agents	
Nitrogen mustard	Chlorambucil, cyclophosphamide, estramustine, ifosfamide, mechlorethamine, melphalan
Ethylenimine derivative	Thiotepa (triethylenethiophosphoramide)
Alkyl sulfonate	Busulfan
Nitrosurea	Carmustine, lomustine, semustine,* streptozocin
Triazene	Dacarbazine
Metal salt	Carboplatin, cisplatin
Antimetabolites	
Antifolates	Methotrexate, raltitrexed (quinazoline antifolate), trimetrexate*
Pyrimidine analogs	Azacitidine,* capecitabine, cytarabine, floxuridine, fluorouracil, gemcitabine
Purine analog	Mercaptopurine, thioguanine, pentostatin, cladribine, fludarabine
Natural products	
Mitotic inhibitor	Vinblastine, vincristine, vindesine,* vinorelbine
Microtubule polymer stabilizer	Docetaxel, paclitaxel (Taxol)
Topoisomerase I inhibitors	Irinotecan, topotecan
Topoisomerase II inhibitors	Etoposide, teniposide
Antibiotics	Bleomycin, dactinomycin, daunorubicin, doxorubicin (Adriamycin), epirubicin, idarubicin, plicamycin, mitomycin, mitoxantrone
Enzyme	Asparaginase
Hormones and hormone antagonists	
Androgen	Fluoxymesterone and others
Corticosteroid	Dexamethasone, prednisone
Estrogen	Diethylstilbestrol
Progestin	Megestrol acetate, medroxyprogesterone acetate
Estrogen antagonist	Raloxifene, tamoxifen, toremifene
Aromatase inhibitor	Aminoglutethimide, anastrozole, letrozole
Androgen antagonist	Bicalutamide, flutamide, nilutamide
Luteinizing hormone–releasing hormone (LHRH) agonist	Leuprolide, goserelin
Thyroid hormones	Levothyroxine, liothyronine

Table 5-1. *(Continued)*

Class and Type	Agents
Miscellaneous agents	
Substituted urea	Hydroxyurea
Methylhydrazine derivative	Procarbazine
Adrenocortical suppressant	Mitotane
Substituted melamine	Altretamine (hexamethyl-melamine)
Acridine dye	Amsacrine*
Bisphosphonates	Pamidronate
Photosensitizing agents	Porfimer
Cytoprotector (reactive species antagonists)	Amifostine, dexrazoxane, mesna
Platelet-reducing agent	Anagrelide
Somatostatin analog	Octreotide
Biologic agents	
Monoclonal antibody	Trastuzumab (Herceptin), rituximab
Interferons	Interferon-α_{2a}, interferon-α_{2b}
Interleukins	Aldesleukin (IL-2), oprelvekin
Myeloid-and erythroid-stimulating factors	Erythropoietin, filgrastim (granulocyte colony-stimulating factor), sargramostim (granulocyte-macrophage colony-stimulating factor)

* Investigational agents, not yet approved by the Food and Drug Administration for general use.

A. **Alkylating agents**
1. **General description.** The alkylating agents are a diverse group of chemical compounds capable of forming molecular bonds with nucleic acids, proteins, and many molecules of low molecular weight. The compounds either are electrophiles or generate electrophiles *in vivo* to produce polarized molecules with positively charged regions. These polarized molecules then can interact with electron-rich regions of most cellular molecules. The cytotoxic effect of the alkylating agents appears to relate primarily to the interaction between the electrophiles and DNA. This interaction may result in substitution reactions, cross-linking reactions, or strand-breaking reactions. The net effect of the alkylating agent's interaction with DNA is to alter the information coded in the DNA molecule. This alteration results in inhibition or inaccurate replication of DNA, with resultant mutation or cell death. One implication of the

mutagenic capability of alkylating agents is the possibility that they are teratogenic and carcinogenic. Because they interact with preformed DNA, RNA, and protein, the alkylating agents are not phase specific, and at least some are cell cycle nonspecific.

2. **Types of alkylating agents**

   a. **Nitrogen mustards.** These compounds produce highly reactive carbonium ions that react with the electron-rich areas of susceptible molecules. They vary in reactivity from mechlorethamine, which is highly unstable in aqueous form to cyclophosphamide, which must be biochemically activated in the liver.

   b. **Ethylenimine derivatives** Triethylenethiophosphoramide (thiotepa) is the only compound in this group that has much clinical use. Ethylenimine derivatives are capable of the same kinds of reactions as the nitrogen mustards.

   c. **Alkyl sulfonates.** Busulfan is the only clinically active compound in this group. It appears to interact more with cellular thiol groups than with nucleic acids.

   d. **Triazines.** Dacarbazine, the only agent of this type, was originally thought to be an antimetabolite because of its resemblance to 5-aminoimidazole-4-carboxamide (AIC). Dacarbazine is now known to act as an alkylator after AIC is cleaved from active diazomethane.

   e. **Nitrosoureas.** The nitrosoureas undergo rapid, spontaneous activation in aqueous solution to form products capable of alkylation and carbamoylation. They are unique among the alkylating agents with respect to being non–cross-resistant with other alkylating agents, being highly lipid soluble, and having delayed myelosuppressive effects (6-to-8 weeks).

   f. **Metal salts.** Cisplatin and carboplatin inhibit DNA synthesis probably through the formation of intrastrand cross-links in DNA. They also react with DNA through chelation or binding to the cell membrane.

B. **Antimetabolites**

   1. **General description.** The antimetabolites are a group of low-molecular-weight compounds that exert their effect by virtue of their structural or functional similarity to naturally occurring metabolites involved in nucleic acid synthesis. Because they are mistaken by the cell for a normal metabolite, they either inhibit critical enzymes involved in nucleic acid syn-

thesis or become incorporated into the nucleic acid and produce incorrect codes. Both mechanisms result in inhibition of DNA synthesis and ultimate cell death. Because of their primary effect on DNA synthesis, the antimetabolites are most active in cells that are actively growing and are largely cell cycle phase specific.

2. **Types of antimetabolites**

   a. **Folic acid analogs.** Methotrexate, the dominant member of this group, and the only one in wide clinical use, inhibits the enzyme dihydrofolate reductase. This inhibition blocks the production of the reduced N-methylenetetrahydrofolate, the coenzyme in the synthesis of thymidylic acid. Other metabolic processes in which there is one carbon unit transfer are also affected but are probably of less importance in the cytotoxic action of methotrexate. Ralitrexed (Tomudex) is a quinazoline antifolate that is an inhibitor of thymidylate synthetase.

   b. **Pyrimidine analogs.** These compounds inhibit critical enzymes necessary for nucleic acid synthesis and may become incorporated into DNA and RNA (e.g., cytarabine, 5-azacitidine).

   c. **Purine analogs.** The specific site of action for the purine analogs is less well defined than for most pyrimidine analogs, although it is well demonstrated that they interfere with normal purine interconversions and thus with DNA and RNA synthesis. Some of the analogs also are incorporated into the nucleic acids. The adenosine deaminase inhibitor pentostatin increases the intracellular concentration of deoxyadenosine triphosphates in lymphoid cells and inhibits DNA synthesis, probably by blocking ribonucleotide reductase. Among the metabolic alterations is nicotinamide adenine dinucleotide (NAD) depletion, which may result in cell death. Cladribine accumulates in cells as the triphosphate, is incorporated into DNA, and inhibits DNA repair enzymes and RNA synthesis. As with pentostatin, NAD levels are also depleted.

C. **Natural products**

   1. **General description.** The natural products are grouped together not on the basis of activity but because they are derived from natural sources. The clinically useful drugs are (a) plant products, (b) fermentation products of various species of the soil fungus *Streptomyces,* and (c) bacterial products.

    2. Types of natural products

        a. Mitotic inhibitors. Vincristine, vinblastine, and their semisynthetic derivatives vindesine and vinorelbine are derived from the periwinkle plant (*Catharanthus roseus*), a species of myrtle. They appear to act primarily through their effect on microtubular protein with a resultant metaphase arrest and inhibition of mitosis.

        b. Podophyllum derivatives. Etoposide and teniposide, semisynthetic podophyllotoxins derived from the root of the May apple plant (*Podophyllum peltatum*), form a complex with topoisomerase II, an enzyme that is necessary for the completion of DNA replication. This interaction results in DNA strand breakage and arrest of cells in late S and early G_2 phases of the cell cycle.

        c. Antibiotics. The antitumor antibiotics are a group of related antimicrobial compounds produced by *Streptomyces* species in culture. Their cytotoxicity, which limits their antimicrobial usefulness, has proved to be of great value in treating a wide range of cancers. All of the clinically useful antibiotics affect the function and synthesis of nucleic acids.

            (1) Dactinomycin, the anthracyclines (doxorubicin, daunorubicin, and idarubicin), and the anthracenedione mitoxantrone cause topoisomerase II–dependent DNA cleavage and intercalate with the DNA double helix.

            (2) Bleomycins cause DNA strand scission. The resulting fragmentation is believed to underlie the drug's cytotoxic activity.

            (3) Mitomycin causes cross-links between complementary strands of DNA that impair replication.

            (4) Plicamycin (mithramycin) complexes with Mg^{2+} to DNA and blocks RNA synthesis.

        d. Enzymes. Asparaginase, the one example of this type of agent, catalyzes the hydrolysis of asparagine to aspartic acid and ammonia and deprives selected malignant cells of an amino acid essential to their survival.

  D. Hormones and hormone antagonists

    1. General description. The hormones and hormone antagonists that are clinically active against cancer include steroid estrogens, progestins, androgens, corticoids and their synthetic derivatives, nonsteroidal synthetic compounds with steroid or steroid-antagonist activity, hypo-thalamic-pituitary analogs, and thyroid hormones. Each agent has diverse effects. Some effects are mediated directly at the cellular level by the drug binding to specific cytoplasmic receptors or by inhibition or stimulation of the production or action of the hormones. These agents may also act by stimulating or inhibiting natural autocrine and paracrine growth factors (e.g., epidermal growth factor, transforming growth factor-α [TGF-α], and TGF-β). The relative role of the various actions of hormones and hormone antagonists are only partially understood and probably vary among tumor types. For estrogen receptor antagonists such as tamoxifen, which when bound to the estrogen receptor ultimately controls the promoter region of genes that affect cell growth, there are a host of modulating factors including some 20 receptor interacting proteins and 50 transcription activating factors as well as many response elements. Other effects are mediated through indirect effects on the hypothalamus and its anterior pituitary-regulating hormones. The final common pathway in most circumstances appears to lead to the malignant cell, which has retained some sensitivity to direct or indirect hormonal control of its growth. An exception to this mechanism is the effect of corticosteroids on leukemias and lymphomas, in which the steroids appear to have direct lytic effects on abnormal lymphoid cells that have high numbers of glucocorticoid receptors.

2. **Types of hormones and hormone antagonists**

a. **Androgens** may exert their antineoplastic effect by altering pituitary function or directly affecting the neoplastic cell.

b. **Antiandrogens** inhibit nuclear androgen binding.

c. **Corticosteroids** cause lysis of lymphoid tumors that are rich in specific cytoplasmic receptors and may have other indirect effects as well.

d. **Estrogens** suppress testosterone production (through the hypothalamus) in males and alter breast cancer cell response to prolactin.

e. **Progestins** appear to act directly at the level of the malignant cell receptor to promote differentiation.

f. **Estrogen antagonists** compete with estrogen for binding on the cytosol estrogen receptor protein in cancer cells. The receptor:hormone complex ultimately controls the promoter region of genes that affect cell growth.

g. **Aromatase inhibitors** are non-steroidal inhibitors of the aromatization of androgens to estrogens. Aminoglutethimide is relatively non selective, having many biochemical sites of inhibition of steroidogenesis. Its use requires corticosteroid replacement. In contrast, the selective aromatase inhibitors, such as anastrozole or letrozole, primarily block the conversion of adrenally-generated androstenedione to estrone by aromatase in peripheral tissues without inhibition of progesterone or corticosteroid synthesis.

h. **Hypothalamic hormone analogs,** such as the luteinizing hormone–releasing hormone (LHRH) agonists leuprolide or goserelin, can inhibit luteinizing hormone and follicle-stimulating hormone (after initial stimulation) and the production of testosterone or estrogen by the gonads.

i. **Thyroid hormones** inhibit the release of thyroid-stimulating hormone (TSH), thus inhibiting growth of well-differentiated thyroid tumors.

E. **Miscellaneous agents** are listed in Table 5-1. Descriptions of specific agents are found in Section III, below.

II. **Clinically useful chemotherapeutic and biologic agents.** Section III of this chapter contains an alphabetically arranged description of the chemotherapeutic and biologic agents that are recognized to be clinically useful. Each drug is listed by its generic name, with other common or trade names included. A brief description is given of the probable mechanism of action, clinical uses, recommended doses and schedules, precautions, and side effects. The role of the biologic agents in the therapy of malignant disease is not as firmly established as it is for chemotherapy, although it is clear that their indications and use will expand greatly as more is learned about cancer cell biology.

A. **Recommended doses: CAUTION.** Although every effort has been made to ensure that the drug dosages and schedules given here are accurate and in accord with published standards, readers are advised to check the product information sheet included in the package of each Food and Drug Administration (FDA)–approved drug. For drugs not yet approved for general use, FDA–National Cancer Institute (NCI) guidelines and any current medical literature should be used to verify recommended dosages, contraindications, and precautions and to review potential toxicity.

B. **Dose selection and designation.** The doses are listed using body surface area (square meters) as the base for nearly all the agents listed. Adult doses from the literature, which are expressed using a weight base, have been converted by multiplying the milligram per kilogram dose by 37 to give the milligram per square meter dose. Doses using a weight base, which have been taken from the pediatric literature, have been converted using a factor of 25. Because many of the drugs are given in combination with other agents, doses most commonly used in popular combinations may also be indicated. These data should not be used as the sole source of information for any of the drugs but rather should be used as a guide to confirm and compare dose ranges and schedules and to identify potential problems.

C. **Drug toxicity: frequency designation.** The designation of the frequency of toxic side effects is indicated as follows (probability of occurrence equals percentage of patients):
1. Universal (90% to 100%)
2. Common (15% to 90%)
3. Occasional (5% to 15%)
4. Uncommon (1% to 5%)
5. Rare ($<1\%$)

These designations are meant only to be guides, and the likelihood of a side effect in each patient depends on that patient's physical and psychologic status; previous treatment; dose, schedule, and route of drug administration; and other concurrent treatment.

D. **Dose modification**
1. **Philosophy.** The optimal dose and schedule of a drug is one that gives maximum benefit with tolerable toxicity. Most chemotherapeutic agents have a steep dose-response curve; therefore, if no toxicity is seen, as a rule, a higher dose should be given to get the best possible therapeutic benefit. If toxicity is great, however, the patient's life may be threatened or the patient may decide that the treatment is worse than the disease and refuse further therapy. How much toxicity the patient and the physician are willing to tolerate depends on the likelihood that more intensive treatment will make a major therapeutic difference (e.g., cure versus no cure) and on the patient's physical and psychological tolerance for adverse effects.

The general grading scheme for all toxicity is as follows:
0—None
1—Mild
2—Moderate
3—Severe
4—Life-threatening
2. **Guidelines**
a. **Nonhematologic toxicity**
(1) **Acute effects.** Acute drug toxicity that is limited to 1 to 2 days and is not cumulative is not usually a cause of

dose modification unless it is of grade 3 or 4, i.e., severe or life threatening [see Common Toxicity Criteria on National Cancer Institute (NCI) Cancer Therapy Evaluation Program (CTEP) home page on the internet at **http://ctep.info.nih.gov/** for individual toxicities and Fig. 3-1 for an example of hematologic toxicity criteria]. Occasionally, repeating a dose that caused intractable nausea and vomiting or a temperature higher than 40°C (104°F) is warranted, but for any other grade 3 or 4 toxicity, the subsequent doses should be reduced by 25% to 50%. If the acute drug effects (e.g., severe paresthesias or abnormalities of renal or liver function) last longer than 48 hours, the subsequent doses should be reduced by 35% to 50%.

A recurrence of the grade 3 or 4 side effects at the reduced doses would be an indication either to reduce by another 25% to 50% or to discontinue the drug altogether. Non–dose-related toxicity, such as anaphylaxis, is an indication to discontinue the offending drug. Lesser degrees of hypersensitivity can often be dealt with effectively by increasing the dose of protective agents (like dexamethasone or diphenhydramine) or slowing the rate of infusion. For some biologic agents, such as herceptin (HER-2/neu directed monoclonal antibody), physiologic effects that look like hypersensitivity reactions occur primarily on first or second doses of treatment and diminish with continued treatment.

(2)   **Chronic effects.** Chronic or cumulative toxicity, such as pulmonary function changes with bleomycin or decreased cardiac function with doxorubicin, is nearly always an indication to discontinue the responsible agent. Chronic or cumulative neurotoxicity due to vincristine, cisplatin, paclitaxel, or other agents may require no dose change, reduction, or discontinuation, depending on the severity of the resultant neurologic dysfunction and the patient's ability to tolerate it.

         b. Hematologic toxicity. The degree of myelosuppression and attendant risk of infection and bleeding that are acceptable depend on the cancer, the duration of the myelosuppression, the goals of therapy, and the general health of the patient. In addition, one must consider the relative benefit of less aggressive or more aggressive therapy. For example, with acute non-lymphocytic leukemia, remission is unlikely unless sufficient therapy is given to cause profound pancytopenia for at least 1 week. Because there is little benefit with lesser treatment, grade 4 leukopenia and thrombocytopenia are acceptable toxicities in this circumstance. Grade 4 myelosuppression is also acceptable when the goal is cure of a cancer that does not involve the marrow, such as testicular carcinoma. With breast cancer, on the other hand, responses are seen with less aggressive treatment, and prolonged pancytopenia may not be acceptable, particularly if chemotherapy is being used palliatively or in an adjuvant setting in which the proportion of patients expected to benefit from chemotherapy is relatively small and excessive toxicity would pose an unacceptable risk. (Whether higher doses might increase cure is currently under investigation.)

         With these caveats in mind, the dose modification schemes shown in Tables 5-2 and 5-3 can serve as a guide to reasonable dose changes for drugs whose major toxicity is myelosuppression. Separate schemes are given for the nitrosoureas and for drugs that have more prolonged myelosuppression.

III. Data for clinically useful chemotherapeutic and biologic agents. *Note:* Although every effort has been made to ensure that the drug dosage and schedules herein are accurate and in accord with published standards, users are advised to check the product information sheet included in the package of each FDA-approved drug and FDA-NCI guidelines for drugs that are not yet approved for general use (see Table 5-1) to verify recommended dosages, contraindications, and precautions.

    Agents that have not yet been approved by the FDA are included, because either they have some demonstrated usefulness or are widely used in investigational studies. As their efficacy and toxicity are more firmly established, it is expected that some will be approved by the FDA for general use, whereas others will remain investigational or be dropped from further study.

Table 5-2.   Dose modifications for myelosuppressive drugs with a nadir[a] at less than 3 weeks

Degree of suppression	ANC (WBC) per μL on day of scheduled treatment[b]		Platelets per μL on day of scheduled treatment	Dose as percentage of immediately preceding cycle
Minimal	≥1,500 (≥3,500)	and	>100,000	100
Mild	1,200–1,500 (3,000–3,500)	or	75,000–100,000	75
Moderate	1,000–1,200 (2,500–3,000)	or	5,000–75,000	50
Severe	<1,000 (<2,500)	or	<50,000	0 (delay 1 wk)

ANC, absolute neutrophil count; WBC, white blood cell.

[a] If the nadir of the ANC is <1,000 per μL and is associated with fever >38.3°C (101°F) or nadir of platelets is <40,000 per μL, decrease dose by 25% in subsequent cycles. If the dose is already to be reduced on the basis of the ANC or platelet count on the day of treatment as per this table, do not reduce further because of the nadir count.

[b] ANC is the preferred parameter if available. If counts are rising at the end of a treatment cycle, it is often appropriate to delay 1 wk and then treat according to the dose modification scheme shown here.

Table 5-3. Dose modifications for myelosuppressive drugs[a] with a nadir at 3 weeks or later

Point in time	ANC (WBC) per µL		Platelets per µL	Dose as percentage of immediately preceding cycle
I. On day of scheduled treatment[b]	>1,800 (>3,500)	and	>100,000	Dose modified for nadir only
	<1,800 (<3,500)	or	<100,000	0[c]
II. At last nadir	>750	and	>75,000	100
	500–750	or	40,000–75,000	75
	<500	or	<40,000	50
III. After 2 wk delay	>1,800 (>3,500)	and	>100,000	Dose modified for nadir only
	1,200–1,800 (2,500–3,500)	or	75,000–100,000	75
	<1,200	or	<75,000	Continue to hold

ANC, absolute neutrophil count; WBC, white blood cell.

[a] Nitrosoureas or other agents with prolonged nadir.

[b] ANC is the preferred parameter to use.

[c] Withhold treatment and repeat count in 2 wk. At 2 wk, treat on basis of lowest dose indicated by nadir (II) or delay (III) section of table.

ALDESLEUKIN

Other names. Interleukin-2 (IL-2), Proleukin.

Mechanism of action. Enhances mitogenesis of T cells, natural killer (NK) cells, and lymphokine-activated killer (LAK) cells; augments cytotoxicity of NK and LAK cells; induces interferon-γ.

Primary indications.
1. Renal cell carcinoma.
2. Melanoma.

Usual dosage and schedule. A wide range of doses and routes (i.v. or s.c.) have been used. Examples are given of moderate- and low-intensity regimens. In any of the schedules, therapy may be stopped prematurely for severe constitutional symptoms or for cardiovascular, renal, hepatic, neurologic, pulmonary, or hematologic toxicity.

1. 600,000 IU/kg (22×10^6 IU/m^2) as a 15-minute i.v. infusion every 8 hours for up to 14 doses on days 1 to 5. Repeat on days 15 to 19. Repeat cycle in 6 to 12 weeks if stable or responding disease.
2. 72,000 IU/kg (2.7×10^6 IU/m^2) i.v. bolus over 15 minutes every 8 hours on days 1 to 5 and 15 to 19. Repeat cycle in 5 to 6 weeks if stable or responding disease.
3. 18 to 22×10^6 IU/m^2 as a 15-minute i.v. infusion daily for 5 days on 2 successive weeks. Repeat every 3 to 6 weeks as tolerated. In some regimens, it is preceded by 3 days with low-dose cyclophosphamide, 350 mg/m^2 i.v. push.
4. 30 to 60×10^6 IU/m^2 i.v. over 10 minutes three times weekly.
5. 9 to 18×10^6 IU/m^2 s.c. for 5 days per week. Repeat weekly for 4 to 6 weeks, then give a 2 to 3 week rest period. For stable or responding disease, repeat for 2 to 3 cycles.
6. 9×10^6 IU/m^2 daily by continuous i.v. infusion on days 1 to 4 (96 hours), together with chemotherapy (cisplatin, vinblastine, dacarbazine) and interferon in melanoma.

Schedules 1, 2, and 6 require hospitalization. Schedules 3, 4, and 5 can be given in an outpatient setting but may require several hours of observation after treatment.

Special precautions. Patients must be carefully monitored after treatment using any of the dosing regimens. Outpatient regimens require that patients have cardiovascular status observed for up to 5 hours, particularly after the first several doses. With higher doses, capillary leak syndrome resulting in hypotension, pulmonary edema, myocardial infarction, arrhythmias, azotemia, and alterations in mental status may occur. Intensive care, controlled volume replacement, and intubation may be required. The lower doses can be given in an outpatient setting.

Toxicity. All are dose dependent.
1. *Myelosuppression.* Uncommon at lower doses, common, but rarely serious at higher doses. Anemia requiring transfusion is common at higher doses. Thrombocytopenia is common at higher doses.
2. *Nausea and vomiting.* Common.
3. *Mucocutaneous effects.* Mucositis is occasional to common. Alopecia is uncommon. Pruritic erythematous rash is common.
4. *Cardiovascular effects.*
    a. Arrhythmias are common and dose-related.

   b. Hypotension is dose-related but is occasionally seen at the lower dose schedules.
   c. Myocardial injury is seen primarily at the higher dose schedules.
   d. Pulmonary edema from capillary leak syndrome is common with intensive dose regimens.
   e. Weight gain is common from edema, particularly in more intensive dose regimens.
5. *Gastrointestinal effects.*
   a. Anorexia is common.
   b. Diarrhea is occasional.
   c. Transient liver function abnormalities, including hyperbilirubinemia, and hypoalbuminemia and elevation of the prothrombin time and partial thromboplastin time are common.
   d. Colonic perforations are rare.
6. *Neuropsychiatric effects.*
   a. Mental status changes are common, with dose-related severity.
   b. Dizziness or light-headedness is common.
   c. Blurry vision and other visual disturbances are occasional.
   d. Seizures are uncommon to rare at lower-dose regimens.
7. *Renal function impairment.* Common but reversible. More frequent laboratory abnormalities include creatinine elevation, hypomagnesemia, acidosis, hypocalcemia, hypophosphatemia, hypokalemia, hypouricemia, and hypoalbuminemia.
8. *Fever.* With or without chills—universal and may be severe.
9. *Bacterial infection.* Occasional. Probably related to chemotactic defect induced in granulocytes.
10. *Myalgias and arthralgias.* Occasional to common.
11. *Malaise and fatigue.* Common and dose related.

Prophylaxis of acute toxicity.
1. Acetaminophen, 650 to 1,000 mg p.o. 1 hour before therapy and every 3 hours for two doses.
2. Cimetidine, 800 mg p.o., or other histamine H_2-receptor antagonist before therapy and daily for duration of treatment.
3. Antiemetics: granisetron, ondansetron, or other $5HT_3$ antagonist, metoclopramide, and prochlorperazine may be used. Do not use dexamethasone.
4. Meperidine, 25 to 50 mg i.v., when chills start after first dose. For subsequent doses, meperidine, 150 mg p.o. 1.5 hours before chills are predicated to start, based on the first treatment.
5. Diphenhydramine, 50 mg p.o. every 3 hours for three doses, may be substituted for meperidine in patients who tolerate the latter drug poorly.
6. Diphenoxylate with atropine (Lomotil), 1 tablet up to six times daily for diarrhea.
7. Hydroxyzine, 25 to 50 mg every 4 to 6 hours for itching.

ALTRETAMINE

Other names. Hexamethylmelamine, Hexalen, HXM.
Mechanism of action. Unknown. Although it structurally resembles the known alkylating agent triethylenemelamine, it has some antimetabolite characteristics.

Primary indication. Carcinoma of the ovary.
Usual dosage and schedule.
1. 260 mg/m^2 p.o. daily in three or four divided doses for 14 or 21 days every 4 weeks when used as a single agent.
2. 150 to 200 mg/m^2 p.o. daily in three or four divided doses for 2 out of 3 or 4 weeks when used in combination.

Special precautions. Concurrent altretamine and antidepressants of the monoamine oxidase (MAO) inhibitor class may cause severe orthostatic hypotension. Cimetidine may increase toxicity.
Toxicity.
1. *Myelosuppression.* Dose-limiting leukopenia and thrombocytopenia are uncommon. Anemia is common.
2. *Nausea and vomiting.* Mild to moderate nausea and vomiting occur in about 30% of patients and are rarely severe. Tolerance may develop.
3. *Mucocutaneous effects.* Alopecia, skin rash, and pruritus are rare.
4. *Miscellaneous effects.*
   a. Peripheral sensory neuropathies are common and may be ameliorated by pyridoxine, but tumor response may be compromised.
   b. Central nervous system (CNS) effects, including agitation, confusion, hallucinations, depression, and Parkinsonian-like symptoms are uncommon with recommended intermittent schedule.
   c. Decreased renal function is occasional.
   d. Increased alkaline phosphatase level is occasional.
   e. Diarrhea is occasional.

AMIFOSTINE

Other name. Ethyol.
Mechanism of action. The prodrug, amifostine, is dephosphorylated to an active free thiol metabolite that can reduce the toxic effects of cisplatin. The differential activity between normal and cancer tissue is thought to be related to higher capillary alkaline phosphatase activity and better vascularity of normal tissue. Pretreatment reduces cumulative renal toxicity from cisplatin.
Primary indications. Patients receiving cisplatin in whom cure or substantial prolongation of survival is not the goal of therapy.
Usual dosage and schedule. 910 mg/m^2 i.v. over 15 minutes once daily starting 30 minutes before chemotherapy.
Special precautions. Hypotension during the infusion. Interrupt the infusion if the decrease in systolic pressure is more than 20% to 25% of the baseline systolic pressure.
Toxicity.
1. *Myelosuppression.* Not increased by amifostine.
2. *Nausea and vomiting.* Common and may be severe.
3. *Mucocutaneous effects.* Skin rash is rare.
4. *Miscellaneous effects*
   a. Flushing and feeling of warmth are occasional.
   b. Chilling and feeling of coldness are occasional.
   c. Dizziness, somnolence, hiccups, and sneezing are occasional.

   d. Allergic reactions are rare.
   e. Hypocalcemia is rare.

AMINOGLUTETHIMIDE

Other names. Cytadren, Elipten, AG

Mechanism of action. Inhibits aromatization and cytochrome P-450 hydroxylating enzymes, thereby blocking the conversion of androgens to estrogens and the biosynthesis of all steroid hormones. This drug causes, in effect, a reversible chemical adrenalectomy.

Primary indications. Breast carcinoma, prostate carcinoma, adrenocortical carcinoma, ectopic Cushing's syndrome.

Usual dosage and schedule. 1000 mg daily in 4 divided doses.

Special precautions. Hydrocortisone must be given concomitantly (particularly for breast cancer) to prevent adrenal insufficiency. Suggested dose is 100 mg daily in divided doses for 2 weeks, then 40 mg daily in divided doses.

Toxicity.
1. *Myelosuppression.* Leukopenia and thrombocytopenia are rare, and if they occur they resolve rapidly when the drug is stopped.
2. *Nausea and vomiting* are occasional and usually mild.
3. *Mucocutaneous effects.* A morbilliform rash is commonly seen during the first week of treatment, but it usually disappears within 1 week.
4. *Hormonal effects.*
   a. Adrenal insufficiency is common without replacement hydrocortisone in patients with normal adrenal glands.
   b. Hypothyroidism is uncommon.
   c. Masculinization is possible.
5. *Neurologic effects.*
   a. Lethargy is common. Although usually mild and transient, it is occasionally severe.
   b. Vertigo, nystagmus, and ataxia is occasional.
6. *Miscellaneous effects.*
   a. Facial flushing is uncommon.
   b. Periorbital edema is uncommon.
   c. Cholestatic jaundice is rare.
   d. Fever is uncommon.

AMSACRINE (Investigational)

Other names. m-AMSA; AMSA.

Mechanism of action. Binds to DNA through intercalation and external binding. Interaction with topoisomerase II to increase DNA strand breakage.

Primary indications. Pediatric and adult acute leukemias.

Usual dosage and schedule.
1. 120 mg/m^2 i.v. over 1–2 hours in 500 ml 5% dextrose and water for 3–5 days.
2. 100 mg/m^2 i.v. over 1–2 hours in 500 ml 5% dextrose and water on days 7, 8, and 9 (in combination regimens).

Special precautions. Use caution if patient is hypokalemic or was given prior anthracycline, as it may potentiate cardiotoxicity. Solution physically incompatible with sodium chloride solutions. Avoid direct contact with skin.

Toxicity.
1. *Myelosuppression.* Universal and dose-limiting.
2. *Nausea and vomiting.* Common.
3. *Mucocutaneous effects.* Mucositis is common and dose-related; occasional skin rash.
4. *Liver.* Common transient liver function abnormalities.
5. *Renal effects.* Rare.
6. *Diarrhea.* Occasional.
7. *Cardiac effects.* Possible. May be affected by prior anthracyclines, e.g., daunorubicin or doxorubicin. Acute arrhythmias particularly in association with hypokalemia.
8. *Neurologic effects.* Seizures, neuropathy, headache, dizziness, CNS depression is uncommon.
9. *Phlebitis and local pain.* Common.

ANAGRELIDE

Other names. Imidazo(2,1-b)quinazolin-2-one, Agrelin.

Mechanism of action. Mechanism for thrombocytopenia unknown but may be due to impaired megakaryocyte function. Inhibitor of platelet aggregation but not at usual therapeutic doses.

Primary indication. Uncontrolled thrombocytosis in chronic myeloproliferative disorders, such as essential thrombocythemia, chronic granulocytic leukemia, and polycythemia rubra vera.

Usual dosage and schedule.
1. 0.5 mg p.o. q.i.d. or 1 mg p.o. b.i.d. Increase by 0.5 mg/d every 5 to 7 days if no response. Maximum daily dose is 10 mg. Maximum single dose is 2.5 mg. Higher doses cause postural hypotension.
2. Alternate dosing schedules:
   a. Elderly: 0.5 mg p.o. daily, increase by 0.5 mg each week.
   b. Abnormal renal or hepatic function: 0.5 mg p.o. b.i.d.

Special precautions. Contraindicated in pregnancy. Use with caution in patients with heart disease. Tachycardia and forceful heartbeat may be exacerbated by caffeine; consumption of caffeine should be avoided for 1 hour before and after anagrelide is taken. Use other drugs that inhibit platelet aggregation (such as nonsteroidal antiinflammatory drugs) with caution. Monitor platelet count every few days during first week, then weekly until the maintenance dose is reached.

Toxicity.
1. *Myelosuppression.* White cell count is none. Anemia is common (36%) but mild. Thrombocytopenic hemorrhage is uncommon (2%).
2. *Nausea and vomiting.* Nausea is occasional (15%), vomiting is uncommon.
3. *Mucocutaneous.* Rash is uncommon (2%). Hyperpigmentation is rare. Sun sensitivity is possible.
4. *Miscellaneous effects.*
   a. Cardiovascular: palpitations (27%), forceful heart beat, and tachycardia are common. Congestive heart failure is uncommon, but fluid retention or edema is common (24%). Tachyarrhythmias (including atrial fibrillation and pre-

mature atrial beats) are occasional. Angina, cardiomyopathy, or other severe cardiovascular effects are rare.
Drinking alcoholic beverages may cause flushing. Higher
than recommended single doses cause postural hypotension. Cardiovascular effects appear to result from vasodilation, positive inotropy, and decreased renal blood flow.

b. Neurologic: headaches are common (44%) and occasionally
are severe; they usually diminish in about 2 weeks. Weakness (asthenia) is common (22%). Dizziness is occasional.

c. Pulmonary: infiltrates are rare but are a reason to stop
anagrelide and treat with steroids.

d. Other gastrointestinal: diarrhea (24%), gas and abdominal pain are common, pancreatitis is rare. Lactase supplementation eliminates diarrhea (anagrelide formulated
with lactose).

ANASTROZOLE

Other name. Arimidex.

Mechanism of action. Decreases estrogen biosynthesis by selective inhibition of aromatase (estrogen synthetase).

Primary indications. Carcinoma of the breast (advanced) with
progression after antiestrogen therapy.

Usual dosage and schedule. 1 mg p.o. daily.

Special precautions. Potential hazard to fetus if given during
pregnancy.

Toxicity.

1. *Myelosuppression.* No dose-related effect.
2. *Nausea and vomiting.* Nausea is occasional, vomiting is uncommon.
3. *Mucocutaneous effects.* Rash is uncommon.
4. *Miscellaneous effects.* Asthenia is common. Musculoskeletal
pain is occasional. Headache is occasional. Arthralgia is occasional. Peripheral edema and weight gain are occasional
(lower than with megestrol). Dyspnea and cough are occasional. Constipation or diarrhea is occasional. Thromboembolic
events are uncommon. Hot flashes are occasional. Hypercalcemia is rare.

ANDROGENS

Other names. Fluoxymesterone (Halotestin), testolactone (Tes-
lac), others.

Mechanism of action. Mechanism of antitumor effects is not
clear.

Primary indications.

1. Breast carcinoma (in combination with other agents).
2. Anemia of myelodysplastic syndromes.

Usual dosage and schedule.

1. *Fluoxymesterone:* 20–40 mg PO daily in 4 divided doses.
2. *Testolactone:* 1000 mg PO daily in 4 divided doses.

Special precautions. Hypercalcemia may occur with initial
therapy.

Toxicity.

1. *Myelosuppression.* None. Erythropoiesis is stimulated.
2. *Nausea and vomiting.* Mild and dose-related.

3. *Mucocutaneous effects.* Acne.
4. *Miscellaneous effects.*
   a. Masculinization—including an increase in facial and body hair, deepening of voice, acne, baldness, and clitoral hypertrophy—is common in females but may be minimized by dose attenuation.
   b. Intrahepatic biliary stasis with hyperbilirubinemia is uncommon but may occur at high androgen doses (17-methyl derivatives only).
   c. Fluid retention may occur, although it is less severe with androgens than with estrogens is occasional.

ASPARAGINASE

Other names. L-Asparaginase, Elspar, pegaspargase, Oncaspar.
Mechanism of action. Hydrolysis of serum asparagine occurs, which deprives leukemia cells of the required amino acid and inhibits protein synthesis. Normal cells are spared because they generally have the ability to synthesize their own asparagine. Pegaspargase is a chemically modified formulation of asparaginase in which the L-asparaginase is covalently conjugated with monomethoxypolyethylene glycol (PEG). This modification increases its half-life in the plasma by a factor of 4 to about 5.7 days and reduces its recognition by the immune system, which allows the drug to be used in patients previously hypersensitive to native L-asparaginase.
Primary indication. Acute lymphocytic leukemia, primarily for induction therapy.
Usual dosage and schedule. Both schedules are usually used in combination with other drugs (see under Special precautions, item 2, below). The schedules listed are only two of many acceptable dosing schedules.
1. L-asparaginase: 6000–18,500 IU/m^2 i.v. daily for up to 14 days.
2. Pegaspargase: 2500 IU/m^2 IM (or i.v.) once every 14 days, in patients who have developed hypersensitivity to native forms of asparaginase.
Special precautions.
1. Be prepared to treat anaphylaxis at each administration of the drug. Epinephrine, antihistamines, corticosteroids, and life-support equipment should be readily available.
2. Giving concurrently with or immediately before vincristine may increase vincristine toxicity.
3. The intramuscular route is preferred for pegaspargase, because of a lower incidence of hepatotoxicity, coagulopathy, and gastrointestinal and renal disorders compared to the intravenous route of administration.
Toxicity.
1. *Myelosuppression.* Occasional.
2. *Nausea and vomiting.* Occasional and usually mild.
3. *Mucocutaneous effects.* No toxicity occurs except as a sign of hypersensitivity.
4. *Anaphylaxis.* Mild to severe hypersensitivity reactions, including anaphylaxis, occur in 20–30% of patients. Such reaction is less likely to occur during the first few days of treatment. It is particularly common with intermittent schedules or re-

peat cycles. If the patient develops hypersensitivity to the *Escherichia coli*-derived enzyme (Elspar), *Erwinia*-derived asparaginase may be safely substituted because the two enzyme preparations are not cross-reactive. Note that hypersensitivity may also develop to *Erwinia*-derived asparaginase, and continued preparedness to treat anaphylaxis must be maintained.

If given IM, asparaginase should be given in an extremity so that a tourniquet can be applied to slow the systemic release of asparaginase should anaphylaxis occur.

Approximately 30% of patients previously sensitive to L-asparaginase will have a hypersensitivity reaction to pegaspargase, while only 10% of those who were not hypersensitive to the native form will have a hypersensitivity reaction to the PEG-modified drug.

5. *Miscellaneous effects.*
   a. Mild fever and malaise are common and occasionally progress to severe chills and malignant hyperthermia.
   b. Hepatotoxicity is common and occasionally severe. Abnormalities observed include elevations of serum glutamic-oxaloacetic transaminase (SGOT), alkaline phosphatase, and bilirubin; depressed levels of hepatic-derived clotting factors and albumin; and hepatocellular fatty metamorphosis.
   c. Renal failure is rare.
   d. Pancreatic endocrine and exocrine dysfunction, often with manifestations of pancreatitis, occasionally occurs. Nonketotic hyperglycemia is uncommon.
   e. CNS effects (depression, somnolence, fatigue, confusion, agitation, hallucinations, or coma) are seen occasionally. They are usually reversible following discontinuation of the drug.

AZACITIDINE (Investigational)

Other names. 5-Azacitidine, 5 aza-C, ladakamycin.

Mechanism of action. A pyrimidine analog antimetabolite that causes interference with nucleic acid synthesis and is incorporated into both DNA and RNA, where it acts as a false pyrimidine.

Primary indication. Acute nonlymphocytic leukemia.

Usual dosage and schedule.
1. 100 mg/m^2 i.v. push q8h for 5 days *or*
2. 150–200 mg/m^2 i.v. daily as continuous infusion for 5 days.

Special precautions. Because of drug instability the dose should be prepared immediately before use and discarded after 8 hours. Infusions should be freshly prepared with Ringer's lactate solution and changed every 8 hours.

Toxicity.
1. *Myelosuppression.* Severe in all patients, with the leukocyte nadir occurring at 12–14 days. Occasionally, suppression is prolonged beyond several weeks.
2. *Nausea and vomiting.* Common. Continuous infusion lessens nausea and vomiting.
3. *Mucocutaneous effects.* Stomatitis and rash is occasional.
4. *Miscellaneous effects.*
   a. Diarrhea is common.

    b. Neurologic problems with muscle pain, weakness, lethargy, and coma is uncommon.

    c. Hepatotoxicity is rare but may be severe.

    d. Transient fever is occasional.

BICALUTAMIDE

Other names. Casodex, ICI 176,334.

Mechanism of action. Competitive inhibitor of androgens at the cellular androgen receptor in the prostate cancer cells.

Primary indication. Carcinoma of the prostate, most often in combination with LHRH agonist.

Usual dosage and schedule. 50 mg daily, in morning or evening.

Special precautions. None.

Toxicity.

1. *Myelosuppression.* None.
2. *Nausea and vomiting.* Uncommon to occasional.
3. *Mucocutaneous effects.* Mild skin rash is occasional.
4. *Miscellaneous effects.*
   a. Secondary pharmacologic effects, including breast tenderness, breast swelling, hot flashes (49%), impotence, and loss of libido are common but reversible after cessation of therapy.
   b. Gastrointestinal effects: diarrhea is uncommon; constipation is occasional.
   c. Elevated liver function tests are uncommon.
   d. Adverse cardiovascular events are similar to those seen with orchiectomy.
   e. Dizziness or vertigo is occasional.

BLEOMYCIN

Other name. Blenoxane.

Mechanism of action. Bleomycin binds to DNA, causes single- and double-strand scission, and inhibits further DNA, RNA, and protein synthesis.

Primary indications.

1. Testis, head and neck, penis, cervix, vulva, anus, and skin carcinomas.
2. Hodgkin's and non-Hodgkin's lymphomas.

Usual dosage and schedule.

1. 10–20 units/m^2 i.v. or IM once or twice a week *or*
2. 30 units i.v. push weekly for 9–12 weeks in combination with other drugs for testis cancer.
3. 60 units in 50 ml of normal saline instilled intrapleurally.

Special precautions.

1. In patients with lymphoma, a test dose of 1 or 2 units should be given IM prior to the first dose of bleomycin because of the possibility of anaphylactoid, acute pulmonary, or severe hyperpyretic responses. If no acute reaction occurs within 4 hours, regular dosing may begin.
2. Reduce dose for renal failure.

Serum creatinine	% of Full dose
2.5–4.0	25
4.0–6.0	20
6.0–10.0	10

3. The cumulative lifetime dose should not exceed 400 units because of the dose-related incidence of severe pulmonary fibrosis. Smaller limits may be appropriate for older patients or those with preexisting pulmonary disease. Frequent evaluation of pulmonary status, including symptoms of cough or dyspnea, rales, infiltrates on chest x-ray film, and pulmonary function studies are recommended to avert serious pulmonary sequelae.
4. Glass containers are recommended for continuous infusion to minimize drug instability.
5. High FiO_2 (fraction of inspired oxygen) (such as might be used during surgery) should be avoided as it exacerbates lung injury, sometimes acutely.

Toxicity.
1. *Myelosuppression.* Significant depression of counts is uncommon. This factor permits bleomycin to be used in full doses with myelosuppressive drugs.
2. *Nausea and vomiting.* Occasional and self-limiting.
3. *Mucocutaneous effects.* Alopecia, stomatitis, erythema, edema, thickening of nail bed, and hyperpigmentation and desquamation of skin are common.
4. *Pulmonary effects.*
    a. Acute anaphylactoid or pulmonary edema–like response is occasional in patients with lymphoma (see Special precautions, above).
    b. Dose-related pneumonitis with cough, dyspnea, rales, and infiltrates, progressing to pulmonary fibrosis.
5. *Fever.* Common. Occasionally severe hyperpyrexia, diaphoresis, dehydration, and hypotension have occurred and resulted in renal failure and death. Antipyretics help control fever.
6. *Miscellaneous effects.*
    a. Lethargy, headache, joint swelling is rare.
    b. IM or SQ injection may cause pain at injection site.

BUSULFAN

Other name. Myleran.
Mechanism of action. Bifunctional alkylating agent. Its effect may be greater on cellular thiol groups than on nucleic acids.
Primary indications.
1. *Standard doses:* chronic granulocytic leukemia.
2. *High doses with stem cell rescue:* acute leukemia, lymphoma.
Usual dosage and schedule.
1. $3–4$ mg/m^2 PO daily for remission induction in adults until the leukocyte count is 50% of the original level, then $1–2$ mg/m^2 daily. Busulfan may be given continuously or intermittently for maintenance.
2. High doses with stem cell rescue—consult specific protocols. Not recommended outside research setting. Typical dose is 1 mg/kg PO q6h for 4 consecutive days.
Special precautions. Obtain complete blood count weekly while patient is on therapy. If leukocyte count falls rapidly to less than $15,000/\mu L$, discontinue therapy until nadir is reached and rising counts indicate a need for further treatment.

Toxicity.
1. *Myelosuppression.* Dose-limiting. A fall in the leukocyte count may not begin for 2 weeks after starting therapy, and it is likely to continue for 2 weeks after therapy has been stopped. Recovery of marrow function may be delayed for 3–6 weeks after the drug has been discontinued. High-dose therapy requires stem cell rescue (e.g., bone marrow transplantation).
2. *Nausea and vomiting.* Rare.
3. *Mucocutaneous effects.* Hyperpigmentation occurs occasionally, particularly in skin creases.
4. *Pulmonary effects.* Interstitial pulmonary fibrosis is rare and is an indication to discontinue drug. Corticosteroids may improve symptoms and minimize permanent lung damage.
5. *Metabolic effects.* Adrenal insufficiency syndrome is rare. Hyperuricemia may occur when the leukemia cell count is rapidly reduced. Ovarian suppression and amenorrhea are common.
6. *Miscellaneous effects.*
   a. Secondary neoplasia is possible.
   b. Fatal hepatovenoocclusive disease with high-dose therapy is occasional.
   c. Seizures after high-dose therapy is occasional.

CAPECITABINE

Other name. Xeloda.

Mechanism of action. An orally administered prodrug that is converted to fluorouracil intracellularly. When this is converted to the active nucleotide, 5-fluoro-2-deoxyuridine monophosphate, it inhibits the enzyme thymidylate synthetase and blocks DNA synthesis. The triphosphate may also be mistakenly incorporated into RNA, which interferes with RNA processing and protein synthesis.

Primary indications. Metastatic breast cancer that is resistant to anthracycline- and paclitaxel-containing chemotherapy regimens. May also be used in patients in whom anthracyclines are contraindicated.

Usual dosage and schedule. 2,500 mg/m^2 p.o. daily with food for 2 weeks, followed by a 1-week rest, given as 3-week cycles. Generally given in two divided doses about 12 hours apart at the end of a meal.

Special precautions. Diarrhea may be severe and require fluid and electrolyte replacement. Incidence and severity may be worse in patients 80 years of age or older.

Toxicity.
1. *Myelosuppression.* Common, but usually mild to moderate with anemia predominating.
2. *Nausea and vomiting.* Common.
3. *Mucocutaneous effects.* Hand-and-foot syndrome is common (45%) and may be severe. Dermatitis is also common (35%). Eye irritation is occasional.
4. *Miscellaneous effects.*
   a. Diarrhea is common (50%); in 13% of patients, it is severe to life-threatening.
   b. Fatigue is common.
   c. Paresthesias are occasional.
   d. Anorexia is occasional to common (20%).

e. Hyperbilirubinemia is common (34%).
f. Fever is occasional.
g. Abdominal pain is occasional to common.
h. Headache or dizziness is occasional.
i. Cardiotoxicity is possible with any fluorinated pyrimidine.

CARBOPLATIN

Other names. Paraplatin, CBDCA.
Mechanism of action. Covalent binding to DNA.
Primary indications. Ovarian, endometrial, and lung cancers, and other cancers in which cisplatin is active.
Usual dosage and schedule.
1. 300–400 mg/m^2 i.v. by infusion over 15–60 minutes or longer, repeated every 4 weeks.
2. *Alternative dosing* uses the area under the curve (AUC): Total dose (mg) = target AUC × (glomerular filtration rate + 25). The target AUC is typically 5–7 depending on previous therapy and concurrent drugs or radiation.
3. Higher doses up to 1600 mg/m^2 divided over several days have been used followed by stem cell rescue (e.g., bone marrow transplantation).

Special precautions. Much less renal toxicity than cisplatin, so there is no need for a vigorous hydration schedule or forced diuresis. Reduce dose to 250 mg/m^2 for creatinine clearance of 41–59 ml/minute, reduce to 200 mg/m^2 for clearance of 16–40 ml/minute.
Toxicity.
1. *Myelosuppression.* Anemia, granulocytopenia, and thrombocytopenia are common and dose-limiting. Red blood cell transfusions may be required. Thrombocytopenia may be delayed (days 18–28).
2. *Nausea and vomiting.* Common; but vomiting (65%) is not as frequent or as severe as with cisplatin and can be controlled with combination antiemetic regimens.
3. *Mucocutaneous effects.* Alopecia is uncommon. Mucositis is rare.
4. *Renal tubular abnormalities.* Elevation in serum creatinine or blood urea nitrogen occurs occasionally. More common is electrolyte loss with decreases in serum sodium, potassium, calcium, and magnesium.
5. *Miscellaneous effects.*
   a. Liver function abnormalities are common.
   b. Gastrointestinal pain is occasional.
   c. Peripheral neuropathies or central neurotoxicity are uncommon.
   d. Allergic reactions are uncommonly seen with rash, urticaria, pruritus, and rarely bronchospasm and hypotension.
   e. Cardiovascular (cardiac failure, embolism, cerebrovascular accidents) are uncommon.
   f. Hemolytic uremic syndrome is rare.

CARMUSTINE

Other names. BCNU, BiCNU, Gliadel wafer (surgically implantable, biodegradable polymer wafer that releases impregnated carmustine from the hydrophobic matrix after implantation.)

Mechanism of action. Alkylation and carbamoylation by carmustine metabolites interfere with the synthesis and function of DNA, RNA, and proteins. Carmustine is lipid soluble and easily enters the brain.

Primary indications.

A. Systemic therapy:
   1. Hodgkin's and non-Hodgkin's lymphomas.
   2. Brain tumors.
   3. Multiple myeloma.
   4. Melanoma.
B. Implantable carmustine-impregnated wafer: Glioblastoma multiforme.

Usual dosage and schedule.

A. Systemic therapy:
   1. 200 to 240 mg/m^2 i.v. as a 30- to 45-minute infusion every 6 to 8 weeks. Dose often is divided and given over 2 to 3 days. Some recommend limiting the cumulative dose to 1,000 mg/m^2 to limit pulmonary and renal toxicity.
   2. Higher doses of up to 600 mg/m^2 have been used with stem cell rescue (e.g., bone marrow or peripheral blood stem cell transplantation).
B. Implantable carmustine-impregnated wafer: Up to 8 wafers, each containing 7.7 mg of carmustine, are applied to the resection cavity surface after removal of the tumor.

Special precautions (systemic therapy). Because of delayed myelosuppression (3 to 6 weeks), do not administer drug more often than every 6 weeks. Await a return of normal platelet and granulocyte counts before repeating therapy. Amphotericin B may enhance the potential for renal toxicity, bronchospasm, and hypotension.

Toxicity.

A. Systemic therapy:
   1. *Myelosuppression.* Delayed and often biphasic, with the nadir at 3 to 6 weeks; it may be cumulative with successive doses. Recovery may be protracted for several months. High-dose therapy requires stem cell rescue.
   2. *Nausea and vomiting.* beginning 2 hours after therapy and lasting 4 to 6 hours, are common.
   3. *Mucocutaneous effects.*
      a. Facial flushing and a burning sensation at the i.v. site may be due to alcohol used to reconstitute the drug; this is common with rapid injection.
      b. Hyperpigmentation of skin after accidental contact is common.
   4. *Miscellaneous effects.*
      a. Hepatotoxicity is uncommon but can be severe.
      b. Pulmonary fibrosis is uncommon at low doses, but its frequency increases at doses higher than 1,000 mg/m^2.
      c. Secondary neoplasia is possible.
      d. Renal toxicity is uncommon at doses of less than 1,000 mg/m^2.
      e. With high-dose therapy, encephalopathy, hepatotoxicity, and pulmonary toxicity are common and dose limiting. Hepatovenooclusive disease also occurs (occasional).

B. Implantable carmustine impregnated wafer: Limited toxicity beyond that expected from craniotomy is seen. Serious intracranial infection was seen in 4% of patients, compared with 1% of placebo-treated patients. Brain edema not responsive to steroids may also be seen in a similar percentage of patients. Abnormal wound healing may occur. Remnants of the wafer may be seen for many months after implantation.

CHLORAMBUCIL

Other name. Leukeran.
Mechanism of action. Classic alkylating agent, with primary effect on preformed DNA.
Primary indications.
1. Chronic lymphocytic leukemia.
2. Low-grade non-Hodgkin's lymphoma.
Usual dosage and schedule.
1. 3–4 mg/m^2 PO daily until a response is seen or cytopenias occur; then, if necessary, maintain with 1–2 mg/m^2 PO daily.
2. 30 mg/m^2 PO once every 2 weeks (with or without prednisone 80 mg/m^2 PO on days 1–5).
Special precautions. Increased toxicity may occur with prior barbiturate use.
Toxicity.
1. *Myelosuppression.* Dose-limiting and may be prolonged.
2. *Nausea and vomiting.* May be seen with higher doses but are uncommon.
3. *Mucocutaneous effects.* Rash is uncommon.
4. *Miscellaneous effects.*
   a. Liver function abnormalities is rare.
   b. Secondary neoplasia is possible.
   c. Amenorrhea and azoospermia is common.
   d. Drug fever is uncommon.
   e. Pulmonary fibrosis is rare.
   f. CNS effects including seizure and coma may be seen at very high doses (>100 mg/m^2).

CISPLATIN

Other names. *cis*-Diamminedichloroplatinum (II), DDP, CDDP, Platinol.
Mechanism of action. Similar to alkylating agents with respect to binding and cross-linking strands of DNA.
Primary indications. Usually used in combination with other cytotoxic drugs.
1. Testis, ovary, endometrial, cervical, bladder, head and neck, gastrointestinal, and lung carcinomas.
2. Soft-tissue and bone sarcomas.
3. Non-Hodgkin's lymphoma.
Usual dosage and schedule.
1. 40–120 mg/m^2 i.v. on day 1 as infusion every 3 weeks.
2. 15–20 mg/m^2 i.v. on days 1–5 as infusion every 3–4 weeks.
Special precautions. Do not administer if serum creatinine level is more than 1.5 mg/dl. Irreversible renal tubular damage may occur if vigorous diuresis is not maintained, particularly with higher doses (>40 mg/m^2) and with additional concurrent

nephrotoxic drugs, such as the aminoglycosides. At higher doses, diuresis with mannitol with or without furosemide plus vigorous hydration are mandatory.

1. An acceptable method for hydration in patients without cardiovascular impairment for cisplatin doses up to 80 mg/m^2 is as follows.
    a. Have patient void, and begin infusion of 5% dextrose in half-normal saline with potassium chloride (KCl) 20 mEq/liter and magnesium sulfate (MgSO$_4$) 1 gm/liter (8 mEq/liter); run at 500 ml/hour for 1.5–2.0 liters.
    b. After 1 hour of infusion, give 12.5 gm of mannitol by i.v. push.
    c. Immediately thereafter start the cisplatin (mixed in normal saline at 1 mg/ml) and infuse over 1 hour through the sidearm of the i.v., while continuing the hydration.
    d. Give additional mannitol (12.5–50.0 gm by i.v. push if necessary to maintain urinary output of 250 ml/hour over the duration of the hydration. If patient gets more than 1 liter behind on urinary output or signs or symptoms of congestive heart failure develop, 40 mg of furosemide may be given.
2. For doses more than 80 mg/m^2 a more vigorous hydration is recommended.
    a. Have patient void, and begin infusion of 5% dextrose in half-normal saline with KCl 20 mEq/liter and MgSO$_4$ 1 gm/liter (8 mEq/liter); run at 500 ml/hour for 2.5–3.0 liters.
    b. After 1 hour of infusion, give 25 gm of mannitol by i.v. push.
    c. Continue hydration.
    d. After 2 hours of hydration, if urinary output is at least 250 ml/hour, start the cisplatin (mixed in normal saline at 1 mg/ml) and infuse over 1–2 hours (1 mg/m^2/minute) through the sidearm of the i.v., while continuing the hydration.
    e. Give additional mannitol (12.5–50 gm by i.v. push) if necessary to maintain urinary output of 250 ml/hour over the duration of the hydration. If patient gets more than 1 liter behind on urinary output or signs or symptoms of congestive heart failure develop, 40 mg of furosemide may be given.
3. For patients with known or suspected cardiovascular impairment (ejection fraction <45%), a less vigorous rate of hydration may be used, provided the dose of cisplatin is limited (e.g., <60 mg/m^2). An alternative is to give carboplatin.

Toxicity.

1. *Myelosuppression.* Mild to moderate, depending on the dose. Relative lack of myelosuppression allows cisplatin to be used in full doses with more myelosuppressive drugs. *Anemia* is common and may have a hemolytic component. Anemia often is amenable to erythropoietin therapy.
2. *Nausea and vomiting.* Severe and often intractable vomiting regularly begins within 1 hour of starting cisplatin and lasts 8–12 hours. Prolonged nausea and vomiting occur occasion-

ally. Nausea and vomiting may be minimized by the use of a combination antiemetic regimen, e.g., dexamethasone, on-danseton or metaclopramide, and lorazepam (see Chap. 33).
3. *Mucocutaneous effects.* None.
4. *Renal tubular damage.* Acute reversible and occasionally irreversible nephrotoxicity may occur, particularly if adequate attention is not given to achieving sufficient hydration and diuresis. Nephrotoxic antibiotics increase risk of acute renal failure.
5. *Ototoxicity.* High-tone hearing loss is common, but significant hearing loss in vocal frequencies occurs only occasionally. Tinnitus is uncommon.
6. *Severe electrolyte abnormalities.* These abnormalities, e.g., marked hyponatremia, hypomagnesemia, hypocalcemia, and hypokalemia, may be seen up to several days after treatment.
7. *Anaphylaxis.* May occur after several doses. Responds to epinephrine, antihistamines, and corticosteroids.
8. *Miscellaneous effects.*
   a. Peripheral neuropathies are clinically significant signs and symptoms are common at cumulative doses <300 mg/m^2.
   b. Hyperuricemia is uncommon, parallels renal failure.
   c. Autonomic dysfunction with symptomatic postural hypotension is occasional.

CLADRIBINE

Other names. 2-Chlorodeoxyadenosine, Leustatin.
Mechanism of action. Deoxyadenosine analog with high cellular specificity for lymphoid cells. Resistant to effect of adenosine deaminase. Accumulates in cells as triphosphate, is incorporated into DNA, and inhibits DNA repair enzymes and RNA synthesis. Also results in NAD depletion. Effect is independent of cell division.
Primary indications. Hairy-cell leukemia, chronic lymphocytic leukemia, and possibly other lymphoid neoplasms.
Usual dosage and schedule.
1. 0.09 mg/kg (3.33 mg/m^2) i.v. daily as a continuous 7-day infusion.
2. 0.14 mg/kg (5.2 mg/m^2) i.v. as a 2-hour infusion daily for 5 days.
3. 0.14 mg/kg (5.2 mg/m^2) s.c. daily for 5 days.
Special precautions. Give allopurinol, 300 mg daily, as prophylaxis against hyperuricemia. Opportunistic infections occur occasionally and should be watched for closely.
Toxicity.
1. *Myelosuppression.* Moderate granulocyte suppression is common. Serious infection is common. Profound suppression of CD4 and CD8 counts is common and often prolonged for over 1 year. Opportunistic infections, including herpes, fungus, and pneumocystic infection, may occur and should be watched for. Some routinely use prophylaxis against one or more of these infections.
2. *Nausea and vomiting.* Mild nausea with decrease in appetite is common, but no vomiting is expected.
3. *Mucocutaneous effects.* Rash is common.
4. *Miscellaneous effects.*

a. Fever, possibly due to release of pyrogens from tumor cells, is common.
b. Headache, myalgia, and arthralgia are occasional to common.
c. Edema and tachycardia are occasional.
d. Cough, shortness of breath, and abnormal breath sounds are occasional.

CORTICOSTEROIDS

Other names. Prednisone, dexamethasone (Decadron), and others.

Mechanism of action. Unknown but apparently related to the presence of glucocorticoid receptors in tumor cells. Mediated in part by *bcl*-2 gene and promotion of apoptotic cell death.

Primary indications.
1. Carcinoma of the breast.
2. Acute and chronic lymphocytic leukemia.
3. Hodgkin's and non-Hodgkin's lymphomas.
4. Multiple myeloma.
5. Cerebral edema.
6. Nausea and vomiting with chemotherapy.

Usual dosage and schedule.
1. *Prednisone:* dose varies with neoplasm and combination. Typical regimen, *except* for acute lymphocytic leukemia, is as follows.
   a. 40 mg/m^2 PO days 1–14 every 4 weeks *or*
   b. 100 mg/m^2 PO days 1–5 every 4 weeks.
2. *Prednisone:* for acute lymphocytic leukemia: 40–50 mg/m^2 PO daily for 28 days.
3. *Dexamethasone:* for cerebral edema: 16–32 mg PO daily to start, then reduce to lowest dose at which symptoms remain controlled.

Special precautions. None.

Toxicity.
1. *Myelosuppression.* None.
2. *Nausea and vomiting.* None.
3. *Mucocutaneous effects.* Acne; increased risk for oral, rectal, and vaginal thrush. Thinning of skin and striae develop with continuous use.
4. *Suppression of adrenal-pituitary axis.* May lead to adrenal insufficiency when corticosteroids are withdrawn. This problem is not common with intermittent schedules.
5. *Metabolic effects.* Potassium depletion, sodium and fluid retention, diabetes, increased appetite, loss of muscle mass, myopathy, weight gain, osteoporosis, and development of cushingoid features. Their frequency depends on dose and duration of therapy.
6. *Miscellaneous effects.*
   a. Epigastric pain, extreme hunger, and occasional peptic ulceration with bleeding may occur. Antacids or inhibitors of acid secretion are recommended as prophylaxis.
   b. CNS effects, including euphoria, depression, and sleeplessness, are common and may progress to dementia or frank psychosis.

    c. Increased susceptibility to infection is common.
    d. Subcapsular cataracts in patients are uncommon but have been seen even when used for prophylaxis and treatment of drug-induced emesis.

CYCLOPHOSPHAMIDE

Other names. CTX, Cytoxan, Neosar.

Mechanism of action. Metabolism of cyclophosphamide by hepatic microsomal enzymes produces active alkylating metabolites. Cyclophosphamide's primary effect is probably on DNA.

Primary indications.
1. Breast, lung, ovary, testis, and bladder carcinomas.
2. Bone and soft-tissue sarcomas.
3. Hodgkin's and non-Hodgkin's lymphomas.
4. Acute and chronic lymphocytic leukemias.
5. Neuroblastoma and Wilms' tumor of childhood.
6. Multiple myeloma.

Usual dosage and schedule.
1. 1000–1500 mg/m^2 i.v. every 3–4 weeks *or*
2. 400 mg/m^2 PO days 1–5 every 3–4 weeks *or*
3. 60–120 mg/m^2 PO daily.
4. High-dose regimens (4–7 gm/m^2 divided over 4 days) are investigational and should only be used with some kind of stem cell rescue (e.g., bone marrow transplantation) and mesna bladder protection.

Special precautions. Give dose in the morning, maintain ample fluid intake, and have patient empty bladder several times daily to diminish the likelihood of cystitis.

Toxicity.
1. *Myelosuppression.* Dose-limiting. Platelets are relatively spared. Nadir is reached about 10–14 days after i.v. dose with recovery by day 21.
2. *Nausea and vomiting.* Frequent with large i.v. doses; less common after oral doses. Symptoms begin several hours after treatment and are usually over by the next day.
3. *Mucocutaneous effects.* Reversible alopecia is common, usually starting after 2–3 weeks. Skin and nails may become darker. Mucositis is uncommon.
4. *Bladder damage.* Hemorrhagic or nonhemorrhagic cystitis may occur in 5–10% of patients treated. It is usually reversible with discontinuation of the drug, but it may persist and lead to fibrosis or death. Frequency is diminished by ample fluid intake and morning administration of the drug. Mesna will protect from this effect.
5. *Miscellaneous effects.*
    a. Immunosuppression is common.
    b. Amenorrhea and azoospermia is common.
    c. Inhibition of antidiuretic hormone is only of significance with very large doses.
    d. Interstitial pulmonary fibrosis is rare.
    e. Secondary neoplasia is possible.
    f. Acute and potentially fatal cardiotoxicity occurs with high-dose therapy. Abnormalities include pericardial effusion, congestive heart failure, decreased electrocardio-

graphic (ECG) voltage, and fibrin microthrombi in cardiac capillaries with endothelial injury and hemorrhagic necrosis.

CYTARABINE

Other names. Cytosine arabinoside, ara-C, Cytosar-U.

Mechanism of action. A pyrimidine analog antimetabolite that, when phosphorylated to arabinosyl-cytosinetriphosphate (ara-CTP), is a competitive inhibitor of DNA polymerase.

Primary indication. Acute nonlymphocytic leukemia.

Usual dosage and schedule.
1. *Induction:* 100–200 mg/m^2 i.v. daily as a continuous infusion for 5–7 days (in combination with other drugs).
2. *Maintenance:* 100 mg/m^2 SQ every 12 hours for 4 or 5 days every 4 weeks (with other drugs).
3. *Intrathecally:* 40–50 mg/m^2 every 4 days in preservative-free buffered isotonic diluent.
4. *High dose:* 2.0–3.0 gm/m^2 i.v. over 1 hour every 12 hours for up to 12 doses.

Special precautions. None for standard doses. High dose, give in *1–3 hour infusion.* Longer infusion enhances toxicity. CNS toxicity is increased in patients with a decreased creatinine clearance.

Toxicity (standard dose only).
1. *Myelosuppression.* Dose-limiting leukopenia and thrombocytopenia occur, with nadir at 7–10 days after treatment has ended and with recovery during the following 2 weeks, depending on the degree of suppression. Megaloblastosis is common.
2. *Nausea and vomiting.* Common, particularly if the drug is given as a push or rapid infusion.
3. *Mucocutaneous effects.* Stomatitis is seen occasionally.
4. *Miscellaneous effects*
   a. Flulike syndrome with fever, arthralgia, and sometimes a rash is occasional.
   b. Transient mild hepatic dysfunction is occasional.

Toxicity (high dose).
1. *Myelosuppression.* Universal.
2. *Nausea and vomiting.* Common.
3. *Mucocutaneous effects.* Occasional to common mucositis.
4. *Neurotoxicity.* Cerebellar toxicity is common, particularly in the elderly, but is usually mild and reversible. However, on occasion it has been severe and permanent or fatal.
5. *Conjunctivitis.* Hydrocortisone 2 drops OU qid for 10 days may ameliorate or prevent keratitis.
6. *Hepatic toxicity with cholestatic jaundice.* Uncommon.
7. *Diarrhea.* Common.

DACARBAZINE

Other names. Imidazole carboxamide, DIC, DTIC-Dome.

Mechanism of action. Uncertain but probably interacts with preformed macromolecules by alkylation. Inhibits DNA, RNA, and protein synthesis.

Primary indications.
1. Melanoma.
2. All soft-tissue sarcomas.
3. Hodgkin's lymphoma.

Usual dosage and schedule.
1. 150–250 mg/m^2 i.v. push or rapid infusion on days 1–5 every 3–4 weeks *or*
2. 400–500 mg/m^2 i.v. push or rapid infusion on days 1 and 2 every 3–4 weeks.
3. 200 mg/m^2 i.v. daily as a continuous 96-hour infusion.

Special precautions.
1. Administer cautiously to avoid extravasation, as tissue damage may occur.
2. Venous pain along the injection site may be reduced by diluting dacarbazine in 100–200 ml of 5% dextrose in water and infusing over 30 minutes rather than injecting rapidly. Ice application may also reduce pain.

Toxicity.
1. *Myelosuppression.* Mild to moderate. This factor allows dacarbazine to be used in full doses with other myelosuppressive drugs.
2. *Nausea and vomiting.* Common and severe but decrease in intensity with each subsequent daily dose. Onset is within 1–3 hours, with duration up to 12 hours.
3. *Mucocutaneous effects.*
    a. Moderately severe tissue damage if extravasation occurs.
    b. Alopecia is uncommon.
    c. Erythematous or urticarial rash is uncommon.
4. *Miscellaneous effects.*
    a. Flulike syndrome with fever, myalgia, and malaise lasting several days is uncommon.
    b. Hepatic toxicity is uncommon.

DACTINOMYCIN

Other names. Actinomycin D, act-D, Cosmegen.
Mechanism of action. Binds to DNA and inhibits DNA-dependent RNA synthesis. Inhibition of topoisomerase II.
Primary indications.
1. Gestational trophoblastic neoplasms.
2. Wilms' tumor, rhabdomyosarcoma, and Ewing's sarcoma of childhood.

Usual dosage and schedule.
1. *Children:* 0.40–0.45 mg/m^2 (up to a maximum of 0.5 mg) i.v. daily for 5 days every 3–5 weeks.
2. *Adults*
    a. 0.40–0.45 mg/m^2 i.v. on days 1–5 every 2–3 weeks.
    b. 0.5 mg i.v. daily for 5 days every 3–5 weeks.

Special precautions.
1. Administer by slow i.v. push through the sidearm of a running i.v. infusion, being careful to avoid extravasation, which causes severe soft-tissue damage.
2. If given at or about the time of infection with chickenpox or herpes zoster, a severe generalized disease may occur that sometimes results in death.

Toxicity.
1. *Myelosuppression.* May be dose-limiting and severe. It begins within the first week of treatment, but the nadir may not be reached for 21 days.
2. *Nausea and vomiting.* Severe vomiting often occurs during the first few hours after drug administration and lasts up to 24 hours.
3. *Mucocutaneous effects.*
   a. Erythema, hyperpigmentation, and desquamation of the skin with potentiation by previous or concurrent radiotherapy are common.
   b. Oropharyngeal mucositis is potentiated by previous or concurrent radiotherapy.
   c. Alopecia is common.
   d. Moderately severe tissue damage occurs with extravasation.
4. *Miscellaneous effects.*
   a. Mental depression is rare.
   b. Hepatovenoocclusive disease, worse with higher doses and shorter schedules, e.g., single dose of 2.5 mg versus 5 days at 0.5 mg/day.

DAUNORUBICIN

Other names. Daunomycin, rubidomycin, DNR, Cerubidine; liposomal daunorubicin, DaunoXome (see next entry).
Mechanism of action. DNA strand breakage mediated by anthracycline effects on topoisomerase II; DNA intercalation; DNA polymerase inhibition.
Primary indications.
1. Acute nonlymphocytic leukemia, acute lymphocytic leukemia.
2. Kaposi's sarcoma (liposomal daunorubicin).
Usual dosage and schedule.
1. 45–60 mg/m^2 i.v. push on days 1, 2, and 3 every 2 weeks as induction therapy for 1 or 2 cycles in combination with other drugs.
2. 45 mg/m^2 i.v. push on days 1 and 2 every 4 weeks as consolidation therapy for 1 or 2 cycles in combination with other drugs.
Special precautions.
1. Administer over several minutes into the sidearm of a running i.v. infusion, taking precautions to avoid extravasation.
2. Do not give if patient has significantly impaired cardiac function (ejection fraction <45%), angina pectoris, cardiac arrhythmia, or recent myocardial infarction.
3. Do not exceed cumulative dosage of 550 mg/m^2 (400 mg/m^2 if given previous radiation therapy that has encompassed the heart).
4. Reduce dose if patient has impaired liver or renal function.

Serum bilirubin (mg/dl)		Serum creatinine (mg/dl)	% of Full dose
1.2–3.0	*or*	–	75
>3.0		>3.0	50

Toxicity.
1. *Myelosuppression.* Dose-limiting pancytopenia with nadir at 1–2 weeks.
2. *Nausea and vomiting.* Occurs on the day of administration in one-half of patients.
3. *Mucocutaneous effects.* Alopecia is common, but stomatitis is rare. Severe local tissue damage may progress to skin ulceration, and necrosis may occur with subcutaneous extravasation.
4. *Cardiac effects.* Potentially irreversible congestive heart failure may occur owing to cardiomyopathy. The incidence is highly dependent on the lifetime cumulative dose, which should not exceed 550 mg/m^2 (400 mg/m^2 if patient was given previous radiotherapy that encompassed the heart). Congestive heart failure may be predicted by serial measurement of left ventricular function or endomyocardial biopsy. Discontinue drug if there is clinical congestive heart failure or if the ejection fraction falls on the radionuclide angiogram,
   a. To less than 45% *or*
   b. To less than 50% if the total decrease is 10% or more (e.g., falls from 59% to 49%).

   If repeat ejection fraction determination shows return of function, drug may be cautiously restarted, but ejection fraction should be measured before each dose. Transient ECG changes are common and are not usually serious.
5. *Miscellaneous effects.*
   a. Red urine caused by the drug and its metabolites is common.
   b. Chemical phlebitis and phlebothrombosis of veins used for injection is common.

DAUNORUBICIN, LIPOSOMAL

Other name. DaunoXome.

Mechanism of action. Daunorubicin, liposomal, which is designed to be protected from removal by the reticuloendothelial system, has a prolonged circulation time compared with unprotected drug. The agent penetrates tumor tissue and releases the active ingredient daunorubicin. The active drug causes DNA strand breakage mediated by anthracycline effects on topoisomerase II; DNA intercalation; and DNA polymerase inhibition.

Primary indications. Kaposi's sarcoma, advanced, human immunodeficiency virus (HIV) associated.

Usual dosage and schedule. 40 mg/m^2 i.v. over 30 to 60 minutes every 2 weeks.

Special precautions.
1. Must be diluted to a concentration of 1 mg/mL with 5% dextrose for injection. Liposomal doxorubicin should be considered an irritant, and care should be taken to avoid extravasation.
2. Do not give if the patient has significantly impaired cardiac function.
3. Do not exceed a lifetime cumulative dose of 550 mg/m^2 (450 mg/m^2 if the patient was given prior chest radiotherapy).
4. Reduce or hold dose in patients with impairment of liver function. A 25% dose reduction is recommended if the

serum bilirubin is 1.2 to 3 mg/dL. One half the normal dose is recommended in patients with serum bilirubin concentration greater than 3 mg/dL.

Toxicity. Effects that are a result of the liposomal doxorubicin have been somewhat difficult to determine with certainty, because most patients have been on several other agents that can result in other drugs that may cause marrow or other toxicity.

1. *Myelosuppression.* Common and dose related. May be severe.
2. *Nausea and vomiting.* Common.
3. *Mucocutaneous effects.* Alopecia is occasional. Stomatitis is occasional.
4. *Miscellaneous effects.*
   a. Cardiac events, including cardiomyopathy or congestive heart failure may occur in treated patients, but appear to be uncommon.
   b. Infusion reactions. Acute infusion-associated reactions with back pain, flushing, and tightness in the chest and throat, alone or in combination, have occurred in approximately 14% of patients treated with liposomal doxorubicin. They usually occur with the first infusion, and are not likely to occur later if the first infusion is given without a reaction. Generally occur during first 5 minutes of the infusion and subside with interruption of the infusion. Some patients tolerate restarting at a lower rate of infusion. Most patients are able to continue therapy.
   c. Fatigue is common.
   d. Diarrhea is common.
   e. Fever is common.
   f. Pain at the injection site is likely after extravasation.

DEXRAZOXANE

Other names. Zinecard, ICRF-187.

Mechanism of action. Probably by means of conversion of dexrazoxane intracellularly to a chelating agent that interferes with iron-mediated free radical generation, which is thought to be responsible, in part, for anthracycline-related cardiomyopathy. Appears to protect against myocardial toxicity without impairment of tumor response.

Primary indications. Prophylaxis of cardiomyopathy in patients who have received a cumulative dose of doxorubicin of 300 mg/m^2 or greater and who are believed would benefit from continued therapy with this drug.

Usual dosage and schedule. 10 mg of dexrazoxane for every 1 mg of doxorubicin, for example, 600 mg/m^2 of dexrazoxane for 60 mg/m^2 of doxorubicin. Repeat whenever doxorubicin is to be repeated. Administered as a slow injection or rapid infusion over 15 to 30 minutes.

Special precautions. None.

Toxicity. Most side effects encountered with dexrazoxane administration are likely to be from the concurrent chemotherapy regimen.

1. *Myelosuppression.* Nadir granulocyte and platelet counts lower than with chemotherapy alone, but duration not prolonged.

2. *Nausea and vomiting.* No increase observed.
3. *Mucocutaneous effects.* No increase observed.
4. *Miscellaneous effects.*
   a. Pain at the injection site is occasional.
   b. Hepatic toxicity is possible.

DOCETAXEL

Other name. Taxotere.

Mechanism of action. Enhanced formation and stabilization of microtubules. Antineoplastic effect may result from nonfunctional tubules or altered tubulin–microtubule equilibrium. Mitotic arrest is seen and is associated with accumulated polymerized microtubules.

Primary indications. Carcinoma of the breast and non–small cell lung cancer.

Usual dosage and schedule. 60–100 mg/m^2 as a 1-hour infusion every 3 weeks.

Special precautions. Severe hypersensitivity reactions with flushing and hypotension with or without dyspnea occur in about 1% of patients (even when premedication is used). Should be used with caution in patients with bilirubin above upper limit of normal (ULN) or other abnormal liver function tests (>1.5 ULN), because of more profound neutropenia.

The following premedication should be given before each course of docetaxel to limit the frequency and severity of hypersensitivity reactions and to reduce the severity of fluid retention: dexamethasone, 8 mg p.o. b.i.d. for 5 days starting 1 day before docetaxel.

Toxicity.
1. *Myelosuppression.* Severe (grade 4) neutropenia is common. Many patients have neutropenic fever.
2. *Nausea and vomiting.* Common, but brief.
3. *Mucocutaneous effects.* Mild mucositis is common; severe mucositis is uncommon. Alopecia is common. Maculopapular eruptions, which may be associated with desquamation, or bullous eruptions from docetaxel occur only occasionally if systemic prophylaxis is used.
4. *Hypersensitivity reactions.* Severe reactions with flushing, hypotension (or rarely hypertension) with or without dyspnea and drug fever are uncommon with use of prophylactic regimen recommended but may be severe.
5. *Miscellaneous effects.*
   a. Fluid retention syndrome is common and cumulative (more commonly after four courses); can be reduced to occasional frequency (6%) by prophylactic steroids; may limit continuing therapy.
   b. Neurologic: mild and reversible dysesthesias or paresthesias are common; more severe sensory neuropathies are uncommon.
   c. Hepatic: reversible increases in transaminase, alkaline phosphatase, and bilirubin.
   d. Local reactions: reversible peripheral phlebitis.
   e. Mild diarrhea is common; severe diarrhea is rare.
   f. Fatigue, weakness (asthenia), and myalgia are common.

DOXORUBICIN

Other names. ADR, Adriamycin, Rubex, hydroxyldaunorubicin.
Mechanism of action. DNA strand breakage mediated by anthracycline effects on topoisomerase II; DNA intercalation; DNA polymerase inhibition.
Primary indications.
1. Breast, bladder, liver, lung, prostate, stomach, and thyroid carcinomas.
2. Bone and soft-tissue sarcomas.
3. Hodgkin's and non-Hodgkin's lymphomas.
4. Acute lymphocytic and acute nonlymphocytic leukemias.
5. Wilms' tumor, neuroblastoma, and rhabdomyosarcoma of childhood.
Usual dosage and schedule.
1. 60–75 mg/m^2 i.v. every 3 weeks. (Or as 96 hours continuous infusion.)
2. 30 mg/m^2 i.v. on days 1 and 8 every 4 weeks (in combination with other drugs).
3. 15–20 mg/m^2 i.v. weekly.
4. 50–60 mg instilled into the bladder weekly for 4 weeks, then every 4 weeks for 6 cycles.
Special precautions.
1. Administer over several minutes into the sidearm of a running i.v. infusion, taking care to avoid extravasation.
2. Do not give if patient has significantly impaired cardiac function (ejection fraction <45%), angina pectoris, cardiac arrhythmia, or recent myocardial infarction.
3. Do not exceed a lifetime cumulative dose of 550 mg/m^2 (450 mg/m^2 if patient was given prior chest radiotherapy or concomitant cyclophosphamide) unless there are known risk modifiers, such as continuous infusion or weekly dosing, and serial measurements of cardiac ejection fraction show minimal change and adequate function.
4. Reduce or hold dose if patient has impaired liver function.
   a. For serum bilirubin of 1.2–3.0 mg/dl: give one-half the normal dose.
   b. For serum bilirubin of more than 3.0 mg/dl: give one-fourth the normal dose.
Toxicity.
1. *Myelosuppression.* Dose-limiting for most patients. Nadir white blood cell (WBC) and platelet counts occur at 10–14 days; recovery by day 21.
2. *Nausea and vomiting.* Mild to moderate in about one-half of patients.
3. *Mucocutaneous effects.*
   a. Stomatitis that is dose-dependent.
   b. Alopecia beginning 2–5 weeks from start of therapy with recovery following completion of therapy is common.
   c. Recall of skin reaction due to prior radiotherapy is common.
   d. Severe local tissue damage possibly progressing to skin ulceration and necrosis if subcutaneous extravasation occurs is common.
   e. Hyperpigmentation of skin overlying veins used for drug injection in which chemical phlebitis has occurred is common.

4. *Cardiac effects.* Potentially irreversible congestive heart failure may occur owing to cardiomyopathy. The incidence is highly dependent on the lifetime cumulative dose, which should not exceed 550 mg/m^2. This limit is lower (450 mg/m^2) if patient has received prior chest radiotherapy or is taking cyclophosphamide concomitantly. Weekly schedule and 96 hours infusions are less cardiotoxic and higher cumulative doses may be tolerable. Congestive heart failure may be predicted by serial measurement of left ventricular function or endomyocardial biopsy. Discontinue drug if there is clinical congestive heart failure or if the ejection fraction falls on the radionuclide angiogram
   a. To less than 45% *or*
   b. To less than 50% if the total decrease is 10% or more (e.g., falls from 59% to 49%).

   If repeat ejection fraction determination shows return of function, drug may be cautiously restarted, but ejection fraction determination should be done before each dose. Transient ECG changes are common and are not usually serious.
5. *Miscellaneous effects.*
   a. Red urine caused by drug and its metabolites is common.
   b. Chemical phlebitis and phlebosclerosis of veins used for injection, particularly if a vein is used repeatedly are common.
   c. Fever, chills, and urticaria are uncommon.

DOXORUBICIN, LIPOSOMAL

Other name. Doxil.
Mechanism of action. Doxorubicin, liposomal, which is designed to be protected from removal by the reticuloendothelial system, has a prolonged circulation time compared with unprotected drug. The agent penetrates tumor tissue and releases the active ingredient doxorubicin. The active drug causes DNA strand breakage mediated by anthracycline effects on topoisomerase II; DNA intercalation; and DNA polymerase inhibition.
Primary indications. Kaposi's sarcoma, advanced, HIV associated.
Usual dosage and schedule. 20 mg/m^2 i.v. infusion over 30 minutes every 3 weeks.
Special precautions. Must be diluted in 250 mL of 5% dextrose for injection.
Toxicity. Effects that are a result of the liposomal doxorubicin have been somewhat difficult to determine with certainty, because most patients have been on several other agents that can result in other drugs that may cause marrow or other toxicity.
1. *Myelosuppression.* Common and dose related. May be severe.
2. *Nausea and vomiting.* Occasional.
3. *Mucocutaneous effects.* Palmar-plantar erythrodysesthesia is uncommon, but may be severe. Alopecia is occasional.
4. *Miscellaneous effects.*
   a. Cardiac events, including cardiomyopathy or congestive heart failure occur in 5% to 10% of patients treated.
   b. Infusion reactions. Acute infusion-associated reactions with flushing, shortness of breath, facial swelling, headache, chills, back pain, tightness in the chest and throat, or hypotension, alone or in combination, have occurred in

approximately 7% of patients treated with liposomal doxorubicin. They usually occur with the first infusion, and are not likely to occur later if the first infusion is given without a reaction. Most resolve over the course of several hours to a day.
c. Asthenia is occasional.
d. Diarrhea is occasional.
e. Fever is occasional.
f. Pain at the injection site is likely after extravasation.

EPIRUBICIN

Other names. 4′Epi-doxorubicin, EPI.
Mechanism of action. DNA strand breakage, mediated by anthracycline effects on topoisomerase II.
Primary indications. Breast carcinoma.
Usual dosage and schedule. 70–90 mg/m² i.v. every 3 weeks administered through the sidearm of a freely flowing i.v. infusion.
Special precautions.
1. Take care to avoid extravasation.
2. Do not exceed a lifetime cumulative dose of 1000 mg/m² (use a reduced dose for patients with prior chest radiotherapy or prior anthracycline or anthracenedione therapy).
Toxicity.
1. *Myelosuppression.* Dose-limiting leukopenia with recovery by day 21.
2. *Nausea and vomiting.* Common.
3. *Mucocutaneous effects.*
   a. Stomatitis that is dose-dependent.
   b. Alopecia beginning approximately 10 days after the first treatment with regrowth when cessation of drug treatment occurs is common but not universal (25–50%).
   c. Severe local tissue damage possibly progressing to skin ulceration and necrosis if subcutaneous extravasation occurs is common.
4. *Cardiac effects.*
   a. Potentially irreversible congestive heart failure may occur owing to cardiomyopathy. The incidence depends on the lifetime dose, which should not exceed 1000 mg/m². This limit is lower if patient has received prior chest radiotherapy or prior anthracycline or anthracenedione therapy. Congestive heart failure may be predicted by serial measurement of left ventricular function or endomyocardial biopsy.
   b. Transient ECG changes are similar in type and frequency to those observed after doxorubicin.
5. *Miscellaneous effects.*
   a. Red-orange urine for 24 hours after injection owing to drugs and its metabolites is common.
   b. Diarrhea is occasional.

EPOETIN

Other names. Recombinant human erythropoietin (rHuEPO), EPO, epoetin-alfa, Epogen, Procrit.

Mechanism of action. Epoetin-alfa is a recombinant glycoprotein that contains 165 amino acids in a sequence identical to that of endogenous human erythropoietin. It has the same biologic activity, inducing erythropoiesis by stimulating the division and differentiation of committed erythroid progenitor cells.

Primary indications.
1. Anemia from chemotherapy in patients with nonmyeloid malignancies.
2. Anemia associated with malignancy, as in multiple myeloma or anemia of chronic disease.
3. Anemia associated with chronic renal failure.
4. Anemia associated with zidovudine therapy in HIV-infected patients.

Usual dosage and schedule.
1. Starting dose is 150 U/kg s.c. three times a week. The dose may be escalated to 300 U/kg s.c. three times a week, after a 4- to 8-week trial at the initial dose, in patients who have not responded satisfactorily.
2. Alternate dose is 40,000 units s.c. once weekly.

Special precautions. Iron supplementation may be beneficial if there is any question of body iron stores. If at any time the hematocrit rises above 40%, hold epoetin injections until the hematocrit falls to 36% or less.

Toxicity.
1. *Myelosuppression.* None. Therapeutic effect is increase in hemoglobin.
2. *Nausea and vomiting.* None.
3. *Mucocutaneous effects.* Rare rashes or hives.
4. *Miscellaneous effects.*
   a. Improved energy level, activity level, and self-rated quality of life scores occur in patients receiving therapy.
   b. Edema is occasional.
   c. Diarrhea is occasional.
   d. Increased cardiovascular blood pressure occurs in about 25% of patients. Hypertension may occur; the risk is greatest in patients with preexisting hypertension. Chest pain is uncommon; edema is occasional.
   e. Seizures are rare.
   f. Influenza-like syndrome is rare to uncommon.
   g. Thrombotic complications are uncommon.

ESTRAMUSTINE

Other name. Emcyt

Mechanism of action. A chemical combination of mechlorethamine and estradiol phosphate, estramustine is designed to selectively enter cells with estrogen receptors, and act as an alkylating agent. May promote microtubule disassembly.

Primary indication. Metastatic prostate carcinoma.

Usual dosage and schedule. 300–600 mg/m^2 PO daily in 2–3 divided doses.

Special precautions. Take with meals and antacids to lessen gastrointestinal disturbances.

Toxicity.
1. *Myelosuppression.* Occurs only occasionally.

2. *Nausea and vomiting.* Commonly seen soon after starting treatment but usually lessens with continued therapy and antiemetics. If persistent and severe, it may be necessary to discontinue the drug.
3. *Mucocutaneous effects.* Rash with fever is rare.
4. *Miscellaneous effects.*
   a. Congestive heart failure—must be watched for in patients with preexisting cardiac disease.
   b. Gynecomastia is occasional.
   c. Vascular (thromboembolism, arterial insufficiency) is uncommon.

ESTROGENS

Other names. Diethylstilbestrol (DES), chlorotrianisene (TACE), diethylstilbestrol diphosphate (Stilphostrol), and others.
Mechanism of action. Suppression of testosterone production via negative feedback on hypothalamus.
Primary indications. Prostate carcinoma.
Usual dosage and schedule.
1. DES, 1–3 mg PO daily.
2. Chlorotrianisene, 12–25 mg PO daily.
3. Diethylstilbestrol diphosphate, 500–1000 mg i.v. daily for 5–7 days, then 250–500 mg i.v. 1 or 2 times weekly.
Special precautions.
1. Acute fluid retention and pulmonary edema are possible, particularly with high-dose i.v. therapy.
2. Hypercalcemia may occur with initial therapy.
Toxicity.
1. *Myelosuppression.* None.
2. *Nausea and vomiting.* Common at the beginning of therapy but diminish or stop with continued treatment. Severity may be lessened by beginning treatment with doses lower than those recommended.
3. *Mucocutaneous effects.* Darkening of nipples is common.
4. *Miscellaneous effects.*
   a. Peripheral edema due to sodium retention is common, but congestive heart failure occurs in fewer than 5% of patients.
   b. Diarrhea is uncommon.
   c. Any patient on estrogens may be at higher risk than normal for thromboemboli. An increase in cardiovascular deaths has been seen in male patients given DES at 5 mg daily for prostate carcinoma.
   d. Increased bone pain, tumor pain, and local disease flare are associated with both good tumor response and tumor progression.
   e. Feminization occurs in male patients.

ETOPOSIDE

Other names. Epipodophyllotoxin, VP-16, VP-16-213, VePesid, Etopophos (etoposide phosphate).
Mechanism of action. Interaction with topoisomerase II produces single-strand breaks in DNA. Arrests cells in late S phase or G_2 phase.

Primary indications.
1. Small cell anaplastic and non–small cell lung carcinomas.
2. Stomach carcinoma.
3. Germ cell cancers.
4. Lymphomas.

Usual dosage and schedule.
1. 120 mg/m^2 i.v. on days 1 to 3 every 3 weeks.
2. 50 to 100 mg/m^2 i.v. on days 1 to 5 every 2 to 4 weeks.
3. 125 to 140 mg/m^2 i.v. on days 1, 3, and 5 every 3 to 5 weeks.
4. 50 mg/m^2 p.o. daily for 21 days. Repeat after 1 to 2 weeks' rest.
5. High-dose therapy (750 to 2,400 mg/m^2) is investigational and should only be used with progenitor cell rescue (e.g., bone marrow or peripheral blood stem cell transplantation).

Special precautions.
1. Administer etoposide as a 30- to 60-minute infusion to avoid severe hypotension. Monitor blood pressure during infusion. Etoposide phosphate may be administered as a 5-minute bolus infusion.
2. Take care to avoid extravasation.
3. Etoposide must be diluted in 20 to 50 volumes (100 to 250 mL) of isotonic saline before use. Etoposide phosphate vials (100 mg) may be reconstituted in 5 to 10 mL (water, saline, or dextrose) to a concentration of 10 or 20 mg/mL.
4. Decrease dose by 50% for bilirubin levels of 1.5 to 3 mg/dL; decrease by 75% for bilirubin levels of 3 to 5 mg/dL; discontinue drug if bilirubin level is more than 5 mg/dL.
5. Decrease dose by 25% for creatinine clearance rate of less than 30 mL/min.

Toxicity.
1. *Myelosuppression.* Dose-limiting leukopenia and less severe thrombocytopenia have a nadir at 16 days with recovery by days 20 to 22.
2. *Nausea and vomiting.* Usually mild to moderate problems in about one third of patients receiving standard doses; common with high-dose therapy. Anorexia is common.
3. *Mucocutaneous effects.*
   a. Alopecia is common.
   b. Stomatitis is uncommon with standard doses; common with high-dose therapy.
   c. Painful rash may occur with high-dose therapy.
   d. Chemical phlebitis is occasional.
4. *Miscellaneous effects.*
   a. Hepatotoxicity is rare.
   b. Diarrhea is uncommon.
   c. Peripheral neurotoxicity is rare.
   d. Allergic reaction is rare.
   e. Hemorrhagic cystitis may occur with high-dose therapy.

FILGRASTIM

Other names. Granulocyte colony-stimulating factor, G-CSF, Neupogen.

Mechanism of action. Promotes growth and differentiation of myeloid progenitor cells. May improve survival and function of granulocytes.

Primary indications.
1. Prophylaxis of granulocytopenia secondary to intensive chemotherapy.
2. Treatment of granulocytopenia secondary to chemotherapy.
3. Granulocytopenia from primary marrow disorders, such as idiopathic neutropenia and aplastic anemia, and myelodysplastic syndrome.
4. Granulocytopenia associated with acquired immunodeficiency syndrome (AIDS) and its therapy.

Usual dosage and schedule.
1. *Adjunct to chemotherapy:* commonly 200–400 µg/m² (5–10 µg/kg) SQ daily, starting no sooner than 24 hours and no later than 4 days after the last dose of chemotherapy, for 10 to 20 days until the neutrophil count exceeds 10,000/µl after the expected nadir. Because of cost factors, vial size, and comparability of effect with "ballpark" doses, some physicians choose to treat patients weighing less than 75 kg with 300 µg daily and patients weighing more than 75 kg with 480 µg daily.
2. *Other purposes:* 40–500 µg/m² SQ, IM, or i.v. daily. Dose and duration are dependent on the purpose of administration.

Special precautions. Use with caution in disorders of myeloid stem cells, since it may promote growth of leukemic cells.

Toxicity.
1. *Myelosuppression.* None (leukocytosis).
2. *Nausea and vomiting.* Rare.
3. *Mucocutaneous effects.* Exacerbation of preexisting dermatologic conditions are occasional; pyoderma gangrenosum is rare.
4. *Miscellaneous effects is* usually mild and short-lived.
   a. Bone pain, musculoskeletal symptoms such as cramps, and back or leg pain is common.
   b. Splenomegaly—with prolonged use.
   c. Exacerbation of preexisting inflammatory or autoimmune disorders is rare.
   d. Mild elevation of lactate dehydrogenase (LDH) and alkaline phosphatase.

FLOXURIDINE

Other name. FUDR

Mechanism of action. A pyrimidine antimetabolite that, when converted to the active nucleotide, inhibits the enzyme thymidylate synthetase.

Primary indications. Hepatic metastasis of gastrointestinal carcinoma, primary hepatic carcinoma.

Usual dosage and schedule. 4.0–6.0 mg/m² as a continuous infusion into the hepatic artery daily for 2 weeks, then off for 2 weeks. Administered via continuous infusion pump.

Special precautions.
1. Reduce dose in patients with compromised liver function.
2. Ulcer-like pain or other significant gastrointestinal symptoms are indications to discontinue intraarterial therapy, as hemorrhage or perforation may occur.

Toxicity.
1. *Myelosuppression.* Uncommon.

2. *Nausea and vomiting.* Uncommon unless the hepatic artery catheter has become displaced and the stomach and duodenum are being infused.
3. *Mucocutaneous effects.*
   a. Stomatitis is an early sign of severe toxicity. It progresses from soreness and erythema to frank ulceration, which may become hemorrhagic in a small number of patients. Esophagitis, proctitis, and diarrhea may also occur.
   b. Partial alopecia is uncommon.
   c. Hyperpigmentation of skin over face, hands, and the vein used for the infusion is occasional.
   d. Maculopapular rash is uncommon.
   e. Sun exposure tends to increase skin reactions.
4. *Miscellaneous effects.*
   a. Neurotoxicity, including headache, minor visual disturbances, and cerebellar ataxia is rare.
   b. Increased lacrimation is uncommon.
   c. Abdominal cramps and pain are common if the catheter is displaced and the stomach and duodenum are being infused. Can progress to frank gastritis or duodenal ulcer.
   d. Liver function abnormalities and jaundice are common when given by hepatic arterial infusion. Dose should be reduced during subsequent cycle.
   e. Sclerosing cholangitis when given by hepatic artery infusion is uncommon.

FLUDARABINE

Other names. FAMP, Fludara.

Mechanism of action. Inhibition of DNA polymerase and ribonucleotide reductase.

Primary indications.
1. Chronic lymphocytic leukemia.
2. Macroglobulinemia.
3. Indolent lymphomas.
4. Acute leukemia (in combination).

Usual dosage and schedule. 25 mg/m^2 i.v. as a 30-minute infusion daily for 5 days. Other dose schedules, usually less intensive, have been used, often in combinations with other drugs. Repeat every 4 weeks.

Special precautions. If there is the potential for tumor lysis syndrome, administer allopurinol and ensure good hydration and close clinical monitoring.

Toxicity.
1. *Myelosuppression.* Granulocytopenia and thrombocytopenia are common but appear to become less common in patients whose disease is responding. Infection, particularly pneumonia, is common during early courses and uncommon after the sixth course.
2. *Nausea and vomiting.* Common (30%) but not usually severe.
3. *Mucocutaneous effects.* Occasional mucositis, rash, no alopecia.
4. *Neurotoxicity.* Uncommon at usual dosage. Somnolence or fatigue, paresthesias, and twitching of extremities may be seen. Severe neurologic symptoms, including visual disturbances, have been common at higher doses than those recommended.

5. *Immune suppression.* Common. Usually seen as a depression in CD4 and CD8 lymphocyte counts. Opportunistic infections may result, and many recommend pneumocystic pneumonia prophylaxis until the CD4 lymphopenia resolves.
6. *Miscellaneous effects.*
   a. Abnormal liver or renal function is rare.
   b. Allergic pneumonitis is occasional to uncommon.
   c. Edema is occasional.
   d. Diarrhea is occasional.
   e. Tumor lysis syndrome is rare.

FLUOROURACIL

Other names. 5-FU, Adrucil, 5-fluorouracil.
Mechanism of action. A pyrimidine antimetabolite that, when converted to the active nucleotide, inhibits the enzyme thymidylate synthetase and thereby blocks DNA synthesis.
Primary indications.
1. Breast, colorectal, anal, stomach, pancreas, esophagus, liver, head and neck, and bladder carcinomas.
2. Basal and squamous cell carcinomas of skin (topically).
Usual dosage and schedule.
1. *Systemic*
   a. 500 mg/m² i.v. on days 1–5 every 4 weeks *or*
   b. 450–600 mg/m² i.v. weekly.
   c. 200–400 mg/m² daily as a continuous intravenous infusion.
   d. 1000 mg/m² daily for 4 days as a continuous i.v. infusion every 3–4 weeks.
2. *Intracavitary:* 500–1000 mg for pericardial effusion; 2000–3000 mg for pleural or peritoneal effusions.
3. *Intraarterial* (liver): 800–1200 mg/m² as a continuous infusion on days 1–4, followed by 600 mg/m² as a continuous infusion on days 5–21.
Special precautions.
1. Reduce dose in patients with compromised liver function.
2. For intraarterial infusion, add 5000 units of heparin to 1 liter of 5% dextrose in water together with the daily dose of fluorouracil. The catheter position should be checked with dye injection every few days to ensure that it has not moved and that the hepatic artery has not thrombosed. Ulcer-like pain or other significant gastrointestinal symptoms are indications to discontinue intraarterial therapy, as hemorrhage or perforation may occur.
3. Precipitation may occur when leucovorin and fluorouracil are mixed in the same bag.
Toxicity.
1. *Myelosuppression.* Dose-limiting with a nadir at 10–14 days after the last dose and recovery by 21 days.
2. *Nausea and vomiting.* May occur but are not usually severe.
3. *Mucocutaneous effects.*
   a. Stomatitis is an early sign of severe toxicity. It progresses from soreness and erythema to frank ulceration, which becomes hemorrhagic in a small number of patients. Esophagitis, proctitis, and diarrhea may also occur.

     b. Partial alopecia is uncommon.
     c. Hyperpigmentation of skin over face, hands, and the veins used for infusion is occasional.
     d. Maculopapular rash is uncommon.
     e. Sun exposure tends to increase skin reactions.
     f. "Hand-foot syndrome" with painful, erythematous desquamation and fissures of palms and soles is common with continuous infusion, occasional with other schedules or combinations.

4. *Miscellaneous effects*
     a. Neurotoxicity, including headache, minor visual disturbances, and cerebellar ataxia is rare.
     b. Increased lacrimation is uncommon.
     c. Cardiac toxicity, including arrhythmias, angina, ischemia, and sudden death is rare. May be more common with continuous infusion and previous history of coronary artery disease.
     d. Hypertriglyceridemia when given in combination with levamisole.

FLUTAMIDE

Other name. Eulexin.
Mechanism of action. Competitive inhibitor of androgens at the cellular androgen receptor in the prostate cancer cells.
Primary indications. Carcinoma of the prostate, most often in combination with LHRH agonists.
Usual dosage and schedule. 250 mg p.o. every 8 hours.
Special precautions. None.
Toxicity.
1. *Myelosuppression.* None.
2. *Nausea and vomiting.* Uncommon to occasional.
3. *Mucocutaneous effects.* Mild skin rash is occasional.
4. *Miscellaneous effects.*
     a. Secondary pharmacologic effects, including breast tenderness, breast swelling, hot flashes, impotence, and loss of libido, are common but reversible after cessation of therapy.
     b. Gastrointestinal effects: diarrhea, flatulence, and mild abdominal pain are common.
     c. Elevated liver function tests are uncommon.
     d. Hypertension is occasional.
     e. Adverse cardiovascular events are similar to those seen with orchiectomy.

GEMCITABINE

Other name. Gemzar.
Mechanism of action. After being metabolized intracellularly to the active diphosphate and triphosphate nucleotides, gemcitabine, a cytidine analog, inhibits ribonucleotide reductase and competes with deoxycytidine triphosphate for incorporation into DNA.
Primary indications.
1. Carcinoma of the pancreas, locally advanced or metastatic.
2. Other carcinomas (investigational).

Usual dosage and schedule. 1,000 mg/m^2 i.v. over 30 minutes once weekly for up to 7 weeks. After 1 week of rest, subsequent cycles are given once weekly for 3 consecutive weeks out of 4.

Special precautions. Prolongation of infusion time beyond 60 minutes increases toxicity.

Toxicity.
1. *Myelosuppression.* Common.
2. *Nausea and vomiting.* Common, but usually not severe.
3. *Mucocutaneous effects.* Alopecia and mucositis are occasional.
4. *Miscellaneous effects.*
   a. Diarrhea is common.
   b. Constipation is occasional.
   c. Transient elevation of serum transaminases and alkaline phosphatase is common.
   d. Mild proteinuria and hematuria is common.
   e. Hemolytic-uremic syndrome is rare (0.25%).
   f. Fever without documented infection is common.
   g. Edema is occasional.
   h. Neurotoxicity: mild paresthesias are occasional.
   i. Dyspnea is occasional.

HYDROXYUREA

Other name. Hydrea.

Mechanism of action. Interferes with DNA synthesis, at least in part by inhibiting the enzymatic conversion of ribonucleotides to deoxyribonucleotides.

Primary indications.
1. Head and neck carcinomas.
2. Chronic granulocytic leukemia; acute lymphocytic and acute nonlymphocytic leukemia with high blast counts.
3. Essential thrombocythemia.
4. Polycythemia rubra vera.
5. Prevention of retinoic acid syndrome in acute promyelocytic leukemia.

Usual dosage and schedule.
1. 800–2000 mg/m^2 PO as a single or divided daily dose *or*
2. 3200 mg/m^2 PO as a single dose every third day (not for leukemias).

Special precautions. The daily dose must be adjusted for blood count trends. Be careful not to change dose too often, because there is a delay in response.

Toxicity.
1. *Myelosuppression.* Occurs at doses of more than 1600 mg/m^2 daily by day 10. Recovery is usually prompt.
2. *Nausea and vomiting.* Common at high doses.
3. *Mucocutaneous effects.* Stomatitis is rare. Maculopapular rash may be seen. Inflammation of mucous membranes caused by radiation may be exaggerated.
4. *Miscellaneous effects.*
   a. Temporary renal function impairment or dysuria is uncommon.
   b. CNS disturbances are rare.
   c. Increased red cell mean corpuscular volume (MCV) is common.
   d. May be leukemogenic.

IDARUBICIN

Other names. 4-Demethoxydaunorubicin, IDA, Idamycin.
Mechanism of action. DNA strand breakage mediated by anthracycline effects on topoisomerase II or free radicals; DNA intercalation; DNA polymerase inhibition.
Primary indications.
1.   Acute nonlymphocytic leukemia.
2.   Blast crisis of chronic granulocytic leukemia.
3.   Acute lymphocytic leukemia.
Usual dosage and schedule. 12–13 mg/m^2 i.v. daily for 3 days (usually in a combination with cytarabine) during induction; 10–12 mg/m^2 i.v. daily for 2 days during consolidation.
Special precautions. Administer over several minutes into the sidearm of a running i.v. infusion, taking care to avoid extravasation. Cardiac toxicity may be less than that with daunorubicin. Maximum dose not yet established. Cumulative doses >150 mg/m^2 have been associated with decreased cardiac ejection fraction.
Toxicity.
1.   *Myelosuppression.* Universal and dose-limiting.
2.   *Nausea and vomiting.* Common.
3.   *Mucocutaneous effects.* Alopecia is common; mucositis is common but usually not severe.
4.   *Hepatic dysfunction.* Common but usually not severe and not clearly due to the idarubicin.
5.   *Renal effects.* Common but usually not clinically significant.
6.   *Other gastrointestinal effects.* Anorexia is common; diarrhea is occasional to common; bleeding is common in one study.
7.   *Cardiac effects.* Uncommon during induction and consolidation (1–5%).
8.   *Tissue damage.* If infiltration occurs is probable.
9.   *Neurologic effects.* Occasional.

IFOSFAMIDE

Other name. Ifex.
Mechanism of action. Metabolic activation by microsomal liver enzymes produces biologically active intermediates that attack nucleophilic sites, particularly on DNA.
Primary indications.
1.   Testicular and lung cancers.
2.   Bone and soft-tissue sarcomas.
3.   Lymphoma.
Special precautions. Must be used with mesna (Mesnex) to prevent hemorrhagic cystitis. Mesna dose is at least 20% of the ifosfamide dose (on a weight basis), administered just prior to (or mixed with) the ifosfamide dose and again at 4 and 8 hours after the ifosfamide to detoxify the urinary metabolites that cause the hemorrhagic cystitis. Higher doses of ifosfamide may require higher doses and longer durations of mesna. Neither mesna nor its only metabolite, mesna disulfide, affect ifosfamide or its antineoplastic metabolites. Mesna disulfide is reduced in the kidney to a free thiol compound, which then reacts chemically with urotoxic metabolites resulting in their detoxification. Vigorous hydration is also required with a minimum of 2 liters of oral or i.v. hydra-

tion daily. Administer as a slow i.v. infusion over a period of at least 30 minutes.

Usual dosage and schedule.

1. 1.2 gm/m^2 i.v. over 30 minutes or more daily for 5 consecutive days every 3 or 4 weeks, usually with other agents. Mesna 120 mg/m^2 is given just before ifosfamide, then mesna 1200 mg/m^2 as a daily continuous infusion is given until 16 hours after the last dose of ifosfamide.
2. 3.6 gm/m^2 i.v. daily as a 4-hour infusion for 2 consecutive days, usually with other agents. Mesna is given at a dose of 750 mg/m^2 i.v. just prior to and at 4 and 8 hours after the start of the ifosfamide.
3. Higher dosage schedules have been used experimentally with up to 14 gm/m^2 being used per course over a 6-day period, with equal or greater doses of mesna.

Toxicity.

1. *Myelosuppression.* Dose-limiting. Platelets are relatively spared. Granulocyte nadirs are commonly reached at 10–14 days, and recovery is seen by day 21. Thrombocytopenia may be seen with higher doses.
2. *Nausea and vomiting.* Common without standard antiemetics.
3. *Mucocutaneous effects.* Alopecia is common; mucositis is rarely seen at standard doses; dermatitis is rare.
4. *Hemorrhagic cystitis.* Common and dose-limiting unless a uroprotective agent such as mesna is used. With mesna, the incidence of hemorrhagic cystitis is 5–10%, and gross hematuria is uncommon. Increasing the duration of mesna may alleviate the problem during subsequent cycles.
5. *Miscellaneous effects.*
    a. CNS toxicity (somnolence, confusion, depressive psychosis, hallucinations, disorientation, and uncommonly seizures, cranial nerve dysfunction, or coma) is occasional with doses in lower range, more common with larger doses.
    b. Infertility is common in men and women, as with other alkylating agents.
    c. Renal impairment is occasional to common. Fanconi syndrome dependent on dose. May be severe acidosis.
    d. Liver dysfunction is uncommon.
    e. Phlebitis is uncommon.
    f. Fever is rare.
    g. Peripheral neuropathy with high-dose therapy is uncommon.

INTERFERON ALPHA

Other names. Roferon-A (interferon alfa-2a, recombinant alpha-A interferon), Intron A (interferon alfa-2b, recombinant alpha-2 interferon).

Mechanism of action. Believed to involve direct inhibition of tumor cell growth and modulation of the immune response of the host, including activation of NK cells, modulation of antibody production, and induction of major histocompatibility antigens.

Primary indications.

1. Chronic myelogenous leukemia.
2. Melanoma (both as adjuvant and metastatic disease therapy).

3. Non-Hodgkin's lymphoma (low grade), mycosis fungoides.
4. Multiple myeloma.
5. Hairy-cell leukemia.
6. Renal cell carcinoma.
7. Other carcinomas in combination with chemotherapy (e.g., fluorouracil in colon carcinoma).
8. Kaposi's sarcoma, HIV associated.
9. Condyloma acuminatum (intralesional).
10. Chronic hepatitis B and C.

Usual dosage and schedule.
1. 3–10 million IU IM or SQ in various schedules. Daily dosing is often used for several weeks or months, followed by 3 times a week dosing.
2. As adjuvant therapy for high risk melanoma, 20 million IU/m² i.v. 5 consecutive days weekly for 4 weeks, then 10 million IU/m² SQ three times weekly for 48 weeks.
3. Investigationally, doses have been higher (up to 50 million IU/m² per dose), usually i.v. at doses higher than 10 million IU/m².

Toxicity.
1. *Myelosuppression.* Common but usually mild to moderate and transient, even with continued therapy.
2. *Nausea and vomiting.* Anorexia occurs in about one-half of all patients, nausea in about one-third, and vomiting in 10%.
3. *Mucocutaneous effects.* Rash, dryness, or inflammation of the oropharynx, dry skin or pruritus, and partial alopecia is occasional to common.
4. *Flu-like syndrome* with fatigue, fever, chills, myalgias, arthralgias, and headache is common to universal with greater severity at higher doses. Tends to diminish with continuing therapy and acetaminophen.
5. *Neurologic effects.*
    a. Peripheral nervous system: occasional paresthesias or numbness.
    b. CNS is uncommon at lower doses, but with higher doses an increased likelihood including headache, somnolence, anxiety, depression, confusion, hallucinations, cerebellar dysfunction, and emotional lability.
6. *General systemic effects.* Fatigue, anorexia, and weight loss is common with chronic administration.
7. *Cardiovascular effects.* Mild hypotension is common but rarely symptomatic. Rarely hypertension, chest pain, arrhythmias.
8. *Infectious effects.* Exacerbation of herpetic eruptions and nonherpetic cold sores is uncommon.
9. *Miscellaneous effects.* Leg cramps, constipation or diarrhea, insomnia, urticaria, hot flashes, coagulation disorders are uncommon.
10. *Metabolic effects and laboratory abnormalities.*
    a. Elevated liver enzymes is common.
    b. Mild proteinuria, increase in serum creatinine is occasional.
    c. Hypercalcemia is occasional.
    d. Hypothyroidism and hyperthyroidism with or without antithyroid antibodies.
    e. Hypertriglyceridemia is rare.

11. Antibody development (binding and neutralizing) occurs more readily with interferon alfa-2a than with interferon alfa-2b. The significance of this is not clear, though it may be associated with the development of clinical resistance in some patients.

IRINOTECAN

Other names. Camptosar, CPT-11.

Mechanism of action. Irinotecan, a semisynthetic derivative of camptothecin, is a potent inhibitor of topoisomerase I, an enzyme essential for effective replication and transcription. It binds to the topoisomerase I—DNA cleavable complex, preventing re-ligation after cleavage by topoisomerase I.

Primary indications. Carcinoma of the colon or rectum.

Usual dosage and schedule. 125 mg/m^2 i.v. over 90 minutes weekly for 4 weeks followed by a 2-week rest to complete one cycle. Doses should be modified upward in the next cycle to 150 mg/m^2 in cases in which there was no toxicity. For severe or worse diarrhea, doses should be held, then modified downward by 25 mg/m^2 during the cycle if there was an increase in stools of 7 to 9 per day and by 50 mg/m^2 if there was an increase in stools of 10 or more. Doses are also held during treatment and reduced in the same and subsequent cycles for severe neutropenia absolute neuliophil count (ANC) <1,000.

Special precautions. Both early and late diarrhea may occur. That which occurs within 24 hours (a cholinergic effect) should be treated with atropine, 0.25 to 1 mg i.v. Late diarrhea should be treated promptly with loperamide (up to 2 mg every 2 hours until the patient is diarrhea free for 12 hours) and prompt fluid and electrolyte replacement as indicated, if the diarrhea becomes severe (increase of 7 or more stools per day) or there is dehydration.

Toxicity.
1. *Myelosuppression.* Neutropenia and anemia are common; thrombocytopenia is uncommon.
2. *Nausea and vomiting.* Common.
3. *Mucocutaneous effects.* Alopecia is common. Stomatitis, rash, and sweating occur occasionally.
4. *Miscellaneous effects.*
    a. Other gastrointestinal.
        (1) Diarrhea is common, often severe. Thirty percent of patients have an increase of more than seven stools daily.
        (2) Anorexia is common.
        (3) Constipation and dyspepsia are occasional.
        (4) Abdominal cramping is common, occasionally severe.
    b. Fever is common, rarely severe.
    c. Headache, back pain, chills, and edema are occasional.
    d. Increase in liver function tests is occasional, rarely severe, except in patients with known liver metastasis.
    e. Dyspnea, cough, or rhinitis is occasional.
    f. Insomnia or dizziness is occasional.
    g. Flushing is occasional.

ISOTRETINOIN

Other names. 13-*cis*-retinoic acid, 13-cRA, Accutane.

Mechanism of action. Binds to cytoplasmic retinoic acid-binding proteins and then is transported to the nucleus where it interacts with nuclear retinoic acid receptors. These then affect expression of the genes that control cell growth and differentiation.

Primary indications.
1. Prevention of second primary cancers in patients with surgically or radiotherapeutically cured head and neck cancer.
2. Treatment of carcinomas of the cervix and skin (in combination with interferon alpha).

Usual dosage and schedule.
1. *Prevention*
   a. 5.6 mg/m² (0.15 mg/kg) PO daily.
   b. 30 mg PO daily.
2. *Treatment:* 40 mg/m² (1 mg/kg) PO daily.

Special precautions. Avoid use in pregnant women because of marked teratogenic potential.

Toxicity.
1. *Myelosuppression.* Rare.
2. *Nausea and vomiting.* Occasional and mild.
3. *Mucocutaneous effects.* Universal, particularly at doses at higher end of range. They include redness, dryness, and pruritus of the skin and mucous membranes; possible vesicle formation; peeling of the skin of the palms and soles; cheilitis; and conjunctivitis. There also may be increased skin photosensitivity (e.g., to sun) and the nails may become brittle. Alopecia is uncommon.
4. *Miscellaneous effects.*
   a. Cataracts and corneal ulcerations or opacities are uncommon.
   b. Musculoskeletal: arthralgias, bone pain, muscle aches are occasional to common; skeletal hyperostosis is common at higher doses (80 mg/m²/day).
   c. Hypertriglyceridemia: mild to moderate elevations are common; marked elevations (>5 times normal) are uncommon. Hypercholesterolemia occurs to lesser degree.
   d. Neurologic: lethargy, fatigue, headache, and mental depression is uncommon; pseudotumor cerebri is rare.
   e. Gastrointestinal: inflammatory bowel disease is rare.
   f. Hepatotoxicity with increased LDH, SGOT, serum glutamic-pyruvic transaminase (SGPT), gamma-glutamyl transpeptidase (GGTP), alkaline phosphatase is occasional.

LETROZOLE

Other name. Femara.

Mechanism of action. Decreases estrogen biosynthesis by selective inhibition of aromatase (estrogen synthetase) in peripheral tissues.

Primary indications. Carcinoma of the breast (advanced) in estrogen responsive postmenopausal women with progression following antiestrogen therapy.

Usual dosage and schedule. 2.5 mg p.o. daily.

Special precautions. Potential hazard to fetus if given during pregnancy.

Toxicity.

1. *Myelosuppression.* No dose related effect.
2. *Nausea and vomiting.* Nausea is occasional, vomiting is uncommon.
3. *Mucocutaneous effects.* Rash is uncommon.
4. *Miscellaneous effects.*
   a. Asthenia is occasional.
   b. Diarrhea is occasional.
   c. Musculoskeletal pain (arthralgia or bone) is occasional to common.
   d. Headache is occasional.
   e. Peripheral edema, weight gain is occasional (lower than with megestrol).
   f. Dyspnea and cough is uncommon to occasional.
   g. Constipation or diarrhea is occasional.
   h. Thromboembolic events are rare.
   i. Hot flushes are occasional.
   j. Hypercalcemia is rare.

LEVAMISOLE

Other name. Ergamisol.

Mechanism of action. Restores immune function, but whether this action is related to the mechanism of potentiation of fluorouracil effect in adjuvant therapy of colon cancer is unknown.

Primary indications. Dukes' C carcinoma of the colon (with fluorouracil).

Usual dosage and schedule. 50 mg PO q8h for 3 days every 2 weeks for 1 year, beginning with first dose of fluorouracil. (Fluorouracil 450 mg/m² i.v. bolus daily for 5 days, then beginning 28 days later 450 mg/m² i.v. bolus weekly.)

Special precautions. Increased bilirubin may require delay of therapy.

Toxicity.

1. *Myelosuppression.* Uncommon.
2. *Nausea and vomiting.* Nausea is common; vomiting is occasional.
3. *Mucocutaneous effects.* Stomatitis and alopecia are uncommon; rash that may be pruritic is occasional.
4. *Miscellaneous effects.*
   a. Dermatitis is occasional.
   b. Fatigue is occasional.
   c. Taste perversion is occasional.
   d. CNS problems (dizziness, somnolence, headache) is uncommon.
   e. Fever and rigors are uncommon.
   f. Musculoskeletal pain is uncommon.
   g. Increased bilirubin and other liver enzymes.
   h. Hypercoagulability leading to venous thrombosis is rare.
   i. Drug interactions with warfarin (increased prothrombin time), phenytoin (increased plasma levels).
   j. Marked elevation of triglyceride levels (with fluorouracil).

LOMUSTINE

Other name. CCNU, CeeNU.

Mechanism of action. Alkylation and carbamoylation by lomustine metabolites interfere with the synthesis and function of DNA, RNA, and proteins. Lomustine is lipid-soluble and easily enters the brain.

Primary indications.
1. Lung and kidney carcinomas.
2. Hodgkin's and non-Hodgkin's lymphomas.
3. Brain tumors.

Usual dosage and schedule. 100–130 mg/m^2 PO once every 6–8 weeks (lower dose used for patients with compromised bone marrow function). Some recommend limiting cumulative dose to 1000 mg/m^2 to limit pulmonary and renal toxicity.

Special precautions. Because of delayed myelosuppression (3–6 weeks), do not treat more often than every 6 weeks. Await a return of normal platelet and granulocyte counts before repeating therapy.

Toxicity.
1. *Myelosuppression.* Universal and dose-limiting. Leukopenia and thrombocytopenia are delayed 3–6 weeks after therapy begins and may be cumulative with successive doses.
2. *Nausea and vomiting.* Begin 3–6 hours after therapy and last up to 24 hours.
3. *Mucocutaneous effects.* Stomatitis and alopecia are rare.
4. *Miscellaneous effects.*
   a. Confusion, lethargy, and ataxia are rare.
   b. Mild hepatotoxicity is infrequent.
   c. Secondary neoplasia is possible.
   d. Pulmonary fibrosis is uncommon at doses of less than 1000 mg/m^2.
   e. Renal toxicity is uncommon at doses of less than 1000 mg/m^2.

LUTEINIZING HORMONE–RELEASING HORMONE ANALOGS

Other names. Leuprolide (Lupron, Lupron depot), goserelin (Zoladex depot).

Mechanism of action. Initial release of follicle-stimulating hormone and luteinizing hormone from the anterior pituitary, followed by diminution of gonadotropin secretion owing to desensitization of the pituitary to gonadotropin-releasing hormone (GnRH) and consequent decrease in the respective gonadal hormones. May also have direct effects on cancer cells, at least in cancer of the breast, in which GnRH-binding sites have been demonstrated.

Primary indications.
1. Metastatic prostate carcinoma.
2. Breast carcinoma in premenopausal and perimenopausal women with metastatic disease (goserelin).

Usual dosage and schedule.
1. Leuprolide depot, 7.5 mg i.m. monthly, 22.5 mg i.m. every 3 months, or 30 mg i.m. every 4 months.
2. Goserelin depot, 3.6 mg s.c. every 4 weeks or 10.8 mg s.c. every 12 weeks. Use only 3.6-mg implant for breast carcinoma.

Special precautions. Worsening of symptoms may occur during the first few weeks.

Toxicity.
1. *Myelosuppression.* Rare, if at all.
2. *Nausea and vomiting.* Occasional.
3. *Mucocutaneous effects.* Erythema and ecchymosis at the injection site, rash, hair loss, and itching are uncommon.
4. *Cardiovascular effects.* Congestive heart failure and thrombotic episodes are uncommon. Peripheral edema is occasional.
5. *Miscellaneous effects.*
    a. Central nervous system: dizziness, pain, headache, and paresthesias are uncommon.
    b. Endocrine: hot flashes are common; decreased libido is common; gynecomastia with or without tenderness is uncommon; impotence is uncommon.
    c. Bone pain, or "flare," is common on initiation of therapy in patients with bony metastasis. This can be minimized by pretreating with flutamide or another androgen antagonist in men with prostate cancer.
    d. Gastrointestinal: anorexia and constipation are uncommon.

MECHLORETHAMINE

Other names. Nitrogen mustard, HN2, Mustargen.
Mechanism of action. Mechlorethamine is a prototype alkylating agent. Its action involves transfer of the alkyl group to amino, carboxyl, hydroxyl, imidazole, phosphate, and sulfhydryl groups within the cell, altering structure and function of DNA (primarily), RNA, and proteins.
Primary indications.
1. Hodgkin's lymphoma.
2. Malignant pleural and, less commonly, peritoneal or pericardial effusions.
3. Cutaneous T cell lymphomas (topically).
Usual dosage and schedule.
1. 6 mg/m² i.v. on days 1 and 8 every 4 weeks (in MOPP regimen for Hodgkin's disease).
2. 8–16 mg/m² by intracavitary injection.
3. 10 mg in 60 ml of tap water applied to entire body surface (avoid eyes).
Special precautions.
1. Administer over several minutes into the sidearm of a running i.v. infusion, taking care to avoid extravasation.
2. Because mechlorethamine is a potent vesicant, extreme care must be exercised while preparing and administering the drug. Gloves and eye glasses are recommended to protect the preparer. If accidental eye contact should occur, institute copious irrigation with normal saline and follow by prompt ophthalmologic consultation. If accidental skin contact occurs, irrigate the affected part immediately with water for at least 15 minutes and follow by 2.6% sodium thiosulfate solution (⅙ M).
3. Mechlorethamine should be used soon after preparation (15–30 minutes) as it decomposes on standing. It *must not* be mixed in the same syringe with any other drug.

Toxicity.
1. *Myelosuppression.* Dose-limiting, with the nadir at about 1 week and recovery by 3 weeks.
2. *Nausea and vomiting.* Universal. They usually begin within the first 3 hours and last 4–8 hours.
3. *Mucocutaneous effects.* Severe painful inflammation and necrosis are likely if extravasation occurs. May be ameliorated if 2.6% thiosulfate solution (⅙ M) is instilled into the area to neutralize active drug, and ice packs are applied locally for 6–12 hours. Maculopapular rash is uncommon.
4. *Miscellaneous effects.*
   a. Phlebitis, thrombosis, or both of the vein used for the injection are common.
   b. Amenorrhea and azoospermia are common.
   c. Hyperuricemia with rapid tumor destruction.
   d. Weakness, sleepiness, and headache are uncommon.
   e. Severe allergic reactions, including anaphylaxis are rare.
   f. Secondary neoplasms are possible.

MELPHALAN

Other names. Phenylalanine mustard, L-sarcolysin, L-PAM, Alkeran.
Mechanism of action. Alkylating agent with primary effect on DNA. Amino acid-type structure may result in cellular transport that is different from other alkylating agents.
Primary indications.
1. Multiple myeloma.
2. Breast and ovarian carcinomas.
Usual dosage and schedule.
1. 8 mg/m^2 PO on days 1–4 every 4 weeks *or*
2. 10 mg/m^2 PO on days 1–4 every 6 weeks *or*
3. 3–4 mg/m^2 PO daily for 2–3 weeks, then 1–2 mg/m^2 PO daily for maintenance.
4. High-dose regimens of 140–200 mg/m^2 i.v. have been used, followed by stem cell rescue (e.g., bone marrow transplantation).
5. 16 mg/m^2 i.v. every 2 weeks × 4, then every 4 weeks.
Special precaution. Myelosuppression may be delayed and prolonged to 4–6 weeks. Reduce i.v. dose by 50% for creatinine >1.5 × normal.
Toxicity.
1. *Myelosuppression.* Dose-limiting; nadir at days 14–21.
2. *Nausea and vomiting.* Uncommon; common with high-dose regimens.
3. *Mucocutaneous effects.* Alopecia, dermatitis, and stomatitis are uncommon; alopecia and mucositis are common with high-dose regimens.
4. *Miscellaneous effects.*
   a. Acute nonlymphocytic leukemia is rare but well documented.
   b. Pulmonary fibrosis is rare.
   c. Diarrhea is common with high-dose regimens.

MERCAPTOPURINE

Other names. 6-Mercaptopurine, 6-MP, Purinethol.
Mechanism of action. A purine antimetabolite that, when converted to the nucleotide, inhibits the formation of nucleotides necessary for DNA and RNA synthesis.
Primary indications. Acute lymphocytic and juvenile chronic granulocytic leukemias.
Usual dosage and schedule.
1. 100 mg/m^2 PO daily if used alone.
2. 50–90 mg/m^2 PO daily if used with methotrexate.
Special precautions.
1. Decrease dose by 75% when used concurrently with allopurinol.
2. Increase interval between doses or reduce dose in patients with renal failure.
Toxicity.
1. *Myelosuppression.* Common but mild at recommended doses.
2. *Nausea and vomiting.* Uncommon.
3. *Mucocutaneous effects.* Stomatitis may be seen with very large doses. Dry, scaling rash is uncommon.
4. *Miscellaneous effects.*
    a. Intrahepatic cholestasis and mild focal centrolobular necrosis with jaundice are uncommon.
    b. Diarrhea is rare.
    c. Hyperuricemia with rapid leukemia cell lysis is common.
    d. Fever is uncommon.

METHOTREXATE

Other names. Amethopterin, MTX, Mexate.
Mechanism of action. Inhibition of dihydrofolate reductase, which results in a block of the reduction of dihydrofolate to tetrahydrofolate. This blockage in turn inhibits the formation of thymidylate and purines, and arrests DNA (predominantly), RNA, and protein synthesis.
Primary indications.
1. Breast, head and neck, gastrointestinal, lung, and gestational trophoblastic carcinomas.
2. Osteosarcomas (high-dose methotrexate).
3. Acute lymphocytic leukemia.
4. Meningeal leukemia or carcinomatosis.
5. Non-Hodgkin's lymphoma.
Usual dosage and schedule.
1. *Gestational trophoblastic carcinoma:* 15–30 mg PO or IM on days 1–5 every 2 weeks.
2. *Other carcinomas:* 40–80 mg/m^2 i.v. or PO 2–4 times monthly with a 7- to 14-day interval between doses.
3. *Acute lymphocytic leukemia:* 15–20 mg/m^2 PO or i.v. weekly (together with mercaptopurine).
4. *Osteogenic sarcoma:* Up to 10 gm/m^2 with leucovorin rescue (high-dose methotrexate). This usage is investigational and should not be applied outside of a research setting.
5. *Intrathecally:* 12 mg/m^2 (not >20 mg) twice weekly.
Special precautions.
1. High-dose methotrexate (>80 mg/m^2) should be administered only by individuals experienced in its use and at institutions where serum methotrexate levels can be readily measured.

2. Intrathecal methotrexate must be mixed in buffered physiologic solution containing no preservative.
3. Avoid aspirin, sulfonamides, tetracycline, phenytoin, and other protein-bound drugs that may displace methotrexate and cause an increase in free drug.
4. Oral anticoagulants, e.g., warfarin, may be potentiated by methotrexate; therefore prothrombin times should be followed carefully.
5. In patients with renal insufficiency it may be necessary to markedly reduce the dose or discontinue methotrexate therapy.
6. Do not give if patient has an effusion, because of "reservoir" effect.

Toxicity.
1. *Myelosuppression.* Occurs regularly, with nadir at 6–10 days after a single i.v. dose. Recovery is rapid.
2. *Nausea and vomiting.* Occasional at standard doses.
3. *Mucocutaneous effects.*
   a. Mild stomatitis is common and a sign that a maximum tolerated dose has been reached. Higher doses may result in confluent or hemorrhagic stomal ulcers and bloody diarrhea.
   b. Erythematous rashes, urticaria, and skin pigment changes are uncommon.
   c. Mild alopecia is frequent.
4. *Miscellaneous effects.*
   a. Acute hepatocellular injury is uncommon at standard doses.
   b. Hepatic fibrosis is uncommon but seen at low chronic doses.
   c. Pneumonitis is rare.
   d. Polyserositis is rare.
   e. Renal tubular necrosis is rare at standard doses.
   f. Convulsions and a Guillain-Barré-like syndrome following intrathecal therapy are uncommon.

MITOMYCIN

Other names. Mitomycin C, Mutamycin.
Mechanism of action. Alkylation and cross-linking by mitomycin metabolites interfere with structure and function of DNA.
Primary indications. Bladder (intravesical), esophagus, stomach, anal, and pancreas carcinomas.
Usual dosage and schedule.
1. 20 mg/m^2 i.v. on day 1 every 4–6 weeks *or*
2. 2 mg/m^2 i.v. on days 1–5 and 8–12 every 4–6 weeks.
3. 10 mg/m^2 i.v. on day 1 every 8 weeks in combination with fluorouracil and doxorubicin for stomach and pancreatic carcinomas.
4. 30–40 mg instilled into the bladder weekly for 4–8 weeks, then monthly for 6 months.

Special precaution. Administer as slow push or rapid infusion through the sidearm of a rapidly running i.v. infusion, taking care to avoid extravasation.
Toxicity.
1. *Myelosuppression.* Serious, cumulative, and dose-limiting. Nadir is reached usually by 4 weeks but may be delayed. Re-

covery is often prolonged over many weeks, and occasionally cytopenia never disappears.
2. *Nausea and vomiting.* Common at higher doses, but severity is usually mild to moderate.
3. *Mucocutaneous effects.*
    a. Stomatitis and alopecia are common.
    b. Cellulitis at injection site if extravasation occurs is common.
4. *Miscellaneous effects.*
    a. Renal toxicity is uncommon.
    b. Pulmonary toxicity is uncommon but may be severe.
    c. Fever is uncommon.
    d. Secondary neoplasia is possible.
    e. Hemolytic-uremic syndrome.

MITOTANE

Other names. *o,p′*-DDD, Lysodren.
Mechanism of action. Suppresses adrenal steroid production, modifies peripheral steroid metabolism, and is cytotoxic to adrenal cortical cells.
Primary indication. Adrenocortical carcinoma.
Usual dosage and schedule. Begin with 2–6 gm PO daily in 3 or 4 divided doses and build to a maximum tolerated daily dose that is usually 8–10 gm, although it may range from 2 to 16 gm. Glucocorticoid and mineralocorticoid replacements during mitotane therapy are necessary to prevent hypoadrenalism. Cortisone acetate (25 mg PO in the a.m. and 12.5 mg PO in the p.m.) and fludrocortisone acetate (0.1 mg PO in the a.m.) are recommended.
Special precautions. Patients who experience severe trauma, infection, or shock should be treated with supplemental corticosteroids. Because of the effect of mitotane on peripheral steroid metabolism, larger than usual replacement doses may be necessary.
Toxicity.
1. *Myelosuppression.* None.
2. *Nausea and vomiting.* Common and may be dose-limiting.
3. *Mucocutaneous effects.* Skin rash occurs occasionally.
4. *CNS effects.* Lethargy, sedation, vertigo, or dizziness in up to 40% of patients; may be dose-limiting.
5. *Miscellaneous effects.* Albuminuria, hemorrhagic cystitis, hypertension, orthostatic hypotension, and visual disturbances are uncommon.

MITOXANTRONE

Other names. Novantrone, dihydroxyanthracenedione, DHAD, DHAQ.
Mechanism of action. DNA strand breakage mediated by anthracenedione effects on topoisomerase II.
Primary indications.
1. Acute nonlymphocytic leukemia.
2. Carcinoma of the breast or ovary.
3. Non-Hodgkin's and Hodgkin's lymphoma.
Usual dosage and schedule.
1. 12–14 mg/m² i.v. as a 5- to 30-minute infusion once every 3 weeks for solid tumors.

2. 12 mg/m^2 i.v. as a 5- to 30-minute infusion daily for 3 days for acute nonlymphocytic leukemia.

Special precautions. Rarely causes extravasation injury if infiltrated. Cardiotoxicity probably less than with doxorubicin; but prior anthracycline, chest irradiation, or underlying cardiac disease increases the risk.

Toxicity.

1. *Myelosuppression.* Universal.
2. *Nausea and vomiting.* Common but less frequent and less severe than with doxorubicin.
3. *Mucocutaneous effects.* Alopecia is common, but its frequency and severity is less than with doxorubicin. Mucositis is occasional.
4. *Cardiac toxicity.* Probably less than with doxorubicin; there is no clear maximum dose, though the risk appears to increase at 125 mg/m^2 cumulative dose.
5. *Miscellaneous effects.*
   a. Local—erythema and swelling with transient blue discoloration if extravasated, but rarely leads to severe skin damage.
   b. Diarrhea is uncommon.
   c. Green or blue discoloration of urine.
   d. Phlebitis is uncommon.

NILUTAMIDE

Other name. Nilandron.

Mechanism of action. Competitive inhibitor of androgens at the cellular androgen receptor in prostate cancer cells. Complements surgical castration.

Primary indications. Metastatic carcinoma of the prostate, in combination with surgical castration.

Usual dosage and schedule. 300 mg p.o. once daily for 30 days, followed by 150 mg once daily thereafter.

Special precautions. Should be restricted to patients with normal liver function test values. A routine chest radiograph should be obtained before therapy and any time that the patient reports new exertional dyspnea or worsening of preexisting dyspnea.

Toxicity.

1. *Myelosuppression.* None.
2. *Nausea and vomiting.* Occasional.
3. *Mucocutaneous effects.* Rash, dry skin, and sweating are uncommon.
4. *Miscellaneous effects.*
   a. Hepatitis is rare (1%).
   b. Interstitial pneumonitis with dyspnea is uncommon (2%). May be higher in patients with Asian ancestry.
   c. Inhibits activity of liver cytochrome P450 isoenzymes and may delay elimination of drugs such as warfarin, phenytoin, and theophylline.
   d. Constipation is uncommon.
   e. Hot flashes are common.
   f. Increased liver function test values are uncommon.
   g. Impaired adaptation to dark is common.

OCTREOTIDE

Other name. Sandostatin.

Mechanism of action. Somatostatin analog that inhibits release of polypeptide hormones, particularly in the pancreas and gut. Slows gastrointestinal transit time. Promotes water and electrolyte absorption, reflecting change from overall secretory to absorptive state.

Primary indications.
1. Carcinoid tumors.
2. Vasoactive intestinal peptide tumors and other amine precursor uptake and decarboxylation tumors.
3. Chemotherapy-induced diarrhea.
4. Acromegaly.

Usual dosage and schedule. 100 to 1,500 µg/day s.c., in two to four divided doses. Doses are usually started at the lower end and titrated upward to the best symptomatic improvement.

Special precautions. Lower doses indicated if severe renal dysfunction (creatinine > 5 mg/dL).

Toxicity.
1. *Myelosuppression.* None.
2. *Nausea and vomiting.* Occasional.
3. *Mucocutaneous effects.* Local site reactions are occasional; other effects are rare.
4. *Endocrine effects.* Hypoglycemia or hyperglycemia is uncommon; hypothalamic pituitary dysfunction is rare.
5. *Other gastrointestinal effects,* including diarrhea, loose stools, or bloating are occasional.
6. *Development of gallstones* is uncommon to common, depending on duration of therapy: incidence is less than 2% if treatment is for 1 month or less; incidence is about 25% if treatment is for 1 year or more.
7. *Bradycardia* and other conduction abnormalities occur in up to 25% of patients with acromegaly who are treated with octreotide.

OPRELVEKIN

Other names. Neumega, Interleukin-11, IL-11.

Mechanism of action. Stimulates proliferation of hematopoietic stem cells and megakaryocyte progenitor cells and induces megakaryocyte maturation, resulting in increased platelet production.

Primary indications. Prevention of severe thrombocytopenia after chemotherapy in patients with nonmyeloid malignancies.

Usual dosage and schedule. 50 µg/kg once daily, starting 6 to 24 hours after completion of chemotherapy. Continue until the postnadir count is ≥50,000 µL. (Treatment for more than 21 days in a row is not recommended.) Next planned cycle of chemotherapy should begin at least 2 days after discontinuation of oprelvekin.

Special precautions. Use with caution in patients with history of trial arrhythmia.

Toxicity.
1. *Myelosuppression.* None. Mild decrease in hemoglobin concentration, predominantly due to increase in plasma volume.
2. *Nausea and vomiting.* None.

3. *Mucocutaneous effects*. Occasional rash, particularly at injection site.
4. *Miscellaneous effects*.
   a. Cardiovascular.
      (1) Atrial arrhythmia (transient) and palpitations is occasional.
      (2) Syncope is occasional. (No anaphylactoid reactions have been observed.)
      (3) Fluid retention with edema or dyspnea on exertion is common, but usually mild to moderate. Not associated with capillary leak syndrome.
   b. Conjunctival injection and mild visual blurring is occasional.

PACLITAXEL

Other name. Taxol.

Mechanism of action. Enhanced formation and stabilization of microtubules. Antineoplastic effect may result from nonfunctional tubules or altered tubulin—microtubule equilibrium. Mitotic arrest is seen and is associated with accumulated polymerized microtubules.

Primary indications.
1. Carcinomas of the ovary, breast, lung, head and neck, bladder, and cervix.
2. Melanoma.
3. Kaposi's sarcoma, acquired immunodeficiency syndrome (AIDS) related.

Usual dosage and schedule.
1. 135 to 225 mg/m² as a 3-hour infusion every 3 weeks.
2. 135 to 200 mg/m² as a 24-hour infusion every 3 weeks.
3. 100 mg/m² as a 3-hour infusion every 2 weeks for the treatment of AIDS-related Kaposi's sarcoma.
4. 80 to 100 mg/m² as a 1-hour weekly infusion.
5. 200 mg/m² as a 1-hour infusion every 3 weeks.

Special precautions. Anaphylactoid reactions with dyspnea, hypotension (or occasionally hypertension), bronchospasm, urticaria, and erythematous rashes may occur as a result of the paclitaxel itself or the Cremophor vehicle required to make paclitaxel water soluble. Such reaction is minimized but not totally prevented by pretreatment with antihistamines and corticosteroids and by prolonging the infusion rate (to 24 hours). Paclitaxel must be filtered with a 0.2-micron in-line filter.

Standard pretreatment regimen.
1. Dexamethasone, 20 mg p.o. 12 hours and 6 hours before treatment. Alternative is dexamethasone, 20 mg i.v. 30 to 60 minutes prior to treatment.
2. Cimetidine, 300 mg i.v. 30 to 60 minutes before treatment (or other histamine H_2-receptor antagonist).
3. Diphenhydramine, 50 mg i.v. 30 to 60 minutes before treatment.

Toxicity.
1. *Myelosuppression.* Granulocytopenia is universal and dose limiting; thrombocytopenia is common; anemia is occasional.
2. *Nausea and vomiting.* Common but usually not severe.

3. *Mucocutaneous effects.* Alopecia is universal; mucositis is occasional at recommended doses.
4. *Hypersensitivity reactions.* Dyspnea, hypotension (or occasionally hypertension), bronchospasm, urticaria, and erythematous rashes are occasionally seen, despite precautions.
5. *Miscellaneous effects.*
    a. Sensory neuropathy is common (30% to 35%).
    b. Hepatic dysfunction is uncommon.
    c. Diarrhea is occasional and mild.
    d. Myalgias and arthralgias are common (25%).
    e. Seizures are rare.
    f. Abnormal electrocardiogram is occasional. If clinically significant bradycardia, stop drug. Restart at slower rate when stable.

PAMIDRONATE

Other name. Aredia.
Mechanism of action. A second-generation bisphosphonate that inhibits resorption of bone. May inhibit osteoclast activity.
Primary indications.
1. Hypercalcemia associated with malignancy.
2. Osteolytic bone metastases of breast cancer.
3. Osteolytic and osteoporotic bone lesions of multiple myeloma.
Usual dosage and schedule.
1. Multiple myeloma: 90 mg i.v. as a 4-hour infusion every month.
2. Breast cancer: 90 mg i.v. as a 2-hour infusion every 3 to 4 weeks.
3. Hypercalcemia of malignancy: 60 to 90 mg i.v. as a 4- to 24-hour infusion. May be repeated every 1 to 8 weeks, as needed.
Special precautions. Potential for renal tubular damage, particularly if infused more rapidly.
Toxicity.
1. *Myelosuppression.* None.
2. *Nausea and vomiting.* Occasional nausea and anorexia.
3. *Mucocutaneous effects.* Occasional infusion site reaction.
4. *Miscellaneous effects.*
    a. Fatigue is occasional.
    b. Laboratory abnormalities are occasional (hypocalcemia, hypokalemia, hypomagnesemia, and hypophosphatemia, particularly at the 90-mg dose).

PENTOSTATIN

Other names. 2'-Deoxycoformycin, Nipent.
Mechanism of action. Inhibition of adenosine deaminase, increase in deoxyadenosine triphosphates, inhibition of methylation reactions.
Primary indications. Hairy-cell leukemia, chronic lymphocytic leukemia, other lymphoid neoplasms, mycosis fungoides.
Usual dosage and schedule. 4 mg/m^2 i.v. push over 1–2 minutes, after hydration with 1 liter of 5% dextrose with 0.5 N saline or equivalent before pentostatin administration and 500 ml after the drug is given. Repeat every 2 weeks. Higher doses with treat-

ment for 1–3 days may be used in chronic lymphocytic leukemia and other lymphoid neoplasms.

Special precautions. Hydration required to ensure urine output of 2 liters daily on the day pentostatin is administered. Patients often are hospitalized for their first drug administration. Allopurinol 300 mg bid is recommended in patients with a large tumor mass. Sedative and hypnotic drugs should be used with caution or not at all because CNS toxicity may be potentiated. Dose reduction or discontinuation needed for renal impairment (creatinine clearance <50 ml/minute).

Toxicity.
1. *Myelosuppression.* Common but severity variable.
2. *Nausea and vomiting.* Common but usually not severe.
3. *Mucocutaneous effects.* Mucositis is rare; skin rashes are occasional to common.
4. *Miscellaneous effects.*
   a. Anorexia is common.
   b. Hepatic dysfunction is occasional.
   c. Diarrhea is uncommon.
   d. Chills and fever are common.
   e. Renal insufficiency is rare at usual doses.
   f. Neuropsychiatric effects. High doses may cause serious neurologic and psychiatric symptoms, including seizures, mental confusion, irritability, and coma.
   g. Cough or other respiratory problems are occasional.
   h. Infections, probably related both to myelosuppression and lymphocytopenia.

PLICAMYCIN

Other names. Mithramycin, Mithracin.
Mechanism of action. Binds to DNA and inhibits DNA-dependent RNA synthesis.
Primary indications.
1. Severe refractory hypercalcemia.
2. Rarely used as antineoplastic agent.
Usual dosage and schedule. 0.6–1.0 mg/m^2 i.v. for 1–3 days, with doses repeated if necessary and tolerated.
Special precautions.
1. Administer as i.v. infusion over 0.5–3.0 hours to reduce severity of gastrointestinal toxicity.
2. Avoid subcutaneous extravasation.
3. Monitor platelet count, prothrombin time, partial thromboplastin time, LDH, SGOT, and blood urea nitrogen (BUN). Discontinue drug if significant abnormality occurs.
Toxicity. High doses, which were used in the past for testicular carcinoma, had severe myelo- and hepatotoxicity.
1. *Myelosuppression.* Dose-related thrombocytopenia is common but usually not severe at doses used for hypercalcemia; leukopenia is not usually significant.
2. *Nausea and vomiting.* Common.
3. *Mucocutaneous effects.*
   a. Blushing of the face followed by a coarsening of skin folds, hyperpigmentation, and possible desquamation is occasional with alternate-day therapy.

b. Stomatitis is common.
c. Papular skin rash is uncommon.
d. Alopecia is uncommon.
4. *Hepatic effects.* Coagulopathy due to clotting factor abnormalities and thrombocytopenia occurs occasionally and may be fatal. Prothrombin time, partial thromboplastin time, SGOT, and LDH must be monitored during therapy.
5. *Miscellaneous effects.*
    a. Diarrhea is common.
    b. CNS toxicity manifested by headache, irritability, and lethargy are dose-dependent.
    c. Phlebitis is uncommon.
    d. Renal effects in more than one-half of patients; some have some abnormality with proteinuria and mild azotemia.
    e. Electrolyte abnormalities (depression of serum calcium, phosphorus, and potassium) are common.

PORFIMER

Other name. Photofrin.
Mechanism of action. Photosensitizing agent. Cellular damage occurs as a result of light-induced radical reactions, including superoxide and hydroxyl radicals.
Primary indications. Obstructing esophageal cancers.
Usual dosage and schedule. 2 mg/kg as a slow i.v. injection over 3 to 5 minutes. This is followed by illumination with laser light 40–50 hours following injection of porfimer. A second course may be given after a minimum of 30 days.
Special precautions. Contraindicated in patients with porphyria, tracheoesophageal or bronchoesophageal fistulas. Contraindicated if tumor is eroding into a major blood vessel. Patients must avoid exposure of skin and eyes to direct sunlight or bright indoor light for 30 days to minimize severe photosensitivity reactions. Sunscreens are of no value.
Toxicity.
1. *Myelosuppression.* None.
2. *Nausea and vomiting.* Occasional to common.
3. *Mucocutaneous effects.* Photosensitivity reaction is occasional to common, particularly if extravasates at injection site. See special precautions above.
4. *Miscellaneous effects.*
    a. Cardiovascular. Atrial fibrillation is occasional. Hypertension, hypotension, or tachycardia is occasional.
    b. Respiratory. Occasional cough, dyspnea, pleural effusion, pneumonia, and respiratory insufficiency have been seen.
    c. Ocular discomfort may be seen, particularly from bright light.
    d. Other gastrointestinal effects, including abdominal pain and constipation, are occasional.
    e. Psychiatric: anxiety, anorexia, confusion, and insomnia are occasional.
    f. Other: occasional asthenia, back pain, chest pain, or other pain. (Chest pain is probably from inflammatory response within area of treatment.)

PROCARBAZINE

Other name. Matulane.

Mechanism of action. Uncertain but appears to affect pre-formed DNA, RNA, and protein.

Primary indications. Hodgkin's and non-Hodgkin's lymphomas.

Usual dosage and schedule. 100 mg/m^2 PO daily for 7–14 days every 4 weeks (in combination with other drugs).

Special precautions. Many food and drug interactions are possible, although their clinical significance may be low.

Drug or food	Possible result
Ethanol	Disulfiram-like reactions: nausea, vomiting, visual disturbances, headache
Sympathomimetics, tricyclic antidepressants, tyramine-rich foods (cheese, wine, bananas)	Hypertensive crisis, tremors, excitation, angina, cardiac palpitations
CNS depressants	Additive depression

Toxicity.

1. *Myelosuppression.* Pancytopenia is dose-limiting. Recovery may be delayed.
2. *Nausea and vomiting.* Frequent during first few days until tolerance develops.
3. *Mucocutaneous effects.*
   a. Stomatitis and diarrhea are uncommon.
   b. Alopecia, pruritus, and drug rash are uncommon.
4. *CNS effects.* Paresthesias, neuropathies, headache, dizziness, depression, apprehension, nervousness, insomnia, nightmares, hallucinations, ataxia, confusion, convulsions, and coma have been reported with varying frequency.
5. *Miscellaneous effects.*
   a. Secondary neoplasia is possible.
   b. Visual disturbances are rare.
   c. Postural hypotension is rare.
   d. Hypersensitivity reactions are rare.
   e. Teratogenesis is strong potential.

PROGESTINS

Other names. Medroxyprogesterone acetate (Provera, Depo-Provera), hydroxyprogesterone caproate (Delalutin), megestrol acetate (Megace).

Mechanism of action. Mechanism of antitumor effects is not clear.

Primary indications. Endometrial and breast carcinomas.

Usual dosage and schedule.

1. Medroxyprogesterone acetate 1000–1500 mg IM weekly or 400–800 mg PO twice weekly.
2. Hydroxyprogesterone caproate 1000–1500 mg IM weekly.
3. Megestrol acetate 80–320 mg PO daily.

Special precautions.

1. Acute local hypersensitivity or dyspnea due to oil in IM preparations is uncommon.
2. Hypercalcemia with initial therapy is occasional.

Toxicity.
1. *Myelosuppression.* None.
2. *Nausea and vomiting.* Rare.
3. *Mucocutaneous effects.* Mild alopecia or skin rash are uncommon.
4. *Miscellaneous effects.*
   a. Mild fluid retention is occasional to common.
   b. Mild liver function abnormalities is occasional; intrahepatic cholestasis may occur.
   c. Menstrual irregularities are common.
   d. Improved appetite, weight gain are common.

RALOXIFENE

Other name. Evista.
Mechanism of action. A selective estrogen receptor modulator that inhibits estrogen effects by competing with estrogen for binding on the cytosol estrogen receptor protein in normal and cancer cells. The receptor—hormone complex ultimately controls the promoter region of genes that affect cell growth. Effects may manifest as estrogen agonistic or antagonistic, depending on the tissue and other modifying factors. Has estrogen-like effects on bone, increasing bone mineral density.
Primary indications.
1. Prevention of osteoporosis in postmenopausal women.
2. Breast cancer prevention in postmenopausal women.
Usual dosage and schedule. 60 mg p.o. daily.
Special precautions. Not recommended as primary cancer preventive agent for most women except under auspices of a controlled clinical trial. May cause fetal harm if administered to a woman. Has not been adequately studied in women with prior history of breast cancer.
Toxicity.
1. *Myelosuppression.* Uncommon and mild.
2. *Nausea and vomiting.* Uncommon.
3. *Mucocutaneous effects.* Rash, sweating, and vaginitis are uncommon.
4. *Miscellaneous effects.*
   a. Thromboembolic events, including deep vein thrombosis, pulmonary embolism, and retinal vein thrombosis, are rare.
   b. Leg cramps are uncommon.
   c. Hot flashes are common.
   d. Lowers total cholesterol and low-density lipoprotein cholesterol.
5. *Carcinogenesis.* No apparent increase in endometrial cancer for up to 39 months.

RALTITREXED

Other name. Tomudex.
Mechanism of action. Raltitrexed is a quinazoline antifolate that is a direct specific inhibitor of thymidylate synthase and thus blocks the conversion of uridylate to thymidylate and consequent DNA synthesis.
Primary indications. Colorectal carcinoma.

Usual dosage and schedule. 3 mg/m^2 i.v. over 15 minutes every 3 weeks.
Special precautions. None.
Toxicity.
1. *Myelosuppression.* Common, but only occasionally severe.
2. *Nausea and vomiting.* Occasional.
3. *Mucocutaneous effects.* Mucositis is occasional and rarely severe.
4. *Miscellaneous effects.*
   a. Diarrhea is occasional.
   b. Elevation of liver transaminase levels is occasional.

RITUXIMAB

Other name. Rituxan.
Mechanism of action. Rituximab is a genetically engineered chimeric (murine and human) monoclonal antibody directed against the CD20 antigen found on the surface of normal cells and in high copy number on malignant B lymphocytes (but not stem cells). The Fab domain of rituximab binds to the CD20 antigen on B lymphocytes and B-cell non-Hodgkin's lymphomas, and the Fc domain recruits immune effector functions to mediate B-cell lysis.
Primary indications. Non-Hodgkin's B-cell lymphoma that is low grade or follicular, CD20 positive, and refractory to conventional therapy.
Usual dosage and schedule. 375 mg/m^2 given as a slow i.v. infusion, initially at a rate of 50 mg/h. If hypersensitivity or other infusion-related events do not occur, escalate in 50 mg/h increments to a maximum of 400 mg/h. Usually takes 4 to 6 hours. Interrupt or slow the infusion rate for infusion-related events. Repeat the dose once weekly for four doses. Premedication with acetaminophen and diphenhydramine may attenuate infusion-related symptoms. Corticosteroids should not be used.
Special precautions. An infusion-related set of symptoms, consisting of fever and chills, with or without true rigors, occurs in most patients during the first infusion. Other hypersensitivity symptoms, including nausea, urticaria, fatigue, headache, pruritus, bronchospasm, dyspnea, sensation of tongue or throat swelling, rhinitis, vomiting, hypotension, flushing, and pain at disease sites, may also be seen. Rarely (< 1 per 1,000 patients) do infusion related events result in a fatal outcome. Hypersensitivity reactions occur within 30 to 120 minutes of starting the infusion and resolve with slowing or interruption of the infusion and with supportive care, including i.v. saline, diphenhydramine, and acetaminophen. The rate of infusion events decreases from 80% during the first infusion to 40% during subsequent infusions.
Toxicity.
1. *Myelosuppression.* Uncommon. However, B-cell depletion occurs in 70% to 80% of patients, with decreased immunoglobulins in a minority of patients. The incidence of infections does not appear to be increased.
2. *Nausea and vomiting.* Occasional, rarely severe.
3. *Mucocutaneous effects.* Pruritus, rash, and urticaria are occasional.
4. *Miscellaneous effects.*

a. Infusion-related hypersensitivity reaction is very common but usually resolves with interrupting or slowing the rate of the infusion and administration of supportive therapy; see special precautions above.
b. Myalgia or dizziness is occasional.
c. Hypotension is occasional but rarely severe.
d. Chest pain, bronchospasm, tachycardia, edema, and postural hypotension are uncommon.
e. Severe angioedema, arrhythmia, and angina are rare.

SARGRAMOSTIM

Other names. Granulocyte-macrophage colony-stimulating factor, GM-CSF, Leukine.
Mechanism of action. Promotes growth and differentiation of myeloid progenitor cells. May improve survival and function of granulocytes, eosinophils, monocytes, and macrophages. Induces release of secondary cytokines (interleukin-1 and tumor necrosis factor).
Primary indications.
1. Acceleration of myeloid recovery and shortening of granulocytopenia secondary to intensive chemotherapy followed by autologous bone marrow transplantation.
2. Granulocytopenia from primary marrow disorders, such as myelodysplastic syndrome or aplastic anemia.
3. Granulocytopenia associated with AIDS and its therapy.
Usual dosage and schedule.
1. *Myeloid reconstitution after autologous bone marrow transplantation:* 250 µg/m^2 i.v. daily as a 2-hour infusion beginning 2–4 hours after the autologous bone marrow infusion and not less than 24 hours after the last dose of chemotherapy or less than 12 hours after the last dose of radiotherapy. Continue for 21 days or until the absolute neutrophil count reaches 20,000/µL.
2. *Bone marrow transplantation failure or engraftment delay:* 250 µg/m^2 daily for 14 days as 2-hour i.v. infusion. If no marrow recovery, may be repeated in 7 days at same or higher dose (500 µg/m^2). Dose and duration are dependent on the response.
3. *Aplastic anemia, myelodysplastic syndrome, and AIDS:* doses may be much lower (50–100 µg/m^2 SQ or IM daily).
Special precautions. Flushing, tachycardia, dyspnea, and nausea occur commonly with the first dose of i.v. therapy; do not infuse for less than 2 hours; longer infusion may help.
Toxicity.
1. *Myelosuppression.* None (leukocytosis).
2. *Nausea and vomiting.* Occasional.
3. *Mucocutaneous effects.* Rash is uncommon; exacerbation of preexisting dermatologic conditions is occasional; mild local reactions at injection site is common.
4. *Miscellaneous effects.* Usually mild and short-lived at standard doses, but with increasing dose, may be more severe.
    a. Bone pain, musculoskeletal symptoms such as cramps, and back or leg pain are common.
    b. Pericarditis, fluid retention, and venous thrombosis are dose-related and uncommon at standard doses.

c. Flulike symptoms (fever, chills, aches, headache) are occasional at standard doses, common at higher doses.

STREPTOZOCIN

Other names. Streptozotocin, Zanosar.

Mechanism of action. Inhibition of DNA synthesis, possibly by interference with pyridine nucleotide synthesis. Streptozocin appears to have some specificity for neoplastic pancreatic endocrine cells. Glucose moiety attached to nitrosourea appears to diminish myelotoxicity.

Primary indications.
1. Pancreatic islet cell and pancreatic exocrine carcinomas.
2. Carcinoid tumors.

Usual dosage and schedule.
1. 1.0–1.5 gm/m^2 i.v. weekly for 6 weeks followed by 4 weeks of observation.
2. 500 mg/m^2 i.v. on days 1–5 every 6 weeks.

Special precautions.
1. A 30- to 60-minute infusion is recommended to reduce local pain and burning around the vein during treatment.
2. Avoid extravasation.
3. Have 50% glucose available to treat sudden hypoglycemia.

Toxicity.
1. *Myelosuppression.* Uncommon and mild.
2. *Nausea and vomiting.* Common and severe. May become progressively worse over 5-day course of therapy.
3. *Mucocutaneous effects.* Uncommon.
4. *Nephrotoxicity.* Renal toxicity is common. Although it is not clearly dose-related, it may limit continued drug use in individual patients. Proteinuria, glucosuria, azotemia, and hypophosphatemia, if persistent or severe, are indications to discontinue therapy. Hydration may ameliorate the problem.
5. *Miscellaneous effects.*
   a. Hypoglycemia: in patients with insulinoma, hypoglycemia may be severe (although transient) owing to a burst of insulin release.
   b. Hyperglycemia is uncommon in normal or diabetic patients, as normal β cells are usually insensitive to streptozocin's effect.
   c. Transient mild hepatotoxicity is occasional.
   d. Second malignancies are possible.

SURAMIN (Investigational)

Other names. Antrypol, Bayer 205, Germanin, Moranyl, Naganol, Naphuride NA.

Mechanism of action. Glycosaminoglycan agonist-antagonist that blocks the binding of growth factors to their receptors. Growth factors affected include platelet-derived growth factor, transforming growth factor-beta (TGF-β), and heparin binding growth factor-2 (also known as basic fibroblast growth factor). Inhibition of DNA polymerases and reverse transcriptase and other proteins. Inhibition of glycosaminoglycan metabolism.

Primary indications.
1. Adrenocortical carcinoma.

2. Prostate carcinoma that is hormone-refractory.
3. Lymphoma that is refractory to standard agents.

Usual dosage and schedule. 350 mg/m^2 by continuous i.v. infusion daily for 7 days after an initial test dose of 200 mg over 10 minutes. The plasma level is then measured, the infusion rate adjusted, and the treatment continued until the plasma level reaches 250–300 µg/ml. The infusion is then stopped for 2 months and the treatment cycle repeated.

Special precautions. Measurement of plasma levels is necessary to achieve the narrow concentration that is therapeutic and not prohibitively toxic. Therapy should be stopped when a steady-state drug level of 300 µg/ml is reached. Because of adrenal suppression, patients require hydrocortisone, 25 mg in the morning and 15 mg at bedtime. All patients should also receive vitamin K 10 mg SQ weekly, to reduce the likelihood of coagulopathy. Prothrombin time must be followed closely, and therapy stopped if prothrombin time exceeds 17.5 seconds.

Toxicity.
1. *Myelosuppression.* Common but usually not severe.
2. *Nausea and vomiting.* Uncommon.
3. *Mucocutaneous effects.* Transient erythematous rash is common.
4. *Adrenocortical insufficiency.* Common.
5. *Neurotoxicity.* Paresthesias are seen commonly and severe polyradiculopathy occasionally. Motor weakness may be seen following termination of therapy. The degree of toxicity appears to be related to the plasma suramin level, with acute serious reactions uncommon at plasma levels of less than 350 µg/ml.
6. *Miscellaneous effects.*
    a. Vortex keratopathy with photophobia, tearing, and blurred vision are common.
    b. Liver function abnormalities are common but reversible.
    c. Coagulopathy is common elevations of the prothrombin time, partial thromboplastin time, and thrombin time, with increased risk of spontaneous bleeding.
    d. Renal effects: proteinuria is common; decrease in creatinine clearance is occasional.
    e. Malaise, fatigue, and lethargy are common after 2–4 months of therapy.

TAMOXIFEN

Other name. Nolvadex.

Mechanism of action. Tamoxifen is a selective estrogen receptor modulator that inhibits estrogen effects by competing with estrogen for binding on the cytosol estrogen receptor protein in cancer cells. This complex is probably transported into the nucleus, where it affects nucleic acid function. It also has effects on cellular growth factors, epidermal growth factors, and TGF-α and TGF-β.

Primary indications.
1. Breast carcinoma.
    a. Metastatic tumors in postmenopausal or premenopausal women with estrogen-receptor—positive (or unknown) tumors.

b. Adjuvant therapy in women with estrogen-receptor—positive (or progesterone-receptor—positive) tumors after primary therapy. Optimal duration of therapy for most women is probably limited to 5 years.
c. Breast cancer prevention in very high risk women.
2. Melanoma, in combination with other drugs (controversial).

Usual dosage and schedule.
1. 10 mg p.o. twice daily.
2. 20 mg p.o. as single daily dose.

Special precautions. Hypercalcemia may be seen during initial therapy. Not recommended as primary cancer preventive agent for most women except under auspices of a controlled clinical trial.

Toxicity.
1. *Myelosuppression.* Uncommon and mild.
2. *Nausea and vomiting.* Occur early in the course of therapy in up to 20% of patients but abate rapidly as therapy is continued.
3. *Mucocutaneous effects.* Cataracts and other eye toxicities have been observed, but effects due to drug are uncommon. Skin rash and pruritus vulvae are uncommon. May cause increase or marked decrease in vaginal secretions and result in difficult or painful intercourse.
4. *Miscellaneous effects.*
   a. Hot flashes are common.
   b. Vaginal bleeding and menstrual irregularity are uncommon to occasional.
   c. Lassitude, headache, leg cramps, and dizziness are uncommon.
   d. Peripheral edema is occasional.
   e. Increased bone pain, tumor pain, and local disease flare (associated both with good tumor response as well as with tumor progression) are occasional.
   f. Diarrhea is occasional.
   g. Slowed progression of osteoporosis.
   h. Reduction in serum cholesterol with favorable changes in lipid profile.
   i. Thromboembolic phenomena are rare.
   j. Liver function test abnormalities are occasional.
5. *Carcinogenesis.* Uterine carcinomas are rare (two to four times the predicted incidence in adjuvant trials).

TENIPOSIDE

Other names. VM-26, Vumon.
Mechanism of action. Topoisomerase II-mediated double-strand DNA breaks. Causes cells cycle transit delay through S phase and arrest at late S/G_2.

Primary indications.
1. Acute lymphocytic leukemia.
2. Neuroblastoma.

Usual dosage and schedule.
1. 165 mg/m^2 i.v. over 30–60 minutes twice weekly for 8–9 doses (with cytarabine).
2. 250 mg/m^2 i.v. over 30–60 minutes weekly for 4–8 weeks (with vincristine and prednisone).

Special precautions.
1. Hypersensitivity reactions usually resolve with interruption of the infusion and often can be prevented with diphenhydramine and hydrocortisone pretreatment. Hypotension is alleviated by prolonging the infusion time. It is a possible vesicant.
2. See package insert for i.v. preparation and administration equipment requirements.

Toxicity.
1. *Myelosuppression.* Common and dose-limiting.
2. *Nausea and vomiting.* Common.
3. *Mucocutaneous effects.* Alopecia and mucositis are common.
4. *Miscellaneous effects.*
    a. Hepatic and renal dysfunction are rare.
    b. Hypersensitivity reactions with urticaria and flushing are occasional. Anaphylaxis is uncommon.
    c. Hypotension is related to drug infusion rate but should be seen only occasionally at the recommended dose schedules.
    d. Secondary leukemias are uncommon.
    e. Diarrhea is common.
    f. Chemical phlebitis is uncommon.

THIOGUANINE

Other names. 6-Thioguanine, 6-TG, Tabloid.

Mechanism of action. A purine antimetabolite that, when converted to the active nucleotide, substitutes for the normal guanine nucleotide in DNA synthesis. Thioguanine also inhibits purine synthesis and conversion reactions.

Primary indication. Acute nonlymphocytic leukemia.

Usual dosage and schedule.
1. *Induction:* 100 mg/m² PO twice daily on days 1–5 (with other drugs).
2. *Maintenance:* 100 mg/m² PO twice daily on days 1–5 every 4 weeks (with other drugs).

Special precautions. None (no dose reduction required for concurrent use of allopurinol).

Toxicity.
1. *Myelosuppression.* Major dose-limiting toxicity.
2. *Nausea and vomiting.* Occasional but not severe.
3. *Mucocutaneous effects.*
    a. Stomatitis and diarrhea, which may necessitate reduction of the dose, are uncommon.
    b. Drug rash is rare.
4. *Miscellaneous effects.* Hepatotoxicity is rare.

THIOTEPA

Other name. Triethylenethiophosphoramide.

Mechanism of action. Alkylating agent similar to mechlorethamine.

Primary indications.
1. Superficial papillary carcinoma of urinary bladder.
2. Malignant peritoneal, pleural, or pericardial effusions.
3. Carcinoma of breast and ovary.
4. Neoplastic meningeal infiltrates.

Usual dosage and schedule.
1. 12 mg/m^2 i.v. bolus every 3 weeks in combination with vinblastine and doxorubicin for breast cancer.
2. 30–60 mg in 40–50 ml water instilled into the bladder and retained for 1 hour. Dose is repeated weekly for 3–6 weeks, then every 3 weeks for 5 cycles.
3. 25–30 mg/m^2 in 50–100 ml saline solution as a single intracavitary injection. Dose may be repeated as tolerated by blood counts.
4. 10–15 mg intrathecally.
5. High-dose therapy using 500–1000 mg/m^2 over 3 days has been used followed by stem cell rescue (e.g., bone marrow transplantation).

Special precaution. Dose should be reduced in patients with impaired renal function, as the drug is primarily excreted in the urine.

Toxicity.
1. *Myelosuppression.* Dose-limiting. Pancytopenia and sepsis may follow intravesical or intracavitary administration. Nadir counts are reached in 1–2 weeks; recovery by 4 weeks is usual.
2. *Nausea and vomiting.* Uncommon.
3. *Mucocutaneous effects.* Uncommon. Thiotepa is *not* a vesicant. Hyperpigmentation of skin occurs at high doses.
4. *Miscellaneous effects.*
    a. Local pain, dizziness, headache, fever are uncommon.
    b. Secondary neoplasms are possible.
    c. Amenorrhea and azoospermia is common.
    d. CNS effects with high-dose therapy.

TOPOTECAN

Other name. Hycamptin.

Mechanism of action. Topotecan, a semisynthetic derivative of camptothecin, is a potent inhibitor of topoisomerase I, an enzyme essential for effective replication and transcription. It binds to the topoisomerase I—DNA cleavable complex, preventing religation after cleavage by topoisomerase I.

Primary indications.
1. Ovarian carcinoma.
2. Small cell and non-small cell carcinoma of the lung.

Usual dosage and schedule. 1.5 mg/m^2 i.v. as a 30-minute infusion daily times five every 3 weeks.

Special precautions. None.

Toxicity.
1. *Myelosuppression.* Universal and dose limiting.
2. *Nausea and vomiting.* Common, but usually mild.
3. *Mucocutaneous effects.* Alopecia is common; stomatitis is occasional but usually mild; skin rash is rare. Diarrhea is occasional.
4. *Miscellaneous effects.*
    a. Fever, headache, fatigue, and weakness are common (15% to 25%) but rarely severe.
    b. Microscopic hematuria is occasional.
    c. Other gastrointestinal symptoms, including diarrhea, constipation, and abdominal pain, occur occasionally.

d. Dyspnea occurs occasionally, but it is uncommon for it to be severe.

TOREMIFENE

Other name. Fareston.
Mechanism of action. A selective estrogen receptor modulator that inhibits estrogen effects by competing with estrogen for binding on the cytosol estrogen receptor protein in cancer cells. The receptor:hormone complex ultimately controls the promoter region of genes that affect cell growth.
Primary indications. Metastatic carcinoma of the breast in postmenopausal women with estrogen receptor positive (or unknown) tumors.
Usual dosage and schedule. 60 mg p.o. daily.
Special precautions. Uncertain whether it has any carcinogenic effect on endometrium as has been observed with tamoxifen. May result in increased prothrombin time in patients taking warfarin (Coumadin). Cytochrome P450 3A4 enzyme inhibitors, such as phenobarbital, phenytoin, and carbamazepine increase the rate of toremifene metabolism, lowering the concentration in the serum.
Toxicity.
1. *Myelosuppression.* Uncommon and mild.
2. *Nausea and vomiting.* Minimal nausea is common early in treatment; vomiting is occasional.
3. *Mucocutaneous effects.* Dry eyes, cataracts are rare. May cause an increase or decrease in vaginal secretions; which may result in difficult or painful intercourse.
4. *Miscellaneous effects.* Hot flashes are common. Sweating is occasional. Vaginal bleeding and menstrual irregularity are occasional. Hypercalcemia is uncommon.

TRASTUZUMAB

Other names. Humanized anti-Her2 antibody, Herceptin.
Mechanism of action. A recombinant humanized monoclonal antibody that targets the extracellular domain of the Her2 growth factor receptor (p185^{Her2}).
Primary indications. Carcinoma of the breast that has overexpression of Her2/neu (c-erbB-2).
Usual dosage and schedule. 4 mg/kg i.v. loading dose over 90 minutes, then 2 mg/kg i.v. over 30 minutes weekly.
Special precautions.
1. During the first infusion, and occasionally during later infusions, a systemic symptom complex similar to that seen with other human monoclonal antibodies is common. This symptom complex consists of mild to moderate chills, fever, asthenia, pain, nausea, vomiting, and headache. These symptoms are generally well managed by temporary slowing or interruption of the infusion and administration of acetaminophen and diphenhydramine.
2. Cardiac dysfunction (cardiac symptoms or an asymptomatic decrease in ejection fraction of 10% or greater) occurs in about 5% of patients treated with trastuzumab alone but in 27% of patients treated with trastuzumab plus anthracycline and in

12% of patients treated with trastuzumab plus paclitaxel. In most cases, this improves with symptomatic therapy. Severe disability or death from cardiac dysfunction occurs in about 1% of patients.

Toxicity.

1. *Myelosuppression.* Uncommon.
2. *Nausea and vomiting.* Occasional to common during first infusion.
3. *Mucocutaneous effects.* Pruritus, rash, or urticaria—frequency uncertain, but can be expected occasionally.
4. *Miscellaneous effects.*
   a. Mild to moderate chills, fever, asthenia, pain, nausea, vomiting, and headache are common, primarily during the first infusion.
   b. Cardiac dysfunction occurs in about 5% of patients treated with trastuzumab alone, but 27% of patients treated with trastuzumab plus anthracycline and in 12% of patients treated with trastuzumab plus paclitaxel. In most cases, this improves with symptomatic therapy.
   c. Chest pain, back pain, dyspnea, and cough are occasional to common.
   d. Diarrhea is occasional.

TRETINOIN

Other names. All-*trans*-retinoic acid, t-RNA, ATRA, Retin-A.

Mechanism of action. Binds to cytoplasmic retinoic acid-binding proteins and then is transported to the nucleus where it interacts with nuclear retinoic acid receptors (RARs). These then affect expression of the genes that control cell growth and differentiation. In acute promyelocytic leukemia, which characteristically has a chromosomal translocation, t(15:17), abnormal mRNA transcripts are seen for RAR-α, the gene for which is on chromosome 17.

Primary indication. Acute promyelocytic leukemia.

Usual dosage and schedule. 45 mg/m^2 PO daily (divided into 2 doses in the morning and 6 hours later) until complete remission, up to a maximum of 90 days.

Special precautions. Avoid use in pregnant women because of marked teratogenic potential. Retinoic acid syndrome (see below) may require mechanical ventilation and dexamethasone 10 mg every 12 hours at the first signs of fever with respiratory distress until resolution of the acute symptoms (often several days). Continuation of retinoid therapy is controversial.

Toxicity.

1. *Myelosuppression.* Rare.
2. *Nausea and vomiting.* Occasional and mild.
3. *Mucocutaneous effects.* Universal, particularly at doses at higher end of range. They include redness, dryness, and pruritus of the skin and mucous membranes; possible vesicle formation; peeling of the skin of the palms and soles; cheilitis; and conjunctivitis. There also may be increased skin photosensitivity (e.g., to sun) and the nails may become brittle. Alopecia is uncommon.
4. *Retinoic acid syndrome.* Leukocytosis, high fever, respiratory distress, diffuse pulmonary infiltrates, pleural or pericardial

effusions with the possibility of impaired myocardial contractility, and hypotension are occasional in patients with acute promyelocytic leukemia (15–25%) (see Chap. 23).

5. *Miscellaneous effects.*
   a. Cataracts and corneal ulcerations or opacities are uncommon.
   b. Musculoskeletal: arthralgias, bone pain, muscle aches are occasional to common; skeletal hyperostosis is common at higher doses (80 mg/m^2/day).
   c. Hypertriglyceridemia: mild to moderate elevations are common; marked elevations (>5 times normal) are uncommon; hypercholesterolemia occurs to lesser degree.
   d. Neurologic: headache is common; lethargy, fatigue, and mental depression are uncommon; pseudotumor cerebri is rare.
   e. Gastrointestinal: inflammatory bowel disease is rare.
   f. Hepatotoxicity with increased LDH, SGOT, SGPT, GGTP, alkaline phosphatase is occasional.
   g. Hyperhistaminemia with shock is rare.

TRIMETREXATE

Other name. TMQ
Mechanism of action. Inhibition of dihydrofolate reductase.
Primary indications.
1. Head and neck squamous cell cancers.
2. Lung carcinoma.
Usual dosage and schedule. 8 mg/m^2 i.v. push daily for 5 days.
Special precautions. None.
Toxicity.
1. *Myelosuppression.* Leukopenia and thrombocytopenia are common.
2. *Nausea and vomiting.* Common but mild to moderate.
3. *Mucocutaneous effects.* Mucositis and skin rash is common (15–25%).
4. *Miscellaneous effects.*
   a. Reversible nephrotoxicity is occasional.
   b. Elevated bilirubin is occasional.
   c. Fatigue is occasional.
   d. Diarrhea is uncommon.
   e. Hypersensitivity is uncommon.

VINBLASTINE

Other name. VLB, Velban, vincaleukoblastine sulfate.
Mechanism of action. Mitotic inhibition with reversible metaphase arrest due to action on microtubular and spindle contractile proteins.
Primary indications.
1. Testicular, gestational trophoblastic, kidney, and breast carcinomas.
2. Hodgkin's and non-Hodgkin's lymphomas.
Usual dosage and schedule.
1. 4–18 mg/m^2 i.v. weekly.
2. 6 mg/m^2 i.v. on days 1 and 15 in combination with doxorubicin, bleomycin, and dacarbazine for lymphomas.

3. 4.5 mg/m^2 i.v. on day 1 every 3 weeks in combination with doxorubicin and thiotepa for breast cancer.

Special precautions. Administer as a slow push, taking care to avoid extravasation.

Toxicity.

1. *Myelosuppression.* Dose-related leukopenia occurs with a nadir at 4–10 days and recovery in 7–10 days. Severe thrombocytopenia is uncommon.
2. *Nausea and vomiting.* Common but not usually severe.
3. *Mucocutaneous effects.*
    a. Extravasation may lead to severe inflammation, pain, and tissue damage. Local infiltration with 1–6 ml of hyaluronidase (150 units/ml) may help.
    b. Mild alopecia is common.
    c. Stomatitis is occasionally severe.
4. *Miscellaneous effects.*
    a. Neurotoxicity manifested by (1) constipation, adynamic ileus, and abdominal pain if very high doses are used; or (2) paresthesias, peripheral neuropathy, and jaw pain with lower doses. Neurotoxicity is less frequent with vinblastine than with vincristine.
    b. Transient hepatitis is uncommon.
    c. Depression, headache, convulsions, and orthostatic hypotension are rare.

VINCRISTINE

Other names. VCR, Oncovin.

Mechanism of action. Mitotic inhibition with reversible metaphase arrest due to drug action on microtubular and spindle contractile proteins.

Primary indications.

1. Breast carcinoma.
2. Hodgkin's and non-Hodgkin's lymphomas.
3. Acute lymphocytic leukemia.
4. Wilms' tumor, neuroblastoma, rhabdomyosarcoma, and Ewing's sarcoma of childhood.
5. Multiple myeloma.

Usual dosage and schedule.

1. 1–2 mg/m^2 (maximum 2.0–2.4 mg) i.v. weekly.
2. 0.4 mg/day as a continuous i.v. infusion on days 1–4.

Special precautions.

1. Administer as a slow i.v. push, taking care to avoid extravasation.
2. Because neurotoxicity is cumulative, neurologic evaluation should be done before each dose and therapy withheld if severe paresthesias, motor weakness, or other severe abnormalities occur. Underlying neurologic problems accentuate vincristine's effect.
3. Reduce dose if liver disease is significant.
4. Stool softeners or high-fiber or bulk diets may avert severe constipation.

Toxicity.

1. *Myelosuppression.* Mild and rarely of clinical significance.
2. *Nausea and vomiting.* Not seen unless paralytic ileus occurs.

3. *Mucocutaneous effects.* Severe local inflammation if extravasation occurs. Alopecia is common.
4. *Neurotoxicity.* Dose-dependent and dose-limiting. Mild paresthesias and decreased deep tendon reflexes are to be expected. More extensive peripheral neuropathies, severe constipation, or ileus are indications to reduce or hold therapy. Autonomic dysfunction with orthostatic hypotension or urinary retention may be seen.
5. *Miscellaneous effects.*
   a. Uric acid nephropathy due to rapid tumor cell lysis and release of uric acid is always a potential problem when therapy is first given.
   b. Syndrome of inappropriate antidiuretic hormone is rare.
   c. Jaw pain is uncommon.

VINDESINE (Investigational)

Other name. VDS.
Mechanism of action. Mitotic inhibition with reversible metaphase arrest due to action on microtubule and spindle contractile protein.
Primary indications.
1. Lung, breast, and esophageal carcinomas.
2. Hodgkin's and non-Hodgkin's lymphomas.
3. Melanoma.
Usual dosage and schedule. 2–3 mg/m^2 i.v. bolus (2–3 minutes) weekly for induction, then every 2 weeks.
Special precautions. Take care to avoid extravasation.
Toxicity.
1. *Myelosuppression.* Leukopenia is common but not usually severe.
2. *Nausea and vomiting.* Occasional.
3. *Mucocutaneous effects.* Alopecia is common.
4. *Neurotoxicity.* Dose-dependent and cumulative, consisting in constipation, paralytic ileus, paresthesia, myalgias, and weakness. Severity is intermediate between vincristine and vinblastine.
5. *Miscellaneous effects.*
   a. Chills and fever are occasional.
   b. Phlebitis is occasional.
   c. Confusion and lethargy are rare.

VINORELBINE

Other name. Navelbine.
Mechanism of action. Binds to tubulin, depolymerizes microtubules causing mitotic inhibition, similar to other vinca alkaloids. Lower affinity for axonal microtubules associated with lower neurotoxicity.
Primary indications.
1. Non–small cell carcinoma of the lung.
2. Metastatic carcinoma of the breast.
Usual dosage and schedule.
1. 30 mg/m^2 i.v. as a 6- to 10-minute rapid infusion weekly when used with a single agent or with cisplatin.
2. 20 to 25 mg/m^2 i.v. as a 6- to 10-minute rapid infusion in various schedules, when used with other myelotoxic agents.

Special precautions. Administer infusion through the side arm of a freely flowing i.v., taking care to avoid extravasation. Reduce dose by 50% for serum bilirubin levels of 2.1 to 3 mg/dL; by 75% for bilirubin levels of more than 3 mg/dL.
Toxicity.
1. *Myelosuppression.* Granulocytopenia is common and dose limiting, with nadir at 7 to 10 days. Thrombocytopenia is uncommon. Anemia is occasional to common.
2. *Nausea and vomiting.* Common, but usually mild to moderate.
3. *Mucocutaneous effects.* Alopecia, mild diarrhea, and stomatitis are occasional. Severe local inflammation can occur with extravasation.
4. *Miscellaneous effects.*
   a. Neurotoxicity: cumulative but reversible constipation and decreased deep tendon reflexes are occasional; paresthesias are uncommon.
   b. Erythema, pain, and skin discoloration at injection site are common; phlebitis at injection site is occasional.
   c. Diarrhea occurs occasionally.

SELECTED READINGS

Chabner BA, Collins JM. *Cancer chemotherapy: principles and practice.* Philadelphia: JB Lippincott Co, 1990;545.

Dorr RT, Van Hoff DD, eds. *Cancer chemotherapy handbook.* Norwalk CT: Appleton & Lange, 1994;1020.

Perry MC, ed. *The chemotherapy source book.* Baltimore: Williams & Wilkins, 1996;1518.

Tannock IF, Hill RP, eds. *The basic science of oncology.* New York: McGraw-Hill, 1998;539.

USP DI oncology drug information. United States Pharmacopeial Convention, Inc. Distributed by Association of Community Cancer Centers, Rockville, MD 1998;517.

High-dose Chemotherapy with Hematopoietic Progenitor Cell and Cytokine Support

David H. Vesole

The first trials of high-dose therapy with hematopoietic stem cell transplantation were initiated in the early to middle 1970s. During the course of the past 25 years, the number of transplantations performed has grown exponentially. According to the International Bone Marrow Transplant Registry (IBMTR), more than 400 institutions worldwide are known to have active transplantation programs, performing more than 25,000 transplantations yearly at an estimated cost of more than $2 billion. In North America, more than 200 transplantation centers perform in excess of 15,000 transplantations yearly; about 70% of all these procedures are autologous. Breast cancer is the most common indication for autologous transplantation: nearly 5,000 transplantations (one third) are performed each year for this indication. With improved supportive care and decreasing costs, the indications for transplantation continue to increase. Select patients can receive high-dose therapy with hematopoietic stem cell transplantation completely as outpatients.

Clinical trials during the past 25 years have demonstrated that high-dose chemotherapy with or without the addition of radiation therapy can result in improved response and overall survival rates for patients with various malignant and nonmalignant diseases. High-dose chemotherapy enables the clinician to exploit the steep dose-response curves observed with many chemotherapeutic agents. The line representing log kill of malignant cells remains linear or slightly curvilinear for many chemotherapeutic agents, particularly for the alkylating agents. Most of the alkylating agents can be dose escalated 4- to 10-fold; some alkylators, such as thiotepa, can be escalated 30-fold when supported with hematopoietic stem cell transplantation. Most nonalkylating agents cannot be dose escalated more than 2-fold; some exceptions include cytarabine (cytosine arabinoside, ara-C), etoposide, mitoxantrone, and paclitaxel (Taxol). Improved supportive modalities, including antibiotics, antiemetics, and hematopoietic cytokines, and the availability of a variety of blood products have improved the safety of high-dose therapy. However, hematopoietic stem cells derived from bone marrow, peripheral blood, or cord blood or by newer *ex vivo* expansion technologies are required to rescue the patient from myeloablative therapy. Thus, the clinician can continue to escalate the doses of chemotherapy or radiation therapy beyond marrow toxicity to the next level of toxicity, the nonhematologic dose-limiting toxicity.

Although dose escalation is possible with hematopoietic stem cell rescue, not all malignancies can be cured with this treatment modality. In some diseases, the doses necessary to achieve complete tumor cell kill exceed the nonmarrow lethal doses of chemotherapy or radiation therapy. In other malignancies, dose escalation beyond the marrow lethal dose results in only modest increases in cell kill. Metastatic melanoma, non–small cell lung cancer, and colon cancer are examples of malignancies that high-dose therapy with hematopoietic stem cell rescue cannot cure.

Even with dose intensification, many patients ultimately suffer disease relapse, which probably results from either failure to eradicate residual tumor cells or, in the case of autotransplantation, the reinfusion of hematopoietic stem cells containing contaminating tumor cells. Using molecular techniques, the latter has been proved to be the case in some hematologic diseases, such as acute myelogenous leukemia (AML). In autologous transplant, which is the predominant modality, newer strategies are being developed to improve outcomes using posttransplantation immunotherapeutic approaches to eradicate minimal residual disease and to decrease potential tumor cell contamination by either positive (stem cell selection) or negative (purging) techniques. These approaches are discussed later.

Allogeneic transplantation provides a source of hematopoietic stem cells that is devoid of contaminating tumor cells. Growing clinical experience supports an immunotherapeutic (graft-versus-tumor) effect of the donor immune system to eradicate minimal residual disease after transplant. This immunoreactivity can be exploited at the time of disease relapse by donor lymphocyte infusions, inducing complete remission in many hematologic malignancies. Unfortunately, transplant-related morbidity and mortality remain problematic because of graft-versus-host disease (GVHD) and prolonged immunosuppression.

I. **Rationale.** The cytocidal effect of chemotherapy in cell culture and animal models follows first-order kinetics. Each treatment kills a set fraction of cancer cells, irrespective of the starting number. The degree of kill in these experimental systems is dose dependent: tumor cell viability decreases in a logarithmic manner, with a linear increase in drug dose. A modest escalation in the dose may result in a much higher fractional kill of tumor cells. Sublethal chemotherapy selects for and encourages development of resistant cells. The use of several chemotherapeutic agents in combination with different mechanisms of action inhibits the development of resistance. In addition, combinations of agents selected for nonoverlapping extramedullary dose-limiting toxicities should be used in maximal doses. Thus, the optimal approach uses the highest possible doses of non–cross-resistant agents with steep dose-response curves as early as possible in the patient's disease course to achieve the highest tumor cell kill and reduce the development of drug resistance. Eradication of tumor (cure) usually requires an 8- to 12-log kill of cancer cells. A complete clinical remission can be obtained with as little as a 4-log cell kill and a partial remission (50% tumor cytoreduction) with as little as a 1- or 2-log kill. Complete remissions are the surrogate short-term markers of potentially successful therapy.

The dosages of many active agents are limited by myelosuppression, even with the use of hematopoietic growth factors. The use of hematopoietic stem cell support allows for increased dosage and combination therapy with agents that would normally produce an unacceptable degree of myelosuppression.

II. **Indications for high-dose therapy with hematopoietic stem cell transplantation**

   A. **Disease.** During the past 10 years, the indications for high-dose therapy and hematopoietic stem cell transplantation have changed markedly, particularly for autologous transplantation. Ten years ago, autologous transplants were performed almost exclusively for non-Hodgkin's lymphoma (NHL) and Hodgkin's disease. Currently, breast cancer is the most common indication for autologous transplant (Fig. 6-1). In addition, a growing number of transplants are being performed for other solid tumors, including ovarian cancer, germ cell cancer, and neuroblastoma. In the hematologic malignancies, transplantations for multiple myeloma are showing the most rapid rise, but the number of autologous transplants performed in patients with AML and chronic myelogenous leukemia (CML) is also increasing. Although most allogeneic transplantations continue to be performed for acute and chronic leukemias, there has been a recent increase in allogeneic transplantations for immunodeficiency disorders, inherited disorders of metabolism, and inherited erythrocyte abnormalities.

   B. **Patient eligibility**

      1. **Host factors.** Autologous transplants can be conducted safely in patients up to 70 years of age if they have adequate performance status, physiologic organ function, and hematopoietic stem cells. For allogeneic transplantation, the usual upper age limit is 55 years, although some centers perform HLA-identical sibling transplants in select patients up to 60 to 65 years of age. For unrelated or mismatched related donors, the usual age limitation is 50 to 55 years.

         For both autologous and allogeneic transplants, patients must meet a minimum physiologic organ function. Common criteria include pulmonary function tests (forced vital capacity, forced expiratory volume, and corrected diffusing capacity) > 50% of predicted; cardiac function with a left ventricular ejection fraction > 40% to 45%; no active infections; liver function tests less than two to four times normal; performance status more than 60% on the Karnofsky scale or < 2 on the Eastern Cooperative Oncology Group (ECOG); scale and serum creatinine level of less than 2 mg/dL. In select dis-

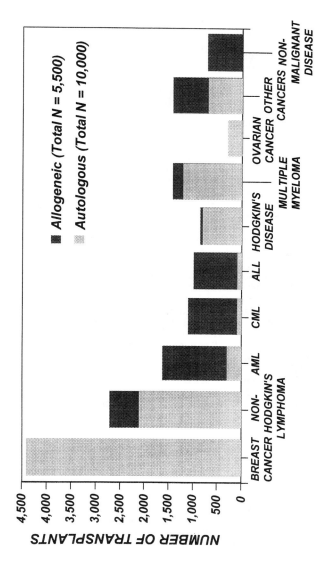

Fig. 6-1.   Indications for blood and marrow transplantation in North America: 1997. (Reprinted with permission from International Bone Marrow Transplant Regents/American Bone Marrow Transplant Regents.

eases, patients with impaired renal function can also be considered for autotransplantation (e.g., multiple myeloma patients treated with high-dose melphalan).

2. **Disease factors.** In general, the patients with malignant disease should show at least a partial response to standard-dose chemotherapy to be considered for high-dose therapy with autologous hematopoietic stem cell transplantation. Some exceptions to this generalization are patients with hematologic malignancies that are refractory to primary chemotherapy and who proceed early in their disease course to transplantation. For example, about 15% to 20% of patients with NHL refractory to induction therapy can achieve durable remissions with transplantation.

III. **Chemotherapeutic agents for dose-intensive strategies.** Agents are chosen for dose intensification based on the steepness and linearity of their dose-response curve; the absence of nonhematologic toxicity that prevents dose-escalation (preferably allowing 5- to 10-fold dose escalation over conventional doses); and, when combined with other agents, a synergistic antitumor effect with a minimum of overlapping nonhematologic toxicity. The doses of alkylating agents are often reduced 20% to 40% when combined, as compared with use as a single agent in high-dose conditioning regimens. There are few randomized trials comparing different preparative regimens. Indeed, in a retrospective study of more than 3,500 women with breast cancer undergoing high-dose therapy and autotransplant, more than 20 different preparative regimens were evaluated by multivariate analysis without identification of a statistically superior regimen. Thus, the choice of chemotherapeutic agents is arbitrary, based largely on anecdotal data, and a matter of personal experience and preference.

Extramedullary toxicities of the most commonly used conditioning agents are listed in Table 6-1. In most cases, drug doses are limited by gastrointestinal toxicity (mucositis, diarrhea) or major organ toxicity (e.g., heart, lung, kidney, or central nervous system [CNS]). When combining drugs in a conditioning regimen, particular attention must be given to overlapping toxicities. Preexisting renal or hepatic insufficiency or both may seriously reduce drug clearance. This can result in higher drug levels and further end-organ toxicity.

A. **Alkylating agents**

1. **BCNU (carmustine)** is a nitrosourea with clinical activity against a number of tumors. It is formulated in a 10% alcohol solution, which may account for the hypotension seen during or shortly after administration. BCNU, which undergoes spontaneous hydrolysis, should be protected from light and is usually administered as a 2-hour infusion. At high dose, pulmonary and hepatic toxicity are dose limiting. Nonhemato-

Table 6-1.   Toxicity of common chemotherapeutic agents

Drug (dose)	Extramedullary dose-limiting toxicity	Other toxicities
BCNU [carmustine] ($300–600$ mg/m^2)	Interstitial pneumonitis	Renal insufficiency, encephalopathy, N/V, VOD
Busulfan ($12–16$ mg/kg)	Mucositis, VOD	Seizures, rash, N/V, hyperpigmentation, pneumonitis
Cyclophosphamide ($120–200$ mg/kg)	Cardiomyopathy	Hemorrhagic cystitis, SIADH, N/V, interstitial pneumonitis
Cytarabine [Ara-C] ($4–36$ g/m^2)	CNS ataxia, mucositis	Pulmonary edema, conjunctivitis, rash, fever, hepatitis
Cisplatin ($150–180$ mg/m^2)	Renal insufficiency, peripheral neuropathy	Renal tubular acidosis, hypomagnesemia, hypokalemia, ototoxicity
Carboplatin ($600–1,500$ mg/m^2)	Ototoxicity, renal insufficiency	Hepatitis, hypo-magnesemia, hypo-kalemia, peripheral neuropathy
Etoposide ($600–2,400$ mg/m^2)	Mucositis	N/V, hepatitis, fever, pneumonia
Ifosfamide ($12–16$ g/m^2)	Encephalopathy, renal insufficiency	Hemorrhagic cystitis
Melphalan ($140–200$ mg/m^2)	Mucositis	N/V, hepatitis, SIADH, pneumonitis
Mitoxantrone ($30–75$ mg/m^2)	Cardiomyopathy	Mucositis
Paclitaxel [Taxol] ($500–775$ mg/m^2)	CNS ataxia, peripheral neuropathy	Anaphylaxis, mucositis
Thiotepa ($500–800$ mg/m^2)	Mucositis	Intertriginous rash, N/V, hyper-pigmentation

CNS, central nervous system; N/V, nausea/vomiting; SIADH, syndrome of inappropriate antidiuretic hormone; VOD, veno-occlusive disease.

logic toxicities are delayed and cumulative. BCNU doses exceeding 300 mg/m^2 are associated with acute or late pneumonitis in at least 20% of patients. Patients should be informed to monitor exercise tolerance; if tolerance diminishes, further evaluation should be performed (chest radiograph, arterial blood gas, pulmonary diffusion capacity). If drug-induced pneumonitis is confirmed, prednisone should be started with a taper over 2 to 3 months. BCNU is also occasionally associated with an increase incidence of veno-occlusive disease (VOD).

2. **Busulfan** has a more marked effect on myeloid cells than lymphoid cells and can cause prolonged aplasia. The major nonhematologic toxicities are VOD of the liver, pneumonitis, and mucositis. Busulfan rapidly enters the CNS and may cause seizures. Patients should receive prophylactic phenytoin (with doses sufficient to achieve therapeutic levels) before initiation of high-dose busulfan, and the phenytoin should be continued for 24 hours after the final dose. At present, busulfan is only available in oral formulation, although an intravenous formulation is in development. If vomiting occurs within half an hour of a dose, or if pill fragments are present in the emesis, most institutions repeat the dose. There is a wide intrapatient and interpatient variation in the absorption and metabolism of busulfan, and some centers perform busulfan pharmacokinetics to tailor busulfan doses.

3. **Cyclophosphamide (Cytoxan)** is probably the most widely used chemotherapeutic agent for dose intensification. Cyclophosphamide requires activation in the liver, but there is no evidence that the P-450 system necessary for that activation is saturated at doses used in intensification. Clearance of cyclophosphamide increases quickly after the first dose, and there is considerable interpatient variability in plasma concentrations with repeated dosing. Total doses as high as 5,000 to 7,000 mg/m^2 divided over 1 to 4 days can be safely administered as 1- to 2-hour infusions each day. Aggressive hydration (hyperhydration) and diuresis or administration of mesna (sodium-2-mercaptoethanesulfonate) as a uroprotectant is necessary to prevent hemorrhagic cystitis (also used for ifosfamide). The dose-limiting toxicities are cardiac and pulmonary. The cardiac effect, some degree of which occurs in up to 25% of patients, is a potentially fatal hemorrhagic myocarditis that may occur acutely or within days or may manifest as heart failure or pericardial effusions as long as 3 to 4 weeks after completion of treatment. The risk of cardiac toxicity is not cumulative, and repeated doses are tolerated in the patients who recover. This toxicity occurs most often in patients who receive more than 200 mg/kg (>7,500 mg/m^2), are older than 50 years, and have a previous history of congestive heart failure. The pulmonary toxicity of cyclophos-

phamide consists of proliferation of atypical type II pneumocytes with fibrosis. It usually manifests clinically within 4 to 6 weeks of therapy as progressive dyspnea, nonproductive cough, hypoxia, and interstitial radiographic changes.

Even at high doses, cyclophosphamide is not myeloablative, and its antitumor effect as a single agent is limited. In autologous transplant, cyclophosphamide, alone or in combination with hematopoietic growth factors, is often used for peripheral blood stem cell (PBSC) mobilization. In allogeneic transplantation, cyclophosphamide is included predominantly as an immunosuppressive agent owing to its lymphocytotoxic effects.

4. **Ifosfamide,** a closely related analog of cyclophosphamide, is also a prodrug that must undergo hepatic metabolism. As with cyclophosphamide, hyperhydration, and/or no protection with mesna, is required to prevent hemorrhagic cystitis. Unlike cyclophosphamide, the dose-limiting toxicity of ifosfamide is toxic encephalopathy manifested as lethargy, confusion, seizures, or stupor. Renal toxicity may also manifest as metabolic acidosis due to accumulation of metabolic by-products resulting in proximal renal tubular acidosis. No definite antitumor advantage of ifosfamide over cyclophosphamide has yet been established.

5. **Melphalan** alkylates target tissues after spontaneous formation of a (nitrogen) mustard-type reactive intermediate *in vivo*. It is administered rapidly in two daily doses of 70 to 100 mg/m^2 or one dose of 140 to 200 mg/m^2. Because less than 15% of the intact drug is excreted renally, melphalan can be administered safely in patients with renal insufficiency. The dose-limiting toxicities are gastro-intestinal toxicity (mucositis, diarrhea) and, less commonly, hepatitis and pneumonitis.

6. **Platinum compounds (cisplatin, carboplatin)** covalently bind to DNA bases and disrupt DNA function. Cisplatin can be escalated only two- to three-fold owing to renal and neurologic toxicity. Cisplatin must be reconstituted in a chloride-containing solution to minimize spontaneous hydrolysis. Aggressive hydration and diuresis with normal saline loading and maintenance of good urine output are required to avoid renal tubular toxicity. Magnesium wasting commonly leads to hypocalcemia and hypokalemia. Peripheral neuropathy and high-frequency hearing loss are potential long-term side effects. Carboplatin has less renal and neurologic toxicities; myelosuppression and hepatic

and gastrointestinal (mucositis and diarrhea) toxicities are more common with carboplatin. Some clinicians use the area under the curve (AUC; Calvert formula) of 20 to 28 for target drug dosing of carboplatin in high-dose preparative regimens.

7. **Thiotepa** has one of the steepest dose-response curves of all the alkylating agents and is not cross-resistant with cyclophosphamide. It, therefore, has been included in many different dose-intensity regimens. Thiotepa penetrates the blood-brain barrier better than most alkylating agents. Mucositis is the dose-limiting toxicity, with CNS toxicity observed only at very high doses. It may increase the risk of hepatic VOD when used with other agents known to have that toxicity.

B. **Nonalkylating and less commonly used agents**

1. **Cytarabine (ara-C)** is an analog of deoxycytidine and has multiple effects on DNA synthesis. It is used in high doses for the treatment of leukemia and in some regimens for NHL. At high dose, cytarabine causes neurologic toxicity, manifested by cerebral and cerebellar dysfunction. Renal dysfunction increases the risk of neurotoxicity substantially. This toxicity may present as dysarthria, gait disturbances, dementia, and coma. These toxicities are usually reversible but may be fatal. If neurologic symptoms develop, the cytarabine should be stopped immediately. Another rare but life-threatening complication is noncardiogenic pulmonary edema. Pulmonary symptoms, when they develop, are often fatal. Ara-C conjunctivitis is responsive to topical steroids, which should be used prophylactically.

2. **Etoposide** is a topoisomerase II inhibitor that shows synergism with platinum compounds. It has high single-agent activity in the treatment of leukemia, lymphomas, and testicular cancer. Its primary nonhematologic toxicities are mucositis, liver toxicity, and hypotension from the lipid formulation if administered rapidly.

3. **Mitoxantrone** is an anthracenedine compound that induces breakage of DNA strands, perhaps through an effect on topoisomerase II. It can be escalated five- to eight-fold above conventional dose. Mucositis and cardiotoxicity are the dose-limiting toxicities, although the latter is minimal compared with the structurally similar anthracyclines daunorubicin and doxorubicin.

4. **Paclitaxel (Taxol)** is a taxane, which stabilizes microtubules leading to mitotic arrest. It has activity against breast and ovarian cancers. One phase I study reported a maximum toler-

ated dose of 725 mg/m². At higher doses, unacceptable CNS, renal, mucosal, and pulmonary toxicities were observed. Peripheral neuropathy was tolerable and not associated with motor weakness. Because paclitaxel is eliminated through hepatic metabolism, hepatic insufficiency can prolong elimination and increase toxicity.

IV. **Total-body irradiation.** Total-body irradiation (TBI) is an integral component of several conditions regimens, particularly for hematologic malignancies requiring allogeneic or autologous transplantation. It has been used since the earliest days of bone marrow transplantation for both immunosuppression (prevention of allograft rejection) and antitumor effect. However, the therapeutic ratio of TBI is small. The usual dosage of TBI is 10 to 14 Gy given in twice or thrice daily doses over 3 to 4 days (e.g., 2 Gy b.i.d. for 3 days). Fractionation (and hyperfractionation) substantially reduces the risk of both interstitial pneumonitis and VOD of the liver. Above that dose, pulmonary, hepatic, and gastrointestinal toxicities become limiting and life-threatening with little therapeutic gain. Acute and chronic toxicities with TBI are summarized in Table 6-2.

V. **Preparative regimens.** During the past 25 years, a large number of intensive preparative (conditioning) regimens requiring hematopoietic stem cell support have been developed. The regimens used for dose intensification are largely empiric, and few have been compared in randomized trials. Important issues, such as optimum combination or doses, the benefit of an "induction" regimen immediately preceding intensification, and the benefit of repeated cycles of dose intensity, have not been rigorously addressed.

A. **Allogeneic transplant.** Preparative regimens must provide effective antitumor activity and suppress host immunity to prevent graft rejection. Commonly used cytotoxic agents include TBI, cyclophosphamide, busulfan, cytarabine, and etoposide. Immunosuppressant agents to reduce the risk of GVHD include steroids, cyclosporine (and cyclosporine analogs, such as tacrolimus), methotrexate, and antithymocyte globulin. Another modality is T-cell depletion of the transplanted cells by monoclonal antibodies, immuno-affinity columns, or immunomagnetic beads. After transplantation of a product that has undergone T-cell depletion, however, patients have an increased risk of graft failure and disease relapse. Therefore, more aggressive regimens are often used in T-cell–depleted patients, including higher doses of TBI, antithymocyte globulin, or a second myeloablative agent (e.g., thiotepa, cytarabine) in addition to cyclophosphamide. Examples of commonly employed preparative regimens using TBI are shown in Table 6-3.

Table 6-2.   Total body irradiation–associated acute and chronic toxicities

System	Acute symptoms and signs	Acute onset	Chronic symptoms and signs	Onset and incidence
Gastrointestinal	Nausea and vomiting, diarrhea	24–48 h	—	—
Hepatic	Venoocclusive disease	6–21 d	—	—
Mucosal tissues	Parotitis, decreased lacrimation, sore throat, mucositis	24–48 h	Sicca syndrome, cataracts	20% with fractionation at 0.5 to 3–4 yr
Endocrine	Acute pancreatitis, steroid-induced hyperglycemia	7–21 d	Gonadal failure, hypothyroidism, delayed bone growth	>90% 40%–55%
Pulmonary	Pneumonitis	1–3 mo	Pulmonary fibrosis	
Renal			Bone marrow transplantation nephropathy	Uncommon
Skin	Erythema, alopecia	5–10 d		
Second malignancies			Secondary leukemia, solid tumors	5%–10% 2% at 10 yr; 7% at 15 yr

Table 6-3.   Common preparative regimens for high-dose therapy with total-body irradiation

Drug	Total dose	Daily dose	Schedule (day)[a]	Indications	Autologous or allogeneic
Single cytotoxic drug regimens					
Cytoxan	120 mg/kg	60 mg/kg	−5, −4	Leukemia, lymphoma, aplastic anemia	Both
TBI	1,200 cGy	200 cGy b.i.d.	−3, −2, −1		
Etoposide	60 mg/kg	60 mg/kg	−3	Leukemia, lymphoma	Allogeneic
TBI	1,320 cGy	120 cGy t.i.d.	−7, −6, −5, −4		
Cytarabine (Ara-C)	36 g/m²	3 g/m² b.i.d.	−9, −8, −7, −6, −5, −4	Leukemia, lymphoma	Allogeneic
TBI	1,200 cGy	200 cGy b.i.d.	−3, −2, −1		
Melphalan	140 mg/m²	140 mg/m²	−4	Leukemia, multiple myeloma	Both
TBI	1,200 cGy	200 cGy b.i.d.	−3, −2, −1		
Combination cytotoxic drug regimens					
Cytarabine (Ara-C)	18 g/m²	3 g/m² b.i.d.	−8, −7, −6	Leukemia, lymphoma	Allogeneic
Cytoxan	90 mg/kg	45 mg/kg	−5, −4		
TBI	1,200 cGy	200 cGy b.i.d.	−3, −2, −1		
Etoposide	60 mg/kg	60 mg/kg	−4	Leukemia, lymphoma	Both
Cytoxan	120 mg/kg	60 mg/kg	−3, −2		
TBI	1,320 cGy	120 cGy t.i.d.	−8, −7, −6, −5[b]		
Thiotepa	10 mg/kg	5 mg/kg	−5, −4	Leukemia, lymphoma	Allogeneic
Cytoxan	120 mg/kg	60 mg/kg	−3, −2		
ATG[c]	120 mg/kg	30 mg/kg	−5, −4, −3, −2		
TBI	1,375 cGy	125 cGy t.i.d.	−9, −8, −7, −6[b]		

[a] Day 0 is day of transplantation, day −5 is 5 days before transplantation, etc.
[b] TBI given twice on this day.
TBI, total-body irradiation; ATG, antithymocyte globulin.

B. **Autologous transplant.** In autologous transplant, non–cross-resistant cytotoxic agents with nonoverlapping extramedullary toxicities are often combined. Combination regimens of two or more agents are generally more effective than single-agent regimens; many of the newer regimens rely on the synergistic effect of alkylating agents with agents such as topoisomerase inhibitors. Immunosuppression is not required. Although TBI is used by some centers as part of the preparative regimen for hematologic malignancies (e.g., lymphoma, multiple myeloma), it is avoided in the treatment of solid tumors (e.g. breast, ovary, testicular) because effective tumoricidal doses exceed extramedullary dose-limiting toxicity. Examples of commonly employed preparative regimens using combination chemotherapy are shown in Table 6-4.

VI. **Hematopoietic stem cells.** Hematopoietic progenitor cells (HPC) are primitive pluripotent stem cells capable of self-renewal and maturation into any of the hema-topoietic lineages and the committed and lineage-restricted progenitor cells. The first observations that lethally irradiated mice could survive after injection of spleen or marrow cells occurred more than 40 years ago. In humans, the first attempts at HPC transplantation began in the early and middle 1970s in recipients of HLA-identical sibling marrow allografts. These initial allogeneic transplants were compromised by severe GVHD. During the subsequent decades, efforts in allogeneic transplantation have been directed toward reducing transplant-related toxicity, decreasing the risk and severity of GVHD perhaps by "minitransplants," and treating relapse with donor lymphocytes. Because technology now permits molecular tagging and tracking of both normal and malignant cells in the blood and marrow, evolving issues in autologous transplant relate to the use of marrow or peripheral blood as a source of HPC and contamination of HPCs by malignant cells. The HPCs have now been characterized in humans to the extent that they can be isolated and expanded *in vitro*.

Hematopoietic recovery after transplantation (termed *engraftment*) is believed to occur in two waves: committed progenitor cells repopulating the marrow within the first month, and the true pluripotent stem cells responsible for the delayed but durable component of hematologic recovery. Quantitation of the number of HPCs necessary to provide hematopoietic reconstitution has evolved during the past 25 years. Flow cytometry has become the gold standard since the surface marker CD34+ was identified in the late 1980s as being present on HPCs. Patients with more than 5×10^6 CD34+ cells/kg recipient weight infused have prompt, predictable, and sustained engraftment. There is a growing consensus that more than 2×10^6 CD34+ cells/kg recipient weight is the minimum number of HPCs associated with granulocyte and platelet recovery (ANC > 500, platelets > 20,000) within 14 days after transplantation. More recently, subsets of CD34+ cells have been identified

Table 6-4. Common preparative regimens for high-dose therapy with total-body irradiation

Drug	Total dose	Daily dose	Schedule (day)	Indications	Autologous or allogeneic
"Big" BU/CY					
Busulfan	16 mg/kg	1 mg/kg q.i.d.	−9, −8, −7, −6	Leukemia, lymphoma	Allogeneic
Cytoxan	200 mg/kg	50 mg/kg	−5, −4, −3, −2		
"Little" BU/CY					
Busulfan	16 mg/kg	1 mg/kg q.i.d.	−7, −6, −5, −4	Leukemia, lymphoma, myeloma, breast cancer	Both
Cytoxan	120 mg/kg	60 mg/kg	−3, −2		
CPB "STAMP I"					
Cisplatin	165 mg/m^2	55 mg/m^2	−6, −5, −4	Breast cancer	Autologous
Cytoxan	5,625 mg/m^2	1,875 mg/m^2	−6, −5, −4		
BCNU	600 mg/m^2	600 mg/m^2	−3		
CTCb "STAMP V"					
Thiotepa	500 mg/m^2	125 mg/m^2	−7, −6, −5, −4	Breast cancer	Autologous
Cytoxan	6 g/m^2	1.5 g/m^2	−7, −6, −5, −4		
Carboplatin	800 mg/m^2	200 mg/m^2	−7, −6, −5, −4		
TC					
Thiotepa	500 mg/m^2	125 mg/m^2	−7, −6, −5, −4	Breast cancer	Autologous
Cytoxan	6 g/m^2	1.5 g/m^2	−7, −6, −5, −4		
CBV					
BCNU	300–600 mg/m^2	300–600 mg/m^2	−6	Hodgkin's disease	Autologous
Etoposide	900–2,400 mg/m^2	300–800 mg/m^2	−6, −5, −4		
Cytoxan	6–7.2 g/m^2	1.5–1.8 g/m^2	−6, −5, −4, −3		

Table 6-4. *(Continued)*

Drug	Total dose	Daily dose	Schedule (day)	Indications	Autologous or allogeneic
BEAM					
BCNU	300 mg/m²	300 mg/m²	−6	Hodgkin's disease, lymphoma	Autologous
Etoposide	800 mg/m²	200 mg/m²	−5, −4, −3, −2		
Cytarabine	800–1,600 mg/m²	200–400 mg/m²	−5, −4, −3, −2		
Melphalan	140 mg/m²	140 mg/m²	−1		
ICE					
Ifosfamide	16 g/m²	4 g/m²	−6, −5, −4, −3	Lymphoma, testicular cancer	Autologous
Carboplatin	1.8 g/m²	600 mg/m²	−6, −5, −4		
Etoposide	1.5 g/m²	500 mg/m² b.i.d.	−6, −5, −4		
BEAC					
BCNU	300 mg/m²	300 mg/m²	−6	Lymphoma, Hodgkin's disease	Autologous
Etoposide	800 mg/m²	200 mg/m²	−5, −4, −3, −2		
Cytarabine	800 mg/m²	200 mg/m²	−5, −4, −3, −2		
Cytoxan	140 mg/kg	35 mg/kg	−5, −4, −3, −2		
MEL					
Melphalan	200 mg/m²	100 mg/m²	−3, −2	Multiple myeloma	Autologous
MCC					
Mitoxantrone	75 mg/m²	25 mg/m²	−8, −6, −4	Ovarian cancer	Autologous
Carboplatin	AUC 28	⅓ total dose	−8, −7, −6 −5, −4		
Cytoxan	120 mg/m²	40 mg/m²	−8, −6, −4		
CBDA/VP					
Carboplatin	2.25 g/m²	750 mg/m²	−6, −5, −4	Testicular cancer	Autologous
Etoposide	2.1 g/m²	700 mg/m²	−6, −5, −4		

AUC, area under the curve (Calvert formula).

on the basis of other cell surface markers, including CD33, CD38, HLA-DR, Thy-1, and Lin, and the ability to stain with the dye rhodamine. The most primitive HPCs can be identified as CD34+, Thy-1+, lin–, CD33–, CD38–, HLA-DR–, and rhodamine–. Only 1% of a bone marrow harvest consists of CD34+ cells with this more primitive pluripotent CD34+ subset comprising less than 0.01%. The most recent advances in stem cell technology use *ex vivo* expansion techniques to increase the number of hematopoietic stem cells for transplantation.

A. **Allogeneic transplant** is used mostly for the treatment of leukemia and other hematologic malignancies. Less than 5% of allogeneic transplant are used for nonmalignant diseases such as aplastic anemia, immunodeficiency syndromes, or hemoglobinopathies. Although most allogeneic transplants consist of bone marrow donation from an HLA-identical sibling, there is a growing use of PBSCs, unrelated bone marrow donors, mismatched family donors, and umbilical cord blood. Until recently, donors were identified by serologic phenotype testing for class I and class II major histocompatibility complex molecules HLA-A, -B, and -DR on lymphocytes. Mendelian inheritance predicts a 25% likelihood of identifying an HLA-identical sibling donor within a family; another 5% of patients have a one-antigen–mismatched family donor. Through the efforts of the National Marrow Donor Program (NMDP), which has HLA typing on more than 2.5 million volunteers, an HLA-compatible unrelated donor can be identified for many patients. Because of HLA polymorphism, most transplant centers now perform genotype analysis that includes HLA-DR, -DQ, and -$DR_{\beta1}$; occasionally, sequencing is required to confirm compatibility. This is particularly important in evaluating potential unrelated donors. Using this technology, an acceptable match can be identified in more than 70% of white patients in the NMDP. In contrast, minorities are greatly under-represented in the NMDP, and the likelihood of identifying an acceptable match for these patients is considerably lower.

Transplant-related mortality rates range from 20% to 30% in HLA-identical sibling transplant recipients and from 40% to 50% in unrelated and mismatched transplant recipients. GVHD is the most common cause of treatment-related mortality, with significant acute GVHD (first 100 days after transplantation) occurring in 10% to 40% of HLA-identical sibling transplant recipients and in more than 40% to 80% of unrelated and mismatched marrow recipients. Chronic GVHD (occurring more than 100 days after transplantation) occurs in about 50% of HLA-identical sibling transplant recipients; the incidence is higher with unrelated donors and mismatched donors. GVHD prophylaxis requires immunosuppression of the donor immune system: a number of modalities are available, usually in combination, including antithymocyte globulin, methotrexate, cyclosporine (and cyclosporine analogs, such as tacrolimus [FK506]), corticosteroids, T-cell depletion of allografts, and monoclonal antibodies (i.e., OKT3). Although the incidence of severe acute and chronic GVHD is lower with T-cell depletion techniques (5% to 20%), there is an increase in graft failure and disease relapse. Recent advances in GVHD prophylaxis has extended the potential donor pool to include partially mismatched donors and haploidentical donors. Another potential donor source is umbilical cord blood. About 300 umbilical cord blood transplantations have been reported worldwide. This source of HPCs is associated with fewer cases of GVHD, but the number of HPCs obtained is limited, as is umbilical cord blood availability. A number of cord blood banks provide storage and donor searches.

A recent trend in allogeneic transplantation is to use hematopoietic growth factor primed or unprimed PBSCs. Sufficient numbers of HPCs can usually be collected in one or two aphereses. The use of PBSC negates the need for a bone marrow harvest and provides a greater number of CD34+ cells than that obtained from bone marrow. This allows for more rapid engraftment. Even though PBSCs contain a log or more T cells than does bone marrow, the incidence of acute GVHD does not appear to be increased. However, recent reports from the M.D. Anderson Cancer Center and other centers suggest that chronic GVHD is higher with PBSC than with bone marrow (80% versus 50%).

B. **Autologous transplants** and the number of centers performing them are increasing at a striking rate. Currently, few centers use autologous bone marrow as the source of HPCs to support high-dose therapy. With the advent of PBSCs and hematopoietic growth factors, the duration of marrow aplasia has been significantly shortened compared with that of autologous bone marrow transplant. Randomized trials have demonstrated that the use of PBSCs has resulted in fewer infectious complications, shorter hospitalizations, and lower costs. Many centers are performing autologous transplants in the outpatient setting.

PBSCs are collected by a process called *leukapheresis*. This is usually coordinated with the transplantation center's blood bank. Patients require insertion of a large-bore central venous catheter before initiation of apheresis. PBSCs can be collected in the steady state or after mobilization by hematopoietic growth factors (e.g., granulocyte colony-stimulating factor [G-CSF] or granulocyte-macrophage colony-stimulating factor [GM-CSF]) with or without chemotherapy (Table 6-5).

Table 6-5. Relative increase in peripheral blood stem cells using different mobilization regimens

Modality	Fold increase
Steady state	1×
Chemotherapy	10–20×
Growth factor alone (G-CSF most common)	10×
Chemotherapy plus growth factor (G-CSF or GM-CSF)	100–1,000×

G-CSF, granulocyte colony-stimulating factor; GM-CSF, granulocyte-macrophage colony-stimulating factor.

Although cyclophosphamide (2 to 7 g/m^2) is the most common single chemotherapeutic agent reported in stem cell mobilization regimens, a number of other agents have been used either alone or in combination with cyclophosphamide or with other agents. As indicated previously, a minimum of 2×10^6 CD34+ cells/kg is necessary for successful engraftment in most patients. Most patients reach their target CD34+ cell goal within five collections. However, in heavily pretreated patients, this minimum requirement is often difficult to achieve. Recent pilot trials indicate that some of the newer hematopoietic growth factors (stem cell factor [SCF], daniplestim, flt-3 ligand), either alone or in combination with other growth factors, increase the yield of CD34+ cells.

PBSC mobilization techniques may also increase the number of tumor cells in the peripheral blood. For example, tumor cells are commonly present in the bone marrow of patients with advanced breast cancer—and may be present even in those with stage I disease. About one fourth of patients with advanced breast cancer have detectable cells in the peripheral circulation; during stem cell mobilization, significantly higher percentages of patients may have detectable tumor cells. Similar findings but with lower rates of contamination have been reported for lymphoma. Essentially all PBSC collections from patients with multiple myeloma contain contaminating tumor cells. Malignant cells contaminating PBSC collections may contribute to relapse after high-dose therapy and autologous transplant.

Efforts to reduce the number of contaminating tumor cells in PBSC autografts have used techniques based on physical, immunologic, and pharmacologic methods. Pharmacologic methods are generally aimed at removing tumor cells from the autograft (purging; negative selection) rather than by enrichment for HPCs. The most common pharmacologic agent is 4-hydroperoxycyclophosphamide. Although promising in pilot trials, the Food and Drug Administration has removed this drug from clinical trials. Physical methods (e.g., density gradients and counterflow centrifugal elutriation) are used less commonly: they use cell size, shape, and density to separate cell populations. The most commonly employed separation techniques use immunologic methodology, most often positive selection for CD34+ cells. An anti-CD34+ cell antibody is bound to a solid phase (e.g., immunoaffinity column, immunomagnetic beads), which binds cells, and then the cells are later released. This results in a 2- to 4-log depletion of contaminating tumor cells. One of the most recent advances in positive selection is the use of sequential columns (anti-CD2 followed by anti-CD34) and by combination of immunologic and physical methods (immunoaffinity columns followed by high-speed flow cytometry). The latter method has been reported to result in a 5- to 7-log depletion of tumor cells.

A new technology to reduce contaminating tumor cells uses *in vitro* culture. Small numbers of HPCs can be expanded 3- to 20-fold *ex vivo* with combinations of cytokines (e.g., IL-3, IL-6, G-CSF, SCF, flt-3, GM-CSF, GM-CSF/IL-3) in large-volume culture or bioreactors. Preliminary results indicate that these expanded cells are capable of complete hematopoietic reconstitution after high-dose therapy. A similar technique using long-term culture permits growth of HPCs while malignant tumor cells are eliminated, allowing for potential autografts in patients with hematologic malignancies, such as CML, who may not be candidates for allogeneic transplantation.

VII. Hematopoietic growth factors and cytokines. More than 20 different cytokines and growth factors are approved or under investigation for use in hematopoietic stem cell transplantation. Colony-stimulating factors shorten the time to bone marrow or PBSC engraftment after high-dose chemotherapy. They act by binding to specific cell surface receptors stimulating proliferation, differentiation, commitment, and selected end-cell functions. Two commercially available hematopoietic growth factors are G-CSF (filgrastim) and GM-CSF (sargramostim). The most common dosages and indications for these growth factors are listed in Table 6-6. For HPC mobilization with growth factors alone, most clinicians start the growth factor on day 1, with initiation of apheresis on day 5. For chemotherapy plus growth factor mobilization, the growth factor is started on the day after completion of the chemotherapy, and apheresis commences when the white blood cell count is more than 1,000. After transplantation, the growth factors are usually started the same day (day 0) or on day 1; growth factor support is continued daily until the absolute neutrophil count is more than 2,000 for a minimum of 1 day.

Several new hematopoietic growth factors are in clinical trials. These growth factors are designed to improve

Table 6-6. Hematopoietic growth factors: Common doses and indications

Growth factor	Clinical indication	Dose
G-CSF[a]	Peripheral blood HPC mobilization	
	With chemotherapy	5–10 μg/kg S.C.
	Without chemotherapy	10–16 μg/kg S.C.
	Hematopoietic recovery after transplantation	5 μg/kg S.C.
GM-CSF[b]	Peripheral blood HPC mobilization	
	With chemotherapy	250 μg/m² S.C.
	Hematopoietic recovery after transplantation	250 μg/m² S.C.
Epoietin	Red blood cell recovery after transplantation	150–300 μ/kg S.C. three times per week

[a] Often rounded off to standard vial size of 300 μg or 480 μg; a common approach is 300 μg for patients who weigh <60 kg, and 480 μg for patients who weigh >60 kg.
[b] Often rounded off to standard vial size of 500 μg.
G-CSF, granulocyte colony-stimulating factor; GM-CSF, granulocyte-macrophage colony-stimulating factor; HPC, hematopoietic progenitor cell.

platelet recovery (IL-11, thrombopoietin, megakaryocyte-derived growth factor), to improve stem cell mobilization in patients who are predicted to be poor mobilizers with G-CSF or GM-CSF (IL-3, daniplestim, stem cell factor), or to enhance dendritic cell proliferation (flt-3 ligand, stem cell factor) as part of immunotherapeutic approaches.

Other cytokines under development or in clinical trials in hematopoietic stem cell transplantation are shown in Table 6-7. Many of these have multiple functions.

VIII. **Toxicities** of dose-intensive regimens can be formidable and life-threatening. They vary considerably with the different preparative regimens, type of transplant (autologous versus allogeneic; related versus unrelated versus mismatched), and the patient's physiologic organ function and performance status. Some of the toxicities associated with transplant preparative regimens are outlined in Tables 6-1 and 6-2. As indicated, some of the toxicities are acute, whereas others are chronic. Stomatitis, esophagitis, and diarrhea can be severe with some regimens. Hepatic, renal, or pulmonary toxicities can occur in 20% to 30% of patients. Most patients require blood product support in the peritransplant period. Central venous catheter infections or thrombosis can be problematic. Most centers use prophylactic antibiotics to prevent bacterial, viral, and fungal infections. One of the most devastating late

**Table 6-7.   Cytokines in
hematopoietic stem cell transplantation**

Cytokine	Clinical application	Proposed mechanism
Interferon-α	Immune modulation Posttransplantation for CML, myeloma, lymphoma	Unknown
Interleukin-2	Immune modulation to prevent posttransplantation relapse	Activates T and natural killer cells
Interleukin-12	Immune modulation after transplantation	Increases Th1 helper T cells
GM-CSF M-CSF	Treatment of fungal infections after transplantation	Enhances macrophage activity

CML, chronic myelogenous leukemia; GM-CSF, granulocyte-macrophage
colony-stimulating factor; M-CSF, macrophage colony-stimulating factor.

toxicities is the development of secondary malignancies:
solid tumors have been reported in 0.7% of patients 5
years after allogeneic transplantation, in 2.2% at 10 years,
and in 6.7% at 15 years. Hematologic disorders, including
myelodysplastic syndrome, lymphoma, and secondary
leukemias, have been variously reported in 5% to 15% of
long-term survivors.

IX. **Response and long-term outcomes.** With a few exceptions, the goal of high-dose therapy with hematopoietic
stem cell transplantation is to cure or substantially prolong good-quality survival. The short-term surrogate
marker for improved survival or cure is complete remission (CR). Partial remission (PR) rarely translates into
important increases in survival and represents only a
1- to 3-log kill of malignant cells. Therefore, partial remission rates have little meaning in dose-intensive regimens. Less than half of patients with advanced malignancy obtain durable remissions with current dose-
intensive regimens, stimulating major research efforts to
eradicate minimal residual disease after transplantation.
The role of dose intensity is covered in disease-related
chapters and is presented only in summary form here.

  A. **Leukemia**
     1. **Acute myelogenous leukemia** is curable in
        15% to 45% of patients with standard chemo-
        therapy. The leukemia-free survival rate is
        highest in patients under 20 years of age and
        lowest in patients over 55 years of age. After
        first relapse, AML is incurable with standard
        therapy. Cytogenetic analysis is critical for de-
        termining which patients are candidates for
        transplantation as consolidation versus consid-

eration at the time of relapse. Patients with favorable AML subtypes, such as FAB-M2 with t (8;21), FAB-M3 with t (15;17) and FAB-M4 with inv (16), have a greater than 75% CR rate and a 50% to 65% 5-year survival rate with standard induction and consolidation therapy. These patients are usually considered for transplantation only at the time of disease relapse. In contrast, patients with the remaining FAB classification (M0, M1, M5, M6, M7) or with M2, M3, or M4 without the favorable cytogenetic marker (or with normal cytogenetics or any other additional chromosomal abnormalities) are often considered for transplantation in the first CR. The probability of leukemia-free survival is 60% in the first CR, 40% in the second or later CR, and 20% in relapse using HLA identical sibling donors (IBMTR data); lower rates are observed with matched unrelated donors or mismatched related donors, usually owing to the increased incidence of GVHD. Data from the Fred Hutchinson Cancer Research Center in Seattle indicate that similar results are obtained in patients undergoing transplant during an untreated early relapse with in those undergoing transplantation in a second CR. About 10% to 20% of patients who fail induction therapy achieve long-term leukemia-free survival with allogeneic transplant. Compared with allogeneic transplant, autologous transplant has lower transplant-related mortality rates because of the absence of GVHD. However, relapse rates approach 50% in most trials. The benefit of autologous transplant, whether purged or unpurged, remains controversial. A recent ECOG trial failed to show any advantage of purged autologous transplant as consolidation therapy for AML over conventional therapy.

2. **Acute lymphoblastic leukemia** (ALL) is curable in 60% to 75% of affected children but in only 20% to 30% of adults. Even in high-risk patients, there are no clinical trials proving that early transplant is beneficial if CR is achieved with standard induction therapy. Because of the rarity of ALL in adults, few institutions have enough patients for randomized trials properly analyzed according to risk factors (e.g., CNS leukemia, high white blood cell count at presentation, male gender, hepatosplenomegaly, Philadelphia chromosome–positive (Ph+) cytogenetics, immunophenotype). Most clinicians agree, even without substantial clinical trial data, that patients with Ph+-positive ALL should proceed to transplant in the first CR.

Patients who undergo transplant as consolidation of first CR have a 50% leukemia-free survival rate, compared with 40% in more than the second CR and 20% in relapse using HLA-identical sibling donors; again, lower rates are observed with alternate donors. The role of autologous transplantation in ALL remains highly controversial.

3. **Chronic myelogenous leukemia** remains the most common indication for allogeneic transplantation. Although interferon therapy alone or with chemotherapy results in major cytogenetic responses in 25% to 40% of patients, with a median duration of survival of more than 7 years, no cures are achieved with this modality. Cure rates approach 70% in patients with CML in chronic phase who receive an HLA-identical sibling transplant within the first year of the disease. Waiting until the development of accelerated phase or blast phase reduces the leukemia-free survival to 35% and 15%, respectively. In the setting of matched unrelated transplant, about 40% of patients are cured when transplantation is performed in chronic phase within the first year. A recent report from Seattle, however, indicates that the use of interferon for more than 6 months results in an increased incidence of acute GVHD in recipients of matched unrelated donor transplants and, subsequently, in lower survival rates than those seen in patients who did not receive interferon therapy. Patients who relapse after transplant may enter a second CR with infusion of donor lymphocytes; success rates as high as 75% have been reported. CML patients without an HLA-compatible sibling or unrelated donor may be considered for autologous transplant. Early results suggest that autologous transplant for CML in chronic phase may prolong survival, especially if some Ph– cells are present after autografting. A number of purging and culture techniques are being investigated to eradicate Ph+ cells for autotransplant.

4. **Chronic lymphocytic leukemia** (CLL) is one of the more recent indications for high-dose therapy with hematopoietic stem cell transplantation. Pilot studies indicate that about 60% of patients with CLL remain in remission after allotransplant at a median follow-up of 3 years, even in refractory disease; this compares with a median survival of less than 12 months using conventional therapy in historical controls. Autotransplants for CLL have had disappointing results, with median leukemia-free survival of less than 12 months.

B. Lymphoma

1. **Hodgkin's disease** is curable with conventional therapy in most patients. Transplantation is an effective modality for primary treatment failure and high-risk patients (e.g., stage IVB), as consolidation, and for patients with disease relapse; long-term disease-free survival is observed in 20% to 30%, 60% to 70%, and 40% to 50%, respectively, for each of these three disease subgroups [Autologous Blood and Marrow Transplant Registry (ABMTR) data]. A variety of preparative regimens have been reported: the BEAM, CBV, and BEAC regimens listed in Table 6-4 are the most commonly employed. In patients receiving nitrosoureas (e.g., BCNU), the clinician must pay particular attention to respiratory symptoms (dry cough, shortness of breath, hypoxia, and interstitial infiltrates on chest radiograph) 4 to 12 weeks after transplant because these symptoms are suggestive of BCNU pulmonary toxicity, a potentially fatal complication that can be reversed with prompt initiation of corticosteroids. There is no survival advantage for allogeneic over autologous transplant, and the former is usually considered only in the setting of excessive bone marrow involvement or inability to collect sufficient PBSCs for autologous transplant.

2. **Non-Hodgkin's lymphoma** is curable with conventional therapy in only 30% to 40% of patients. Less than 10% of relapsed patients achieve long-term survival with conventional salvage therapy. The early transplant trials were conducted in patients with intermediate-grade lymphoma with disease relapse or disease that was refractory to secondary salvage therapy. In this setting, the survival rate was only about 20%. Cure rates of 30% to 50% were reported in patients who received high-dose therapy with autotransplant earlier in the disease course. A randomized trial comparing high-dose therapy with autologous transplant to standard salvage therapy (DHAP) in patients with chemotherapy-sensitive first relapse proved conclusively that high-dose therapy was the superior treatment (46% versus 12% 5-year event-free survival rate). About 15% to 35% of patients with primary refractory disease achieve durable remission with high-dose therapy. When transplantation was used as consolidation therapy, a recent randomized French trial of patients with aggressive NHL did not show significant differences in 3-year or disease-free survivals. However, a recent Italian trial indicated that high-risk patients (group 2

or 3 in the International Prognostic Index) with intermediate-grade lymphoma treated with high-dose therapy and autologous transplantation as consolidation had superior outcomes compared with patients treated with standard induction therapy (70% to 85% disease-free survival rates at 5 years). A randomized ECOG trial is currently open to resolve these conflicting observations. Allogeneic transplantation does not appear to be superior to autologous transplantation in treating intermediate-grade lymphomas. Although fewer relapses are observed after allogeneic transplant, presumably because of a graft-versus- lymphoma effect, the transplant-related mortality offsets the lower relapse rate.

Low-grade NHL accounts for about one third of all lymphomas. These lymphomas are usually extensive at diagnosis and follow an indolent clinical course of 5 to 10 years with or without aggressive therapy. Some centers are treating patients in the first CR with high-dose therapy and autologous transplant. The most favorable results have been observed in patients with minimal disease at the time of transplant whose hematopoietic stem cells are polymerase chain reaction negative for bcl-2. This is usually accomplished by *in vitro* bone marrow purging with monoclonal antibody cocktails. However, because of the brevity of the follow-up in most of these reports, the benefit of high-dose therapy with autologous transplant remains uncertain. More recently, pilot trials using allogeneic transplant have been reported. This approach has the advantage of the absence of contaminating tumor cells and a graft-versus-lymphoma effect. The pilot trial data indicate a 50% to 60% disease-free survival rate 2 to 3 years after transplant.

One area of controversy is mantle cell lymphomas. These are aggressive intermediate-grade lymphomas with a median survival of about 2 years using conventional therapy. There is currently no definite evidence of a survival advantage using autologous or allogeneic transplant for primary refractory disease, relapsed disease, or after the second CR. Small pilot trials support the use of high-dose therapy with autologous transplant as consolidation for the first CR.

Because most patients with NHL relapse even after high-dose therapy, current emphasis is focused on posttransplant immunotherapy to eradicate minimal residual disease. This includes low-dose IL-2, interferons, idiotype-specific vaccines, and dendritic cell vaccines.

C. **Plasma cell dyscrasias**
  1. **Multiple myeloma** is an incurable B-cell malignancy that constitutes 10% of all hematologic malignancies. With standard therapy, the median survival is 30 to 36 months. A randomized trial comparing high-dose therapy with autologous transplant to standard chemotherapy demonstrated a superior outcome in the high-dose therapy arm (overall survival time, 57 months versus 42 months). A National Cancer Institute (NCI) High Priority Intergroup Trial (S9321) is comparing early versus late transplant to determine the optimal timing of transplants. Even with autotransplant, there is no plateau in the survival curves, indicating that cure is unlikely. Allogeneic transplant, in contrast, may be curative in 20% to 25% of patients but is associated with extremely high transplantation-related mortality rates, approaching 40% to 50% in most reports. About 50% of patients who achieve CR with allotransplant eventually relapse. Some of these patients may achieve a second CR with donor leukocyte infusions by a graft-versus-myeloma effect.
  2. **Primary amyloidosis** is a plasma cell dyscrasia associated with light-chain deposition in one or more organ systems. With standard therapy, the median survival time is 18 to 24 months, less than 1 year for patients with cardiac amyloidosis. Recent reports from Boston University and the Mayo Clinic indicate that high-dose therapy with autotransplantation can effect high remission rates and improve survival rates. An ECOG trial is now open to evaluate this modality.
D. **Solid tumors.** High-dose chemotherapy with autologous hematopoietic reconstitution is an accepted modality for the treatment of various solid tumors that show a steep dose-response curve. The optimal patient population, timing of high-dose therapy, and drug regimens are under investigation.
  1. **Breast cancer** remains a controversial disease in terms of high-dose therapy with autologous transplantation. In metastatic disease, a single randomized trial comparing tandem transplant to standard therapy reported superior CR, disease-free, and overall survival rates. However, this was a small study of only 90 patients, with considerable concerns about methodology and the extent of dose intensity in both arms. An NCI-sponsored randomized intergroup trial (PBT-101) comparing high-dose therapy with standard therapy closed in December 1997; the results of this study will be available in 1999. In general, patients who demonstrate chemotherapy-sensitive disease

(PR or CR) after four to six cycles of salvage therapy are considered candidates for high-dose therapy as consolidation. CR is achieved in more than 50% of patients, compared with 5% to 10% of patients using standard salvage therapy. Based on single-institution trials, about 20% to 30% of patients remain disease free at a median follow-up of 3 to 5 years. It is uncertain how many of these patients will remain disease free and may be cured. Favorable prognostic features include chemotherapy-sensitive disease, a single metastatic site, no prior adjuvant chemotherapy, hormone receptor positive, long interval between primary disease and recurrence (>1 year), and absence of CNS or liver disease. Evaluation of more than 20 different preparative regimens in a multivariate analysis failed to identify a single superior regimen; the most common regimens are STAMP I and STAMP V (see Table 6-4). Pilot trials using multicycle high-dose chemotherapy with autologous transplant have been disappointing.

The most rapidly growing indication for high-dose therapy with autotransplant is high-risk breast cancer. Peters and colleagues first reported the superior outcome of high-dose therapy with autotransplant, and compared to historical control patients treated with conventional therapy, in patients with 10 or more positive (cancer-involved) axillary lymph nodes. In the initial report, a 72% disease-free survival was reported at 3.3 years (70% at 5 years in a follow-up report) in the transplant group, compared with 25% to 35% in historical controls treated with standard therapy. To confirm these observations, two NCI-sponsored randomized trials have recently been completed comparing high-dose therapy with autotransplant to standard therapy.

Even less data are available to evaluate the efficacy of high-dose therapy and autologous transplant in patients with four to nine involved lymph nodes. Historical control data indicate a 5-year disease-free survival rate ranging from 40% to 50%. Data from the Autologous Blood and Marrow Transplant Registry (ABMTR) indicate a 3-year disease-free survival rate of about 60% in patients with stage II or III breast cancer. The disease-free survival rate approaches 70% in patients with hormone receptor–positive disease who receive posttransplant tamoxifen and radiation therapy to the chest wall and axilla. An NCI-sponsored randomized trial comparing intensive sequential chemotherapy with high-dose therapy for patients with four to nine involved lymph nodes is open for accrual.

2. **Ovarian cancer,** like breast cancer, is sensitive to conventional-dose chemotherapy. Therefore, trials of dose-escalated chemotherapy with hematopoietic stem cell rescue have been pursued. The largest single-institution study was reported from Loyola University. In the 100 patients with recurrent ovarian carcinoma completing high-dose therapy with autologous transplant, the median progression-free survival (PFS) and overall survival (OS) rates were 7 and 13 months, respectively. In the 20 patients with the most favorable features (platinum chemosensitivity and less than 1 cm residual disease), the PFS and OS were 19 and 30 months, respectively. The ABMTR reported the results of 422 patients with ovarian cancer completing high-dose therapy with autologous transplant; with a median follow-up of 29 months, the PFS and OS were 8 months and 14 months, respectively. Favorable prognostic factors included younger age (less than 48 years), good performance status, platinum-sensitive disease, and first CR or PR. The best results were observed in patients in the first CR or PR after one chemotherapy regimen (PFS and OS of 10 months and 30 months, respectively).

   Two pilot trials evaluating high-dose therapy with autologous transplant as consolidation therapy for previously untreated advanced-stage ovarian cancer have demonstrated promising results. One trial reported 5-year PFS and OS rates of 51% and 60%, respectively; the other reported 5-year PFS and OS rates of 24% and 60%, respectively, with a median survival of 30 months. This compares favorably with historical control data showing a 20% to 30% 5-year survival rate with conventional therapy. The NCI is currently sponsoring a phase III clinical trial to compare standard therapy with high-dose therapy in previously untreated patients with chemotherapy-sensitive ovarian cancer (GOG 164). The Southwest Oncology Group (SWOG 9106) has undertaken a phase II trial comparing two different high-dose chemotherapy regimens in relapsed patients with platinum-sensitive disease.

3. **Germ cell cancers** are chemotherapy-sensitive malignancies that afflict young people. Patients with advanced-stage disease who fail to achieve CR to initial platinum-based standard therapy have a poor prognosis: their long-term disease-free survival rate is less than 5%. High-dose therapy with autotransplantation results

in a disease-free survival rate of 5% to 20%. A second group of patients who are potential candidates for transplantation includes the 10% of patients who relapse after achieving CR. Although salvage therapy produces a more than 50% response rate, only 20% to 30% of these patients achieve durable remissions. High-dose therapy with autotransplantation results in a 30% to 50% long-term disease-free survival rate for patients with responsive relapse. For resistant relapse, the long-term disease-free survival rate after autotransplant is 5% to 20%. One of the current areas of interest is the selection of high-risk patients for high-dose therapy with autotransplant as consolidation.

4. **Small cell lung cancer** is a chemosensitive malignancy with a long-term disease-free survival rate of about 20% at 2 years in patients with limited disease. Nearly 150 transplants have been reported to the ABMTR for small cell lung cancer. The largest experience has been reported by the Boston group, with a 2-year disease-free survival of 50% in nearly 80 patients. The SWOG is planning a multi-institutional trial to confirm these results.

E. **Other diseases** in which high-dose therapy with transplantation has reported efficacy include aplastic anemia (AA) and myelodysplastic syndromes (MDS). AA has a guarded prognosis because of the risk of infection and fatal hemorrhage. The 1-year survival rate for severe AA is less than 20%. Allogeneic transplantation results in a long-term survival rate ranging from 50% to 90%. Favorable prognostic factors are younger age (<16 years), no prior transfusions, short interval from diagnosis to transplant, and no evidence of infection. The preparative regimen consists of immunosuppressive agents: cyclophosphamide alone or with antithymocyte globulin or with TBI. Patients who do not have a compatible sibling donor may be considered for a matched unrelated donor transplantation. About 15% to 30% of patients survive with engraftment.

MDS is a clonal disorder of HPCs. There is no effective standard therapy for this disorder. Allogeneic transplantation can produce long-term disease-free survivors: about 40% of patients younger than 40 years but only 15% to 20% of patients older than 40 years. A recent report from Europe claimed a 28% 2-year disease-free survival for MDS patients undergoing autologous transplant. Again, age was a critical prognostic feature, with a 2-year disease-free survival rate of 39% in patients younger than 40 years compared with 25% in patients older than 40 years. The median follow-up in this study of 55 patients was only 10 months; longer follow-up is required to confirm these preliminary findings.

One of the newest areas of clinical interest is autoimmune diseases. Although predominantly published as case reports, there appears to be clinical improvement or stabilization in disease parameters after high-dose therapy with autologous transplant for multiple sclerosis, systemic lupus erythematosus, scleroderma, and rheumatoid arthritis. Preparative regimens focus on immunosuppression with cyclophosphamide with TBI or antithymocyte globulin.

X. **Future directions.** As we approach the new millennium, the field of high-dose therapy is evolving into *ex vivo* HPC expansion, gene therapy, improved CD34+ selection techniques, mini-transplants, improved GVHD prophylaxis and treatment, improvement in safety of matched unrelated and mismatched donor transplants, DNA and idiotype vaccines, dendritic cell recruitment and transplantation, novel hematopoietic growth factors, and post-transplant immunotherapy to eradicate minimal residual disease.

SELECTED READINGS

Anderson JE, Litzow MR, Appelbaum FR, et al. Allogeneic, syngeneic, and autologous bone marrow transplantation for Hodgkin's disease: the 21-year Seattle experience. *J Clin Oncol* 1993;11:2342–2350.

Armitage JO, Antman KH, eds. *High-dose cancer therapy: pharmacology, hematopoietins, stem cells.* 2nd ed. Baltimore: Williams & Wilkins, 1995;929.

Attal M, Harousseau JL, Stoppa AM, et al. A prospective, randomized trial of autologous bone marrow transplantation and chemotherapy in multiple myeloma. *N Engl J Med* 1996;335:91–97.

Bezwoda WR, Seymour L, Dansey RD. High-dose chemotherapy with hematopoietic rescue as primary treatment for metastatic breast cancer: a randomized trial. *J Clin Oncol* 1995;13:2483–2489.

Brenner MK, Rill DR, Moen RC, et al. Gene-marking to trace origin of relapse after autologous bone-marrow transplantation. *Lancet* 1993;341:85–86.

Burt RK, Deeg HJ, Lothian ST, Santos GW, eds. *On call in . . . Bone Marrow Transplantation.* Austin: RG Landes Co, 1996.

Collins RH Jr., Shpilberg O, Drobyski WR, et al. Donor leukocyte infusions in 140 patients with relapsed malignancy after allogeneic bone marrow transplantation. *J Clin Oncol* 1997;15:433–444.

Forman SJ, Blume KG, Thomas ED, eds. *Bone marrow transplantation.* Boston: Blackwell Scientific Publications, 1994.

Freedman AS, Gribben JG, Neuberg D, et al. High dose therapy and autologous bone marrow transplantation in patients with follicular lymphoma during first remission. *Blood* 1996;88:2780–2786.

Gianni AM, Bregni M, Siena S, et al. High-dose chemotherapy and autologous bone marrow transplantation compared with MACOP-B in aggressive B-cell lymphoma. *N Engl J Med* 1997;336:1290–1297.

Kernan NA, Bartsch G, Ash RC, et al. Retrospective analysis of 462 unrelated marrow transplants facilitated by the National Marrow Donor Program (NMDP) for treatment of acquired and congenital disorders of the lymphohematopoietic system and congenital metabolic disorders. *N Engl J Med* 1993;328:593–602.

Lazarus HM. Hematopoietic progenitor cell transplantation in breast cancer: current status and future directions. *Cancer Invest* 1998;16:102–126.

Peters WP, Ross M, Vredenburgh JJ, et al. High-dose chemotherapy and autologous bone marrow support as consolidation after standard-dose adjuvant therapy for high-risk primary breast cancer. *J Clin Oncol* 1993;11:1132–1143.

Philip T, Guglielmi C, Hagenbeek A, et al. Autologous bone marrow transplantation as compared with salvage chemotherapy in relapses of chemotherapy-sensitive non-Hodgkin's lymphoma. *N Engl J Med* 1995;333:1540–1545.

Rowe JM, Ciobann N, Ascensao J, et al. Recommended guidelines for the management of autologous and allogeneic bone marrow transplantation. *Ann Intern Med* 1994;120:143–158.

Schmitz N, Dreger P, Zander A, et al. Results of a randomized, controlled, multicentre study of recombinant human granulocyte colony-stimulating factor (filgrastim) in patients with Hodgkin's disease and non-Hodgkin's lymphoma undergoing autologous bone marrow transplantation. *Bone Marrow Transplant* 1995;15:261–266.

Stiff PJ, Bayer R, Kerger C, et al. High-dose chemotherapy with autologous transplantation for persistent/relapsed ovarian cancer: a multivariate analysis of survival for 100 consecutively treated patients. *J Clin Oncol* 1997;15:1309–1317.

Thomas ED, Clift TA. Indications for marrow transplantation in chronic myelogenous leukemia. *Blood* 1989;73:861–864.

Zittoun RA, Mandelli F, Willemze R, et al. Autologous or allogeneic bone marrow transplantation compared with intensive chemotherapy in acute myelogenous leukemia. *N Engl J Med* 1995;332:217–223.

Chemotherapy of
Human Cancer

Carcinomas of the Head and Neck

Ronald C. DeConti

Achievement of a management plan resulting in long-term control or cure for many patients with carcinomas of the head and neck remains an elusive, only partially realized goal for head and neck surgeons, radiation oncologists, and medical oncologists. Important gains in understanding the natural history of these neoplasms have been made, and the individual achievements of irradiation, surgical techniques, and chemotherapy have been stressed. However, only recently have these modalities been combined to form new treatment plans, and any increased benefit to the patient that might result from this multidisciplinary effort is now being explored.

This discussion focuses on the squamous cell carcinomas of the lining of the upper aerodigestive tract, which extends from the lip to the esophagus. These tumors account for about 5% of the new cancer cases seen in the United States each year. Excluded from this discussion are the melanomas, lymphomas, and sarcomas (which also occur in this area) as well as carcinomas of the thyroid, esophagus, and salivary glands. A cross-sectional view of the anatomic regions and the relative frequency of cancer occurring in each area are shown in Fig. 7-1. The large number of potential tumor sites and some difficulty in determining the exact site of origin have led to broad use of these larger subdivision terms in an attempt to avoid confusion and to group the related sites. Table 7-1 lists major sites within each of these anatomic subdivisions.

I. **Common and divergent characteristics.** Carcinomas of the head and neck are frequently considered together by students, generalists, and medical oncologists as though they represent a single therapeutic problem. A number of factors promote this concept.
   A. **Similarities.** In the United States, more than 90% of all lesions are squamous cell carcinomas, and these lesions occur predominantly in men (3:1). Most patients share common demographic and epidemiologic risk factors. The incidence of head and neck cancer increases with the use of alcohol and tobacco and with advancing age. Head and neck cancers occur in continuity, one with another, and it is occasionally difficult to determine the precise site of origin in the close confines of the complicated interrelated structures comprising the oral cavity, pharynx, larynx, and sinuses. Furthermore, patterns of spread are similar, with local failure, local recurrence, and regional node failures predominating. For carcinomas originating at most sites, spread below the clavicle is unusual, occurring in only a few patients, usually as pulmonary involvement. Bone lesions, usually the result of local

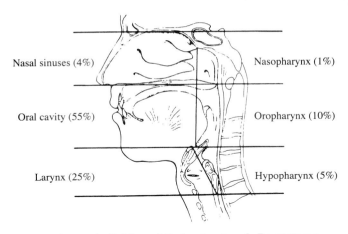

Fig. 7-1. Anatomic divisions of the head and neck. Percentages indicate the relative frequency of carcinoma in these regions.

Table 7-1. Upper aerodigestive tract sites

Region	Area	Site
Oral cavity	—	Lip
		Buccal mucosa
		Lower alveolar ridge
		Upper alveolar ridge
		Retromolar trigone
		Floor of mouth
		Hard palate
		Oral tongue
Pharynx	Nasopharynx	Posterior wall
		Lateral wall
	Oropharynx	Faucial arch
		Tonsillar fossa and tonsil
		Base of tongue
		Pharyngeal wall
	Hypopharynx	Piriform fossa
		Postcricoid area
		Posterior wall
Larynx	Supraglottis	Ventricular band
		Arytenoid
		Epiglottis
	Glottis	True vocal cords
	Subglottis	Subglottis
Paranasal sinuses		Antrum
		Nasal cavity
		Ethmoid
		Sphenoid
		Frontal

extension involving the mandible or floor of the skull, are not uncommon, although widespread bone metastases are unusual. A few patients develop hepatic metastases. Inanition, oral ulceration, fistula formation, respiratory difficulty, and aspiration characterize the late course of the disease. Recurrence after primary treatment usually occurs within 18 months, and patients who are not cured usually die within 3 years of diagnosis.

B. Differences. For the surgeon or radiation oncologist, the differences among carcinomas at different sites may be more significant than the similarities. Certainly, presenting signs and symptoms differ markedly. For example, patients with an anterior tongue lesion may describe pain, sensation of mass, and limited motion of the tongue. Hoarseness, dysphagia, or sore throat may predominate in patients with carcinoma of the larynx. More importantly, differences in location influence the frequency of nodal spread and the chances for contralateral node involvement. These factors frequently determine the optimal treatment plan.

II. Primary treatment. A discussion of the specific variations in primary treatment choices for the multitude of sites where head and neck carcinomas occur is beyond the scope of this chapter. In general, early lesions in most locations are suitable for treatment by surgery or irradiation, and the therapeutic choice is usually made by considering the complications of each treatment, that is, the deformities of definitive surgery or the complications of irradiation. With increasing failure rates and the likelihood of pathologic, if not clinical, lymph node involvement as tumor bulk increases, clinicians have begun to investigate combined-modality approaches. Radiation can be used electively before operation or postoperatively after a microscopic assessment of regional nodes provides the opportunity for postsurgical pathologic staging. Many studies now report improved local and regional node control after such multimodality approaches. Although substantial progress has been made in improving end results for early-stage lesions at many sites and in decreasing the morbidity and deformity from the treatment, the outcome for tumors in advanced stages remains poor: For stage III disease, the 3- to 5-year survival rate is 25% to 60%. For stage IV disease, long-term survival rates of 10% to 30% have been reported.

III. Staging. Any consideration of outcome in relation to treatment relies heavily on detailed pretreatment assessment of the extent of the tumor.

A. TNM classification. A complex site-specific staging system has been devised by the American Joint Committee on Cancer. This system incorporates a TNM classification to identify, clinically and pathologically, the size of the primary tumor (T), the presence and extent of regional node metastases (N), and the presence of distant metastases (M). Table 7-2 outlines the

Table 7-2.   TNM staging system for carcinomas of the oral cavity

Primary tumor

TX	No available information on primary tumor
T0	No evidence of primary tumor
Tis	Carcinoma *in situ*
T1	Greatest diameter of tumor ≤2 cm
T2	Greatest diameter of tumor >2–4 cm
T3	Greatest diameter of tumor >4 cm
T4	Invasion to adjacent structures such as antrum, pterygoid muscles, base of tongue, or skin of neck

Regional nodal status

NX	Nodes cannot be assessed
N0	No clinically positive node
N1	Single clinically positive ipsilateral node ≤3 cm in diameter
N2	Single clinically positive ipsilateral node >3–6 cm; or multiple clinically positive nodes, none >6 cm; or bilateral or contralateral nodes, none >6 cm
N3	Metastasis in a lymph node >6 cm in greatest dimension

Distant metastasis

MX	Not assessed
M0	No (known) distant metastasis
M1	Distant metastasis present

TNM system for carcinoma of the oral cavity. For lesions of the nasopharynx, hypopharynx, and larynx, fixation or anatomic extensions are substituted for tumor size when determining the extent of the primary lesion.

B. Stages. The stage grouping for head and neck cancers is shown in Table 7-3. Stages I and II are determined by the size of the tumor in the absence of nodal involvement or distant metastases. Stage III includes

Table 7-3.   Stage grouping for carcinomas of the oral cavity, pharynx, larynx, and paranasal sinuses

Stage	Groups
I	T1, N0, M0
II	T2, N0, M0
III	T3, N0, M0
	T1 or T2 or T3, N1, M0
IV	T4, N0 or N1, M0
	Any T, N2 or N3, M0
	Any T, any N, M1

both large tumors and tumors of any size with early regional node involvement. Stage IV lesions may be huge with local extension or may be of any size with distant metastatic disease. This stage grouping has been uniformly applied to each tumor site to demonstrate gradations in prognosis.

IV. **Chemotherapy**

A. **Prognostic factors.** Whether chemotherapy is considered for the treatment of advanced recurrent head and neck cancer or for preoperative induction treatment, a number of similar, single prognostic variables have now been clearly identified (Table 7-4).

1. **Stage of carcinoma.** Small lesions with minimal regional node involvement respond better than the massive tumors of stage IV. Patients with stage IV disease due to bulky lymph nodes commonly get little benefit from treatment. Response rates are lowest for stage IV disease with pulmonary or visceral metastases. Because patients with head and neck cancers have an increased risk of developing second primary neoplasms, the finding of distant metastases in the absence of primary or regional node recurrence suggests this possibility.

2. **State of health.** Both poor Eastern Cooperative Oncology Group (ECOG) performance status (see Table 3-2 in Chapter 3) and weight loss of more than 5% have been found to affect prognosis adversely. It is still unclear whether aggressive attempts to improve nutrition or restore cellular immunity with hyperalimentation result in gains in the response and survival rates.

3. **Prior treatment.** Many studies have reported the adverse effect of prior radiation therapy on

Table 7-4. Factors prognostic for response to chemotherapy

Favorable	Unfavorable
Stage III	Stage IV
No metastasis	Pulmonary metastasis
ECOG performance status 0–1	ECOG performance status 2–3
No weight loss	Weight loss
Normal immune mechanism	Impaired delayed hypersensitivity
Prior surgery	Prior irradiation
Long disease-free interval	Short disease-free interval
No prior chemotherapy	Prior chemotherapy
Combination chemotherapy	Single-agent chemotherapy
Poorly differentiated tumor	Well-differentiated tumor
Nasopharynx	Other sites

ECOG, Eastern Cooperative Oncology Group.

response to chemotherapy. This effect has usually been attributed to an impaired tumor blood supply, a large tumor burden, and poor patient performance status. The failure to respond to irradiation and a rapid relapse after radiation therapy have also been shown to affect response rates adversely.

B. **Pretreatment assessment.** The extent of evaluation required to determine the suitability of a patient for chemotherapy depends, to a considerable degree, on the intent of therapy and type of program to be employed. The major organ systems affected by the antineoplastic drugs under consideration are bone marrow, lungs, and kidneys. Any pretreatment assessment should consider not only careful evaluation of the size and extent of tumor but also the presence of comorbid disease processes involving these organ systems. A careful history, review of systems, physical assessment, and routine laboratory data may provide clues in these areas.

1. **Bone marrow function.** Chronic alcoholism and malnutrition or the effect of the tumor on glutition and appetite may contribute to the high incidence of folate deficiency seen in this population. Because of the additive effect of this deficiency and the inhibition of folate metabolism by methotrexate, there is often increased sensitivity to even small doses of methotrexate, which manifests as marked clinical toxicity.

2. **Pulmonary function.** Chronic obstructive pulmonary disease is common in this group of patients. Moderate to severe pretreatment reductions in timed forced expiratory volumes may be reduced further with treatment with bleomycin. If clinical assessment suggests impaired pulmonary reserve and bleomycin is to be part of the treatment program, pretreatment pulmonary function studies should be performed.

3. **Renal function.** Both cisplatin and methotrexate affect renal function. The major cumulative toxicity of cisplatin is renal. Unfortunately, there may be considerable impairment of renal function before the serum creatinine concentration rises; cisplatin doses of 80 to 120 mg/m^2 require serial determination of creatinine clearance to assess the cumulative effects of the drug on renal function.

Limited renal excretion of methotrexate prolongs the duration of a high serum concentration, which in turn extends the duration of impaired DNA synthesis for normal as well as neoplastic tissues. Weekly intravenous methotrexate is usually given to patients with advanced disease after it is established that the serum creatinine level is normal. A careful clinical assessment at the time of each subsequent dose is probably a more reliable indicator of actual and potential methotrexate toxicity than are serial determinations of creatinine in this situation. Most episodes of serious methotrexate toxicity relate to a failure to appreciate intercurrent events that limit excretion of these relatively low doses of the drug. The most common of these toxicities is probably dehydration, which is related to progressive disease, increasingly poor oral intake, nausea and vomiting, or mucositis that may have been caused by prior drug treatment. Third-space reservoirs created by pleural effusions or ascites may lead to delayed clearance, prolonged serum drug levels, and increased toxicity. The addition of any drug that further alters renal clearance of methotrexate may tip the balance toward serious toxicity. Aspirin and other nonsteroidal antiinflammatory agents, probenecid, sulfonamides, phenytoin, cefoxitin, and gentamicin may decrease methotrexate clearance and increase toxicity. Careful patient assessment at intervals with these considerations in mind helps to avoid these pitfalls.

C. **Single-agent responses.** Methotrexate, bleomycin, fluorouracil, cisplatin, carboplatin, and doxorubicin (Adriamycin) have been studied extensively as individual agents for head and neck carcinomas. More recently, ifosfamide, the taxanes, and vinorelbine have been shown to have activity. Most combinations derive from these agents.

  1. **Methotrexate.** In efforts to improve its therapeutic index, methotrexate has been more extensively investigated for the management of head and neck cancer than any other solid tumor.

  a. **Intravenous methotrexate** in doses of 40 to 60 mg/m^2 weekly is probably the most widely accepted conventional single-agent treatment for this group of tumors. Treatment with methotrexate results in objective response in 25% to 50% of patients, 7% to 10% of which are complete responses. Responses may occur after 1 to 2 weeks but usually require 4 to 6 weeks to become evident. Median response durations range from 2 to 6 months. Responders survive significantly longer than nonresponders. Treatment is usually given on an outpatient basis, and drug-related mortality is less than 4%.

  b. **Intraarterial infusions of methotrexate** either alone or with systemic leucovorin have been used in an attempt to improve drug concentrations in tumor tissue and to improve the therapeutic index of treatment. Although these techniques have resulted in marginally superior response rates, the lack of a single predominant blood supply to most tumors, the technical difficulties of the procedure, and the morbidity of problems with clot, embolus, and infection have precluded widespread adoption of this approach; it is not recommended for general use.

c. **Leucovorin rescue** has made possible the use of moderate (240 to 500 mg/m^2) to high (1 to 3 g/m^2) doses of methotrexate in attempts to improve response rates. Although individual investigators have reported favorable rates with decreased morbidity using these higher doses of methotrexate, the duration of response is not increased, and two comparative trials have demonstrated no advantage of these treatment approaches over weekly intravenous methotrexate. The need for hydration, urinary alkalinization, and careful monitoring of renal clearance and the high cost of treatment have been important factors in limiting general use of this approach, and it is not recommended outside a research setting.

2. **Bleomycin** attracted interest for treatment of head and neck cancers because of its generally mild myelosuppressive effects and the potential for its application in combination with myelosuppressive chemotherapy. Bleomycin, 10 to 30 units/m^2, is usually given weekly, biweekly, or on a 5-day-per-month schedule by intramuscular and intravenous injections. These approaches are convenient for outpatient use. Tumor response rarely occurs at cumulative doses of less than 200 units/m^2, and response most often requires a total dose of 300 units/m^2. These doses usually produce significant mucosal toxicity. Response rates range between 15% and 25% and are generally inferior in duration to those achieved with methotrexate. The mucosal toxicity that accompanies the use of bleomycin is generally more frequent and severe than that produced with the use of a weekly methotrexate schedule.

3. **Cisplatin.** Cisplatin, 40 to 60 mg/m^2 i.v., is given on an every-3-week schedule. Higher doses result in an increased risk of renal toxicity unless special precautions are taken. Doses of 80 to 120 mg/m^2 may be tolerated if preceded by hydration and accompanied by mannitol adminis-

tration (with or without furosemide) for diuresis to protect renal function (see Chapter 5). The effectiveness of the selective serotonin receptor antagonists (ondansetron [Zofran] and granisetron [Kytril]) in control of nausea and vomiting in the first 24 hours after therapy has increased patients' tolerance to cisplatin and has made it considerably easier to administer an intermediate dose of this drug on an outpatient basis. Cisplatin produces objective tumor responses in about 25% of patients, many of whom were treated previously with other antineoplastic drugs. Occasionally, dramatic tumor responses occur, although the frequency of complete remission is still low. Its major side effects are severe nausea and vomiting (which may be more of a problem after 24 hours than in the first 24 hours, during which serotonin receptor antagonists offer better protection), tinnitus, occasional high-tone deafness, peripheral neuropathy, and most significantly, renal toxicity (with progressive loss in creatinine clearance in some patients).

4. **Carboplatin.** An analog of cisplatin that produces minimal renal toxicity, little peripheral neuropathy, and less emesis, carboplatin has a favorable toxicity profile that gives it considerable practical utility in head and neck cancer. Doses of 360 to 400 mg/m^2, usually divided in three daily doses and repeated at 4-week intervals, have resulted in response rates approaching those of cisplatin. Its ease of administration and favorable therapeutic index recommend its use for palliation. Prolonged thrombocytopenia can be dose limiting. Adoption of the Calvert formula to determine dose may improve both tolerance and efficacy.

5. **5-Fluorouracil.** 5-Fluorouracil (5-FU) may be of somewhat greater value for oral cavity lesions than other agents; it has an overall 15% response rate. Use by infusion was popularized by a small phase II study demonstrating a much higher response rate, which has not been duplicated. However, most combinations with 5-FU have used the drug this way. Attempts to improve response rates using leucovorin in conjunction with 5-FU have not yet demonstrated long-term value.

6. **Ifosfamide.** Phase II studies have shown encouraging response rates of 20% to 42% for ifosfamide, with mesna used as a uroprotector in both bolus and infusion schedules.

7. **Taxanes.** Both paclitaxel and docetaxel have shown high response rates in phase II trials.
   a. **Paclitaxel**, 250 mg/m^2 every 3 weeks with granulocyte colony-stimulating factor

(G-CSF) support, achieved responses of 40% of advanced head and neck cancers in an ECOG phase II trial. Other schedules and doses are under investigation; a 3-hour infusion every 3 weeks has been found to be tolerable and convenient for outpatient therapy.

  b. **Docetaxel** has been shown to produce response rates of 32% to 50% in small phase II trials. A dose of 100 mg/m^2 i.v. administered over 1 hour every 3 weeks was used to achieve these results.

 8. **Other drugs**

  a. **Anthracyclines** appear to be of little overall value except in nasopharyngeal cancer, in which both doxorubicin and mitoxantrone have shown responses in about 25% of patients.

  b. **Vinca alkaloids.** Vincristine and vinblastine achieve low response rates. Vinorelbine appeared promising in early trials.

  c. **Gemcitabine** has shown modest activity (18% response rate) in phase II trials to date.

  d. **Topoisomerase inhibitors** have shown little activity.

  e. **Retinoids** have not yet been shown to be effective in advanced disease.

  f. **Numerous biologic response modifiers** have been studied but have not demonstrated any value in clinical practice.

D. **Combination chemotherapy responses.** Multiple attempts have been made to improve single-agent response rates with combination chemotherapy. A number of studies using methotrexate, bleomycin, fluorouracil, cisplatin, and carboplatin in a variety of schedules have been reported. More recently, phase II combination investigations include ifosfamide and paclitaxel (Taxol).

  The ECOG, in a comparison of methotrexate, bleomycin, and cisplatin versus weekly methotrexate, demonstrated a clear-cut advantage for combination chemotherapy. Forty-eight percent of patients with advanced disease responded to an outpatient program using methotrexate, bleomycin, and cisplatin, compared with 35% using methotrexate alone. Complete remissions were achieved in 16% of patients receiving combination chemotherapy and in 8% treated with methotrexate alone. The median duration of response was the same in both treatment groups, and no survival advantage was demonstrated for the combination treatment. Although neither response rate is exceptional, the careful randomization and stratification procedures used lend weight to the result.

Combinations of cisplatin or carboplatin and fluorouracil or methotrexate demonstrate like outcomes: improved response rates but no overall gain in survival. Phase II studies with newer agents, usually combined with cisplatin, suggest similar results. Comparative assessments of the quality of life or of symptom scores have rarely been performed.

E. **Combined-modality treatment.** Attempts to increase tumor destruction with drugs before definitive therapy or together with radiation therapy are not new, although developments in combination chemotherapy reawakened enthusiasm for this approach.

1. **Drugs before irradiation or surgery (neoadjuvant therapy)**

    a. **Methotrexate.** In several small, single-institution studies, methotrexate in moderate and high doses with leucovorin rescue was given for several doses or cycles before irradiation or surgery. These schedules produced response rates of about 75% and avoided the problems of oral mucositis and ulceration reported by the older studies of concomitant chemotherapy with radiotherapy. No data are available to permit comparisons of these rescue programs with weekly methotrexate schedules.

    b. **Combination chemotherapy.** A number of combination drug therapy programs have been developed as initial treatment for advanced locoregional disease. These programs were intended either to reduce tumor bulk and allow more effective radiotherapy or to improve resectability of advanced lesions. In general, the programs use high-dose cisplatin in conjunction with hydration and diuretics (see Chapter 5) combined with either bleomycin or fluorouracil and administered by intravenous infusion for 3 to 5 days. Vincristine is frequently included, and methotrexate is usually omitted. These programs produce high response rates (67% to 94%). Complete clinical disappearance of tumor is achieved in 19% to 28% of patients, and partial response is achieved in 48% to 74%. After one to three cycles of drug treatment, surgery, irradiation, or both follow. The number of patients with advanced locoregional disease who were made disease free was higher than expected based on pretreatment staging expectations. Improvement in survival is limited to those patients who achieved complete response.

    The achievements and limitations of this plan of therapy are outlined in Table 7-5. In

Table 7-5. Achievements of induction or neoadjuvant chemotherapy for patients with head and neck cancers

Major tumor regressions occur in 60% to 90% of patients with locally advanced disease.

Complete clinical regression occurs in 20% to 50%.

Response rates increase with the number of cycles given, up to three.

Pathologic complete regressions are confirmed in 25% to 60% of patients with clinical complete responses.

Treatment does not adversely affect surgical or radiation therapy complications.

Drug response appears to predict response to irradiation.

Complete responders may achieve locoregional disease control with radiation therapy and avoid surgery.

Quality of life may be improved for patients with tumors in some sites by organ preservation.

Frequency of distant metastasis as cause of treatment failure is reduced.

Complete responders have longer survival.

Overall survival is unchanged.

general, neoadjuvant therapy best remains in the context of a clinical investigation.

The most important demonstration of the value of neoadjuvant or induction chemotherapy relates to organ preservation. Trials stimulated by the high response rates achieved by these treatments have shown the ability to preserve the larynx and voice. The best known trial (VA 268) showed that laryngeal preservation was possible in 64% of patients who received induction chemotherapy followed by radiation therapy, with survival rates comparable to those for patients treated with laryngectomy and radiation therapy. Survival was not compromised in patients who received chemotherapy. Long-term survival was the same, with evidence of preservation of voice and presumed maintenance of quality of life.

2. **Concurrent chemotherapy and radiotherapy.** Bleomycin, fluorouracil, methotrexate, and cisplatin have been administered synchronously with radiation therapy in attempts to demonstrate synergistic effects. Most uncontrolled studies suggested improved tumor responses and some gain in survival for patients with unresectable disease. Although randomized trials have found improvement in the initial response or disease-free survival rate, gains in overall survival have been difficult to document. Two studies demonstrated benefit for oral cavity

primary lesions with concurrent bleomycin or fluorouracil. Enhanced mucositis has been a common limitation of combined treatment.

Cisplatin appears attractive as an agent for concurrent therapy because of its radiosensitizing properties, established activity, and paucity of mucosal toxicity. Weekly dosing of cisplatin during radiotherapy resulted in higher response rates but no overall difference in complete response or survival rate compared with radiotherapy alone. When cisplatin was given as a 100-mg/m^2 bolus every 3 weeks with concurrent radiation therapy in a Radiation Therapy Oncology (RTOG) trial, improvement in the number of complete responders and 4-year survival rates was suggested.

A randomized intergroup trial has recently demonstrated improved survival in nasopharyngeal carcinoma with that same schedule of cisplatin together with radiation therapy compared with radiation therapy alone. After radiation therapy, patients also received two cycles of cisplatin and 5-FU.

Because combination chemotherapy has been demonstrated to be more effective than single-agent therapy, studies are now focusing on combination chemotherapy together with radiation therapy. Because of the more severe local and systemic toxicities that can be associated with these regimens, attempts have been made to modify radiation therapy scheduling to facilitate the administration of combined-modality therapy while avoiding intolerable toxicity. Newer studies are evaluating split-course schedules and rapid alterations of chemotherapy and radiation therapy as well as hyperfractionated radiation. Preliminary results suggest improved short-term tumor control and a survival advantage despite increased toxicity. This subject continues as an active and promising area of clinical investigation, and patients should be encouraged to participate in these trials.

3. **Drugs as posttreatment adjuvants.** Whereas the most recent emphasis in head and neck cancer has been on achieving gains in early tumor control, little attention has been paid to the potential of postoperative or postirradiation adjuvant drug therapy studies. Suggestive phase II data have not been confirmed in larger, randomized phase III comparisons. Reasons for negative results include small sample size, inadequate therapy, poor patient compliance, and statistical analysis based on intention to treat. Posttreatment adjuvant therapy remains investigational.

F. Selected treatment plans. Four types of drug treatment programs are displayed in Table 7-6.
  1. Cytoreductive induction treatment
   a. Selection of patients. This treatment is designed to reduce tumor bulk before surgery or radiation therapy in patients with advanced-stage disease and no prior therapy. The induction treatment regimen is intended for hospitalized patients after assessment of the extent of the tumor and an evaluation to exclude comorbid disease processes that might unacceptably increase the risks of treatment.
   b. Administration
    (1) Cisplatin plus 5-fluorouracil. Oral hydration is begun the evening before treatment. On the morning of treatment, an intravenous infusion of 5% dextrose in 0.5 N saline with potassium chloride, 20 mEq/L, and magnesium sulfate, 1 g/L, is begun at a rate of 200 mL/h. One of a number of intensive regimens to alleviate nausea and vomiting should be begun (see Chapter 27). Furosemide, 40 mg i.v., and mannitol, 12.5 g i.v., are given after the first liter. Immediately thereafter, if the patient is voiding freely, cisplatin, 100 mg/m^2, is added to a calibrated solution set and infused intravenously over a 30-minute period. 5-FU, 1,000 mg/m^2, is divided between 2 liters of 5% dextrose in 0.5 N saline, with potassium chloride, 20 mEq/L, given every 24 hours. A continuous infusion of 5-FU is maintained for 5 days, usually with an infusion pump. The necessity for additional diuretics is judged by the extent of nausea and vomiting, the urinary volume, and evidence of congestive heart failure. If adequate oral intake has not been resumed, additional intravenous fluids may be given. An infusion pump may be used to help ensure an even rate of flow.

The patient may be discharged after completion of the treatment course, depending on drug tolerance and the ability to eat and drink. An interim clinic visit before a second induction course is recommended as a safeguard. A second course of treatment is planned on day 22 but should be administered only after hematologic

Table 7-6.   Selected drug treatment programs in head and neck cancer

Intent	Suitability	Scheme
Cytoreductive induction treatment	Advanced stage, no prior treatment	**CF** Cisplatin 100 mg/m^2 i.v. on day 1 with induced diuresis, *and* Fluorouracil 1,000 mg/m^2/d as 24-h infusion on days 1–5 Cycle repeats in 3–4 wk
Concurrent radiotherapy	Advanced stage, no prior treatment	**Daily radiation therapy** Cisplatin 100 mg/m^2 i.v. on day 1 with induced diuresis repeat day 22, 43 **Split-course radiation therapy** Cisplatin 75 mg/m^2 i.v. on day 1 with induced diuresis, *and* Fluorouracil 1,000 mg/m^2 as 24-h infusion on days 1–4 Cycle repeats in 4 weeks Radiotherapy 30 Gy/15 fractions begun on day 1 Evaluate at week 9: CR or unresectable—repeat third chemotherapy cycle with 30 Gy/15 fractions; PR, stable, and resectable—have surgery with a third cycle of chemotherapy and radiotherapy (30 Gy/15 fractions) 2–6 wk after operation
Palliation	Any prior treatment	Either cisplatin 20 mg/m^2 i.v. on days 1–5 *or* Carboplatin AUC 6 on day 1, *and* Fluorouracil 800 mg/m^2 on days 1–5 by ambulatory infusion pump Cycle repeats in 3–4 wk Paclitaxel (Taxol) 175 mg/m^2 as 3-h infusion on day 1 with steroid premedication Cisplatin 75 mg/m^2 i.v. on day 1 with induced diuresis Cycle repeats in 3 wk
Palliation	Prior treatment and contraindications to combination drugs	Methotrexate 40–60 mg/m^2 i.v. weekly Paclitaxel (Taxol) 175–200 mg/m^2 i.v. every 3 wk with steroid premedication

CR, complete response; PR, partial response.

values and serum creatinine levels are normal. If tumor regression is continuing on day 43 after two cycles of treatment, a third cycle may be considered, although the cumulative risks of renal and pulmonary toxicity increase with continued treatment. At this point, irradiation, surgery, or both should be considered once again.

2. **Concurrent chemotherapy and conventional fraction radiation therapy.** Cisplatin, 100 mg/m², is given with appropriate hydration, diuresis, and antiemetics on days 1, 22, and 43 of radiation therapy, with attention to the cautions of cisplatin therapy. This is a relatively straightforward plan with no added mucosal toxicity.

3. **Concurrent chemotherapy and split-course radiotherapy.** With this program, the dose of cisplatin is reduced to 75 mg/m², and fluorouracil infusion duration is limited to 4 days. The plan of therapy is outlined in Table 7-6. Treatment is administered with hydration and antiemetics as described in a previous section.

   Careful attention to fluid and nutritional support during possible periods of intense mucositis is necessary. In potentially operable patients, a decision for surgery is usually made after two courses of chemotherapy.

4. **Combination chemotherapy for advanced recurrent disease.** The approach to advanced recurrent disease is based on prior treatment and the perceived ability of the patient to tolerate intensive chemotherapy.

   a. **Cisplatin plus 5-fluorouracil (CF).** With advanced recurrent disease, two courses of treatment with CF (see Section IV.F.1 and Table 7-6) may be elected, followed by an intermittent program with lower doses of drug.

   b. **Ambulatory infusion.** An alternative treatment choice uses three to five daily doses of cisplatin or one dose of carboplatin together with continuous-infusion 5-FU administered using an ambulatory infusion pump. Either cisplatin, 20 mg/m²/day i.v. for 5 days, or carboplatin, area under the curve (AUC) 6 on day 1 only as a short infusion, can be combined with 5-FU, 800 mg/m²/day for 5 days as a continuous infusion. Dividing the dosage of cisplatin eliminates the need for aggressive hydration, shortens and simplifies the chemotherapy procedures, and promotes outpatient usage of these regimens.

    c. **Paclitaxel and Cisplatin. Paclitaxel (Taxol),** 175 mg/m^2, is administered as a 3-hour infusion in 500 to 1,000 mL of D5W or 0.9% sodium chloride after premedication with steroids (see Chapter 5) to avoid possibilities of shock. Thirty to sixty minutes before treatment, the patient is premedicated with 50 mg i.v. diphenhydramine and 300 mg i.v. cimetidine. Additional hydration is given during this period before cisplatin treatment. Mannitol, 12.5 g i.v. is given first, then **cisplatin**, 75 mg/m^2 i.v., is infused over 30 to 60 minutes. After cisplatin infusion, an additional 25 g of mannitol is given, followed by 2 liters of D5½ N saline plus 20 mEq/L of potassium chloride over several hours. Furosemide, 40 mg i.v., is given if necessary. Less aggressive rates of hydration may be necessary in older patients to prevent the development of congestive heart failure and pulmonary edema. Antiemetics are given as described previously.

5. Methotrexate alone for advanced disease

    a. **Selection of patients.** With a number of increased response rates reported for drug combinations compared with methotrexate alone, single-agent methotrexate should probably be reserved for the following selected patients:

- Patients in relapse after induction treatment programs without methotrexate
- Patients who refuse treatment with cisplatin or Taxol
- Patients whose neuropathy excludes a cisplatin treatment program
- Patients whose reliability and follow-up opportunities are poor

    b. **Treatment plan.** The usual starting dose of methotrexate is 40 mg/m^2; if advanced age, nutritional status, anemia, borderline renal function, or other factors suggest sensitivity of normal tissues to methotrexate might be increased, the initial dose may be reduced to as low as 20 mg/m^2. Blood cell counts are done weekly, and if there is no evidence of mucositis or myelosuppression, the dose is escalated to a maximum of 60 mg/m^2. Most patients tolerate this treatment with minimal nausea and vomiting. A few require antiemetics. Careful attention to oral hydration may be helpful for preventing or reducing the severity of mucositis (see Chapter 27). Candidiasis is common and, if present, should be treated with nystatin (Mycostatin) or another antifungal agent. If mucositis or myelosuppression occurs, treatments are delayed until they clear and blood cell counts are normal. Six to eight weeks of therapy may be necessary to achieve a response.

V. Problems in supportive care

A. **Support systems.** The population of patients with head and neck cancer includes many elderly men—often social reprobates, recluses, heavy smokers and drinkers, and occasionally frank derelicts. They are frequently divorced or separated from their families, and many live alone, often in reduced circumstances. Lack of family, friends, resources, and initiative are often impediments to adequate care, especially in advanced-disease situations in which close follow-up, regular clinic visits, and adherence to treatment schedules are important. These patients desperately need a primary caregiver to be in the home or closely allied with the home to promote their well-being and optimal use of medical care and to derive advantage from the health care delivery system. Social service, ministerial help, American Cancer Society patient programs (such as I Can Cope), patient support groups, Alcoholics Anonymous, and other social care groups should be enlisted to help the patient cope with illness. Smoking cessation programs may be appropriate for those with early cancers that may be cured.

B. **Nutrition.** Gradual, progressive weight loss and inanition are common factors in the relentless illness of many patients. Their nutrition is generally inadequate, and repetitive efforts at reinforcing the need for a high-calorie diet, as free of alcohol as possible, must be given. Depending on the location of the tumor and the particular problems with swallowing, efforts need to be extended on a regular basis to ensure adequate patient nutrition. Many patients, or their families, need to be instructed in the use of blended foods, high-protein supplements, or both. Some patients benefit from the use of a pediatric feeding tube when deformities in the anatomy prevent adequate swallowing. In selected patients, feeding by a gastrostomy tube may be appropriate, especially early in the patient's clinical course when it is hoped that it may be only a temporary expedient. Most patients benefit from any attempts at oral hyperalimentation. The role of intravenous hyperalimentation is not clear and needs to be considered early in the management course during the perioperative or radiation therapy period when induction treatment is taking place. Its role for patients with advanced disease state is still unclear. Efforts to maintain nutrition must be reinforced at every opportunity with the family, the caregiver, and the patient. Dietary advice or consultation with a dietetic department should be sought.

C. **Mouth care.** An important problem for some patients with head and neck cancer is mouth care. Many patients have difficulty with secretions. Xerostomia may be produced by radiation therapy and may require treatment with artificial saliva. An additional agent that may be helpful is pilocarpine, 5 to 10 mg given orally three times daily with water. At the opposite extreme, patients with posterior tongue lesions may have edema and swelling that precludes adequate swallowing, and the pooling of secretions and subsequent aspiration becomes a problem. These patients may benefit from the use of suction to drain their secretions. Cleansing mouthwash may be appropriate (see Chapter 27), and efforts at dental hygiene need to be maintained. Radiation-induced bone necrosis or fistulas need to be cleaned or débrided and occasionally packed with toothpaste or other material to promote comfort. Dental consultation is helpful in many patients, particularly before radiation therapy.

D. **Hypothyroidism.** Weakness, apathy, listlessness, and weight loss may develop insidiously in patients subjected to thyroid irradiation or resection. Such symptoms may mistakenly be construed as suggesting disease relapse.

E. **Hypercalcemia.** Hypercalcemia is common in patients with epidermoid carcinoma of the head and neck. As many as 23% of patients with advanced recurrent head and neck cancers may experience hypercalcemia before their death. In general, this phenomenon accompanies late-stage recurrent tumor, often with little evidence of bone involvement. Dehydration, all too common in these patients, may be a precipitating factor; in many patients, hypercalcemia is mild and easily controlled with hydration, saline diuresis, or both. Although hydration, saline diuresis, or reduction in tumor (achieved with irradiation, drug therapy, or surgery) frequently reverses this phenomenon, a few patients require pamidronate for adequate treatment (see Chapter 30). If patients have advanced disease without the hope of substantial palliation, consideration can also be given to withholding treatment for hypercalcemia and allowing the patient to die a natural, more comfortable death than might occur if the hypercalcemia were treated and the patient were obligated to die of locally progressive disease.

F. **Aspiration pneumonia.** The anatomic deformities induced by surgery, recurrent tumor, or both make patients with head and neck cancer highly susceptible to aspiration of pooled secretions. Fever, tachycardia, tachypnea, rales, and infiltrates in the lung are usual findings and are often confused with primary bacterial pneumonia. Knowledge of the aspiration or observation of the event may be the only decisive method of proving the diagnosis. Immediate recognition of aspiration should be followed by treatment with steroids, antibiotics, or both.

G. **Granulocytopenia and infection.** There is always an urgent need to identify pulmonary and other infections quickly in the presence of drug-induced granulocytopenia. The mortality due to pneumonia and sepsis is high in this situation. Appropriate cultures are needed in an effort to document infection and help distinguish the problem from aspiration. Fever in a granulocytopenic patient should be treated promptly with broad-spectrum antibiotics without awaiting results of blood or sputum cultures (see Chapter 28). In selected situations, the use of G-CSF may reduce the duration of granulocytopenia and ameliorate infections.

VI. **Cancer prevention.** No discussion of treatment of head and neck cancer would be complete without mention of efforts in cancer prevention. Clearly, alcohol and tobacco use are synergiologic epidemiologic factors in the development of these neoplasms, and all patients should be encouraged in behavior modification and other cessation programs.

Recent evidence suggests that isotretinoin (13-*cis*-retinoic acid) can both clinically improve and histologically mature oral leukoplakia and erythroplakia. Further, the incidence of second head and neck cancers and second primary lung cancers appears to be reduced by this treatment. Although the optimal dose is not yet established, 5.6 mg/m^2/day given orally appears to be a relatively safe and probably effective dosage. This represents a new and challenging area for research.

SELECTED READINGS

Adelstein DJ, Sharran VM, Earle AS, et al. Simultaneous versus sequential combined technique therapy for squamous cell head and neck cancer. *Cancer* 1990;65:1685–1691.

Al-Kourainy K, Kish J, Ensley J, et al. Achievement of superior survival for histologically negative versus histologically positive clinically complete responders to cisplatin combination in patients with locally advanced head and neck cancer. *Cancer* 1987;59:233.

Al-Sarraf M, LeBlanc M, Giri PG, et al. Chemoradiotherapy vs. radiotherapy in patients with advanced nasopharyngeal cancer: phase III randomized Intergroup study 0099. *J Clin Oncol* 1998;16:1310–1317.

Al-Sarraf M, Pajak TF, Marcial VA, et al. Concurrent radiotherapy and chemotherapy with cisplatin in inoperable squamous cell carcinoma of the head and neck: an RTOG study. *Cancer* 59:259–265, 1987.

American Joint Committee on Cancer. *AJCC cancer staging manual.* 5th ed. Philadelphia: Lippincott-Raven, 1997:294.

Department of Veterans Affairs Laryngeal Cancer Study Group. Induction chemotherapy plus radiation compared with surgery plus radiation in patients with advanced laryngeal cancer. *N Engl J Med* 1991;324:1685–1690.

Merlano M, Benasso M, et al. Five-year update of a randomized trial of alternating radiotherapy and chemotherapy compared with radiotherapy alone in treatment of unresectable squamous cell carcinoma of the head and neck. *J Natl Canc Inst* 1996;88(9):583–589.

Murphy BA. New drug therapy for squamous carcinoma of the head and neck. *Curr Opin Oncol* 1996;8(3):221–226.

Carcinoma of the Lung

Joan H. Schiller

Carcinoma of the lung is responsible for more than 155,000 deaths each year in the United States. This represents one third of all deaths due to cancer and more than the number of deaths due to breast, colon, and prostate cancers combined. The incidence of the disease continues to rise, particularly in women and blacks, and thus is likely to present a significant public health problem for years to come.

Lung cancer consists of four major histologic types: adenocarcinoma, squamous cell carcinoma, large cell carcinoma, and small cell carcinoma. Because of the unique biologic features of small cell lung cancer (SCLC), its staging and treatment differ radically from the other three types of lung cancer, which collectively are called non–small cell lung cancer (NSCLC). Thus, these two groups are addressed in two separate sections.

I. **Etiology.** Lung cancer is predominantly a disease of smokers. Eighty percent of lung cancer occurs in active or former smokers, and an additional 5% of cases are estimated to occur as a consequence of passive exposure to tobacco smoke. Tobacco smoke causes an increased incidence of all four histologic types of lung cancer, although adenocarcinoma (particularly the bronchoalveolar variant) is also found in nonsmokers. Other risk factors for lung cancer include exposure to asbestos or radon. Familial factors, such as activity of carcinogen-metabolizing hepatic enzyme systems (e.g., 4-debrisoquine hydroxylase), may also play a role in determining an individual's propensity to develop lung cancer.

II. **Molecular biology**. Numerous genetic changes have been associated with lung tumors. Most common among these include activation or overexpression of the myc family of oncogenes in SCLC and NSCLC and of K-ras oncogene in NSCLC, particularly adenocarcinoma. Inactivation or deletion of the p53 and retinoblastoma tumor-suppressor genes, and a recently identified tumor-suppressor gene on chromosome 3p (the FHIT gene), have been found in 50% to 90% of patients with SCLC. Abnormalities of p53 and 3p have been associated with 50% to 70% of cases of NSCLC. The clinical significance of p53 mutations is unclear; early studies suggested that p53 mutations imparted a negative prognosis, but subsequent studies have refuted this, and even suggested the contrary. The K-ras mutation is more frequently found in smokers, those with adenocarcinoma, and those with poorly differentiated tumors. It is also associated with poor prognosis.

III. **Screening**. Three U.S. randomized screening studies failed to detect an impact on mortality of screening high-risk patients with chest radiographs or sputum cytology, although earlier-stage cancers were detected in the screened groups. At this time, routine screening for lung cancer is not recommended.

IV. **Non–small cell lung cancer**. The prognosis and treatment of NSCLC are dependent primarily on stage of disease at the time of diagnosis. Although histologic differences (adenocarcinoma versus large cell carcinoma versus squamous cell carcinoma) among the NSCLCs affect their natural history and presentation, these differences are of relatively little importance in determining patient management.

A. **Staging.** The current TNM staging classification is shown in Table 8-1. The stage grouping (Table 8-2) was updated in 1997 to reflect a need for greater specificity in staging and greater homogeneity of outcome within stages. The major differences in the new stage grouping are (a) stages I and II are divided into IA and IB, and IIA and IIB, respectively; (b) stage T3, N0, M0 is moved to IIB; and (c) satellite pulmonary nodules within the same lobe of the primary tumor are classified as T4 (nodules within another lobe on the ipsilateral side are M1).

B. **Pretreatment evaluation.** The diagnosis of lung cancer is usually made by bronchial biopsy or percutaneous needle biopsy. Although the disease is usually discovered on chest radiographs, a computed tomography (CT) scan of the chest is necessary to evaluate the extent of the primary disease, mediastinal extension or lymph adenopathy, and the presence or absence of other parenchymal nodules in patients in whom surgical resection is a consideration. CT of the upper abdomen is performed to look for asymptomatic hepatic or adrenal metastases. Bone scans should be obtained for the patient with bone pain, chest pain, or an elevated calcium or alkaline phosphatase level. Head CT is not routinely done in the absence of central nervous system (CNS) signs or symptoms. Preoperative mediastinoscopy and biopsy are recommended for mediastinal lymph nodes greater than 1 cm on CT scan.

Pulmonary function testing is necessary before definitive surgery. Increased postoperative morbidity is associated with a predicted postoperative 1-second forced expiratory volume of less than 800 to 1,000 mL; a preoperative maximum voluntary ventilation less than 35% of predicted; a carbon monoxide diffusing capacity less than 60% of predicted; and an arterial oxygen pressure (Po_2) of less than 60 mm Hg or a carbon dioxide pressure (Pco_2) of more than 45 mm Hg.

C. **Management**

1. **Stage I disease.** Lobectomy is the treatment of choice for stage I NSCLC, with cure rates of 60% to 80% reported. Within stage I, patients with T2, N0 disease do not fare as well as those with T1, N0 cancers. In about 20% of patients

Table 8-1. TNM definitions

Primary tumor

TX	Tumor proven by the presence of malignant cells in broncho-pulmonary secretions but not visualized roentgenographically or bronchoscopically, or any tumor that cannot be assessed as in a retreatment staging
T0	No evidence of primary tumor
Tis	Carcinoma *in situ*
T1	A tumor that is 3 cm or less in greatest dimension, surrounded by lung or visceral pleura, and without evidence of invasion proximal to a lobar bronchus at bronchoscopy
T2	A tumor more than 3 cm in greatest dimension, or a tumor of any size that either invades the visceral pleura or has associated atelectasis or obstructive pneumonitis extending to the hilar region. At bronchoscopy, the proximal extent of demonstrable tumor must be within a lobar bronchus or at least 2 cm distal to the carina. Any associated atelectasis or obstructive pneumonitis must involve less than an entire lung
T3	A tumor of any size with direct extension into the chest wall (including superior sulcus tumors), diaphragm, or the mediastinal pleura or pericardium without involving the heart, great vessels, trachea, esophagus, or vertebral body, or a tumor in the main bronchus within 2 cm of the carina without involving the carina
T4	A tumor of any size with invasion of the mediastinum or involving the heart, great vessels, trachea, esophagus, vertebral body or carina or presence of malignant pleural effusion; a satellite nodule within the same lobe

Nodal involvement

N0	No demonstrable metastasis to regional lymph nodes
N1	Metastasis to lymph nodes in the peribronchial or the ipsilateral hilar region, or both, including direct extension
N2	Metastasis to ipsilateral mediastinal lymph nodes or subcarinal lymph nodes, or both
N3	Metastasis to contralateral mediastinal lymph nodes, contralateral hilar lymph nodes, ipsilateral or contralateral scalene or supraclavicular lymph nodes

Distant metastasis (M)

MX	Cannot be assessed
M0	No distant metastasis
M1	Distant metastasis, including pulmonary nodule not in the same lobe as the primary tumor

Table 8-2.   1997 Revisions to the International Staging Classification for Lung Cancer

Stage	TNM subset	5-yr survival rate (%) Clinical stage	5-yr survival rate (%) Pathologic stage
IA	T1, N0, M0	61	67
IB	T2, N0, M0	38	57
IIA	T1, N1, M0	34	55
IIB	T2, N1, M0	24	39
	T3, N0, M0		
IIIA	T3, N1, M0	9	25
	T1–3, N2, M0		
IIIB	T4, any N, M0	13	23
	Any T, N3, M0		
IV	Any T, any N, M1	1	

From Mountain. *Chest* 1997; 111:1710–1717.

with medical contraindications to surgery but with adequate pulmonary function, high-dose radiotherapy results in cure. No role of adjuvant chemotherapy for stage I NSCLC has been identified. Patients with a resected stage I NSCLC are at high risk for the development of second lung cancers (about 2%–3% per year).

2. **Stage II disease.** Treatment of stage II NSCLC is surgical resection. Although the role of neoadjuvant chemotherapy is under investigation, it cannot be routinely recommended until the results of randomized clinical trials confirm clinical benefit. The subset of T3, N0 disease has a different natural history and treatment strategy than stage III N2 disease and thus has been moved to stage II. Patients with peripheral chest wall invasion should undergo resection of the involved ribs and underlying lung. Chest wall defects are then repaired with chest wall musculature or Marlex mesh and methylmethacrylate. Postoperative radiotherapy is often given. Five-year survival rates as high as 50% have been reported.

3. **Locally advanced (stage IIIA and IIIB) disease.** Treatment of locally advanced NSCLC is one of the most controversial issues in the management of lung cancer. Treatment options include surgery for less advanced disease, or radiotherapy, either of which has been given with or without chemotherapy for control of micrometastases. Interpretation of the results of clinical trials involving patients with locally

advanced disease has been clouded by a number of issues, including changing diagnostic techniques, different staging systems, and heterogeneous patient populations that may have disease that ranges from "nonbulky" stage IIIA (clinical N1 nodes, with N2 nodes discovered only at the time of surgery or mediastinoscopy), to "bulky" N2 nodes (enlarged adenopathy clearly visible on chest radiographs, or multiple nodal level involvement), to clearly inoperable stage IIIB disease.

   a.   **Nonbulky stage IIIA (and selected stage II) disease.** The primary treatment of stage II disease is surgical resection. Two randomized studies conducted by the Lung Cancer Study Group examined the issue of postoperative adjuvant chemotherapy for stage II and stage IIIA disease. In general, these studies demonstrated an improvement in disease-free survival for patients receiving postoperative chemotherapy, with overall survival bordering on statistical significance. A randomized intergroup study has recently been completed to define further the role of postoperative chemotherapy in patients with resected stage II or IIIA NSCLC; patients were randomized to receive either radiotherapy plus chemotherapy (cisplatin, 60 mg/m^2 i.v. on day 1, and etoposide, 120 mg/m^2 i.v. on days 1 to 3 every 4 weeks for four cycles) or radiotherapy alone. Until these results are available, postoperative adjuvant chemotherapy for this group of patients cannot be routinely recommended. Postoperative radiotherapy has been shown to reduce local recurrences after resection of stage II or III squamous cell carcinoma of the lung but does not prolong survival.

   b.   **Pancoast tumors.** Pancoast tumors are upper-lobe tumors that adjoin the brachial plexus and are frequently associated with Horner's syndrome or shoulder and arm pain; the latter is due to rib destruction, involvement of the C-8 or T-1 nerve roots, or both. Treatment consists of a combined-modality approach with radiotherapy and surgery. Five-year survival rates range from 25% to 50%. Combined preoperative chemotherapy and radiotherapy is being studied.

   c.   **Bulky stage IIIA (N2) and stage IIIB.** The optimal treatment for bulky stage IIIA and stage IIIB disease is also controversial. Current investigational efforts are directed at identifying the optimal combined-modality approach, involving treatments directed at local control of the disease (surgery or radiotherapy) and micrometastatic disease (chemotherapy). Possibilities include radiotherapy only, preoperative chemotherapy, or chemotherapy plus radiotherapy.

(1) Preoperative chemotherapy plus surgery. There have been four small randomized studies involving surgery with or without preoperative chemotherapy; two are positive and two are negative. All involve 50 to 60 patients, and all report response rates of 35% to 62% after induction chemotherapy.

A European study compared preoperative chemotherapy (mitomycin, ifosfamide, and cisplatin for three courses) followed by surgery, versus surgery without preoperative chemotherapy for patients with stage IIIA disease. (All patients also received postoperative mediastinal radiotherapy after surgery.) Thirty patients in each treatment arm were evaluated; the median survival time was 26 months for patients receiving preoperative chemotherapy plus surgery, compared with 8 months for patients treated with surgery alone. Chemotherapy induced responses in 18 (60%) of 30 patients.

Investigators at the M.D. Anderson Cancer Center randomized patients to surgery or three cycles of cyclophosphamide, etoposide, and cisplatin followed by surgery and three cycles of postoperative chemotherapy. The median survival time of the 32 patients randomized to the surgery-alone group was 11 months, compared with 64 months in the 28 patients randomized to the combined-modality arm.

Two negative randomized trials have also been reported. The Lung Cancer Study Group randomized 57 patients to preoperative radiation therapy or preoperative MVP (mitomycin, vinblastine, cisplatin) chemotherapy in patients with technically unresectable stage IIIA and IIIB NSCLC; no survival difference was observed.

The Cancer and Leukemia Group B randomized 47 patients with N2 NSCLC to preoperative and postoperative cisplatin plus etoposide or preoperative and postoperative radiotherapy. Although the study was terminated early because of poor accrual, there was no statistically significant difference in survival.

These four studies have several important differences that should be noted. The two positive studies were single-institution studies and generally included less advanced patients than the two negative studies. The role of surgery in the management of advanced stage IIIA patients is being investigated in a randomized intergroup trial. All patients receive 45 Gy of induction radiotherapy plus two cycles of cisplatin and etoposide; they are subsequently randomized to surgery or boost radiotherapy plus an additional two cycles of chemotherapy.

(2) Chemotherapy plus radiation therapy. Chemotherapy plus radiotherapy is the treatment of choice for patients with bulky or inoperable stage III disease. Two randomized studies have demonstrated an improvement in median and long-term survival with cisplatin, 100 mg/m^2 i.v. on days 1 and 29, and vinblastine, 5 mg/m^2 on days 1, 8, 15, 22, and 29, followed by radiation therapy on day 50 (60 Gy over a 6-week period) versus radiotherapy alone. Active areas of investigation include proper sequencing of thoracic radiation therapy and chemotherapy (concurrent versus sequential), choice of chemotherapy, fractionation, and treatment fields.

4. Stage IV disease

    a. Issues regarding treatment. Chemotherapy improves survival in patients with metastatic NSCLC (about 10% 1-year survival rate in untreated patients versus 35% to 40% 1-year survival rate with treatment). It reduces symptoms, and a study on cost-effectiveness demonstrated a cost benefit for chemotherapy compared with supportive care. However, median survival is still poor (9 to 10 months), and thus a discussion must ensue with the patient regarding possible benefits, chance of response, and quality of life with treatment. Because chemotherapy is not curative, goals for treatment should include palliation of symptoms and a modest improvement in survival.

The principal factors predicting response to chemotherapy and survival are performance status and extent of disease. Patients with a poor performance status (Eastern Cooperative Oncology Group [ECOG] performance status of 2 to 4) are unlikely to respond to treatment, and they tolerate the therapy poorly; thus, they probably should not be treated. Favorable prognostic factors include no weight loss, female sex, normal serum lactic dehydrogenase level, and no bone or liver metastases. Chemotherapy is administered for six to eight cycles, or until disease progression is documented.

b. **First-line chemotherapy.** Chemotherapy for metastatic NSCLC should be a platinum-based regimen. Recent meta-analysis of large randomized trials indicated that survival is most often improved with platinum-based therapy and that combination regimens improve survival compared with single agents. Although a direct comparison of cisplatin-based therapies and carboplatin-based therapies is limited, most of the data suggest that cisplatin and carboplatin may have comparable efficacy.

Several new agents have recently been found to have activity in metastatic NSCLC (Table 8-3). The ECOG recently compared cisplatin and etoposide to two different paclitaxel (Taxol)-containing regimens: cisplatin and high-dose paclitaxel, (250 mg/m^2 over 24 hours) with growth factor support, vs. cisplatin and low-dose paclitaxel. The response rate of the etoposide plus cisplatin arm was 12%, compared with 31% and 26% in the high-dose and low-dose paclitaxel arms, respectively. Median survival times were 7.4 months, 10.1 months, and 9.6 months, and the 1-year survival rates were 31%, 40%, and 37%, respectively.

Although having only modest activity as a single agent, vinorelbine (Navelbine) produces a survival advantage and higher response rates when combined with cisplatin than does cisplatin alone. The Southwestern Oncology Group (SWOG) compared cisplatin alone with cisplatin plus weekly vinorelbine. The median survival was 6 months and 8 months, respectively,

Table 8-3. Common chemotherapy regimens for metastatic non–small cell lung cancer

Regimens evaluated in phase III trials

Cisplatin plus paclitaxel	
Cisplatin	75 mg/m² i.v. on day 1
Paclitaxel	135 mg/m² i.v. on day 1 over 24 hours
	Repeat cycle every 3 weeks.
Cisplatin plus vinorelbine	
Cisplatin	100 mg/m² i.v. on day 1
Vinorelbine	25 mg/m² weekly
	Repeat cycle every 4 weeks

Regimens evaluated in phase II trials

Carboplatin plus paclitaxel	
Carboplatin	Area under the curve (AUC) of 6, day 1
Paclitaxel	225 mg/m² i.v. on day 1
	Repeat cycle every 3 weeks
Cisplatin plus gemcitabine	
Cisplatin	100 mg/m² i.v. on day 1 or 2 or 15
Gemcitabine	1,000 mg/m² i.v. on days 1, 8, and 15
	Repeat each cycle every 28 days
Cisplatin plus docetaxel	
Cisplatin	75 mg/m² i.v. on day 1
Docetaxel	75 mg/m² i.v. on day 1
	Repeat each cycle every 21 days

and 1-year survival was 16% and 35%, respectively.

c. **New agents.** Several new agents have recently completed or are currently undergoing evaluation in the Food and Drug Administration (FDA) drug-approval process for NSCLC. These new drugs or drug combinations have been reported to result in response rates of 30% to 50% and 1-year survival rates of 35% to 50% in phase II studies, but are only now being evaluated in comparative randomized phase III studies. Because of their widespread usage and availability, they are also listed in Table 8-3.

d. **Second-line chemotherapy.** There have been no randomized trials evaluating second-line regimens in patients who have failed first-line therapy. In phase II trials involving highly selected patients, docetaxel and gemcitabine have been reported to have activity. Given the phase II nature of these studies and the heterogeneous patient populations, impact on survival cannot be ascertained.

e. **Isolated brain metastases.** In patients with controlled disease outside of the brain who have an isolated cerebral metastasis in a resectable area, resection followed by whole-brain radiotherapy is superior to whole-brain radiotherapy alone.

V. **Small cell carcinoma.** SCLC differs from NSCLC in a number of important ways. First, it has a more rapid clinical course and natural history, with the rapid development of metastases, symptoms, and death. Untreated, the median survival time for patients with local disease is typically 12 to 15 weeks, and for those with advanced disease, 6 to 9 weeks. Second, it exhibits features of neuroendocrine differentiation in many patients (which may be distinguishable histopathologically) and is associated with paraneoplastic syndromes. Third, unlike NSCLC, SCLC is exquisitely sensitive to both chemotherapy and radiotherapy, although resistant disease often develops. Because of the rapid development of distant disease and its extreme sensitivity to the cytotoxic effects of chemotherapy, this mode of therapy forms the backbone of treatment for this disease.

A. **Staging.** Because of the propensity of this disease to metastasize so quickly and the fact that micrometastatic disease is presumed to be present in all patients at the time of diagnosis, this disease is usually classified into either a local or an extensive stage. Local disease is typically defined as disease that can be encompassed within one radiation port, usually considered limited to the hemithorax and to regional nodes, including mediastinal and ipsilateral supraclavicular nodes. Extensive-stage disease is usually defined as disease that has spread outside those areas.

B. **Pretreatment evaluation.** Common sites of metastases for SCLC include the brain, liver, bone marrow, bone, and CNS. For this reason, a complete staging work-up consists of a complete blood cell count; liver function tests; CT of the brain, chest, and abdomen; a bone scan; and bone-marrow aspiration and biopsy. However, this complete staging work-up should not be undertaken unless the patient is a candidate for combined-modality treatment with chest radiation and chemotherapy, the patient is being evaluated for a clinical study, or the information is helpful for prognostic reasons. If the patient is not a candidate for combined-modality treatment or a clinical study, stopping the staging at the first evidence of extensive-stage disease is usually appropriate.

C. **Prognostic factors.** As in NSCLC, the major pretreatment prognostic factors are stage, performance status, and bulky disease. Hepatic metastases also confer a poorer prognosis. If the patient's initial poor performance status is due to the underlying malignancy, these symptoms often disappear quickly with treatment, resulting in a net improvement in quality of life. However, major organ dysfunction from non-malignant causes often results in an inability of the patient to tolerate chemotherapy.

D. Therapy. A number of combination chemotherapeutic regimens are available for SCLC (Table 8-4). However, no clear survival advantage has been demonstrated for any one regimen over another. With these chemotherapy regimens, overall response rates of 75% to 90% and complete response rates of 50% for localized disease can be anticipated. For extensive-stage disease, overall response rates of about 75% and complete response rates of 25% are common. Despite these high response rates, however, the median survival time remains about 14 months for limited-stage disease and 7 to 9 months for extensive-stage disease. Less than 5% of patients with extensive-stage disease survive more than 2 years.

1. **Dose intensity.** A recent dose intensity meta-analysis of chemotherapy in SCLC, which evaluated doses not requiring bone marrow transplantation support, showed no consistent correlation between dose intensity and outcome. Clinical trials evaluating the role of mar-

Table 8-4.   Chemotherapy regimens for small cell lung cancer

Cisplatin based

EP

Etoposide	120 mg/m² i.v. on days 1–3, *or*
	120 mg/m² p.o. b.i.d. on days 1–3
Cisplatin	60 mg/m² i.v. on day 1
or	
Cisplatin	25 mg/m² i.v. on days 1–3
Etoposide	100 mg/m² i.v. on days 1–3
	Repeat cycle every 3 wk

Carboplatin based

Carboplatin	300 mg/m² i.v. on day 1
Etoposide	100 mg/m² i.v. on days 1–3
or	
Carboplatin	100 mg/m² i.v. on days 1–3
Etoposide	120 mg/m² i.v. on days 1–3
	Repeat cycle every 4 wk

Adriamycin based

CAV

Cyclophosphamide	1,000 mg/m² i.v. on day 1
Doxorubicin (Adriamycin)	45–50 mg/m² i.v. on day 1
Vincristine	1.4 mg/m² i.v. on day 1
	(maximum, 2 mg)
	Repeat cycle every 3 wk

row ablative doses of chemotherapy with subsequent progenitor cell replacement (e.g., autologous bone marrow transplantation) are ongoing.

2. **Alternating therapy and consolidation chemotherapy.** Use of alternating non–cross-resistant chemotherapy regimens has been explored because of the mathematic model created by Goldie and Coldman that predicts improved tumor response when more chemotherapy agents of different mechanisms are used concurrently and early. Despite the mathematic model, randomized trials of alternating chemotherapy regimens versus standard regimens have not consistently yielded significant improvements in survival. The lack of benefit may represent, not a failure of the Goldie-Coldman model, but rather the lack of two totally non–cross-resistant chemotherapy regimens.

3. **Duration of therapy.** Most randomized studies do not show a survival benefit for prolonged administration of chemotherapy. Several studies have demonstrated no survival benefit of prolonged first-line treatment over treatment on relapse. The optimal duration of treatment for SCLC is 4 to 6 months.

4. **New agents.** The topoisomerase inhibitor topotecan has a 40% response rate as a single agent in previously untreated, extensive-stage SCLC. Paclitaxel also has been reported to have a 34% to 41% response rate in two phase II studies. The role of both of these agents as first-line therapy in combination with other drugs awaits the outcome of ongoing randomized studies.

5. **Second-line therapy.** No curative regimens for patients with recurrent disease have been identified. Oral etoposide, 50 mg/m^2/day for 21 days, resulted in a 45% response rate in 22 patients with recurrent disease, 18 of whom had prior intravenous etoposide treatment. The median duration of response, however, was only 4 months. Etoposide, 37.5 mg/m^2 p.o. on days 1 through 14, when combined with ifosfamide, 1.2 g/m^2 i.v. on days 1 to 4, and cisplatin, 20 mg/m^2 i.v. on days 1 to 4, resulted in a 61% response rate in 18 patients with a 25-week median survival time, although significant toxicities were reported.

Topotecan has a 20% to 40% response rate in patients with *sensitive* SCLC (those patients who relapsed 2 or more months after their first-line therapy), with a median survival of 22 to 27 weeks. For patients with *refractory* disease (progressed through or within 3 months of com-

pletion of first-line therapy), the response rate
in phase II studies is only between 3% and 11%.
Median survival is about 20 weeks. Preliminary
results of a randomized trial comparing topotecan, 1.5 mg/m^2/day $\times$ 5, with CAV (cyclophosphamide, doxorubicin [Adriamycin], and vincristine) in patients who relapsed or progressed
2 or more months from completion of first-line
chemotherapy have been reported. There was
no difference in response rates, duration of
response, or survival between the two groups.

E. **Chemotherapy plus chest irradiation.** Numerous
studies have been done with chemotherapy and
thoracic radiotherapy for patients with limited-stage
SCLC. Conflicting results have been attributed to differences in chemotherapy regimens and different
schedules integrating chemotherapy and thoracic radiation (concurrent, sequential, and "sandwich" approach). Two recent meta-analyses concluded that
thoracic irradiation does result in a small but significant improvement in survival and major control of the
disease in the chest, although no conclusions could be
made regarding the optimal sequencing of chemotherapy and thoracic radiation. Preliminary analysis of an
intergroup trial involving concurrent conventional
once-daily fractionation (180 cGy/fraction; five fractions per week for 5 weeks; total dose of 45 Gy) and cisplatin (60 mg/m^2 day 1) plus etoposide (120 mg/m^2/day
for 3 days) demonstrated a 42% 2-year survival rate.
In one randomized trial, early administration of thoracic irradiation in the combined-modality therapy of
limited-stage SCLC was superior to late or consolida-
tive thoracic irradiation.

F. **Prophylactic cranial irradiation.** Numerous trials have demonstrated that prophylactic brain irradiation does not enhance survival but does decrease
the risk of brain metastases without a decrease in
mental function.

VI. **Palliation**

A. **Radiotherapy.** Palliative radiotherapy is often
helpful in controlling the pain of bone metastases or
neurologic function in patients with brain metastases. Chest radiotherapy may help control hemoptysis, superior vena cava syndrome, airway obstruction, laryngeal nerve compression, and other local
complications.

B. **Pleural effusions.** Common sclerosing agents include tetracycline (no longer available), doxycycline,
talc, and bleomycin. The disadvantage of bleomycin
is its cost; talc, although effective, had the disadvantage of requiring a thoracoscopy and general anesthesia for insufflation. Comparative randomized trials are ongoing.

C. **Brachytherapy.** For patients with bronchial obstruction who have received maximum external-beam

radiotherapy, the use of high-dose endobronchial irradiation may be of temporary benefit.

D. **Cachexia.** Megestrol acetate, 160 mg to 800 mg daily, may improve the appetite of some patients.

E. **Chemotherapy.** In randomized trials involving both NSCLC and SCLC patients, chemotherapy has been shown to reduce the incidence of cancer-related symptoms such as pain, cough, hemoptysis, and shortness of breath.

F. **Colony-stimulating factors.** Filgrastim (granulocyte colony-stimulating factor) decreases the incidence of neutropenic fevers, the median duration of neutropenia, days of hospitalization, and days of antibiotic treatment in patients with extensive-stage SCLC. However, as discussed previously, the clinical benefit of maintaining a dose-intense approach in the treatment of SCLC patients has not been established.

Caution must be exercised when using colony-stimulating factors in patients receiving combined-modality treatment with both chemotherapy and thoracic irradiation. A randomized study by the SWOG found that patients receiving sargramostim (granulocyte-macrophage colony-stimulating factor) and chemotherapy with concurrent thoracic irradiation had a significant increase in thrombocytopenia over patients receiving concurrent chemotherapy and radiation therapy without growth factor.

SELECTED READINGS

Arriagada R, et al. Randomized trial on prophylactic cranial irradiation (PCI) for patients (pts) with small cell lung cancer (SCLC) in complete remission (CR). *Proc Am Assoc Clin Oncol* 1994;13:334.

Bonomi P, Kim K, Chang A, et al. Phase III trial comparing etoposide (E), cisplatin (C) versus Taxol (T) with cisplatin-G-CSF (G) versus Taxol-cisplatin in advanced nonsmall cell lung cancer: an Eastern Cooperative Group (ECOG) trial. *Proc Am Soc Clin Oncol* 1996; 15:382.

Crawford J, Ozer H, Stoller R, et al. Reduction by granulocyte-colony stimulation factor of fever and neutropenia induced by chemotherapy in patients with small-cell lung cancer. *N Engl J Med* 1991; 325:164–170.

Dillman RO, Herndon J, Seagren SL, Eaton WL Jr, Green MR. Improved survival in stage III non-small cell lung cancer: seven-year follow-up of CALGB 8433. *JNCI* 1996;88:1210.

Eddy DM. Screening for lung cancer. *Ann Intern Med* 1989;111:232.

Elias AD, Herndon J, Kumar P, Sugarbaker D, Green MR, for the Cancer & Leukemia Group B. A phase III comparison of "best local-regional therapy" with or without chemotherapy (CT) for stage IIIA T1-3N2 non-small cell lung cancer (NSCLC): preliminary results.

Faylona E, Loehrer P, Ansari R, et al. Phase II Study of daily oral etoposide plus ifostomide plus cisplatin for previously treated recurent small-cell lung cancer: A Hoosier Oncology Group Trial. *J Clin Oncol* 1995;1209–1214. *Proc Am Assoc Clin Oncol* 1997;16:448a.

Giaccone G, Dalesio O, McVie GJ, et al. Maintenance chemotherapy in small cell lung cancer: long-term results of a randomized trial. *J Clin Oncol* 1993;11:1230–1240.

Holmes EC, Gail M, for the Lung Cancer Study Group. Surgical adjuvant therapy for stage II and III adenocarcinoma and large-cell undifferentiated carcinoma. *J Clin Oncol* 1986;4:710.

Jaakkimainen L, Goodwin PJ, Pater J, et al. Counting the costs of chemotherapy in a National Cancer Institute of Canada randomized trial in nonsmall cell lung cancer. *J Clin Oncol* 1990;8:1301–1309.

Johnson D, et al. Cisplatin (P) and etoposide (E) and concurrent thoracic radiotherapy (TRT) administered once versus twice daily for limited-stage (LS) small cell lung cancer (SCLC): preliminary results of an intergroup trial. *Proc Am Soc Clin Oncol* 1994;13:333.

Klasa R, Murray N, Coldman A. Dose-intensity meta-analysis of chemotherapy regimens in small-cell carcinoma of the lung. *J Clin Oncol* 1991;9:499.

Le Chevalier T, Brisgand D, Douillard JY, et al. Randomized study of vinorelbine and cisplatin vs. vindesine and cisplatin vs. vinorelbine alone in advanced nonsmall-cell lung cancer: results of a European multicenter trial including 612 patients. *J Clin Oncol* 1994;12:360–367.

Lilenbaum R, Green R. Novel chemotherapeutic agents in the treatment of nonsmall cell lung cancer. *J Clin Oncol* 1993;11:1391.

Lung Cancer Study Group. Effects of post-operative mediastinal radiation on completely resected stage II and stage III epidermoid cancer of the lung. *N Engl J Med* 1986;315:1377.

Marino P, Preatoni A, Cantoni A, et al. Single-agent chemotherapy versus combination chemotherapy in advanced non-small cell lung cancer: a quality and meta-analysis study. *Lung Cancer* 1995;13:1.

Mountain CF. Revisions in the International System for Staging Lung Cancer. *Chest* 1997;111(6):1486.

Murray N, Coy P, Pater J, et al. Importance of timing for thoracic irradiation in the combined modality treatment of limited-stage small-cell lung cancer. *J Clin Oncol* 1993;11:336.

Neal CR, Amdur RJ, Mendenhall WM, et al. Pancoast tumor: radiation therapy alone vs. preoperative radiation and surgery. *Int J Radiat Oncol Biol Phys* 1991;21:651–660.

Non-Small Cell Lung Cancer Collaborative Group. Chemotherapy in non-small cell lung cancer: a meta-analysis using updated data on individual patients from 52 randomized clinical trials. *Br Med J* 1995;311:899.

Pignon JP, Arriagada R, Ihde DC, et al. A meta-analysis of thoracic radiotherapy for small-cell lung cancer. *N Engl J Med* 1992;327:1618–1624.

Rosell R, Gomez-Codina J, Camps C, et al. A randomized trial comparing preoperative chemotherapy plus surgery with surgery alone in patients with non-small-cell lung cancer. *N Engl J Med* 1994;330:153–158.

Sandler A, et al. A phase II study of daily oral VP-16 plus ifosfamide plus cisplatin (poVIP) for previously treated recurrent small cell lung cancer (SCLC): a Hoosier Oncology Group trial. *Proc Am Soc Clin Oncol* 1994;13:327.

Sause W, Scott C, Taylor S, et al., for the Radiation Therapy Oncology Group (RTOG) 88-08 and ECOG 3488. Preliminary results of a phase III trial in regionally advanced, unresectable non-small cell lung cancer. *JNCI* 1995;87:198.

Schiller JH, et al. Topotecan (T) versus (vs) cyclophosphamide (C), doxorubicin (A), and vincristine (V) for the treatment (tx) of Patients (pts) with recurrent small cell lung cancer (SCLC): a phase III study. *Proc Am Soc Clin Oncol* 1996;14:2345–2352.

Wagner H Jr, Lad T, Piantadosi S, et al. Randomized phase 2 evaluation of preoperative radiation therapy and preoperative chemotherapy with mitomycin, vinblastine, and cisplatin in patients with technically unresectable stage IIIA and IIIB non-small cell cancer of the lung. *Chest* 1994;106[Suppl 6]:348S–354S.

Walker-Renard P, Vaughan L, Sahn S. Chemical pleurodesis for malignant pleural effusions. *Ann Intern Med* 1994;120:56.

Warde P, Payne D. Does thoracic irradiation improve survival and local control in limited-stage small-cell carcinoma of the lung? A meta-analysis. *J Clin Oncol* 1992;10:890.

Wozniak AJ, Crowley JJ, Balcerzak SP, et al. Randomized trial comparing cisplatin with cisplatin plus navelbine in the treatment of advanced non-small-cell lung cancer: a Southwest Oncology Group study. *J Clin Oncol;* 1998;16(7): 2459–2465.

Carcinomas of the Gastrointestinal Tract

John C. Marsh

Cancers of the gastrointestinal (GI) tract (esophagus, stomach, small and large intestines) account for nearly 13% of all cases of cancer in the United States and for about 15% of cancer deaths. Colon cancer is by far the most common of these malignancies, with cancer of the rectum, stomach, esophagus, and small intestine occurring with decreasing frequency. Surgery continues to be the principal curative modality, but irradiation and chemotherapy have increasingly important roles and, in certain adjuvant situations, may improve the cure rate produced by surgery. Chemotherapy alone is not curative in patients with overt metastatic disease. Drugs produce objective remissions in only 15% to 40% of patients. However, there is little question that meaningful palliation and an increase in survival can be achieved in patients who respond to chemotherapy. Controlled clinical trials, often by interinstitutional cooperative groups, have been useful in defining the natural history and therapeutic benefit of various treatment modalities. Participation in such clinical trials should be encouraged.

I. Carcinoma of the esophagus
A. General considerations and aims of therapy

1. **Epidemiology.** Cancer of the esophagus has been predominantly of the squamous cell (epidermoid) variety and represents about 1% of the cases of cancers in the United States. Risk factors include heavy tobacco and alcohol use. It is more common in men than women and occurs more often in blacks than in whites. The average patient is in his or her 60s at presentation. In certain parts of China, epidermoid esophageal cancer is the most common kind of cancer, which is thought to be related to dietary habits of the region and perhaps a consequence of fungal contamination of pickled vegetables. Other predisposing factors for esophageal cancer include achalasia, a history of lye burns of the esophagus, and prior epidermoid carcinomas of the aerodigestive tract.

   In recent years, the incidence of adenocarcinoma of the esophagus (along with adenocarcinoma of the proximal stomach) has increased greatly. By the mid-1980s, it accounted for about one third of all esophageal cancer cases among white men and in some institutions is approaching 60% of newly diagnosed cancers of the esophagus. Adenocarcinoma is predominantly a disease of middle-aged white men, is less strongly associated with alcohol and tobacco use, and is frequently associated with Barrett's esophagus (epithelial metaplasia of the lower esophagus), which is sometimes seen with reflux esophagitis. The rate of increase of adenocarcinomas of the esophagus and gastric cardia during the 1970s and 1980s exceeded that of any other cancer, including lung cancer, non-Hodgkin's lymphoma, and melanoma. The cause of this impressive increase is not known, although recent epidemiologic studies have implicated obesity, which has been increasing in the U.S. population during the past few decades. This may in turn be associated with epithelial metaplasia in the esophagus (Barrett's esophagus). Adenocarcinomas of the esophagus tend to involve the lower third of that organ, whereas the middle third is the most common site for the epidermoid variety. Optimal chemotherapy for the two histologic types of esophageal cancer is not known to be different, with little or no difference in response rate in most series. It has been suggested, however, that a lower expression of thymidylate synthase in squamous cell carcinoma than in adenocarcinoma may make the former more sensitive to fluorouracil-based chemotherapy.

2. **Clinical manifestations and pretreatment evaluation.** Carcinoma of the esophagus is usually associated with progressive and persistent dysphagia. Pain, hoarseness, weight loss, and chronic cough are unfavorable manifestations that indicate spread to regional structures (e.g., mediastinal nodes), recurrent laryngeal nerve, or fistula formation between the esophagus and the airway. The most common sites of metastasis are regional lymph nodes (which may include cervical, supraclavicular, intrathoracic, diaphragmatic, celiac axis, or periaortic), the liver, and the lungs.

Diagnosis is usually made by barium swallow, endoscopy, and biopsy or lavage cytology. Staging should be based on chest radiographic appearance, computed tomography (CT) scan of the abdomen and chest, and careful physical examination of the cervical and supraclavicular nodes. Endoscopic esophageal ultrasound is still investigational but may be useful in assessing the depth of tumor invasion. The preoperative staging of esophageal cancer is still inadequate, owing to the inability to evaluate lymph nodes accurately. Bronchoscopy should be done for upper- and middle-third tumors, and a bone scan is useful in patients with bone pain or tenderness. Survival is related to pathologic stage, which can only be defined surgically (Table 9-1).

3. **Treatment and prognosis.** The primary treatment of stage I and II carcinoma of the esophagus is surgical resection. About half of esophageal cancers are operable, and half of these are resectable. Patients with more advanced disease (stage III) are best treated, at least initially, with nonsurgical means, usually a combination of radiation therapy and chemotherapy. In patients who respond to such treatment, the carcinoma may subsequently be operable, whereas patients with metastatic disease to the liver, lung, or bone are best treated with systemic therapy. Palliative feeding procedures, such as with a jejunostomy or gastrostomy tube, may be useful if subsequent surgical resection is not to be done. The overall median survival time is less than 1 year, and the overall 5-year survival rate is 5% to 10%. The prognosis is related to the size of the lesion, the depth of penetration of the esophagus, and nodal involvement. Current controlled

Table 9-1. TNM stages for carcinoma of the esophagus

Primary tumor

Tis	Carcinoma *in situ*
T1	Invades lamina propria or submucosa
T2	Invades muscularis propria
T3	Invades adventitia
T4	Invades adjacent structures

Regional lymph nodes

N0	No nodal metastasis
N1	Regional node metastasis

Distant metastasis

M0	None
M1	Present

Stage grouping

0	Tis, N0, M0
I	T1, N0, M0
IIA	T2 or T3, N0, M0
IIB	T1 or T2, N1, M0
III	T3, N1, M0
	T4, any N, M0
IV	Any T, any N, M1

Modified from American Joint Committee on Cancer. *AJCC Staging Manual,* 5th ed. Philadelphia: Lippincott-Raven, 1997.

clinical trials are helping to evaluate the relative roles of chemotherapy, radiation, and surgery in all stages of the two predominant histologic types. Most emphasis has been on preoperative ("neoadjuvant") combined-modality treatment, with few supporting data available for postoperative treatment, although the concept is being evaluated as more patients survive initial combined-modality therapy. This is important because many patients who achieve good local control have disease recurrence in distant sites subsequent to surgery.

B. Treatment of advanced (metastatic) disease. Various agents with modest activity when used alone are available. These include cisplatin, fluorouracil, bleomycin, paclitaxel, methotrexate, mitomycin, vinorelbine, and doxorubicin. Response rates range from 15% to 30% and are usually brief. Most data are for epidermoid carcinoma, the exception being paclitaxel, which appears equally effective in both histologic types. The most active drugs appear to be cisplatin, paclitaxel, and fluorouracil. Patients with no history of prior chemotherapy are more likely to respond than those who have had previous treatment. Single agents are less helpful than combination chemotherapy because of their lower response rates and brief duration of response. Cisplatin-based regimens have been most extensively tested. Among the most active are the following:

1. **Cisplatin + fluorouracil + interferon-α**
    a. Cisplatin, 100 mg/m^2 i.v. on day 1
    b. Fluorouracil, 750 mg/m^2/day as a continuous i.v. infusion on days 1 to 5,
    c. Interferon-α, 3×10^6 units s.c. daily on days 1 to 28.

        Repeat every 28 days. Give cisplatin on every other cycle after the first three cycles.

        The response rate in a small series was 73% for squamous cell carcinoma and 33% for adenocarcinoma with a median response duration of 29 weeks.

2. **Paclitaxel + cisplatin**
    a. Paclitaxel, 200 mg/m^2 i.v. over 24 hours,
    b. Cisplatin, 75 mg/m^2 i.v.,
    c. Granulocyte colony-stimulating factor (G-CSF), 300 μg s.c. daily for 10 days.

        Repeat every 21 days. After cycle 3, give cisplatin every other cycle.

        This regimen is active in adenocarcinoma and perhaps in squamous cell carcinoma; overall, 10 of 20 patients responded.

3. **Second-line therapy** may be chosen from the following single agents: methotrexate, 40 mg/m^2 i.v. weekly; bleomycin, 15 units/m^2 i.v. twice

weekly; vinorelbine, 25 mg/m² i.v. weekly; or mitomycin, 20 mg/m² i.v. every 4 to 6 weeks.

C. **Combined-modality treatment for potentially curable patients.** The poor results with immediate surgery, due in part to inadequate staging techniques, have focused attention for some years on preoperative combined-modality treatment with radiation therapy, chemotherapy, or both, followed by surgery (or in some instances, not followed by surgery). This approach is controversial, because of uncertainty of staging and lack of definitive, randomized clinical trials. Aggressive staging, including endoscopic ultrasound, CT scanning, and laparoscopy, often combined with jejunostomy feeding tube placement for nutritional support if needed, is being used increasingly. The two different histologies present in some series can also confuse interpretation. Patients with stage II and III disease are often treated in this fashion.

Radiation therapy, as either a preoperative or postoperative adjunct to surgery, has not improved overall survival in most series. Radiation therapy alone has 5-year survival rates ranging from 0% to 10%. Combined-modality treatment has been superior. In a randomized trial comparing radiotherapy alone with radiotherapy plus chemotherapy in 121 patients, 88% of whom had squamous cell cancer, the Radiation Therapy Oncology Group reported a 5-year survival rate of 27% for the combined-modality group and 0% for the radiation therapy group. Median survival times were 14.1 and 9.3 months, respectively. Most patients had stage T2 disease and were node negative by CT scanning. Combined chemotherapy and radiotherapy is, therefore, a reasonable approach for patients who refuse surgery or whose disease is unresectable for anatomic or physiologic reasons, particularly those with epidermoid carcinoma.

1. **Radiation therapy + fluorouracil + cisplatin.**

   a. Radiation therapy, 200 cGy/day for 3 weeks, 5 days weekly; then 2 additional weeks to the boost field for a total of 5,000 cGy, *and*

   b. Fluorouracil, 1,000 mg/m²/day by continuous infusion for 4 days on weeks 1, 5, 8 and 11, with cisplatin, 75 mg/m² i.v. at 1 mg/min on the first day of each course. Reduce fluorouracil for severe diarrhea or stomatitis, and cisplatin for severe neutropenia or thrombocytopenia.

   c. Surgery, when it can be done, is probably appropriate because most patients treated with chemotherapy and radiotherapy still have residual tumor. Even though a high proportion, 25% in many series, have complete pathologic responses at surgery, the preoperative identification of these patients is not accurate. A recent randomized trial from Ireland of 113 patients with adenocarcinoma of the esophagus has shown a 3-year survival rate of 32% for patients treated with preoperative chemotherapy with fluorouracil and cisplatin and with radiotherapy followed by surgery, compared with 6% for patients treated with surgery alone. Similarly, a recent study from the University of Michigan of 100 patients (75% adenocarcinoma) has shown a 3-year survival rate of 32% for combined-modality treatment, compared with 15% for surgery alone, with a reduction in local recurrence in the combined group (19% versus 39%). Optimal results may involve all three major treatment modalities, with at least some of the chemotherapy being given concurrently with radiation therapy. Better preoperative treatments are being defined in phase II trials, incorporating such agents as paclitaxel, and postoperative chemotherapy is also being evaluated. The following may be used in potentially resectable patients:

2. **Cisplatin + fluorouracil + radiotherapy (Dublin regimen)**
   a. Fluorouracil, 15 mg/kg (555 mg/m^2) i.v. over 16 hours daily, days 1 to 5 *and*
   b. Cisplatin, 75 mg/m^2 i.v. infused over 8 hours on day 7 after 1 full day of hydration. Repeat both drugs at 6 weeks.
   c. Radiotherapy, 40 Gy in 15 fractions over 3 weeks, beginning on the first day of chemotherapy.
   d. Surgery is done 8 weeks after beginning treatment, blood counts permitting.

3. **Fluorouracil + cisplatin + vinblastine + radiotherapy (Michigan regimen)**
   a. Vinblastine, 1 mg/m^2 i.v. on days 1 to 4 and 17 to 20 of radiotherapy *and*
   b. Cisplatin, 20 mg/m^2/day by continuous i.v. infusion on days 1 to 5 and 17 to 21 of radiotherapy *and*
   c. Fluorouracil, 300 mg/m^2/day by continuous i.v. infusion on days 1 to 21 of radiotherapy *and*
   d. Radiotherapy is 45 Gy in 15 fractions (300 cGy b.i.d.) for 3 weeks.
   e. Surgery is done at 6 weeks.

D. **Supportive care.** Esophagitis during a combined-modality treatment program is nearly universal, and nutritional support frequently is required, preferably using alimentation by feeding tube placed by enterostomy. Peripheral alimentation is difficult with the continuous chemotherapy administration. Gastrostomy tubes are to be avoided, because of the usual requirement for a gastric pull-up after resection of the esophageal tumor.

E. **Follow-up studies.** For patients with potentially curative therapy, history and physical examination may be done every 1 to 3 months for 1 year, then every 3 to 4 months for 2 years. Chest radiographs should be evaluated every 3 to 4 months for 2 years and then annually. A CT of the abdomen and chest should be obtained at the end of combined-modality treatment, every 6 months for 2 years, and then annually for a total of 5 years. Most disease recurrences occur within that time.

II. **Gastric carcinoma**

  A. **General considerations and aims of therapy**

  1. **Epidemiology.** The incidence of stomach cancer has decreased dramatically in the United States since the beginning of the century, although it has stabilized in the last 20 years. The leading cause of cancer death in 1930, it now ranks 12th. No improvement has been seen, however, in 5-year survival rates, which range from 5% to 16%. The only curative modality at present is surgery. The male-to-female ratio is 2:1. Stomach cancer is still the leading cause of cancer deaths among men in Japan and is also common in China, Finland, Poland, and Chile. A high rate of chronic gastritis and intestinal metaplasia of the stomach is associated with a high incidence of gastric cancer. *Helicobacter pylori* has been implicated in such changes and in gastric cancer, particularly the more distal "intestinal" type, as well as in peptic ulcer. Although the incidence in the United States has decreased, the location of gastric cancers has migrated proximally. Cancers in the fundus of the stomach have increased from 14% of gastric cancers in 1950 to 24% at present. Nearly half the stomach cancers occurring in white men are located proximally.

  2. **Clinical manifestations and evaluation.** The most common symptoms are weight loss, abdominal pain, nausea, vomiting, changes in bowel habits, fatigue, anorexia, and dysphagia. The diagnosis generally is made by endoscopy and biopsy, although barium swallow is frequently helpful. Endoscopic ultrasonography is increasingly used; it is more accurate in gauging the depth of the cancer in the gastric wall than in determining nodal involvement. Metastases are to the liver, pancreas, omentum, esophagus, and bile ducts by direct extension and to regional and distant lymph nodes, such as those in the left supraclavicular area. Pulmonary and bone metastases are a late finding. Staging of suspected gastric cancer should be based on CT

scans of the chest, abdomen, and pelvis and on liver function tests. Tumor markers, such as CEA, CA 19-9, and CA 72-4, may be useful for subsequent assessment of the response to therapy. Prognosis is reflected by accurate staging (Table 9-2). The new revised staging method classifies patients according to the number of pathologically involved regional lymph nodes. The groupings are 1 to 6, 7 to 15, and more than 15 involved lymph nodes; surgically staged patients resected for cure have 5-year survival rates of 46%, 30%, and 10%, respectively.

Table 9-2.   TNM stages for carcinoma of the stomach

Primary tumor

Tis	Carcinoma *in situ*
T1	Invades lamina propria or submucosa
T2	Invades muscularis propria or subserosa
T3	Penetrates serosa (visceral peritoneum)
T4	Invades adjacent structures

Regional lymph nodes

N0	No nodal metastasis
N1	Metastasis in 1–6 regional lymph nodes
N2	Metastasis in 7–15 regional lymph nodes
N3	Metastasis in more than 15 regional lymph nodes

Distant metastasis

M0	None
M1	Present

Stage grouping

0	Tis, N0, M0
IA	T1, N0, M0
IB	T1, N1, M0
	T2, N0, M0
II	T1, N2, M0
	T2, N1, M0
	T3, N0, M0
IIIA	T2, N2, M0
	T3, N1, M0
	T4, N0, M0
IIIB	T3, N2, M0
IV	T4, N1, M0
	T1, N3, M0
	T2, N3, M0
	T3, N3, M0
	T4, N2, M0
	T4, N3, M0
	Any T, any N, M1

Modified from American Joint Committee on Cancer. *AJCC Staging Manual,* 5th ed. Philadelphia: Lippincott-Raven, 1997.

3. **Treatment and prognosis.** Most stomach cancers are adenocarcinomas. Important prognostic factors include tumor grade and gross appearance. Diffusely infiltrating lesions are less likely to be cured than sharply circumscribed, nonulcerating lesions. The presence of regional lymph node involvement or involvement of contiguous organs in the surgical specimen indicates an increased likelihood of recurrence, as does the presence of dysphagia at the time of diagnosis. Patients with proximal lesions or lesions requiring total, rather than distal subtotal, gastrectomy are also at greater risk.

B. **Treatment of advanced (metastatic, locally unresectable, or recurrent) disease**

1. **Single agents** with activity include epirubicin, mitomycin, doxorubicin, cisplatin, etoposide (VP-16), fluorouracil, irinotecan (CPT-11), hydroxyurea, the taxanes, and the nitrosoureas. Single agents have low response rates (15% to 30%), brief durations of response, and few complete responses, and they have little impact on survival.

2. **Combinations of drugs** are more widely used than single agents, largely because of higher response rates, more frequent complete responses, and the theoretical potential of longer survival. A controlled trial (1985) of fluorouracil alone versus fluorouracil plus doxorubicin (Adriamycin) (FA) versus fluorouracil, doxorubicin, and mitomycin (FAM), however, failed to show a survival benefit for the combinations, which were more costly and toxic. Response rates, which were measurable in only about half the patients, were higher with the combinations. New combinations are continually being reported, with the initial results generally being higher than those found in subsequent confirmatory studies or randomized trials. Some epirubicin regimens from Europe appear to be active, but that agent is not routinely available in the United States. The combination of cisplatin and irinotecan has been reported to be active (48% response rate and 10-month median survival time) in a small Japanese study. Drug combination therapy has been shown to improve median survival by about 6 months in patients with metastatic disease, compared with the best supportive care in four small, randomized trials.

   a. **ELF.** The ELF (leucovorin, etoposide, and fluorouracil) regimen was designed to be less toxic than the regimen of etoposide, doxorubicin, and cisplatin (EAP), and in the hands of its originators, it appears to be as effective. Initial experience suggested a response rate of about 50%, with an 11-month month median survival. The regimen is as follows:

(1) Leucovorin, 300 mg/m^2 as a 10-minute i.v. infusion, *followed by*

(2) Etoposide, 120 mg/m^2 as a 50-minute i.v. infusion, *followed by*

(3) Fluorouracil, 500 mg/m^2 i.v. as a 10-minute infusion.

All agents are given on days 1, 2, and 3. The course is repeated in 21 to 28 days.

b. **FAMTX.** This regimen compared favorably to FAM in a large European clinical trial and to EAP in the United States. Response rates were 41% and 33% in the two studies, with median survival times of 10.5 and 7.3 months, respectively. The need for leucovorin "rescue" of methotrexate makes it rather cumbersome.

Before methotrexate administration, hydrate with 1 liter of isotonic sodium bicarbonate (1.4% bicarbonate) (urine pH must be higher than 7.0.) Infuse 2 liters of an identical solution over 24 hours after methotrexate is given. The regimen is as follows:

(1) Methotrexate, 1.5 g/m^2 by i.v. bolus infusion after the hydration and urine alkalinization, day 1 *and*

(2) Fluorouracil, 1.5 g/m^2 by i.v. bolus infusion starting 1 hour after the end of the methotrexate infusion *and*

(3) Leucovorin, 15 mg/m^2 orally starting 24 hours later on day 2, given every 6 hours for 3 days or until the methotrexate level is less than 2×10^{-8} molar. If the methotrexate level is more than 2.5×10^{-6} at 24 hours, increase leucovorin dose to 30 mg/m^2 every 6 hours for 96 hours.

(4) Doxorubicin, 30 mg/m^2 i.v. on day 15 if the white blood cell count (WBC) is more than 3,000/µL or the absolute neutrophil count (ANC) is more than 1,500/µL and the platelet count is more than 70,000/µL. The cycle is repeated every 4 weeks.

Renal function must be normal and blood levels of methotrexate should be monitored with this regimen.

c. **Hydroxyurea + leucovorin + fluorouracil + cisplatin.** A large phase II study of this regimen in France has reported a response rate of 62% and median sur-

vival time of 11 months. The regimen is as
follows:
  (1) Hydroxyurea, 1.5 to 2 g p.o. on days 0,
         1, 2, *and*
  (2) Leucovorin, 200 mg/m^2 i.v. as a 2-hour
         infusion on days 1 and 2, *before*
  (3) Fluorouracil, 400 mg/m^2 i.v. bolus
         and 600 mg/m^2 by 22-hour infusion
         on days 1 and 2, *then*
  (4) Cisplatin, 80 mg/m^2 i.v. on day 3
         every other cycle.
         The cycle is repeated every 14 days.
  C. Adjuvant therapy. Despite numerous trials of post-
      operative chemotherapy following potentially cura-
      tive gastric resection, its value is uncertain. Until
      benefit is shown, there is no specific role for adjuvant
      chemotherapy after surgery. An intergroup study is
      evaluating the role of postoperative radiotherapy and
      chemotherapy (fluorouracil + leucovorin).
  D. Follow-up studies. Reasonable follow-up studies for
      patients in remission after surgery consist of history
      and physical examination every 3 months for 3 years,
      every 6 months for 2 years, and then annually. Com-
      plete blood cell count and liver function tests may be
      done on the same schedule. Abdominal CT and chest
      radiographs should be done annually. Endoscopy
      should be done if new symptoms develop.
  E. Combined-modality therapy. Radiotherapy re-
      duces the frequency of local recurrence in patients
      with potentially curative gastric resection. A large
      number of patients have locally unresectable or in-
      completely resectable disease, and it has been known
      for some time that fluorouracil used in conjunction
      with radiotherapy adds to the survival of such pa-
      tients compared with radiotherapy alone, so long as
      they have no evidence of metastatic disease and have
      disease that can be encompassed by a treatment port.
      It is not clear that radiation therapy added to che-
      motherapy is better, in terms of survival, than chemo-
      therapy alone. However, although the role of radia-
      tion therapy in the management of gastric cancer is
      yet to be defined, the large number of local recur-
      rences seen in this disease suggest a potential value.
      Thus, it seems appropriate to treat such patients at
      the present time with a combined-modality regimen.
      Although there is no standard regimen, a reasonable
      regimen is as follows:
      1. Radiotherapy, 45 Gy at 180 cGY/day to the
          tumor (or tumor bed) and nodal chains daily for
          5 days weekly × 5 weeks
      2. Chemotherapy, started on the first or second
          day of radiotherapy
          a. Leucovorin, 20 mg/m^2 i.v. bolus on days 1
              to 4.
          b. Fluorouracil, 400 mg/m^2 i.v. bolus on days
              1 to 4, each dose given after the leucovorin.

The chemotherapy is repeated at the same daily dose for 3 days on week 5 of radiotherapy.

3. Continuing chemotherapy. After a 4- to 5-week rest to allow recovery of the WBC count to more than 3,500/µL and platelet count to more than 150,000/µL, treat with *either*

  a. Leucovorin, 20 mg/m² i.v. bolus on days 1 to 5, and fluorouracil, 425 mg/m² i.v. bolus on days 1 to 5, each dose given after the leucovorin. Repeat for two to four cycles. *or,*

  b. **ELF** (see Section II.B.2.a) for at least two cycles.

  Continuation of either regimen should depend on response and tolerance.

  The use of preoperative, or neoadjuvant, chemotherapy is somewhat in vogue at the present time, owing to some encouraging responses and apparent conversion of unresectable tumors to resectable ones by the administration of multidrug combinations. This approach is still under investigation.

F. Complications. Hematologic and GI toxicities from the chemotherapy may be accentuated by concurrent radiotherapy. If the complications are sufficiently severe, chemotherapy, radiotherapy, or both should be withheld until improvement. Consideration is given to treating at reduced doses. Hematopoietic growth factors may be of benefit in preventing severe infections secondary to neutropenia, but their use has not yet resulted in improved survival.

G. Treatment of refractory disease. If the patient's disease recurs or progresses with the recommended regimens, it is reasonable to consider combinations containing drugs not previously administered, or any of the single agents mentioned in Section II.B.1.

III. Cancer of the small intestine

A. Carcinoid tumors. Carcinoid tumors are the most common tumors of the appendix and ileum. They may develop in other parts of the GI tract but much less commonly. The usual histologic criteria of malignancy are not always applicable. Invasion and evidence of distant spread are more useful prognostic features.

In one series, the 60% of patients with intestinal carcinoids that were still confined to the wall of the gut had a 5-year survival rate of 85%, whereas those with tumors invading the serosa or beyond had a 5% survival rate at 5 years. Patients in the latter group were nearly always symptomatic, whereas patients in the former group were not. (Their tumors were discovered at surgery for appendicitis or other causes.) Tumors of the appendix are usually benign by these criteria, whereas those of the ileum are more often invasive. Surgical resection is the definitive therapy.

1. **Carcinoid syndrome.** About 10% of patients with carcinoid tumors have the carcinoid syndrome, which includes diarrhea, abdominal cramps, malabsorption, and flushing. With tumors of intestinal origin, liver metastases are nearly always present. Serotonin is thought to be responsible for the abdominal symptoms. Its metabolite 5-hydroxyindoleacetic acid (5-HIAA) is excreted in large quantities in the urine and is a useful marker of disease activity. The symptoms may respond to simple antidiarrheal therapy. The flushing caused by the syndrome has been attributed to bradykinin, formed by the interaction of kallikrein (produced by the tumor) with a plasma protein. If simple symptomatic measures do not suffice, the best treatment is the synthetic, long-acting somatostatin analog octreotide acetate (Sandostatin). This agent, injected at a dose of 50 to 150 µg s.c. every 6 to 12 hours, effectively decreases the secretion of serotonin and other gastroenteropancreatic peptides, such as insulin or gastrin. It has been helpful in ameliorating the symptoms of carcinoid tumors (e.g., flushing and diarrhea). There are even modest objective antitumor effects. The excretion of 5-HIAA is reduced by octreotide, so patients receiving it can no longer be followed accurately with this marker.

2. **Treatment of advanced carcinoid tumors**
   a. **Effective agents.** Doxorubicin, fluorouracil, mitomycin, cyclophosphamide, methotrexate, interferon-α, and streptozotocin have been shown to have some activity in this disease. A major advantage of using streptozotocin in combination is its relative lack of myelotoxicity. Response rates for combinations of fluorouracil and streptozotocin, or for streptozotocin and cyclophosphamide, in treating carcinoids of various kinds are 25% to 35%; the overall response rate for patients with tumors of intestinal origin is 41%. A median duration of response of 7 months may be expected, and patients with a good performance status have the greatest likelihood of response. Tumor response correlates well with reduction of 5-HIAA excretion. Some reports have indicated responses with interferon-α, including responses in some patients previously treated with chemotherapy, although these responses are usually transient. When the disease is confined to the liver, it

is sometimes possible to achieve good palliation with hepatic artery embolization.

b. Recommended regimens

(1) Streptozotocin, 500 mg/m^2 i.v. on days 1 to 5, and fluorouracil, 400 mg/m^2 i.v. on days 1 to 5. Repeat the course every 6 weeks if the disease has responded or is stable, *or*

(2) If the patient does not respond, doxorubicin, 60 mg/m^2 i.v. every 3 weeks, can be given with appropriate monitoring of cardiac function and leukocyte count, *or*

(3) Interferon-α, 3 to 6 million U/day i.m.

c. Precautions. Treatment of carcinoid tumors may precipitate or exacerbate the carcinoid syndrome during the first days of treatment, and the serotonin antagonists cyproheptadine and methysergide, as well as octreotide, should be available.

B. Adenocarcinomas. Adenocarcinomas of the small intestine are so uncommon that there is no large chemotherapy experience to report. Survival of patients with small intestinal cancer is a function of stage (Table 9-3). There is a modest response rate of metastatic disease to FAM, and this is a reasonable first choice. It is not clear what the response would be to current first-line colon cancer regimens.

Fluorouracil, 600 mg/m^2 i.v. on days 1, 8, 29, and 36,

Doxorubicin, 30 mg/m^2 i.v. on days 1 and 29,

Mitomycin, 10 mg/m^2 i.v. on day 1.

IV. Cancer of the large intestine

A. General considerations and aims of therapy. Taken together, cancers of the colon and rectum are by far the most frequent malignancies of the GI tract, and they account for the most deaths. Fewer than half of patients found to have large bowel cancers are cured by surgery, although it is still the only curative modality available. There have been some advances in early diagnosis and in techniques of surgery, but nationwide mortality figures have not really changed appreciably. In some institutions, the relative incidence of colon cancer is increasing, whereas the incidence of rectal cancer is decreasing. Local recurrence is much more common for rectal cancer (40% to 50%). About half of large bowel cancer recurrences are in the liver.

1. Staging. The most commonly used staging system is the Dukes staging system or its modifications. This system classifies the tumor in terms of the extent to which it penetrates the bowel wall and involves regional lymph nodes. Dukes A lesions are confined to the mucosa and submucosa and are associated with a 5-year

Table 9-3.   TNM stages for carcinoma of the small intestine

Primary tumor

Tis   Carcinoma *in situ*
T1   Invades lamina propria or submucosa
T2   Invades muscularis propria
T3   Invades through the muscularis propria into the subserosa or
      into nonperitonealized perimuscular tissue with extension
      2 cm or less
T4   Perforates visceral peritoneum or directly invades other organs
      or structures

Regional lymph nodes

N0   No nodal metastasis
N1   Regional node metastasis

Distant metastasis

M0   None
M1   Present

Stage grouping

0   Tis, N0, M0
I   T1 or T2, N0, M0
II   T3 or T4, N0, M0
III   Any T, N1, M0
IV   Any T, any N, M1

Modified from American Joint Committee on Cancer. *AJCC Staging Manual,*
5th ed. Philadelphia: Lippincott-Raven, 1997.

survival rate of more than 80%. Dukes B1 lesions penetrate the muscularis but do not reach the serosa; patient survival rates are 60% to 80%. Dukes B2 lesions penetrate to the serosa or through it into the pericolic fat; patient survival rates range from 40% to 70%. Dukes C lesions indicate nodal involvement. If the serosa has not been penetrated (in the Astler-Coller modification of the Dukes system), it is called a C1 lesion, with an associated 35% to 60% 5-year survival rate; the C2 lesions are through the serosa and are associated with a 15% to 30% survival rate. Dukes D lesions have distant metastases at the time of initial staging, and there are virtually no 5-year survivors. This pathologic staging method is helpful for selecting patients who are at sufficiently high risk to justify adjuvant therapy, such as chemotherapy or irradiation. The TNM system for colorectal cancer is being used increasingly (Table 9-4), but the Dukes classification is still more popular. The many modifications of the Dukes system support the argument that the TNM sys-

**Table 9-4.   TNM stages for
carcinoma of the colon and rectum**

Primary tumor

Tis   Carcinoma *in situ* and intramucosal (within lamina propria)
T1   Invades through muscularis mucosa into submucosa
T2   Invades muscularis propria
T3   Invades through muscularis propria into subserosa or
       non-peritonealized pericolic or perirectal tissues
T4   Invades adjacent organs or structures or perforates visceral
       peritoneum

Regional lymph nodes

N0   No nodal metastasis
N1   Metastasis in 1 to 3 regional nodes
N2   Metastasis in 4 or more regional nodes

Distant metastasis

M0   None
M1   Present

Stage grouping		Dukes'
0	Tis, N0, M0	—
I	T1 or T2, N0, M0	A
II	T3 or T4, N0, M0	B
III	Any T, N1, N2, M0	C
IV	Any T, any N, MI	

Modified from American Joint Committee on Cancer. *AJCC Staging Manual,*
5th ed. Philadelphia: Lippincott-Raven, 1997.

tem should be used to avoid confusion. Staging is most accurately done at surgery. Abdominal, chest, and pelvic CT are helpful for preoperative assessment of extrabowel involvement and for postsurgical follow-up, but the findings may be falsely negative when small peritoneal implants are present. Bone scans are seldom needed, except for assessment of bone pain, because bone metastases occur rather late in the course of the disease.

2. **Serum carcinoembryonic antigen** (CEA) level may parallel disease activity, although it is not increased in all patients with colon cancer. It is worth measuring preoperatively and, if elevated, postoperatively, because failure of an elevated value to return to normal may signify incomplete removal of the tumor. Likewise, a serial rise in CEA values after an initial fall to normal indicates recurrence. CEA values may also be an indicator of response during chemotherapy treatment, with a fall signifying improvement and a rise heralding progression

of tumor. Patients who have a normal serum CEA level preoperatively may still demonstrate an elevated CEA value at the time of recurrence. A rising CEA level is an indication for careful reevaluation with CT and possibly laparoscopy because some patients may have isolated, resectable, and thus potentially curable metastases.

B. Treatment of advanced disease

  1. Effective agents and combinations. For more than 30 years, fluorouracil has been the standard agent in the treatment of advanced colorectal disease not amenable to surgical or radiotherapeutic control. Response rates have varied widely, but a generally agreed-on figure is 20%. Several combinations of other agents with fluorouracil have been reported to have improved response rates and, in some instances, improved survival. They include leucovorin, methotrexate, interferon-α, and cisplatin. The methotrexate + fluorouracil and leucovorin + fluorouracil combinations have been shown to be superior to fluorouracil alone in controlled trials. Moderate-dose methotrexate requiring leucovorin rescue combined with fluorouracil has produced excellent survival in our experience, but only when the fluorouracil and methotrexate are separated by a 24-hour interval (compared to 1 hour). The best of these regimens remains to be determined by controlled studies. Continuous infusion of fluorouracil for varying periods of time has been evaluated but is not clearly superior to the bolus fluorouracil regimens with modulation.

  Recently, irinotecan (CPT-11, Camptosar) has been shown to be the most active agent since fluorouracil to be used in metastatic colon cancer. The response rate after progression on fluorouracil is in the range of 15% to 20% and is currently the second-line treatment of choice. Its activity as a first-line agent is 15% to 30%, and responses are at least as durable as with fluorouracil. Preliminary data on the combination of irinotecan + fluorouracil + leucovorin are encouraging, and a large randomized trial comparing each drug alone to the combination is in progress.

  A number of other new agents are also in development, including the thymidylate synthase inhibitors capecitabine, uracil-ftorafur (UFT), and raltitrexed (Tomudex) and a cisplatin analog, oxaliplatin. Some of these have recently been approved for use in colorectal cancer.

2. **Liver metastasis.** If the patient's disease is primarily in the liver, the response rate with intravenous fluorouracil alone is only about 10%. Intermittent hepatic artery infusion with fluorouracil, which is associated with a response rate of about 50%, should also be considered. Continuous infusion with floxuridine (FUdR), either by continuous external infusion with permanent catheters or by an implanted or portable pump, has also been used, with response rates averaging 50%. The impact on survival is controversial.

3. **Recommended regimens**
   a. **Fluorouracil + leucovorin.** Leucovorin, 20 mg/m^2, i.v., is followed by fluorouracil, 425 mg/m^2 i.v. The combination is given daily for 5 days. Courses are repeated at 4 and 8 weeks and every 5 weeks thereafter.
   b. **Irinotecan**, 125 mg/m^2 as a 90-minute i.v. infusion with appropriate potent antiemetics. Any diarrhea should be treated aggressively with loperamide, 4 mg p.o., then 2 mg every 2 hours after each loose stool. Treatment is given weekly for 4 weeks with a 2-week rest; then the cycle is repeated.
   c. **Fluorouracil + methotrexate + leucovorin.** Methotrexate, 200 mg/m^2 i.v., is given over 30 minutes after hydration with 1,500 mL 5% dextrose in 0.5N saline. At 24 hours, fluorouracil, 600 mg/m^2 i.v. bolus, is given, followed by leucovorin, 10 mg/m^2 (to the nearest 5 mg) p.o. every 6 hours × 6. The regimen is repeated every 2 weeks.
   d. **Fluorouracil + leucovorin** by 24-hour continuous infusion. Fluorouracil, 2,600 mg/m^2, and leucovorin, 500 mg/m^2, are given concurrently by 24-hour continuous i.v. infusion weekly. The drugs are administered using two separate infusion pumps to prevent the catheters from being blocked by "stones." The fluorouracil dose is lowered to 2,100 mg/m^2 for grade 3 hematologic or GI toxicity.
   e. **Hepatic artery infusion.** The catheter must be carefully positioned by an experienced angiographer through the axillary or femoral artery. A continuous i.v. heparin infusion of 5,000 U/day is given with fluorouracil, 800 mg/m^2/day for 4 days, then 600 mg/m^2 for a maximum of 17 days as tolerated. Weekly doses of 600 mg/m^2 i.v. can then be given to maintain whatever response has occurred, or the hepatic artery infusion can be repeated in the hospital in 4

to 6 months if the intravenous therapy does not prevent relapse. The position of the catheter must be checked twice weekly.

For the implanted pump, the initial dose of floxuridine is 0.2 to 0.3 mg/kg/day in heparinized saline given for 2 weeks, alternating with 2 weeks of heparinized saline without floxuridine. Heparin is used in a dose of 200 U/mL. Most patients can tolerate a daily floxuridine dose of 0.15 to 0.20 mg/kg for repeated cycles of 14 days every 4 weeks. Dexamethasone in a dose of 20 mg in the infused mixture is often used to treat or prevent the biliary sclerosis that sometimes accompanies such treatment.

C. **Adjuvant chemotherapy**
 1. **Colon cancer.** The combination of fluorouracil and levamisole given for 1 year improves the disease-free as well as the overall survival of patients with node-positive (Dukes C), resectable colon cancer, but not the survival of patients with stage B2 disease. For a time, this regimen was the standard of care in node-positive patients. Recent data indicate that 6 months of fluorouracil plus low-dose leucovorin is equally effective and is probably less toxic and less expensive. It is not yet clear whether patients with stage B2 disease should be treated. Certain patients can be identified as high risk by various biologic markers, and strong consideration should be given to treating them with adjuvant therapy, even though definitive proof of efficacy is lacking. Other active agents, such as irinotecan, may find a role in adjuvant therapy. A European study has reported the efficacy of the murine monoclonal antibody 17-1A as an adjuvant in colorectal cancer, with results similar to those achieved by chemotherapy. Confirmatory U.S. studies are in progress.

Although historical data support the use of postoperative radiotherapy for locally advanced colon cancer (Dukes B3 or C3, or any T4 lesion), there are as yet no controlled clinical trials that confirm its efficacy. Chemotherapy with fluorouracil should probably be incorporated into the regimen and used for a total of 6 months after radiation therapy.

The recommended adjuvant regimen for node-positive patients (stage III) is as follows:
   a. Leucovorin, 20 mg/m^2 i.v., and fluorouracil, 425 mg/m^2 i.v., daily × 5 on weeks 1, 5, 9, 14, 19, and 24.
 2. **Rectal cancer**
   a. **Preoperative irradiation.** Several studies have shown that preoperative irradiation benefits patients with rectal cancer,

although there are disadvantages in terms of accuracy of staging, delay before surgery, incomplete knowledge of the extent of tumor for treatment planning, and inappropriate administration of radiation to patients with early (Dukes A or B1) or advanced (Dukes D) lesions. Possible advantages include downstaging of tumor, improved sphincter preservation, improved resectability, and earlier initiation of systemic therapy. Better preoperative staging includes the use of magnetic resonance imaging (MRI) and endorectal ultrasound. Clinical trials are ongoing.

  b. **Postoperative irradiation, with and without chemotherapy.** Several controlled clinical trials have shown convincingly that radiation therapy alone reduces local recurrence but has little or no effect on overall survival. Fluorouracil-based chemotherapy added to radiation therapy is superior to either modality alone in terms of both local control and distant disease, thus improving overall survival. The optimal administration of fluorouracil during radiation therapy appears to be by protracted venous infusion (PVI), requiring a port and ambulatory pump, rather than by bolus. Whether the chemotherapy that does not accompany radiation therapy should be by bolus or PVI, along with the roles of levamisole and leucovorin, is being addressed by current clinical trials.

  The recommended adjuvant regimen for Dukes B2 or C rectal cancers is as follows:
  (1) Fluorouracil, 500 mg/m^2 i.v. bolus daily on days 1 to 5 and days 36 to 40.
  (2) Radiation therapy, 4,500 cGy in 180-cGy fractions over 5 weeks, with tumor boost of 540 to 900 cGy, beginning on day 64.
  (3) Fluorouracil, 225 mg/m^2/day by PVI throughout the period of radiation therapy, days 64 to 105.
  (4) Fluorouracil, 500 mg/m^2 i.v. bolus daily, on days 134 to 138 and days 169 to 173.

D. **Follow-up.** In the asymptomatic patient, follow-up after treatment includes history and physical examination every 3 months for 3 years, then every 6 months for 2 years. CEA, complete blood cell count, examination of stool for occult blood, and liver function tests are appropriately done at the same intervals. Colonoscopy should be done annually for 3 years, and may then be decreased in frequency to every 3 years if no polyps are found. Annual chest x-ray studies are appropriate. CT of the abdomen, pelvis, or chest should probably not be done routinely except to evaluate symptoms or a rising CEA level, which can indicate recurrent but sometimes resectable disease.

E.   **Complications of therapy or disease.** The complications of chemotherapy are those attributable to the individual drugs. Myelosuppression, nausea, vomiting, and diarrhea are common and may require dose modification and symptomatic treatment. Radiation complications are similar and also include dysuria, tenesmus, and rectal discharge of blood or mucus. Phenazopyridine (Pyridium) is useful in treating dysuria, and loperamide (Imodium) or diphenoxylate (Lomotil) is recommended for diarrhea. If toxicity is substantial (grade 3 or 4) during radiotherapy, a treatment delay of at least 1 week is warranted. During chemotherapy with fluorouracil-based regimens, mild diarrhea (grade 1) may be treated symptomatically. Moderate diarrhea (grade 2 or 3) is an indication for dose reduction by 50%, and severe diarrhea (grade 3 or 4) is an indication for stopping chemotherapy for 1 week or longer. Dehydration is a real risk with grade 3 or 4 diarrhea, and intravenous hydration may be necessary. Octreotide, 50 to 100 µg t.i.d., may help to alleviate severe diarrhea. Oral mucositis can often be prevented on subsequent courses without dose reduction by holding ice in the mouth for 20 minutes before, during, and after the intravenous bolus of fluorouracil. Nausea is usually not severe with fluorouracil regimens and usually responds to prochlorperazine or dexamethasone. Hematopoietic growth factors are seldom warranted for the mild neutropenia that is observed with bolus fluorouracil therapy.

F.   **Treatment of refractory disease.** No satisfactory treatment exists for the patient whose disease progresses on the regimens listed previously for metastatic disease. Some patients with liver disease failing intravenous therapy may respond to fluorouracil or floxuridine given as a hepatic artery infusion. The combination of cyclophosphamide + methotrexate + vincristine has produced some responses, but response rates are of the order of 10% and are usually brief. The regimen is as follows:

1.   Cyclophosphamide, 300 mg/m^2 i.v. weekly, *and*
2.   Vincristine, 1.4 mg/m^2 i.v. weekly (maximum dose, 2 mg), *and*
3.   Methotrexate, 25 mg/m^2 i.v. weekly.

We also have occasionally seen responses with single-dose mitomycin, 15 to 20 mg/m^2 i.v. every 6 weeks.

V. **Cancer of the anal canal.** These cancers, constituting only 1% to 3% of all cases of large bowel cancer, were historically treated by abdominoperineal resection with about a 50% cure rate. They have been seen more commonly in women. However, in recent years, there is an increase of these cancers in men, particularly homosexuals. The human papillomavirus has been implicated in some patients, and anal warts are sometimes seen as well. Patients infected with the human immunodeficiency virus (HIV) also have an increased incidence of anal cancer.

A. **Local disease.** It has been found that combined-modality treatment with chemotherapy and irradiation is curative in 75% to 80% of patients and thus allows avoidance of abdominoperineal resection with retention of anal function. The following regimen is recommended:

1. Radiotherapy, 4,500 cGy in 25 fractions (5 weeks), *and concurrently*

2. Fluorouracil, 1,000 mg/m^2 by continuous i.v. infusion daily $\times$ 4 days (days 1 to 4 and 29 to 32), *and*

3. Mitomycin, 10 mg/m^2 i.v. on days 1 and 29

A biopsy should be done 4 weeks after radiation therapy. If negative, no further treatment is needed. If positive, consider an additional 900 cGy (5 fractions) and a 4-day course of fluorouracil, 1,000 mg/m^2 by continuous i.v. infusion on days 1 to 4, and cisplatin, 100 mg/m^2 i.v. on day 2. If the biopsy is persistently positive, an abdominoperineal resection is appropriate.

B. **Metastatic disease.** For metastatic disease, the following regimen is recommended:

1. Mitomycin, 10 mg/m^2 i.v. every 4 weeks $\times$ 2, then every 10 weeks, *and*

2. Doxorubicin, 30 mg/m^2 i.v. every 4 weeks $\times$ 2, then every 5 weeks, *and*

3. Cisplatin, 60 mg/m^2 i.v., every 4 weeks $\times$ 2, then every 5 weeks.

SELECTED READINGS

Al-Sarraf M, Martz K, Herskovic A, et al. Progress report of combined chemoradiotherapy versus radiotherapy alone in patients with esophageal cancer: an Intergroup study. *J Clin Oncol* 1997;15: 277–284.

Ardalan B, Chua L, Tian E, et al. A phase II study of weekly 24-hour infusion with high-dose fluorouracil with leucovorin in colorectal carcinoma. *J Clin Oncol* 1991;9:625–630.

Blot WJ, Devesa SS, Kneller RW, et al. Rising incidence of adenocarcinoma of the esophagus and gastric cardia. *JAMA* 1991;265: 1287–1289.

Boku N, Ohtsu A, Shimada Y, et al. Phase II study of a combination of CDDP and CPT-11 in metastatic gastric cancer: CPT-11 study group for gastric cancer [Abstract]. *Proc Am Soc Clin Oncol* 1997;16:264.

Conti JA, Kemeny NE, Saltz LB, et al. Irinotecan is an active agent in untreated patients with metastatic colorectal cancer. *J Clin Oncol* 1996;14:709–715.

Costa F, Ilson D, Forastiere A, et al. Phase II study of paclitaxel and cisplatin in patients with advanced adenocarcinoma and squamous cell carcinoma of the esophagus [Abstract]. *Proc Am Soc Clin Oncol* 1997;16:262.

Flam MS, John MJ, Mowry PA, et al. Definitive combined modality therapy of carcinoma of the anus: a report of 30 cases including results of salvage therapy in patients with residual disease. *Dis Colon Rectum* 1987;30:495–502.

Gastrointestinal Tumor Study Group. Prolongation of disease-free interval in surgically treated rectal cancer. *N Engl J Med* 1985;312:1465–1472.

Haller DG, Catalano PJ, Macdonald JS, Mayer RJ. Fluorouracil (FU), leucovorin (LV) and levamisole (LEV) adjuvant therapy for colon cancer: four-year results of INT-0089 [Abstract]. *Proc Am Soc Clin Oncol* 1997;16:265.

Ilson DH, Sirott M, Saltz L, et al. A phase II trial of interferon alfa-2a, 5-fluorouracil, and cisplatin in patients with advanced esophageal carcinoma. *Cancer* 1995;75:2197–2202.

Kelsen D, Atiq OT, Saltz L, et al. FAMTX versus etoposide, doxorubicin and cisplatin: a random assignment trial in gastric cancer. *J Clin Oncol* 1992;10:541–548.

Leichman L, Nigro N, Vaitkevicius VK, et al. Cancer of the anal canal: model for preoperative adjuvant combined modality therapy. *Am J Med* 1985;78:211–215.

Louvet C, deGramont A, Beerblock K, et al. Hydroxyurea, leucovorin, fluorouracil and cisplatin: final results of a large multicenter phase II study in advanced gastric cancer [Abstract]. *Proc Am Soc Clin Oncol* 1997;16:264.

Marsh JC, Bertino JR, Katz KH, et al. The influence of drug interval on the effect of methotrexate and fluorouracil in the treatment of metastatic colorectal cancer. *J Clin Oncol* 1991;9:371–380.

Moertel CG, Hanley JA. Combination chemotherapy trials for metastatic carcinoid tumor and the malignant carcinoid syndrome. *Cancer Clin Trials* 1979;2:327–334.

Neugut AI, Marvin MR, Rella VA, Chabot JA. An overview of adenocarcinoma of the small intestine. *Oncology* 1997;11:529–536.

O'Connell MJ, Laurie JA, Kahn M, et al. Prospectively randomized trial of postoperative adjuvant chemotherapy in patients with high-risk colon cancer. *J Clin Oncol* 1998;16:295–300.

O'Connell MJ, Martenson JA, Wieand HS, et al. Improving adjuvant therapy for rectal cancer by combining protracted-infusion fluorouracil with radiation therapy after curative surgery. *N Engl J Med* 1994;331:502–507.

Poon MA, O'Connell MJ, Moertel CG, et al. Biochemical modulation of fluorouracil: evidence of significant improvement of survival and quality of life in patients with advanced colorectal carcinoma. *J Clin Oncol* 1989;7:1407–1418.

Reed ML, Vaitkevicius VK, Al-Sarraf M, et al. The practicality of chronic hepatic artery infusion therapy of primary and metastatic hepatic malignancies: ten-year results of 124 patients in a prospective protocol. *Cancer* 1981;47:402–409.

Roder JD, Bottcher K, Busch R, et al. Classification of regional lymph nodes metastasis from gastric carcinoma. *Cancer* 1998;82:621–631.

Rothenberg ML, Pazdur R, Rowinsky EK, et al. A phase II multicenter trial of alternating cycles of irinotecan (CPT-11) and fluorouracil/LV in patients with previously untreated metastatic colorectal cancer (CRC) [Abstract]. *Proc Am Soc Clin Oncol* 1997;16:266.

Rougier P, Bugat R, Douilllard JY, et al. Phase II study of irinotecan in the treatment of advanced colorectal cancer in chemotherapy-naïve patients and patients pretreated with fluorouracil-based chemotherapy. *J Clin Oncol* 1997;15:251–260.

Shepard KV, Levin B, Karl RC, et al. Therapy for metastatic colorectal cancer with hepatic artery infusion chemotherapy using a subcutaneous implanted pump. *J Clin Oncol* 1985;3:161–169.

Sirott MN, Kelsen D, Johnson B, et al. a-Interferon (INF), 5-fluorouracil (FU), and cisplatin (CDDP): an active regimen in advanced adenocarcinoma (ADENOCA) and squamous cell carcinoma (SCC) of the esophagus [Abstract]. *Proc Am Soc Clin Oncol* 1992;11:172.

Urba S, Orringer M, Turrisi A, et al. A randomized trial comparing surgery to preoperative concomitant chemoradiation plus surgery in patients with resectable esophageal cancer: updated analysis [Abstract]. *Proc Am Soc Clin Oncol* 1997;16:277.

Vaughn DJ, Haller DG. Adjuvant therapy for colorectal cancer: past accomplishments, future directions. *Cancer Invest* 1997;15:435–447.

Walsh TN, Noonan N, Hollywood D, et al. A comparison of multimodal therapy and surgery for esophageal adeno-carcinoma. *N Engl J Med* 1996;335:462–467.

Wilke H, Preusser P, Fink U, et al. High dose folinic acid/etoposide/5-fluorouracil in advanced gastric cancer-a phase II study in elderly patients or patients with cardiac risk. *Invest New Drugs* 1990;8: 65–70.

Willett CG, Tepper JE, Shellito PC, Wood WC. Indications for adjuvant radiotherapy in extrapelvic colonic carcinoma. *Oncology* 1989;3:25–31.

Carcinomas of the Pancreas, Liver, Gallbladder, and Bile Ducts

David J. Schifeling

Carcinomas of the pancreas, liver, and biliary passages account for about 2% of all cases of cancer and for 5% of all cancer-related deaths in the United States. Virtually all patients with these cancers die from this disease. However, advances in molecular biology are expected to lead to earlier diagnosis and improved treatment.

I. **Adenocarcinoma of the pancreas**
    A. **Epidemiology and etiology.** Pancreatic cancer occurred with increasing incidence during the past several decades and currently is the fifth leading cause of cancer-related deaths in the United States. Risk factors for pancreatic cancer include age, male sex, race (Polynesians, blacks), and tobacco exposure. It is rare before 30 years of age, and the incidence rises throughout life, with peak occurrence during the seventh decade. Smokers have 1.6 to 3.9 times the risk of developing pancreatic cancer compared with nonsmokers. Pancreatitis is commonly associated with carcinoma of the pancreas in pathologic specimens. Whether patients with chronic pancreatitis are at greater risk for developing pancreatic cancer is uncertain. Patients with familial pancreatitis appear to have a greater risk. Diabetes mellitus is often discovered just before the diagnosis of pancreatic cancer, but patients with diabetes mellitus do not have a greater risk of pancreatic cancer. Hereditary pancreatic cancer has been observed in rare families with an autosomal site-specific pattern, in families with BRCA-2 mutations, and in hereditary nonpolyposis colorectal cancer (HNPCC) families.
    B. **Presenting signs and symptoms.** Pain is the most common presenting symptom. It occurs in three fourths of patients with carcinoma of the head of the pancreas and in virtually all patients with carcinoma of the body or tail. Usually, the pain is a dull ache in the epigastrium that radiates to the right upper quadrant when the tumor is in the head of the pancreas or to the left upper quadrant when the tumor is in the body or tail. It may be an atypical sharp or intermittent epigastric pain, or it may be located in the lumbar region of the back. As many as one fifth of patients present with nonspecific symptoms, including weight loss, anorexia, nausea, vomiting, and constipation. Seventy percent of patients with carcinoma of the head of the pancreas have

jaundice, whereas fewer than 15% of patients with carcinoma of the pancreatic body have jaundice. Physical findings are generally associated with advanced carcinomas and include weight loss, hepatomegaly, and abdominal mass.

C. **Diagnostic evaluation.** Ultrasonography and computed tomography (CT) demonstrate masses in the pancreas or dilation of the pancreatic duct or the common bile duct. Sensitivity and specificity of CT are about 90%, whereas sensitivity and specificity of ultrasonography are somewhat less. Both tests detect relatively large mass lesions of the pancreas and usually miss 1- to 2-cm carcinomas. Endoscopic retrograde cholangiopancreatography (ERCP) demonstrates subtle ductal abnormalities; sensitivity and specificity are in excess of 90%. Endoscopy-directed biopsies of pancreatic ducts have diagnosed tumors smaller than 1- to 2-cm in diameter. Percutaneous transhepatic cholangiography may be performed if ERCP is unsuccessful and yields similar information. Percutaneous fine-needle aspiration of suspicious abnormalities identified on CT scan can confirm the diagnosis of pancreatic cancer, with 80% to 90% sensitivity and 100% specificity.

D. **Laboratory tests.** CA 19-9 is a cell surface glycoprotein associated with pancreatic cancer. Rising serum levels may be a useful early indicator of recurrent or progressive disease.

E. **Staging and preoperative evaluation**
1. **Staging.** The primary tumor, regional lymph nodes, and potential sites of metastatic disease must be carefully assessed (Table 10-1). CT of the abdomen assesses the primary site, regional lymph nodes, and liver. Chest radiographs screen for metastatic disease in the chest. Routine laboratory studies and physical examination screen for other sites of involvement.
2. **Preoperative evaluation.** Preoperative evaluation should be performed stepwise from least

Table 10-1.   TNM staging for pancreatic cancer

Stage	Definition
I	T1 (tumor ≤2 cm), T2 (tumor >2 cm, confined to pancreas), N0, M0
II	T3 (tumor extends to duodenum, bile duct, or peri-pancreatic tissue), N0, M0
III	T1–3, N1, M0
IVA	T4 (tumor extends to stomach, spleen, colon, or adjacent large vessels), N0–1, M0
IVB	T1–4, N0–1, M1

N1, any nodal metastases; M1, any distant metastases.
American Joint Committee on Cancer. *AJCC staging manual,* 5th ed. Philadelphia: JB Lippincott, 1997.

invasive to most invasive as indicated by the clinical situation. Preoperative evaluation can be stopped when metastatic disease or definite evidence for unresectable locoregional spread is identified. All patients should undergo CT. If no hepatic metastasis or major blood vessel involvement is identified, then arteriography can be performed to assess major blood vessel involvement and tumor blood supply. If no major blood vessel involvement is identified, then laparoscopy can be used to identify small metastases in the liver or peritoneum. Laparoscopy identifies metastatic disease in 40% of patients with pancreatic cancer who have had negative findings on CT and arteriogram. In one series, nearly 80% of cancers were resectable when all tests, including laparoscopy, were negative. After negative CT and arteriography alone, only 15% to 20% of pancreas cancers were resectable at laparotomy.

F. Primary therapy

   1. Surgery. Three fourths of patients with pancreatic cancer are operative candidates, but only 15% to 20% have resectable tumors. Patients without evident metastatic cancer or major blood vessel involvement, whose performance status permits operative intervention, are candidates for curative surgery. Five to 10% of the patients resected for cure survive 5 years. Surgical bypass procedures may also palliate obstructive jaundice and gastric outlet obstruction. Endoscopic stent placement may palliate obstructive jaundice.

   2. Radiation therapy. External-beam radiation therapy can palliate unresectable carcinomas. It may also be used as a surgical adjuvant in combination with chemotherapy. Great care and expertise must be exercised to plan the radiation fields. These fields must encompass known disease without excessive involvement of adjacent normal tissue. Surgical clips placed at laparotomy or laparoscopy can guide treatment.

   3. Combined-modality therapy

      a. Resected carcinomas. On the basis of a randomized study by the Gastrointestinal Tumor Study Group (GITSG), postoperative combined-modality therapy is recommended for patients with resected carcinoma of the pancreas. The GITSG demonstrated that postoperative adjuvant radiotherapy (split-course in their study) plus fluorouracil is better than adjuvant radiotherapy alone. On the basis of the demonstrated benefit of prolonged infusion of fluorouracil or fluorouracil modulated by leucovorin in colon and rectal carcinomas, both of these approaches have been safely combined with radiotherapy (40 to 50 Gy in standard fractionation) in pancreatic cancer. The recommended treatments have the advantage of avoiding split-course radiotherapy. Recommended regimens are as follows:

(1) Fluorouracil, 225 mg/m² by continuous i.v. infusion throughout radiation therapy or 300 mg/m² by continuous i.v. infusion 5 days per week during radiation therapy, *or*

(2) Fluorouracil, 425 mg/m² by i.v. push 1 hour after leucovorin, 20 mg/m² by i.v. push daily for 4 days during the first week of radiation therapy and for 3 days during the fifth week of radiation therapy, *or*

(3) Fluorouracil, 500 mg/m² by i.v. push midway during a 2-hour infusion of leucovorin, 500 mg/m² weekly for the first 6 weeks of radiation therapy.

At the completion of combined-modality therapy, chemotherapy should be continued for 6 months using weekly intravenous-push fluorouracil or a modulated fluorouracil regimen. Two-year and 5-year survival rates similar to the 43% and 25% rates seen in the combined-modality groups in the GITSG trials may be anticipated, although this has not yet been adequately tested.

b. **Localized unresectable carcinoma.** A series of randomized trials conducted by the GITSG demonstrated superior survival of patients with localized but unresectable pancreatic cancer when treated with combined-modality therapy, compared with patients treated with radiation therapy or chemotherapy alone. These clinical trials also used split-course radiation therapy. As discussed in Section F.3.a, current clinical trials do not support a specific combined-modality treatment program. However, 60 Gy of radiation should be delivered in a single course of external-beam radiation to gross tumor, and 40 to 50 Gy to microscopic cancer. Chemotherapy may be given by any of the regimens noted in Section F.3.a. After completion of combined-modality therapy, chemotherapy should be continued for 6 months using bolus fluorouracil or a modulated fluorouracil regimen. In the GITSG trials, the median survival time was 10 months in the combined-modality group, compared with 5 months in the radiotherapy-alone group. Specialized modes of administration of the radiation therapy may be considered, including intraoperative radiotherapy to boost the dose to the gross tumor or conformational radiation therapy to minimize the dose to surrounding tissues while delivering maximum dose to the tumor. Quality-of-life studies have not been reported.

G. **Chemotherapy of metastatic disease.** Patients with pancreatic cancer are often poor candidates for chemotherapy because of severe weight loss, poor performance status, severe pain, lack of measurable or evaluable disease, and the presence of jaundice or hepatic involvement, which may interfere with clearance of therapeutic agents. However, two recent randomized clinical trials demonstrated survival and quality-of-life benefits to chemotherapy in selected patients with advanced pancreatic cancer.

1. **Single agents.** A number of single agents have demonstrated activity (Table 10-2), although no agent has demonstrated consistent complete and partial response rates of 20% or greater using CT to measure response. Gemcitabine (2′,2′-defluorodeoxycytidine), a nucleoside analog, has been accepted as first-line therapy for

Table 10-2.   Single-agent chemotherapy in pancreatic cancer

Drug	No. of patients	Complete plus partial response rate range (%)	Clinical benefit[a] range (%)
Gemcitabine	158	5.4–11	17.2–27
Fluorouracil	237	0–12.5[b]	5–50
Mitomycin	44	27[c]	NA
Streptozocin	27	11[c]	NA
Doxorubicin	28	8[c]	NA
Ifosfamide	113	6–22	NA
Irinotecan (CPT-11)	95	9–10	NA
Topotecan	62	0–10	NA
Docetaxol	30	20	NA

[a] Sustained (≥4 wk) improvement of one of the following parameters without worsening of any of the others: performance status, composite pain measurement (average pain intensity and narcotic analgesic use) or weight.
[b] Studies reported with response evaluation by computed tomography.
[c] Studies reported before routine use of computed tomography.
NA, not available.

metastatic pancreatic cancer in patients with adequate performance status, based on two phase II trials and one phase III trial. These trials demonstrated modest antitumor activity (complete and partial response rates, 5.4% to 11%), whereas "clinical benefit" was observed in about one quarter of patients. *Clinical benefit* was defined as sustained (more than 4 weeks) improvement of one of the following parameters without worsening of any of the others: performance status, composite pain measurement (average pain intensity and narcotic analgesic use), and weight. Bolus fluorouracil had a 0% objective response rate and 5% clinical benefit rate in the randomized trial with gemcitabine. Although response rates with modulated fluorouracil regimens have been poor, responses in CT-monitored studies are better with modulated fluorouracil than with bolus fluorouracil.

2. **Combination chemotherapy.** Combination chemotherapy has been investigated (Table 10-3). The most commonly used regimens are fluorouracil + doxorubicin + mitomycin (FAM) and streptozocin + mitomycin + fluorouracil (SMF), with response rates reported between 13% and 43%. These and other combination regimens have not shown an advantage over single-agent therapy.

3. **Current recommendations.** Single-agent therapy with gemcitabine, 1,000 mg/m^2 i.v. weekly for 7 weeks followed by 1 week rest, then 4-week cycles of 3 weekly doses followed by 1 week rest, is recommended for patients with metastatic pancreatic cancer and with an Eastern Cooperative Oncology Group (ECOG) performance status of 0 to 2, who are not eligible for clinical trials. Toxicity is generally modest with moderate myelosuppression, with neutropenia and anemia, mild to moderate nausea,

Table 10-3. Combination chemotherapy for carcinoma of exocrine pancreas

Regimen	Dosages
SMF	Streptozocin, 1 g/m^2 i.v. on days 1, 8, 29, and 36 Mitomycin, 10 mg/m^2 i.v. on day 1 Fluorouracil, 600 mg/m^2 i.v. on days, 1, 8, 29, and 36 Repeat cycle every 8 weeks
FAM	Fluorouracil 600 mg/m^2 i.v. on days 1, 8, 29, and 36 Doxorubicin (Adriamycin), 30 mg/m^2 i.v. on days 1 and 29 Mitomycin, 10 mg/m^2 i.v. on day 1 Repeat cycle every 8 weeks

an influenza-like syndrome that includes low-grade fever and malaise, minimal alopecia, and occasional rash. If the tumor does not respond or progresses after initial response to gemcitabine, treatment with fluorouracil in a modulated or weekly bolus regimen or mitomycin, 20 mg/m² i.v. on day 1 every 4 to 6 weeks, could be considered. Because of the limited effectiveness of current therapy, participation in clinical trials should be encouraged, especially with phase II trials of new agents or combinations.

II. **Malignant islet cell carcinomas**
  A. **Epidemiology and natural history.** Islet cell neoplasms occur in about 1 in 100,000 people per year. Eighty percent of these tumors secrete one or more hormones excessively: most commonly insulin or gastrin; less commonly glucagon, serotonin, or adrenocorticotropic hormone (ACTH); and rarely vasoactive intestinal peptides (VIP), growth hormone-releasing hormone (GHRH), or somatostatin. Twenty percent are nonfunctional. Islet cell tumors may occur with the multiple endocrine neoplasia type I (MEN-I) syndrome. In families with this autosomal dominant syndrome, 80% of affected members develop islet cell tumors, most commonly gastrinoma (54%), insulinoma (21%), glucagonoma (3%), or VIPoma (1%). Other endocrine manifestations of MEN-I include parathyroid hyperplasia, pituitary adenomas (often a prolactinoma), and occasionally adrenal or thyroid adenomas. About one fourth of gastrinomas are associated with MEN-I. Eighty to 90% of gastrinomas occur in the head of the pancreas. Insulinomas are equally common in the head, body, and tail. Gastrinomas tend to be multiple small tumors, whereas insulinomas tend to be single tumors and glucagonomas and VIPomas single large tumors. The median age of patients is in the sixth decade. There are no sex or race associations.

  Islet cell tumors generally present with symptoms caused by hormone hypersecretion, most commonly fasting hypoglycemia, or the Zollinger-Ellison syndrome, followed by others. VIPomas are associated with episodic severe secretory diarrhea with hypokalemia, hypochlorhydria, and metabolic acidosis. Classically, glucagonomas are associated with necrolytic migratory erythema, mild diabetes, severe muscle wasting, and marked hyperaminoaciduria.

  Sixty percent of gastrinomas are malignant. Histologic appearance and tumor size do not predict malignancy; only the presence of metastatic disease confirms malignancy. Ninety percent of malignant gastrinomas have liver metastases. Other sites of spread include abdominal nodes, peritoneum, bone, and lung. Median survival from time of diagnosis of metastatic disease is about 2.5 years. Only 10% of insulinomas are malignant. They are usually larger than 2.5 cm, whereas benign insulinomas are generally smaller than 2.5 cm. Most glucagonomas and VIPomas are malignant (60% to 80%).

B. Treatment of advanced disease

    1. Endocrine syndromes. The first goal of treatment must be to control endocrine syndromes.

        a. Gastric acid suppression. The H^+-K^+-ATPase inhibitors omeprazole and lansoprazole successfully control gastric acid secretion in all patients with gastrinoma. Optimal doses must be individualized and periodically reevaluated. Gastric acid secretion in the hour preceding the next dose of omeprazole or lansoprazole should be less than 10 mEq in patients who have had no previous gastric surgery and less than 5 mEq in those who have had an acid-reducing procedure. The starting dose is 60 mg/day with both agents. Doses greater than 80 mg/day should be divided.

        b. Insulin suppression. Diazoxide, 3 to 8 mg/kg/day p.o. divided in three doses (e.g., 50 to 150 mg p.o. t.i.d.), is the therapy of choice for hypoglycemia associated with insulinoma when dietary measures fail. A diuretic should be given with diazoxide to prevent water retention.

        c. Octreotide acetate (Sandostatin). Octreotide acetate is a somatostatin analog that inhibits gut hormone secretion. It is generally useful for carcinoid and VIPoma syndromes and is possibly useful for controlling symptoms in patients with glucagonomas, GHRH tumors, and gastrinomas. In patients with unresectable insulinoma, it can reduce insulin secretion by 50% and return blood glucose levels to normal. However, it must be initiated cautiously in patients in the hospital because profound hypoglycemia may occur. The usual starting dose of octreotide is 50 µg s.c. b.i.d.; thereafter, the dose and frequency of injections can be increased to 100 µg t.i.d.

    2. Chemotherapy for advanced islet cell tumors. Streptozocin is the most active single agent, with a 50% response rate. It is a nonmyelosuppressive nitrosourea with diabetogenic effects in animals. Doxorubicin is also an active agent. The combination of streptozocin and doxorubicin was demonstrated to have a superior response rate (69%), time to tumor progression (20 months), and survival time (2.2 years) than the combination of streptozocin and fluorouracil or single-agent chlorozotocin in a North Central Cancer Treatment Group study. This combination is recommended as first-line chemotherapy.

  a. Streptozocin, 500 mg/m^2 i.v. on days 1 to 5, and doxorubicin 50 mg/m^2 i.v., on days 1 and 22. Repeat every 6 weeks.

  Renal impairment occurs in about 30% of patients receiving a streptozocin-based regimen; about one third of those with renal insufficiency have creatinine levels higher than 2 mg/dL. Nausea and vomiting occur in about 60% of patients. Leukopenia occurs in about 75%, but only 10% have a white blood cell count of less than 1,000/μL. Stomatitis is uncommon. Liver function test abnormalities may also occur. Deaths caused by treatment are rare.

  b. α-Interferon may diminish excess hormone secretion and induce shrinkage of tumors; some trials have reported 50% response rates. This agent can be used after chemotherapy failure.

III. Ampullary carcinomas. In up to 80% of people, the common bile duct and main pancreatic duct empty into a common channel, the ampulla of Vater. Periampullary carcinomas can be classified according to their site of origin. Type I tumors originate in the ampulla of Vater or the duodenal portion of the common bile duct. Type II carcinomas are duodenal tumors involving the ampulla of Vater. Type III are mixed ampullary—periampullary carcinomas, and type IV are pancreatic head carcinomas involving the ampulla. Type IV tumors carry a much worse prognosis and should be distinguished from the ampullary or periampullary carcinomas. Types I to III periampullary and ampullary carcinomas generally can be extirpated surgically. Large tumors require a Whipple resection, whereas local excision may be curative for small tumors. The overall 5-year survival rate is 40% to 50% for patients with types I to III carcinomas. The roles of irradiation and chemotherapy are uncertain. Tumors larger than 2 cm in diameter should be treated as adenocarcinoma of the pancreas.

IV. Carcinoma of the bile ducts (cholangiocarcinoma)

  A. Epidemiology and natural history. The incidence of primary biliary tree carcinoma is about 2 per 100,000 population. Men are affected more commonly than women. Tumors occur most often in late-middle-aged and elderly patients. They are associated with cholelithiasis, ulcerative colitis, obesity, liver flukes, and exposure to thorium oxide (Thorotrast). Patients present with obstructive jaundice, except for the occasional patient with a carcinoma identified at laparotomy for cholelithiasis. About half of bile duct tumors are located proximally. Ten percent have multicentric involvement of the bile ducts. Local invasion is common. Liver involvement occurs in nearly half of these patients. Surgical cure is uncommon. Bypass procedures or intubation of the biliary tree may offer palliation to patients whose tumors cannot be resected. Radiation therapy may relieve proximal obstruction without intubation or a bypass procedure. Combined-modality therapy with radiation and fluorouracil should be considered in patients with an unresectable but localized cancer.

B. Chemotherapy for advanced disease. Few reports are available for this unusual tumor, but its response rate to fluorouracil, alone or in combination with streptozocin, is about 10%. Outside the context of a clinical trial, one of the following regimens is recommended:

1. Fluorouracil, 500 mg/m^2 i.v. push on days 1 to 5 every 4 weeks or 500 mg/m^2 i.v. weekly, *or*
2. Fluorouracil, 400 mg/m^2 i.v. on days 1 to 5, and streptozocin, 500 mg/m^2 i.v. on days 1 to 5. Repeat every 6 weeks.

V. Carcinoma of the gallbladder

A. Epidemiology and natural history. Carcinomas of the gallbladder are seen predominantly in late-middle-aged and elderly women, with the highest incidence in Native Americans and the populations of central and eastern Europe and Israel. The areas of high frequency also report a high incidence of cholelithiasis. Patients with "porcelain" or calcified gallbladders identified on radiographs have a 12% to 62% risk of cancer. Carcinoma of the gallbladder most commonly presents with pain, nausea and vomiting, and weight loss. Jaundice occurs in only one third of patients. Anorexia, abdominal distention, pruritus, and melena occur in some patients. One percent of patients undergoing cholecystectomy are found to have carcinoma of the gallbladder. Overall survival is poor; less than 5% of patients who undergo resection survive 5 years. When the tumor is histologically confined to the mucosa or submucosa, survival rates of 64% at 5 years and 44% at 10 years have been reported. Gallbladder carcinomas may invade locally into the bile ducts, liver, pancreas, stomach, or duodenum. They also may spread to regional lymph nodes and distantly to liver.

B. Chemotherapy for advanced disease. Few reports are available for review. Seven (18%) of 40 patients responded to fluorouracil. Seven (28%) of 25 patients responded to mitomycin. Four (31%) of 14 patients treated with fluorouracil + doxorubicin + mitomycin responded. Choices of therapy are as follows:

1. Fluorouracil, 500 mg/m^2 i.v. on days 1 to 5 every 4 weeks or 500 to 600 mg/m^2 i.v. weekly, *or*
2. FAM, a three-drug combination of fluorouracil, 600 mg/m^2 i.v. on days 1, 8, 29, and 36, plus doxorubicin (Adriamycin), 30 mg/m^2 i.v. on days 1 and 29, plus mitomycin, 10 mg/m^2 i.v. on day 1. Repeat every 8 weeks.

Although there may be a slightly improved response rate with FAM, the toxicity is significant, and no survival or quality-of-life benefit has been demonstrated.

VI. Primary carcinoma of the liver

A. **Epidemiology.** Primary carcinoma of the liver is rare in the United States. There are fewer than 10,000 new patients annually, accounting for less than 2% of all malignancies. However, it is the leading cause of cancer death in parts of Africa and Asia. Ninety percent of primary carcinomas of the liver are hepatocellular carcinomas or hepatoma; the remaining carcinomas include cholangiocarcinomas (about 7%), hepatoblastomas, angiosarcomas, and other sarcomas. Histologic subsets of hepatocellular carcinoma have been recognized. Fibrolamellar carcinomas occur in young patients and are more likely to be resectable and cured. Hepatocellular carcinomas are more common in men than women. The peak occurrence is during the sixth decade, with the highest incidence during the ninth decade.

There appear to be three major factors associated with hepatocellular carcinoma: (a) viral hepatitis B and C; (b) alcohol abuse; and (c) aflatoxin exposure. Seventy-five percent of patients with hepatocellular carcinoma have concomitant cirrhosis, and 4% to 20% of patients with cirrhosis have hepatocellular carcinoma at autopsy, depending on the population studied. Among the patients with hepatocellular carcinoma, 15% to 80% have hepatitis B surface antigenemia. In China, the incidence of hepatocellular carcinoma parallels the incidence of hepatitis B infection. The introduction of an effective hepatitis B vaccine may reduce the risk of hepatocellular carcinoma in these areas. In Africa, the increased risk appears to be related to exposure to aflatoxin, which is produced by the fungi *Aspergillus flavus* and *Aspergillus parasiticus* during improper food storage. Three to 27% of patients with long-standing hemochromatosis develop hepatocellular carcinoma. Anabolic steroids have also been associated with hepatocellular carcinoma. Tumors induced by anabolic steroids may retain hormone dependence and regress after withdrawal of the steroid.

B. **Presentation.** Patients with primary carcinoma of the liver commonly complain of right upper quadrant pain, abdominal distention, or weight loss. The pain is usually dull or aching but may be acute and radiate to the right shoulder. Fatigue, loss of appetite, and unexplained fever may occur. Patients with underlying cirrhosis may present with hepatic decompensation: new ascites, variceal bleeding, jaundice, or encephalopathy. Rarely, patients present with paraneoplastic syndromes: erythrocytosis is most common; hypercalcemia, hyperthyroidism, and carcinoid syndrome have been described. Physical findings include nodular hepatomegaly with an arterial bruit and hepatic rub. Extrahepatic spread occurs in about 50% of patients during the course of the illness. Twenty percent of patients have lung metastases.

C. **Diagnostic evaluation and screening.** α-Fetoprotein levels are elevated in 70% of patients and associated with a poor prognosis. Ultrasonography and CT have a high sensitivity when lesions are larger than 2 cm; however, small lesions are frequently missed. Magnetic resonance imaging is generally equivalent to CT but at a greater cost. Fine-needle aspiration with cytology or biopsy usually confirms the diagnosis. Serial α-fetoprotein measurements every 3 to 4 months and liver ultrasound every 4 to 6 months should be considered in high-risk patients with hepatitis B antigenemia or with hepatitis C and cirrhosis. Patients with hepatitis C without cirrhosis and patients with hemochromatosis should be considered for less intensive screening.

D. **Staging** (Table 10-4). Staging procedures should include a chest radiograph, CT of the abdomen, a complete blood cell count, a blood chemistry profile, and an α-fetoprotein measurement. If these do not disclose unresectable cancer or sites of metastatic cancer, then CT of the chest and arteriogram (upper abdominal and hepatic) should be performed to guide surgical intervention and further screening for extrahepatic involvement.

Table 10-4. TNM staging for hepatocellular cancer

Stage	Definition
I	T1 (solitary tumor ≤2 cm without vascular invasion), N0, M0
II	T2 (solitary tumor ≤ 2 cm with vascular invasion; or multiple tumors in the same lobe that are all ≤2 cm and without vascular invasion; or a solitary tumor >2 cm without vascular invasion), N0, M0
IIIA	T3 (solitary tumor >2 cm with vascular invasion; or multiple tumors in the same lobe that are all ≤2 cm with vascular invasion; or multiple tumors, any of which are >2 cm in the same lobe with or without vascular invasion), N0, M0
IIIB	T1–3, N1 (regional nodes involved), M0
IVA	T4 (multiple tumors involving more than one lobe or a major branch of the portal or hepatic veins), N0, M0
IVB	Any T, any N, M1

Modified from American Joint Committee on Cancer. *AJCC staging manual,* 5th ed. Philadelphia: JB Lippincott; 1997.

E. **Primary therapy.** At presentation, 25% of patients with hepatocellular carcinoma have potentially resectable lesions. At laparotomy, only 10% to 12% are resected. Operative mortality is 10% to 30%. Cirrhosis and advanced lesions are the factors limiting resection. Long-term survival is achieved in 15% to 30% of patients whose tumors are resected. Recurrences appear in liver, regional lymph nodes, lungs, and bone. Liver transplantation may permit resection of small tumors in patients with advanced cirrhosis, and survival is similar or better than that seen after resection without transplantation. Percutaneous ethanol injection can also control selected patients' tumors.

F. **Therapy of advanced hepatocellular carcinoma**

1. **Single agents.** Numerous single agents have been tested in primary hepatocellular carcinoma: alkylating agents, antimetabolites, plant alkaloids, and cisplatin have been ineffective. Doxorubicin, 60 mg/m^2 i.v. every 21 days, is recommended. This regimen results in a partial response rate of about 16%.

2. **Combination chemotherapy and other modes of treatment.** Combination chemotherapy has not had better success than single agents. Hepatic artery infusion has been studied and appears to have an increased response rate compared with intravenous chemotherapy. Similarly, chemoembolization has been employed. To date, no survival advantage has been proved for intraarterial therapy or chemoembolization. Immunotherapy has not shown promise in hepatocellular carcinoma. Irradiation has had a limited role in treating liver tumors because of hepatic intolerance to radiation.

SELECTED READINGS

Burris HA, Moore MJ, Andersen J, et al. Improvements in survival and clinical benefit with gemcitabine as first-line therapy for patients with advanced pancreas cancer: a randomized trial. *J Clin Oncol* 1997;15:2403–2413.

Collier J, Sherman M. Screening for hepatocellular carcinoma. *Hepatology* 1998;27:273–278.

Figueras J, Jaurrieta E, Valls C, et al. Survival after liver transplantation in cirrhotic patients with and without hepatocellular carcinoma: a comparative study. *Hepatology* 1997;25:1485–1489.

Gastrointestinal Tumor Study Group. Further evidence of effective adjuvant combined radiation and chemotherapy following curative resection of pancreatic cancer. *Cancer* 1987;59:2006–2010.

Glimelius B, Hoffman K, Sjoden PO, et al. Chemotherapy improves survival and quality of life in advanced pancreatic and biliary cancer. *Ann Oncol* 1996;7:593–600.

Howard TJ. Pancreatic adenocarcinoma. *Curr Probl Cancer* 1996; 20:281–328.

Jensen RT, Fraker DL. Zollinger-Ellison syndrome: advances in treatment of gastric hypersecretion and the gastrinoma. *JAMA* 1994; 271:1429–1435.

Kalser MH, Ellenberg SS. Pancreatic cancer: adjuvant combined radiation and chemotherapy following curative resection. *Arch Surg* 1985;120:899–903.

Lencioni R, Pinto F, Armillotta N, et al. Long-term results of percutaneous ethanol injection therapy for hepatocellular carcinoma in cirrhosis: a European experience. *Eur Radiol* 1997;7:514–519.

Moertel CG, Gunderson LL, Mailliard JA, et al. Early evaluation of combined fluorouracil and leucovorin as a radiation enhancer for locally unresectable, residual, or recurrent gastrointestinal carcinoma. *J Clin Oncol* 1994;12:21–27.

Moertel CG, Hahn RG, O'Connell MS. Therapy of locally unresectable pancreatic carcinoma: a randomized comparison of high dose (6000 rads) radiation alone, moderate dose radiation (4000 rads- 5-fluorouracil), and high dose radiation- 5-fluorouracil. Gastrointestinal Tumor Study Group. *Cancer* 1981;48:1705–1710.

Moertel CG, Lefkopoulo M, Lipsitz S, Hahn RG, Klaassen D. Streptozocin-doxorubicin, streptozocin-fluorouracil, or chlorozotocin in the treatment of advanced islet-cell carcinoma. *N Engl J Med* 1992;326:519–523.

Palmer KR, Kerr M, Knowles G, Cull A, Carter DC, Leonard RCF. Chemotherapy prolongs survival in inoperable pancreatic carcinoma. *Br J Surg* 1994;81:882–885.

Schifeling DJ, Konski AA, Howard JM, Dobelbower RR, Merrick HW, Skeel RT. Radiation therapy and 5-fluorouracil modulated by leucovorin for adenocarcinoma of the pancreas. *Int J Pancreatol* 1992;12:239–243.

Schnall SF, Macdonald JS. Chemotherapy of adenocarcinoma of the pancreas. *Semin Oncol* 1996;23:220–228.

Shutze WP, Sack J, Aldrete JS. Long-term follow-up of 24 patients undergoing radical resection for ampullary carcinoma, 1953 to 1988. *Cancer* 1990;66:1717–1720.

Stabile BE. Islet cell tumors. *Gastroenterologist* 1997;5:213–232.

Tsukuma H, Hiyama T, Tanaka S, et al. Risk factors for hepatocellular carcinoma among patients with chronic liver disease. *N Engl J Med* 1993;328:1797–1801.

Warshaw AL, Gu ZY, Wittenberg J, Waltman AC. Preoperative staging and assessment of resectability of pancreatic cancer. *Arch Surg* 1990;125:230–233.

Carcinoma of the Breast

Roland T. Skeel

I. **Natural history, evaluation, and modes of treatment**
   A. **Epidemiology and etiology.** Carcinoma of the breast gave way to carcinoma of the lung as the most common cause of cancer deaths among women in the United States in 1986. Nonetheless, in 1998, more than 180,000 new cases of breast cancer were diagnosed, and there were nearly 44,000 women who died from this cancer. The incidence of breast cancer varies widely among different populations. Women in western Europe and the United States have a higher incidence than women in most other parts of the world, possibly in part because of the high intake of animal protein and fat. Although discrete causes of breast cancer cannot be identified in individual women, many factors increase a woman's risk of developing the disease. Among the strongest of the risk factors is family history, particularly if more than one family member has developed breast cancer at an early age. Genetic linkage analysis has let to the discovery of dominant germline mutations in two tumor-suppressor genes, BRCA-1 and BRCA-2, localized to chromosomes 17 and 13, respectively, which are associated with a high risk of female breast cancer as well as ovarian cancer (BRCA-1 and BRCA-2), male breast cancer (BRCA-2), and other cancers. Although these mutations account for less than 10% of all cases of breast cancer and probably for only 25% to 30% of inherited cases, families with both breast and ovarian cancers have nearly a 50% chance of having BRCA-1 mutations. Carriers of these genes face up to a 55% to 70% lifetime risk of breast cancer, depending on familial history, perhaps the specific mutation, and other cellular genes that may modify penetrance. Other less common or less well-defined genetic mutations may be present in other familial breast cancers. Additional factors that increase breast cancer risk are early menarche, late age at birth of first child, and prior benign breast disease (particularly if there is a high degree of benign epithelial atypia). Present use of birth control pills appears to have a small effect on the risk of developing breast cancer (relative risk, 1.24); risk from prior use diminishes over time. Although breast cancer may occur among men, such cases represent fewer than 1% of all breast cancers and are infrequently seen in most hospitals.
   B. **Detection, diagnosis, and pretreatment evaluation**
      1. **Screening.** Because more lives can be saved if breast cancer is diagnosed at an early stage,

many programs have been designed to detect small, early cancers. Monthly breast self-examination for all women after puberty and yearly breast examinations by a physician or other trained professional after a woman is 30 years of age are recommended. Mammography, when done on a regular basis, can reduce mortality due to breast cancer by 30% in women older than 50 years. The benefit for women aged 40 to 50 years has been more difficult to demonstrate. Mammography is recommended at age 40 years as a baseline, once every 1 to 2 years between the ages of 40 and 50 years (depending on risk factors and the recommending organization), and yearly after 50 years of age. An upper age of effectiveness is not established. Although each method for early detection can be of some help in finding early lesions that can be successfully removed before metastasis has occurred, mammography is capable of detecting the smallest and therefore the most curable lesions. Thus, despite the high cost of screening mammography ($75 to $140 in many areas of the United States), it is highly recommended that the above guidelines be followed. Mammography has clearly led to the discovery of many earlier cancers and sharply increased the discovery of preinvasive cancers (ductal carcinoma *in situ* [DCIS]).

2. **Presenting signs and symptoms.** Although increasing numbers of nonpalpable cancers are being found by mammography, breast cancer is still most often discovered by a woman herself as an isolated, painless lump in the breast. If the mass has gone unnoticed, ignored, or neglected for a time, there may be fixation to the skin or underlying chest wall, ulceration, pain, or inflammation. Some early lesions present with discharge or bleeding from the nipple. At times, the primary lesion is not discovered, and the woman presents with symptoms of metastatic disease, such as pleural effusion, nodal disease, or bony metastases. About half of all lesions are in the upper outer quadrant of the breast (where most of the glandular tissue of the breast is). About 20% are central masses, and 10% are in each of the other quadrants. One quarter of all women with breast cancer have axillary node metastasis at the time of diagnosis, although this is less common when the primary tumor has been detected by screening mammography or other screening method.

3. **Staging.** Carcinoma of the breast is staged according to the size and characteristics of the primary tumor (T), the involvement of regional

lymph nodes (N), and the presence of metastatic disease (M). An abridged version of the commonly used TNM classification of breast cancer
is shown in Table 11-1, and the stage grouping
is outlined in Table 11-2. Although preliminary
staging is commonly done before surgery, definitive staging that can be used for prognostic and
further treatment planning purposes usually
must await postsurgical pathologic evaluation
when the primary tumor size and the histologic
involvement of the lymph nodes are established.

Table 11-1.   Abridged TNM classification of breast cancer

Primary tumor

Tis	Carcinoma *in situ:* intraductal carcinoma, lobular carcinoma *in situ,* or Paget's disease of the nipple with no tumor
T1	Tumor ≤2 cm
T1mic	≤0.1 cm
T1a	>0.1–0.5 cm
T1b	>0.5–1 cm
T1c	>1–2 cm
T2	Tumor >2 to 5 cm
T3	Tumor >5 cm
T4	Any size with extension to chest wall or skin (chest wall includes ribs, intercostal muscles, and serratus anterior muscle, but not pectoral muscles)
T4a	Extension to chest wall
T4b	Edema, skin ulceration, or satellite skin nodules confined to same breast
T4c	Both (T4a and T4b) criteria
T4d	Inflammatory carcinoma

Nodal involvement: Pathologic

pN0	No regional lymph node metastasis
pN1	Metastasis to movable ipsilateral axillary nodes
pN1a	Only micrometastasis (≤0.2 cm) (prognosis of patients with pN1a is similar to that of patients with pN0)
pN1b	Macrometastasis (>0.2 cm)
i	To one to three nodes, any >0.2 cm, all <2 cm
ii	To four or more nodes, any >0.2 cm, all <2 cm
iii	Extension of tumor (<2 cm) beyond capsule of node
iv	Any metastatic focus ≥2 cm
pN2	Fixed metastasis to ipsilateral axillary nodes
pN3	Metastasis to ipsilateral internal mammary nodes

Distant metastasis

M0	None known
M1	Metastases present, including to ipsilateral supraclavicular lymph nodes

Table 11-2. **Stage grouping of breast cancer**[a]

Stage	Description
0	Tis, N0, M0
I	T1, N0, M0
IIA	T0–1, N1, M0
	T2, N0, M0
IIB	T2, N1, M0
	T3, N0, M0
IIIA	T0–2, N2, M0
	T3, N1–2, M0
IIIB	T4, any N, M0
	Any T, N3, M0
IV	Any T, any N, M1

[a] Patients are staged in the highest group possible for their composite TNM. For example, a patient with T1a, N2, M0 would have stage IIIA disease because of the N2 status.

In up to 30% of patients with palpable breast masses (not found by mammography), but without clinical evidence of axillary lymph node involvement, the histologic evaluation of the nodes reveals cancer. In patients with negative nodes by routine histologic evaluation, serial sectioning may reveal microscopic cancer deposits in additional patients. Tumor cell detection using immumocytologic evaluation of the bone marrow may also be of prognostic value. In a somewhat smaller number, nodes that clinically appear positive contain no cancer when examined histologically.

4. **Diagnostic evaluation**
   a. **Before biopsy**, the woman should have a careful **history,** during which attention should be paid to risk factors, and a **physical examination,** with a focus not only on the involved breast but also on the opposite breast, all regional lymph node areas, the lungs, bone, and liver. This examination should be followed by bilateral mammography to help assess the extent of involvement and to look for additional ipsilateral or contralateral disease.
   b. **Excisional or core needle biopsy of the primary lesion** is performed, and the specimen is given intact (not in formalin) to the pathologist, who can divide the specimen for histologic examination, hormone receptor assays, flow cytometric measurements of ploidy and the percentage of cells in the S phase, or other specialized tests.

   c. **After confirmation of the histology,** the patient is evaluated for possible metastatic disease.

   (1) **Mandatory studies** include a chest radiograph, complete blood count, blood chemistry profile, and estrogen and progesterone receptor assays on the primary breast carcinoma and grossly cancerous nodal tissues.

   (2) **Other studies,** including radionuclide scan of the bones, skeletal survey (usually obtained only if the radionuclide scan is positive), and computed tomography scan of the liver (abdomen) are optional unless the history, physical examination, or blood studies suggest a poor prognosis or point to specific organ involvement. A carcinoembryonic antigen assay is also performed often. Additional studies that may impart clinically useful prognostic information include evaluation of the ploidy of the malignant cells and their DNA synthesis rate (percentage in S phase) and the content of other markers, such as the c-erbB-2 (Her-2) oncogene and its protein product, p53 mutations, or cathepsin D.

5. **Histology.** About 75% to 80% of all breast cancers are infiltrating ductal carcinomas, and 10% are infiltrating lobular carcinomas; these two types have similar biologic behavior. The remainder of the histologic types of invasive breast carcinoma may have a somewhat better prognosis but are usually managed more according to the stage than to the histologic type.

C. **Approach to therapy**

1. **Prevention.** Until recently, it was unknown whether any preventive measures would be effective in reducing the incidence of breast cancer. Two trials using selective estrogen receptor modulators (SERMs) have demonstrated that 3 to 5 years of preventive treatment with these agents reduces the rate of cancer development over the short term. Women at increased risk because of family history, age, and other risk factors, who are treated with tamoxifen, 20 mg/day, were found to have a 45% reduction in the rate of occurrence of invasive breast cancer compared with women treated with placebo. Noninvasive disease was also decreased. Raloxifene, 60 or 120 mg/day, also appears to reduce the risk of breast cancer in postmenopausal women (who had osteoporosis and a standard or reduced risk

of breast cancer), with a relative risk of 0.26. Raloxifene may have a lower risk of the development of endometrial cancer than tamoxifen. Effects on survival, when used in breast cancer prevention, have not yet been demonstrated for either agent. A trial underway is comparing these two agents.

The approach to management of women at very high risk because of family history or known suppressor gene mutations is in evolution. Increased surveillance, such as increasing the frequency of mammography to every 6 months, has been suggested as a reasonable conservative approach. Bilateral oophorectomy after childbearing age has been recommended, particularly for the BRCA-1 mutations, because of the inadequacy of methods to screen for ovarian cancer. Prophylactic mastectomy may be preferred by some women, but there remains some risk of breast cancer in residual breast glandular tissue, and the irreversible loss of nipple sensation may be distressing to some women. The role of SERMs in patients with these mutations is uncertain, in part because most cancers found in this situation are estrogen- and progesterone-receptor negative.

2. **Surgery** has been and remains the most frequently used mode of primary therapy for most women with carcinoma of the breast. The role of surgery in the primary management of carcinoma of the breast has been evolving with a **trend to lesser surgery (e.g., wide local excision)** together with axillary node dissection. Complete axillary node dissection may become unnecessary when the reliability of **sentinel node identification,** removal, and histologic assessment is established with greater certainty. This technique may spare many women the additional surgical procedure of axillary node dissection and its attendant risk of arm edema and dysethesias. The **lumpectomy and axillary node evaluation (or removal) are followed by radiotherapy** to control the microscopic cancer remaining in the breast. Depending on the stage of the cancer, additional radiotherapy may be used to treat upper internal mammary nodes. For most women, this therapy yields therapeutic results that are as good as **modified radical mastectomy** without the need for amputating the breast and its attendant physical deformity and psychological trauma.

Although many women and their physicians are opting for lesser surgery, some version of the modified radical mastectomy is still more commonly performed in most areas of the

United States; in this operation, the breast, pectoralis fascia (with or without the pectoralis minor muscle), and lymph nodes are removed. There are wide geographic variations in the use of breast-conserving surgery throughout the United States. For most women, operations more extensive than the modified radical mastectomy are probably of no benefit, and lesser operations that are not combined with radiotherapy are insufficient in terms of providing important prognostic information regarding the status of the axillary lymph nodes and controlling the local disease (40% of women treated with excisional biopsy alone have recurrence in the ipsilateral breast).

For patients who have had mastectomy, reconstruction is being done with increasing frequency. It may be done at the time of mastectomy or delayed for a period (usually 1 to 2 years). Options include insertion of a silicone or saline implant or transposition of a rectus muscle flap. Neither procedure has resulted in worsening of the prognosis from the breast cancer or a significant increase in the difficulty in detecting local recurrences.

3. **Radiotherapy's** role in the management of carcinoma of the breast has been expanded since the early 1970s. Radiotherapy is now commonly used in conjunction with excisional biopsy of varying degree as part of the primary therapy. In this circumstance, the radiotherapy is commonly delivered using external-beam therapy to the entire breast with a boost of therapy to the tumor bed using either external-beam therapy or implantation of radioactive substances. Radiotherapy may also be given after mastectomy in women who have a high likelihood of local recurrence, and it is highly effective in preventing the reappearance of disease in the treated fields. In some circumstances it may also improve survival. Local recurrences and distant metastases also are frequently treated successfully with radiotherapy. This mode of treatment is particularly critical to the management of painful bony lesions or sites of impending pathologic fracture.

4. **Chemotherapy and endocrine therapy** are used to reduce the likelihood of recurrence in early disease and to treat more advanced disease with or without distant metastasis. Endocrine therapy may consist in surgical, radiotherapeutic, or chemotherapeutic ablation or inhibition of the ovaries or adrenal glands; or it may consist of additive therapy with antiestrogens, aromatase inhibitors, progestins, androgens, or

luteinizing hormone–releasing hormone (LHRH) agonists. Endocrine therapy is generally ineffective (as sole therapy) for the treatment of metastatic disease in patients with low levels of estrogen and progesterone receptors in the cancer cells and is increasingly effective as the level of receptors rises. The best responses can be expected in women in whom the estrogen receptor level is high and progesterone receptors are present. Chemotherapy is apparently equally effective regardless of the level of hormone receptors in the cancer cell. Other factors, such as Her-2/neu (c-erbB-2), may also affect responsiveness to hormonal therapy (tamoxifen), with patients overexpressing this oncogene not faring as well. There is no established role for hormonal therapy or chemotherapy for DCIS, though there may be an emerging role for antiestrogen therapy in the prevention of invasive disease.

5. **Multimodal therapy** has had a more beneficial impact on carcinoma of the breast than on any other common cancer affecting adults.

    a. **Postoperative chemotherapy or hormonal therapy** (including ovarian ablation in premenopausal women) for women with a high risk of recurrence owing to positive axillary nodes (i.e., nodes containing cancer) is selected on the basis of the hormone receptor status of the tumor and also on the menopausal status and age of the woman. Most node-positive patients benefit from adjuvant therapy, with a decrease in the annual rates of recurrence by 25% to 40% and of death by 15% to 30%.

        Studies have shown that many women with negative nodes also benefit from adjuvant chemotherapy or hormonal (tamoxifen) therapy. Although the percentage decrease in mortality is similar to that for node-positive women, the lower baseline mortality for node-negative women results in less absolute benefit per 100 women treated. Current clinical trials use tumor size, hormone receptor status, DNA synthesis rate (percentage of cells in S phase), and other factors to aid in determining the patients, among those with negative nodes, who are most likely to relapse and thus most likely to benefit from adjuvant therapy.

    b. **Radiotherapy** to the breast and nodal areas after excisional biopsy or quadrantectomy of the breast cancer is as effective a treatment as mastectomy in terms of local recurrence and survival. For most patients, it is not only equivalent but preferable treatment because of the preservation of the breast.

   c. **Consultation** with a surgeon, radiotherapist, and medical oncologist is critical once the diagnosis of carcinoma is highly suspected or histologically confirmed. It is important to have all of these oncology specialists see the patient before final decisions regarding therapy are made, so the primary physician and the patient can have opinions from several perspectives about optimal management.

     It is critical to have the patient (and her family if she desires) share in the therapy decisions after hearing the options, the relative advantages and disadvantages of each option, and the recommendations of the consultants. The patient should be given an opportunity to hear why the recommended treatment is thought by the physicians to be best and to decide whether that is acceptable to her.

D. Prognosis. There is a broad spectrum in the biologic behavior of breast carcinoma from aggressive, rapidly fatal, inflammatory carcinoma to relatively indolent disease with late-appearing metastasis and survival time of 10 to 15 years. The likelihood of relapse and survival are influenced by the stage of the disease and the hormone receptor status at diagnosis, pathologic characteristics of the tumor, measures of proliferative activity of the cancer cell, oncogene and tumor suppressor gene (tumor) expression or amplification (c-erbB-2, c-myc, p53), and age and general health of the patient.

  1. **Stage.** Axillary node involvement and the size of the primary tumor are major determinants of the likelihood of survival.

    a. **Nodes.** In one large National Surgical Adjuvant Breast Project study, before the use of modern adjuvant therapy, 65% of all patients who underwent radical mastectomy survived 5 years, and 45% survived 10 years. When no axillary nodes were positive, the 5-year survival rate was nearly 80% and the 10-year survival rate 65%. If any axillary nodes were positive, the 5-year survival rate was less than 50% and the 10-year survival rate 25%. If four or more nodes were positive, the 5-year survival rate was 30% and the 10-year survival rate less than 15%. Since that time (1975), there has been improvement, with 5-year survival rates of 87% for stage I, 75% for stage II, 45% for stage III, and 13% for stage IV breast cancer.

      b. **Primary tumor.** Patients with large primary tumors do not do as well as patients with small tumors, irrespective of the nodal status, although patients with large primary tumors are more likely to have node involvement. Tumors that are fixed to the skin or to the chest wall do worse than those that are not. Patients with inflammatory carcinomas have a particularly poor prognosis, with a median survival time of less than 2 years and a 5-year survival rate of less than 10% in some series. Aggressive initial chemotherapy may improve the outlook for some patients.

   2. **Estrogen and progesterone receptors.** Patients without estrogen or progesterone receptors (or with very low levels) are twice as likely to relapse during the first 2 years after diagnosis as those who are receptor positive. This observation is true for both premenopausal and postmenopausal patients within each major node group (0, 1 to 3, and 4 or more).

   3. **Other prognostic factors** are emerging as independent prognostic factors, particularly for node-negative cancers, and include the percentage of cells in DNA synthesis (low percentage in S phase better than high percentage) and the ploidy of the breast cancer cells (diploid better than aneuploid). Additional tumor markers that may have predictive value include c-erbB-2, cathepsin D, c-myc oncogene amplification, and p53 suppressor gene expression.

II. Chemotherapy and endocrine therapy

  A. General considerations and aims of therapy. Carcinoma of the breast is responsive to many cytotoxic chemotherapeutic agents, hormonal agents, and other endocrine manipulations.

   1. **Endocrine therapy** is presumed to be effective because the breast cancer tissue retains some of the endocrine sensitivity of the normal breast tissue. In premenopausal women, if the breast cancer growth is supported by estrogen production from the ovary, antiestrogen therapy, removal of endogenous estrogen by oophorectomy, or suppression of estrogen production using an LHRH agonist logically results in regression of the cancer, at least those tumor cells that are dependent on the estrogen. (The dependent cells seem to be those that have the estrogen receptors.) Other mechanisms of action of the antiestrogen tamoxifen include inhibition of the epithelial growth factor, transforming growth factor-α (TGF-α), and stimulation of the epithelial inhibitory factor TGF-β. Complicating the anticipated interactions of

SERMs further are the presence of different classes of estrogen receptors, different ligands, many receptor-interacting proteins, a host of transcription-activating factors, and several response elements.

2. **Chemotherapy.** As with other cancers, the basis for the effectiveness of cytotoxic drugs in the treatment of carcinoma of the breast is not completely understood. It is clear, however, that combinations of drugs are considerably more effective than single agents (although how many is enough is not as certain), and nearly all treatment programs use the drugs in various combinations. In addition to their cytotoxic effects, chemotherapeutic agents may induce menopause in premenopausal women, thus affecting estrogen production as well as killing cells directly.

3. **Biologic therapy.** With the development of the humanized anti-Her-2 antibody, (Trastuzumab, Herceptin) and Her-2 peptide vaccines, biologic therapy of breast cancer has become a reality. Although it appears that these modes of therapy will have a role in the armamentarium of the oncologist, the degree to which biologic therapy will have an impact on survival and quality of life in patients with breast cancer is uncertain. Nevertheless, the possibilities for biologic therapy have now been demonstrated, and further developments are certain to emerge in the next 5 years.

4. **Aims of therapy** differ depending on the stage of disease being treated.

   a. **For early disease**, the aim is to eradicate micrometastases to render the patient free of disease and prevent recurrence. If eradication of cancer cells cannot be achieved, long-term suppression is desirable. Coincident with this aim is the goal of avoiding unnecessarily excessive drug-induced toxicity, both short- and long-term. Of particular theoretical concern is the possibility of second cancers arising many years after the completion of chemotherapy. Thus, a goal of investigational studies has been to try to determine the minimum therapy that is effective for preventing the maximum number of recurrences in any given clinical situation. If micrometastases cannot be eradicated, long-term suppression is also a reasonable goal of therapy. This may in fact be what is accomplished by tamoxifen and other SERMs and the reason that chronic (5 years) therapy is needed.

   b. **For advanced disease**, the aim is usually to reduce the tumor burden temporarily

and the resultant disability in order to alleviate the patient's symptoms, improve
performance, and prolong meaningful survival. Whereas long-term toxicity is not
usually of great import, short-term toxicity
is a major area of concern for both physician and patient because the aim of therapy is to improve how the patient feels
(quality of life) as well as to prolong survival time.

B. **Effective agents** for treating carcinoma of the breast
can be found among the alkylating agents, antimetabolites, natural products (antibiotics, vinca
alkaloids, and taxanes), hormones, hormone antagonists, and biologic agents.

1. **Among the cytotoxic drugs,** the most commonly used agents include doxorubicin (Adriamycin), cyclophosphamide, methotrexate, fluorouracil, paclitaxel, docetaxel, vinorelbine
(Navelbine), thiotepa, mitoxantrone, and vincristine. Each of these agents has a response
rate of 20% to 40% when used as a single agent.
Because combinations are so much more effective (60% to 80% response rate) than single
agents, these drugs are rarely used alone.

2. **Among the hormones and antihormones,**
the most commonly used agents are tamoxifen
(the other SERMs toremifene and raloxifene
are not as widely used), aromatase inhibitors
(anastrozole and letrozole), various progestins
(e.g., megestrol acetate), aminoglutethimide,
fluoxymesterone, the LHRH agonists (leuprolide and goserelin), and prednisone. These
agents are most often used alone but may be
used in combination with cytotoxic drugs or sequentially with cytotoxic drugs; prednisone is
used less commonly than in previous years and
is used only with cytotoxic agents.

3. **Biologic agents** are new in the armamentarium of effective agents in breast cancer.
Trastuzumab (Herceptin) has demonstrated efficacy, and the demonstration of the capability
of Her-2 peptide vaccines to elicit T-cell immunity may presage an additional effective biologic therapy in breast cancer.

4. **Radiotherapy** should generally be delayed
until the completion of adjuvant chemotherapy
to decrease the frequency of distant recurrence,
particularly in women with positive nodes or
other unfavorable prognostic indicators.

C. **Treatment of early disease.** Standard treatment of
early disease depends on primary tumor size, nodal
status, menopausal status of the patient, hormone receptor status of the tumor, and other tumor characteristics. Because there is not yet optimal therapy for

any subset of women with breast cancer, the patient and her physician should be encouraged to participate in a clinical trial. If none is available or the patient declines, Table 11-3 can be used as a guide for assessing risk. Table 11-4 may be used as a guide to select the type of therapy, depending on stage of disease, menopausal state, age, receptor status, and other risk factors.

1. **Cytotoxic therapy** is recommended for all premenopausal and most postmenopausal women with positive nodes, irrespective of hormone receptor status. It should also be used in higher-risk premenopausal and postmenopausal women with negative nodes, particularly if they have negative hormone receptors. We are less inclined to use cytotoxic therapy in the adjuvant treatment of older women (over 70 years of age with comorbid conditions, over 80 years of age without comorbid conditions), particularly if they are hormone receptor positive and are at lower risk. How much, if any, cytotoxic therapy adds to anti-estrogen (tamoxifen) therapy in lower-risk node-negative, hormone receptor–positive patients is

Table 11-3.   Prognostic factors for assessing risk of recurrence of breast cancer

Value	Parameter
Nodal status	Risk increases with presence of metastasis and numbers of nodes involved
Tumor size	Risk increases with tumor size independent of nodal status
Estrogen and progesterone receptors	Positive receptors confer better prognosis
Age	Complex factor. Women aged 45 to 49 years have best prognosis, with increasing likelihood of deaths from their breast cancer in older and younger age groups
Morphology	Higher nuclear grade, higher histologic grade, tumor necrosis, peritumoral lymphatic vessel invasion, increased microvessel density tumors have worse prognosis
DNA content and proliferative capacity	Tumors that are diploid and have low S-phase fraction do better than those that are aneuploid or have a high S-phase fraction (by flow cytometry)
Oncogene expression	Her-2/neu (c-erbB-2) and c-myc amplification have possible association with earlier relapse and shorter survival

Table 11-4.   Systemic adjuvant therapy for breast cancer—guidelines

Tumor category	Premenopausal women	Postmenopausal women[a]	
		≤80 yr	>80 yr
Node positive			
ER and/or PR positive	CT with TAM or oophorectomy	TAM with or without CT	TAM
ER and PR negative	CT	CT	None or CT
Node negative			
ER and PR indeterminate because tumor too small ER and/or PR positive	None	None	None
≤2 cm			
Low risk[b]	None	None	None
High risk	CT plus TAM	TAM	TAM
>2 cm	CT plus TAM	TAM with or without CT	TAM
ER and PR negative	CT	CT	None

[a] Comorbid conditions may modify decision to treat and choice of therapy.

[b] Based on factors such as size <1 cm, low histologic grade, or a low percentage (<6%–10% of cells in S phase (see Table 11-3). CT, chemotherapy AC (doxorubicin [Adriamycin] plus cyclophosphamide) for four cycles; CAF (cyclophosphamide, doxorubicin, fluorouracil); CMF (cyclophosphamide, methotrexate, fluorouracil); CMFP (cyclophosphamide, methotrexate, fluorouracil, prednisone) for six cycles; other chemotherapy may be of equal or better efficacy (such as AC followed by paclitaxel); ER, estrogen receptor; PR, progesterone receptor; TAM, tamoxifen (for 5 yr, alone or after completion of chemotherapy).

not established. We use AC (doxorubicin [Adriamycin] and cyclophosphamide) more commonly in women with a higher risk of recurrence, and CMF (cyclophosphamide, methotrexate, and fluorouracil) more in those who have lesser risks (e.g., are node negative), who have comorbid conditions, or in whom cardiac risk of doxorubicin is deemed important. There may be a slight advantage to doxorubicin-based regimens (AC or CAF [cyclophosphamide, doxorubicin, and fluorouracil]) in terms of disease-free or overall survival, but the difference, if present, is small, and the toxicity is greater. There appears to be an advantage in node-positive women to the sequential use of AC followed by paclitaxel (Taxol). Longer follow-up studies are needed to determine whether this should become standard for all women with node-positive disease. Moderate escalation of the doses of the standard chemotherapy regimens does not appear to be of benefit in improving survival. Whether very-high-dose chemotherapy with autologous bone marrow or peripheral blood progenitor cell reinfusion will fulfill the promise of improving the survival of women at very high risk of recurrence will be determined with certainty only after analysis of recently completed and ongoing clinical trials. The recommended regimens are as follows:

a. **AC**

Doxorubicin, 60 mg/m² i.v. push through a rapidly running i.v., *and*

Cyclophosphamide 600 mg/m² i.v.

Repeat every three weeks for four cycles.

b. **CAF**

Cyclophosphamide, 100 mg/m²/day p.o. on days 1 to 14 (given as a single daily dose), *and*

Doxorubicin, 30 mg/m² i.v. push on days 1 and 8, through the side arm of a free-flowing i.v. infusion of normal saline, *and*

Fluorouracil, 500 mg/m² i.v. push on days 1 and 8.

Repeat every 28 days for 6 cycles.

c. **CMF(P)**

Cyclophosphamide, 100 mg/m² p.o. on days 1 to 14, *and*

Methotrexate, 40 mg/m² i.v. on days 1 and 8, *and*

Fluorouracil, 600 mg/m² i.v. on days 1 and 8, *with or without*

Prednisone, 40 mg/m² p.o. on days 1 to 14, during the first three cycles only.

Repeat cycle every 28 days for six cycles.

d. **Dose modifications** are outlined in Table 11-5.

Table 11-5.   Dose modification for chemotherapy of breast carcinoma

Dysfunction			Percentage of full dose
Hematologic toxicity ANC (WBC)/µL on day of scheduled treatment		Platelets/µL on day of scheduled treatment	Dose as percentage of immediately preceding cycle
≥1,800 (≥3,500)	*and*	>100,000	100
1,500–1,800 (3,000–3,500)	*or*	75,000–100,000	75 (see note)
1,000–1,500 (2,500–3,000)	*or*	50,000–75,000	50
<1,000 (<2,500)	*or*	<50,000	0 (delay 1 wk)

Note: Absolute neutrophil count (ANC) is the preferred parameter if available. Some use 100 dosing for ANC 1500–1800. If counts are rising at the end of a treatment cycle, it is often appropriate to delay 1 or even 2 wk and then treat according to the dose modification scheme shown here. If the ANC is <1,000/µL and is associated with fever >38.3°C (101°F) or the nadir platelet count is <40,000/µL, decrease dose by 25% in subsequent cycles. If the nadir white blood cell (WBC) count is >3,500/µL and the platelet count is >125,000/µL, increase the dose by 25 percent.

Renal dysfunction (serum creatinine, mg/dL)	Percentage of full dose to use		
	M	T	Others
<1.5	100	100	100
1.5–2	50	75	100
2–3.5	0	50	100
>3.5	0*	0*	0*

Hepatic dysfunction (serum bilirubin, mg/dL)	A, VLB, VCR	C, M, F, T
<1.5	100	100
1.5–3	50	100
3.1–5	25	100
>5	0[a]	0[a]

Hemorrhagic cystitis	Discontinue cyclophosphamide and substitute melphalan 4 mg/m^2 p.o. on days 1–5 of each cycle.
Gastrointestinal toxicity	For debilitating vomiting or diarrhea, reduce doses of C, M, F, and A by 25% for one cycle. For severe mucositis (ulcerations that inhibit eating), reduce subsequent F, M, and A by 50%. Reescalate if possible.

continued

Table 11-5. *(Continued)*

Cardiotoxicity	Discontinue doxorubicin.
Hypercorticism	If side effects such as hypertension, severe insomnia, psychosis, or uncontrolled diabetes occur, reduce or stop prednisone.
Neurotoxicity	Reduce vincristine, vinblastine, or vinorelbine dose by 50% for moderate paresthesias or severe constipation. Discontinue for severe paresthesias, decreased strength, difficulty walking, cranial nerve palsies, etc.
Hypersensitivity reactions	See guidelines for paclitaxel, docetaxel, and other individual drugs.

[a] Safe guidelines cannot be given, and expert evaluation is required before therapy is applied.
A, doxorubicin (Adriamycin); C, cyclophosphamide; F, fluorouracil; M, methotrexate; T, thiotepa; VCR, vincristine; VLB, vinblastine.

e. **A minimal effective dose and duration of drugs** are required for therapy of micrometastases to be effective. If women are arbitrarily given less therapy than they can tolerate, their likelihood of remaining disease free appears to be less than those who are given full doses of the drugs. This observation has led to the recommendation that if postoperative chemotherapy is to be given, doses should be as high as the patient can tolerate and should be continued for the entire planned period of therapy.

2. **Tamoxifen**, 10 mg p.o. b.i.d. (or 20 mg once daily), is recommended in hormone receptor–positive women with positive nodes. It should be continued for 5 years. Longer durations do not improve survival and may increase complications, such as endometrial carcinoma and thromboembolism. It is also beneficial in hormone receptor–positive premenopausal and postmenopausal women with negative nodes who are not determined to be at low risk of recurrence. Although there were earlier suggestions that tamoxifen was of benefit to older (over 70 years) women irrespective of receptor status, this seems less likely now. In patients who are receptor positive and receive cytotoxic chemotherapy, tamoxifen appears to have an added benefit. It has a relatively low risk in the adjuvant setting, and our current recommendations generally include

tamoxifen where it is indicated in addition to chemotherapy in Table 11-4.

3. **Response to therapy.** It is impossible to determine whether individual patients have responded to treatment for micrometastatic disease unless they relapse because there are no parameters to measure. The effectiveness of such treatment must therefore depend on population studies. Because breast cancer may have a long natural history, and the disease may recur after 5 to 10 years, it is critical to defer final conclusions regarding any study until at least 5 years and preferably 10 years have passed. It is possible to make some observations, however, regarding the benefits of this kind of multimodal therapy.

   a. **Chemotherapy** improves both disease-free and overall survival in all groups of patients. Although the proportional reduction in death rate is similar for both high- and low-risk patients (e.g., node-positive and node-negative), the absolute benefit is greater for those at higher risk of recurrence and death.

   b. **Tamoxifen** (and probably other SERMs) improves disease-free and overall survival in most estrogen receptor–positive patients. Although the proportional reduction in death rate is similar for both high- and low-risk patients (e.g., node-positive and node-negative), the absolute benefit is greater for those at higher risk of recurrence and death.

   c. **Chemotherapy plus tamoxifen** is better than chemotherapy alone in many estrogen receptor–positive patients. Relative benefits depend on disease status, likelihood of recurrence, and perhaps other factors, such as Her-2 (c-erbB-2) status (confers less benefit with tamoxifen alone).

   d. **In node-negative women,** because the likelihood of recurrence is lower, the absolute survival benefit is less and must be weighed against the toxicity of any proposed therapy.

D. **Treatment of advanced disease** is undergoing continuing evolution with the aim of improving the quality and duration of remissions and survivals. In patients with bony metastasis or cerebral metastasis, radiotherapy usually is an important component in the management, and a radiotherapist should participate in planning the patient's treatment. Regardless of the role of radiotherapy, however, chemotherapy or endocrine therapy is generally indicated in patients who have advanced disease.

1. **Endocrine therapy** is indicated in women who have had a positive test for estrogen or progesterone receptors in their tumor tissue. It is not generally recommended as the sole therapy for women who have low receptor levels or have previously been shown to be unresponsive to hormonal manipulation. It is also not appropriate therapy for women with brain metastasis, lymphangitic pulmonary metastasis, or other dire visceral disease, such as extensive liver metastasis, in which a slow response could jeopardize survival. For **premenopausal women,** oophorectomy still may the treatment of choice, but few women opt for this, given the effectiveness of medical therapies. The LHRH analogs goserelin and leuprolide can achieve the equivalent of a medical oophorectomy. This treatment may be combined with tamoxifen. **For postmenopausal women,** tamoxifen or another SERM is the initial treatment of choice. After failure of tamoxifen, either an aromatase inhibitor (anastrozole or letrozole) or a progestin (megestrol) is used as a secondary agent, provided there has been evidence of responsiveness to the primary hormonal therapy. Adrenal suppression with aminoglutethimide is less commonly used because of greater side effects but is still effective.

   Commonly used regimens are as follows:

   Tamoxifen, 10 mg p.o. twice daily or 20 mg p.o. daily (alternative–toremifene, 60 mg p.o. daily).

   Anastrozole, 1 mg p.o. daily (alternative–letrozole, 2.5 mg p.o. daily).

   Megestrol acetate, 40 mg p.o. q.i.d.

   Aminoglutethimide, 250 mg p.o. q.i.d.; hydrocortisone, 100 mg p.o. in divided doses daily for the first 2 weeks, then 40 mg p.o. in divided doses daily. Fludrocortisone, 0.05 to 0.1 mg p.o. may be given daily or every other day if there is evidence of salt wasting.

   Fluoxymesterone, 10 mg p.o. b.i.d.

2. **Cytotoxic combination chemotherapy** is used as the first treatment for advanced disease, in hormone receptor–negative patients, and at times in patients with several organs involved because the responses are more rapid and the rate of response is greater when drugs are used in combination than when endocrine therapy is used alone. For patients over 65 years of age, however, initiation of hormone therapy alone may be justified, with cytotoxic therapy being reserved for patients who have failed one or more hormonal treatments.

a. **Primary therapy.** Although several regimens have been shown to be effective, CAF, AC, and CMF(P) are the most commonly used as initial therapy. With the discovery of the effectiveness of paclitaxel in the treatment of breast cancer, this drug is also included as first-line therapy, often with doxorubicin. If the patient has not failed adjuvant therapy within 6 months of receiving a doxorubicin-containing regimen, and it is not contraindicated because of recent myocardial infarction, congestive heart failure, or reduced left ventricular ejection fraction, doxorubicin is commonly employed in initial therapy. If doxorubicin cannot be used, then either paclitaxel or CMF is used.

(1) **CAF**

Cyclophosphamide, 100 mg/m^2 p.o. on days 1 to 14, *and*

Doxorubicin, 30 mg/m^2 i.v. on days 1 and 8, *and*

Fluorouracil, 500 mg/m^2 i.v. on days 1 and 8.

Repeat the cycle every 4 weeks.

(2) **AC**

Doxorubicin, 60 mg/m^2 i.v. push through a rapidly running i.v., *and*

Cyclophosphamide, 600 mg/m^2 i.v.

Repeat every three weeks.

When the cumulative doxorubicin dose reaches 550 mg/m^2, substitute methotrexate 40 mg/m^2.

(3) **CMFP**

Cyclophosphamide, 100 mg/m^2 p.o. on days 1 to 14, *and*

Methotrexate, 40 mg/m^2 i.v. on days 1 and 8, *and*

Fluorouracil, 600 mg/m^2 i.v. on days 1 and 8, *and*

Prednisone, 40 mg/m^2 p.o. on days 1 to 14, during the first three cycles only.

Repeat the cycle every 4 weeks.

(4) **Doxorubicin plus paclitaxel** with or without filgrastim (Neupogen)

Doxorubicin, 50 to 60 mg/m^2 i.v., *followed in 4 hours by*

Paclitaxel, 150 mg/m^2 i.v. over 24 hours (or alternatively, over 3 hours), *and*

Filgrastim, 300 μg/day s.c. starting 24 hours after the end of chemotherapy, for 10 days.

Limit the number of cycles of doxorubicin to six (300 to 360 mg/m^2) to limit enhanced cardiotoxicity from the combination. Alternatively, paclitaxel administered over 3 hours on day 2 may also limit cardiotoxicity. Left ventricular ejection fraction should be monitored when the doxorubicin dose reaches 300 mg/m^2.

b. **Secondary therapy** depends on what treatment the patient has had previously. If the patient relapses while on CMF or CMFP treatment or within 6 months after finishing CMF treatment for micrometastatic disease, it is not likely that these drugs used in combination can be helpful in achieving a second remission. Because doxorubicin is among the most effective agents against breast carcinoma, it should be used in any combination in this situation. One of the regimens listed previously may be used. Additional choices include the following:

Paclitaxel, 150 to 175 mg/m^2 i.v. over 3 hours every three weeks, *or*

Docetaxel, 60 to 100 mg/m^2 i.v. over 1 hour every 3 weeks (premedication with oral corticosteroids such as dexamethasone, 8 mg b.i.d., for 5 days starting one day prior to starting docetaxel is necessary to reduce the severity of fluid retention and hypersensitivity reactions) or

Vinorelbine, 30 mg/m^2 i.v. over 6 to 10 minutes weekly.

Other agents with activity include mitomycin, gemcitabine, mitoxantrone, and the investigational agents dibromodulcitol, epirubicin, and vindesine. If fluorouracil has not been used in previous regimens, using it with leucovorin may be effective.

3. **Dose modifications** are outlined in Table 11-5.
4. **Response to therapy**
   a. **Endocrine therapy.** Of patients who are estrogen receptor negative, fewer than 10% have a response to either additive or ablative endocrine therapy. Among estrogen receptor–positive patients, about 60% have a partial, or better, response to either additive or ablative endocrine therapy. Responses to endocrine therapy tend to last longer than responses to cytotoxic chemotherapy, frequently lasting 12 to 24 months.
   b. **Cytotoxic chemotherapy** produces responses in 60% to 80% of patients regard-

less of their estrogen receptor status. The responses to therapy at times are durable, but the median duration in most studies is less than 1 year.

E. **Dose-intensive therapy** with peripheral blood stem cell or bone marrow transplantation replacement for carcinoma of the breast remains controversial, although it is commonly used both in academic medical centers and community hospitals. The complete remission rates in metastatic disease after intensive combination chemotherapy are in the range of 50%, compared with 5% to 10% after standard therapy. Unfortunately, most of these complete remissions are not durable, with about 20% of patients alive and free of disease at 6 to 7 years. The overall 5-year survival rate is in the range of 40% to 50%, however, which is better than the 20% 5-year survival rate that would be expected with standard therapy. It is clear that only patients with chemotherapy-sensitive disease have substantial benefit to dose- intensive therapy. Thus, it is important to demonstrate responsiveness to standard treatment (such as with four cycles of AC) before subjecting a patient to the rigors and high cost of dose-intensive therapy. Despite one randomized trial showing benefit, many experts are unconvinced, and it is probably best to defer judgment pending completion of larger randomized trials of high-dose therapy with bone marrow transplantation versus standard therapy in metastatic disease. There is no clearly best dose-intensive regimen, although the STAMP-V regimen has been popular and relatively easy to administer (see Chapter 6). Several randomized trials are evaluating the use of dose-intensive therapy in the adjuvant setting. The promise for benefit here may be greater, given the improvement in survival that is seen using standard adjuvant chemotherapy, but final judgment must await the analysis of results from the ongoing trials.

F. **Complications of therapy.** Acute toxicities are primarily hematologic and gastrointestinal. Subacute toxicities include alopecia, hemorrhagic cystitis, hypertension, edema, and psychoneurologic abnormalities. Chronic or long-term toxicities may be cardiac or neoplastic. Dose modifications for the more common problems are given in Table 11-5. These guidelines are designed to be helpful in selecting a course of therapy that will be effective with the least risk of life-threatening toxicity. Because of individual differences, toxicities that are worse than expected may occur, and the responsible physician must always be alert to special circumstances that dictate further attenuation of the drug doses. The drug data listed in Chapter 5 should be consulted for the individual toxicities, precautions, and toxicity prevention measures for each drug.

Adjuvant tamoxifen therapy also has consequences. These include a two-fold to four-fold increase in endometrial cancer and an increase in thromboembolic disease. Hot flashes are common but can be ameliorated in some women using a progestin, such as megestrol, 20 mg b.i.d., or a clonidine patch (Catapres-TTS-1). There are also beneficial effects of tamoxifen on lipid profiles, the rate of osteoporosis, and possibly the rate of myocardial infarction.

SELECTED READINGS

Albain K, Green S, Osborne K, et al. Tamoxifen (T) versus cyclophosphamide, Adriamycin and 5-FU plus either concurrent or sequential T in postmenopausal, receptor (+), node (+) breast cancer: a Southwest Oncology Group phase III intergroup trial (SWOG-8814, INT-0100). *Proc Am Soc Clin Oncol* 1997;16:A-450, 128a.

American Joint Committee on Cancer. *AJCC cancer staging manual,* 5th ed. Philadelphia: Lippincott-Raven, 1997:294.

Auquier A, Rutqvist LE, Host H, et al. Post-mastectomy megavoltage radiotherapy: the Oslo and Stockholm trials. *Eur J Cancer* 1992; 28(2–3):433–437.

Ayash LJ, Wheeler C, Fairclough D, et al. Prognostic factors for prolonged progression-free survival with high-dose chemotherapy with autologous stem-cell support for advanced breast cancer. *J Clin Oncol* 1995;13(8):2043–2049.

Benner SE, Clark GM, McGuire WL. Review: steroid receptors, cellular kinetics, and lymph node status as prognostic factors in breast cancer. *Am J Med Sci* 1988;296:59–66.

Bezwoda WR, Seymour L, Dansey RD: High-dose chemotherapy with hematopoietic rescue as primary treatment for metastatic breast cancer: a randomized trial. *J Clin Oncol* 1995;13(10):2483–2489.

Bonadonna G, Valagussa P. Adjuvant systemic therapy for resectable breast cancer. *J Clin Oncol* 1985;3:259–275.

Bianco AR, DeLaurentis, M, Carlomango C, et al. 20 Year update of the Naples GUN Trial of adjuvant breast cancer therapy: evidence of interaction between c-erbB-2 expression and tamoxifen efficacy. *Proc Am Soc Clin Oncol* 1998;17:97a.

Buzdar AU, Hortobagyi GN, Frye D, et al. Bioequivalence of 20-mg once-daily tamoxifen relative to 10-mg twice-daily tamoxifen regimens for breast cancer. *J Clin Oncol* 1994;12:50–54.

Clark GM, McGuire WL. Prediction of relapse or survival in patients with node-negative breast cancer by DNA flow cytometry. *N Engl J Med* 1989;320:627–633.

Cobleigh MA, Vogel CL, Tripathy D, et al. Efficacy and safety of Herceptin (humanized anti-HER2 antibody) as a single agent in 222 women with HER2 overexpression who relapsed following chemotherapy for metastatic breast cancer. *Proc Am Soc Clin Oncol* 1998;17:97a.

Collaborative Group on Hormonal Factors in Breast Cancer: breast cancer and hormonal contraceptives: collaborative reanalysis of individual data on 53,297 women with breast cancer and 100,239 women without breast cancer from 54 epidemiological studies. *Lancet* 1996;347(9017):1713–1727.

Cummings SR, Norton L, Ekert D, et al. Raloxifene reduces the risk of breast cancer and may decrease the risk of endometrial cancer in post-menopausal women: two-year findings from the multiple outcomes of raloxifene evaluation (MORE) trial. *Proc Am Soc Clin Oncol* 1998;17:2a.

Disis ML, Grabstein KJ, Sleath PR, Cheever MA. HER-2/neu peptide vaccines elicit T cell immunity to the HER-2/neu protein in patients with breast and ovarian cancer. *Proc Am Soc Clin Oncol* 1998;17:97a.

Early Breast Cancer Trialists' Collaborative Group. I. Systemic treatment of early breast cancer by hormonal, cytotoxic, or immune therapy: 133 randomised trials involving 31,000 recurrences and 24,000 deaths among 75,000 women. *Lancet* 1992;339:1–15.

Early Breast Cancer Trialists' Collaborative Group. II. Systemic treatment of early breast cancer by hormonal, cytotoxic, or immune therapy: 133 randomised trials involving 31,000 recurrences and 24,000 deaths among 75,000 women. *Lancet* 1992;339:71–85.

Early Breast Cancer Trialists' Collaborative Group. Effects of radiotherapy and surgery in early breast cancer: an overview of the randomised trials. *N Engl J Med* 1995;333(22):1444–1455.

Early Breast Cancer Trialists' Collaborative Group. Tamoxifen for early breast cancer: an overview of the randomised trials. *Lancet* 1998;351:1451–1467.

Eddy DM. High-dose chemotherapy with autologous bone marrow transplantation for the treatment of metastatic breast cancer. *J Clin Oncol* 1992;10:657–670.

Fisher B, Slack N, Katrych D, Wolmark N. Ten year follow-up results of patients with carcinoma of the breast in a cooperative clinical trial evaluating surgical adjuvant chemotherapy. *Surg Gynecol Obstet* 1975;140:528–534.

Fisher B, Redmond C, Fisher ER, Caplan R. Relative worth of estrogen or progesterone receptor and pathologic characteristics of differentiation as indicators of prognosis in node-negative breast cancer. *J Clin Oncol* 1988; 6:1076–1087.

Fisher B, Redmond C, Jimitrov NV, et al. A randomized clinical trial evaluating sequential methotrexate and fluorouracil in the treatment of node negative breast cancer who have estrogen negative tumor. *N Engl J Med* 1989;320:473–478.

Fisher B, Costatino J, Redmond C, et al. A randomized trial evaluating tamoxifen in the treatment of patients with node-negative breast cancer who have estrogen-receptor positive-tumors. *N Engl J Med* 1989;320:479–484.

Fisher B, Redmond C, Poisson R, et al. Eight-year results of a randomized clinical trial comparing total mastectomy and lumpectomy with or without irradiation in the treatment of breast cancer. *N Engl J Med* 1989;320:822–828.

Fisher B, Redmond C, Legault-Poisson S, et al. Postoperative chemotherapy and tamoxifen compared with tamoxifen alone in the treatment of positive-node breast cancer patients aged 50 years and older with tumors responsive to tamoxifen: results from the National Surgical Adjuvant Breast and Bowel Project B-16. *J Clin Oncol* 1990;8(6):1005–1018.

Fisher B, Costatino JP, Redmond CK, Fisher ER, Wickerham DL, Cronin WM, et al. Endometrial cancer in tamoxifen-treated breast cancer patients: findings from the National Surgical Adjuvant Breast and Bowel Project (NSABP) B-14. *JNCI* 1994;86:527–537.

Fisher B, Dignam J, Bryant J, et al. Five versus more than five years of tamoxifen therapy for breast cancer patients with negative lymph nodes and estrogen receptor-positive tumors. *JNCI* 1996; 88(21):1529–1542.

Fisher B, Dignam J, Mamounas EP, et al. Sequential methotrexate and fluorouracil for the treatment of node-negative breast cancer patients with estrogen receptor-negative tumors: eight-year results from National Surgical Adjuvant Breast and Bowel Project (NSABP) B-13 and first report of findings from NSABP B-19 comparing methotrexate and fluorouracil with conventional cyclophosphamide, methotrexate, and fluorouracil. *J Clin Oncol* 1996; 14(7):1982–1992.

Fisher B, Costantino JP, Wickerham DL, et al. Surgical adjuvant breast and bowel project P–1 Study. *J Natl Cancer Inst* 1998; 90:1371–1388.

Fowble BL, Solin LJ, Schultz DJ, Goodman. Ten year results of conservative surgery and irradiation for stage I and II breast cancer. *Int J Radiat Oncol Biol Phys* 1991;21:269–277.

Gail MH, Brinton LA, Byar DP, et al. Projecting individualized probabilities of developing breast cancer for white females who are being examined annually. *JNCI* 1989;81:1879–1886.

Gasparini G, Weidner N, Bevilacqua P, et al. Tumor microvessel density, p53 expression, tumor size, and peritumoral lymphatic vessel invasion are relevant prognostic markers in node-negative breast carcinoma. *J Clin Oncol* 1994;12:454–466.

Goldberg RM, Loprinzi CL, O'Fallon JR, et al. Transdermal clonidine for ameliorating tamoxifen-induced hot flashes. *J Clin Oncol* 1994;12:155–158.

Goldhirsch A, Glick JH, Gelber RD, Senn H-J. Meeting highlights: international consensus panel on the treatment of primary breast cancer. *JNCI* 1998;90:1601–1608.

Henderson IC, Berry D, Demetri G, et al. Improved disease-free and overall survival from the addition of sequential paclitaxel but not from the escalation of doxorubicin dose level in the adjuvant chemotherapy of patients with node-positive breast cancer. *Proc Am Soc Clin Oncol* 1998;17:101a.

Hudis C, Riccio L, Seidman A, et al. Lack of increased cardiac toxicity with sequential doxorubicin and paclitaxel. *Cancer Invest* 1998; 16(2):67–71.

Hutchins L, Green S, Ravdin D, et al. CMF versus CAF with and without tamoxifen in high-risk node-negative breast cancer patients and a natural history follow-up study in low-risk node-negative patients: first results of intergroup trial INT 0102. *Proc Am Soc Clin Oncol* 1998;17:1a.

Ingle JN, Krook JE, Green SJ, et al. Randomized trial of bilateral oophorectomy versus tamoxifen in premenopausal women with metastatic breast cancer. *J Clin Oncol* 1986;4:178–185.

Mansour EG, Gray R, Shatila AH, et al. Survival advantage of adjuvant chemotherapy in high-risk node-negative breast cancer: ten-year analysis—an intergroup study. *J Clin Oncol* 1998;16:3486–3492.

McGuire WL, Tandon AK, Allred DC, Chamness GC, Clark GM. How to use prognostic factors in axillary node-negative breast cancer patients. *JNCI* 1990;82:1006–1015.

Nattinger AB, Gottlieb MS, Veum J, Yahnke D, Goodwin JS. Geographic variation in the use of breast-conserving treatment for breast cancer. *N Engl J Med* 1992;326:1102–1107.

Osbone CK. Tamoxifen in the treatment of breast cancer. *N Engl J Med* 1998;339:1609–1618.

Peters WP, Ross M, Vredenburgh JJ, et al. High-dose chemotherapy and autologous bone marrow support as consolidation after standard-dose adjuvant therapy for high-risk primary breast cancer. *J Clin Oncol* 1993;11:1132–1143.

Pickle LW, Johnson KA. Estimating the long-term probability of developing breast cancer. *JNCI* 1989;81:1854–1855.

Pritchard KI, Paterson AH, Paul NA, et al. Increased thromboembolic complications with concurrent tamoxifen and chemotherapy in a randomized trial of adjuvant therapy for women with breast cancer. *J Clin Oncol* 1996;14(10):2731–2737.

Ravdin PM, Green S, Albain KS, et al. Initial report of the SWOG biological correlative study of c-erbB-2 expression as a predictor of outcome in a trial comparing adjuvant CAFT with tamoxifen alone. *Proc Am Soc Clin Oncol* 1998;17:97a.

Rivkin SE, Green S, Metch B, et al. Adjuvant CMFVP vs tamoxifen vs concurrent CMFVP and tamoxifen for postmenopausal, node-positive, and estrogen receptor-positive breast cancer patients: a Southwest Oncology Group study. *J Clin Oncol* 1994;12:2078–2085.

Rosen PP, Groshen S, Saigo PE, Kinne DW, Hellman S. Pathological prognostic factors in stage I (T1 N0 M0) and stage II (T1 N1 M0) breast carcinoma: a study of 644 patients with median follow-up of 18 years. *J Clin Oncol* 1989;7:1239–1251.

Rosen PP, Groshen S, Kinne DW, Norton L. Factors influencing prognosis in node-negative breast carcinoma: analysis of 767 T1N0M0/T2N0M0 patients with long-term follow-up. *J Clin Oncol* 1993;11:2090–2100.

Rutqvist LE, Mattsson A. Cardiac and thromboembolic morbidity among postmenopausal women with early-stage breast cancer in a randomized trial of adjuvant tamoxifen. *JNCI* 1993;85:1398.

Sigurdsson H, Baldetorp B, Borg A, et al. Indicators of prognosis in node-negative breast cancer. *N Engl J Med* 1990;322:1045–1053.

Slamon DJ, Godolphin W, Jones LA, et al. Studies of HER-2/neu proto-oncogene in human breast and ovarian cancer. *Science* 1989;244:707–712.

Slamon D, Leyland-Jones B, Shak S, et al. Addition of Herceptin (humanized anti-HER2 antibody) to first line chemotherapy for HER2 overexpressing metastatic breast cancer (HER2-/MBC) markedly increases anticancer activity: a randomized multinational controlled phase III trial. *Proc Am Soc Clin Oncol* 1998;17:98a.

Sledge GW, Neuberg D, Ingle J, et al. Phase III trial of doxorubicin vs. paclitaxel vs. doxorubicin + paclitaxel as first-line therapy for metastatic breast cancer: an intergroup trial. *Proc Am Soc Clin Oncol* 1997;16:1a.

Taylor SG 4th, Gelman RS, Falkson G, Cummings FJ. Combination chemotherapy compared to tamoxifen as initial therapy for stage IV breast cancer in elderly women. *Ann Intern Med* 1986;104:455–461.

Tormey DC, Weinberg VE, Holland JF, et al. A randomized trial of five and three drug chemotherapy and chemoimmunotherapy in women with operable node positive breast cancer. *J Clin Oncol* 1983;1:138–145.

Van Dam FSAM, Schagen SB, Muller MJ, et al. Impairment of cognitive function in women receiving adjuvant treatment for high-risk breast cancer: high-dose versus standard-dose chemotherapy. *JNCI* 1998;90:210–218.

Veronesi U, Saccozzi R, Del Vecchio M, et al. Comparing radical mastectomy with quadrantectomy, axillary dissection, and radiotherapy in patients with small cancers of the breast. *N Engl J Med* 1981;305:6–11.

Zujewski J, Liu ET. The 1998 St. Galen's consensus conference: an assessment. *JNCI* 1998;90:1587–1589.

Gynecologic Cancer

C. O. Granai, Walter H. Gajewski, and Robert D. Legare

I. **Carcinoma of the cervix.** Cervical cancer is the most common female malignancy worldwide but ranks only 10th in the United States. The 70% reduction in cervical cancer deaths in the United States in the last 30 years is largely the result of effective screening by Papanicolaou's (Pap) smear, which identifies disease while preinvasive. Nevertheless, there will be an estimated 13,700 new cases and 4,900 deaths from invasive cervical cancer in the United States this year. Cervical cancer correlates with sexual intercourse at an early age, multiple sex partners, high parity, human papillomavirus infection (particularly types 16 and 18), human immunodeficiency virus infection, and cigarette smoking. The established relationship with sexual and social behavior permits squamous cancer of the cervix to be categorized as a sexually or socially transmitted disease and thus is theoretically preventable.

A. **Pathology and patterns of spread**

1. **Histology.** More than 80% of cervical cancers are of the squamous cell histologic type. The other 20% are principally adenocarcinomas. Squamous cell cancer arises from the exocervix, whereas adenocarcinoma is from the columnar epithelium of the endocervix. Less common cervical malignancies also occur, each having unique biologic behaviors. For example, adenosquamous and adenoid cystic carcinomas are aggressive tumors and thus have a relatively poor prognosis. Adenoid basal and verrucous cancers behave in the opposite fashion. More virulent yet is the infrequent small cell cancer of neuroendocrine origin, which sometimes presents with confusing paraendocrine symptoms. Lymphomas, carcinomas, melanomas, and primary sarcomas (e.g., embryonal rhabdomyosarcomas, leiomyosarcomas, malignant mixed müllerian tumors) also develop on the cervix. Finally, not all neoplasms on the cervix are primary from that site. Metastasis to the cervix can arise from the uterus, breast, colon, and kidney. Discussed here are the management principles pertaining to squamous cell cancer only.

2. **The continuum of neoplasia.** Cervical neoplasia is a disease continuum, spanning from mild dysplasia (cervical intraepithelial neoplasia type I [CINI]) to invasive cancer. Not uncommonly, preinvasive neoplasia, particularly that of low grade, spontaneously stabilizes or

resolves, but rapid, unpredictable progression to malignancy can also occur. The next step beyond the highest degree of preinvasive neoplasia is microinvasion. Expert opinions differ on what parameters best define this lesion. Fundamental to all concepts of microinvasion, however, is localized, readily resectable disease without or with very low risk of metastases.

Unlike squamous neoplasia, in which there is a clear-cut histologic demarcation (the basement membrane) beyond which the invasion becomes obvious, there are no equivalent histologic boundaries within the cervical stroma by which to delineate degrees of glandular (*adeno*) neoplasia. This makes diagnostic distinctions between preinvasion, microinvasion, and true invasion more precarious with glandular histologies.

3. **Spread pattern.** Expanding through the cervical stroma, the squamous cancer extends onto the vagina and uterus and laterally into the paracervical and parametrial soft tissues, ultimately to involve the pelvic sidewall and obstruct the ureters. Direct extension into the bladder or rectum is uncommon. While invading the stroma, the cancer can enter lymphatic vessel spaces, with consequent spread to the obturator and iliac lymph nodes and ascension to the aortic and supraclavicular groups. Hematogenous dissemination is found in 10% of patients. Distant sites of metastases include the lungs, mediastinum, bone, and liver.

B. **Diagnosis and staging**
   1. **Clinical manifestations.** Because of effective screening, many diagnoses of cervical cancer are made before the onset of symptoms. However, intermenstrual bleeding, postcoital bleeding (classic, but uncommon), postmenopausal bleeding, and vaginal discharge can result from friable, ulcerated, often necrotic cervical epithelium. Pelvic, lumbosacral, gluteal, and back pains are worrisome symptoms for advanced disease (e.g., nodal metastasis). Hematuria or rectal bleeding rarely occur but suggest organ involvement.
   2. **Diagnosis.** The diagnosis of cervical cancer can be proved only by biopsy, not by Pap smear. Although the correlation between Pap smear (cytology) and biopsy (histology) results is good (60% to 85%), cytology *per se* is insufficient for diagnosing any degree of cervical neoplasia, let alone malignancy. Practically, an abnormal Pap smear should be considered a "red flag," a warning of possible neoplasia, thus demanding further investigation (e.g., colposcopy and biopsy).

Although most cervical neoplasia is identified through abnormal Pap smears, any gross cervical lesions should be sampled for biopsy.

3. **Staging** (Table 12-1). In contrast to ovarian and endometrial cancers, which are staged surgically, cervical cancer is staged clinically. Recent changes in staging of early disease have attempted to better stratify stage IB disease. The most important determinant of stage in cervical cancer is the clinical examination, with particular emphasis on the pelvic and rectal examination. Chest x-ray studies and evaluation of the ureters using computed tomography (CT) are also done. In clinically early disease, cystoscopy and proctoscopy are neither helpful nor cost-effective.

C. **Treatment**
   1. **Early clinical disease**
      a. **Stage IA.** Stage IA1 disease can be treated by either cone biopsy, simple total hysterectomy, or modified radical hysterectomy. Theoretically, the same option exists for stage IA2 disease, but the recurrence rate is higher after cone biopsy compared with radical surgery. To the extent it exists, the extra risk inherent in pursuing a minimalistic treatment strategy (i.e., cone biopsy) must be assumed by the well-informed patient, who typically makes the choice because of the strong desire to preserve fertility.
      b. **For stages IB and IIA** disease, either a radical hysterectomy with pelvic lymphadenectomy or radical radiation therapy (whole pelvis plus brachytherapy) can be used. Both approaches produce comparable 5-year survival rates. Surgery, however, offers certain advantages: less long-term morbidity, ovarian conservation, better posttreatment sexual function, and surgicopathologic staging permitting risk stratification.
      c. **Risk stratification.** Nodal metastasis significantly worsens prognosis. In stage IB cervical cancer, factors correlating with pelvic node involvement are lesion size, tumor grade, vascular and lymphatic space invasion (VSI), parametrial extension, and depth of stromal invasion. Microvessel counts are also being investigated as risk predictors. High-risk patients identified by surgical staging are candidates for adjuvant treatment, preferably on protocol. Recent Gynecologic Oncology Group (GOG) trials showed decreased recurrence rates

**Table 12-1.   1995 FIGO staging
(Montreal) for carcinoma of the cervix uteri**

Stage grouping	Definition
I	The carcinoma is strictly confined to the cervix (extension to the corpus should be disregarded).
IA	Invasive cancer identified only microscopically. All gross lesions even with superficial invasion are stage IB cancers. Invasion is limited to measured stromal invasion with maximum depth of 5 mm and no wider than 7 mm.
IA-1	Measured invasion of stroma no greater than 3 mm in depth and no wider than 7 mm.
IA-2	Measured invasion of stroma greater than 3 mm, no greater than 5 mm, and no wider than 7 mm. The depth of invasion should not be more than 5 mm, taken from the base of the epithelium, either surface or glandular, from which it originates. Preformed space involvement (vascular or lymphatic) should not alter the staging but should be specifically recorded to determine whether it should affect treatment decisions in the future.
IB	Clinical lesions confined to the cervix or preclinical lesions greater than those of stage IA.
IB-1	Clinical lesions no greater than 4 cm in size.
IB-2	Clinical lesions greater than 4 cm in size.
II	The carcinoma extends beyond the cervix but has not extended to the pelvic wall. The carcinoma involves the vagina but does not extend as far as the lower third.
IIA	No obvious parametrial involvement.
IIB	Obvious parametrial involvement.
III	The carcinoma has extended to the pelvic wall. On rectal examination, there is no cancer-free space between the tumor and the pelvic wall. The tumor involves the lower third of the vagina. All cases with a hydronephrosis or nonfunctioning kidney are included unless they are known to be due to other causes.
IIIA	No extension to the pelvic wall.
IIIB	Extension to the pelvic wall and/or hydronephrosis or nonfunctioning kidney.
IV	The carcinoma has extended beyond the true pelvis or has clinically involved the mucosa of the bladder or rectum. A bullous edema as such does not permit a case to be allotted to stage IV.
IVA	Spread of the growth to adjacent organs.
IVB	Spread to distant organs.

among patients with two or more high-risk factors who received postoperative radiotherapy with sensitizing chemotherapy. The matter still remains controversial, however.

d. **Special cases.** The optimal therapy for the bulky cervical cancer (stage IB2) is controversial. Neoadjuvant (upfront) chemotherapy followed by either radical surgery or radiation therapy is being used by some as an alternative approach to primary radical radiation therapy (external and implants) in managing the difficult lesions.

Other special cases of cervical cancer include cervical cancer and neoplasia occurring during pregnancy, carcinoma of the cervical stump after supracervical hysterectomy, the unexpected finding of cancer after "benign hysterectomy," cervical cancer and a coexisting pelvic mass or pelvic inflammatory disease, cervical cancer and ureteral obstruction, and cervical cancer and acquired immunodeficiency syndrome (AIDS). Each of these complex situations needs appropriate, often unique, interventions (or no intervention) in the context of the actual tumor biology, anatomic circumstances, and the specific patient.

2. **Advanced disease**

   a. **Stage IIB to IVA cervical cancers**, by default, have been managed by radical radiation therapy. The modest 5-year survival rates reported vary with stage and institution but generally range from 20% to 60%. Sensitizing chemotherapy in conjunction with radiation may enhance efficacy overall. With stage IVA disease, barring evidence of distant or unresectable disease, cure is also occasionally possible using ultraradical surgery (i.e., primary pelvic exenteration).

   b. **Stage IVB** disease is essentially incurable. Accordingly, treatment is individualized and palliative.

   c. **Chemotherapy** in advanced disease, using either single agents or combinations, can produce short-term responses. Cisplatin has been considered the most active single agent; other drugs that demonstrate a response rate of 15% or more include paclitaxel (Taxol), irinotecan (CPT-11), carboplatin, bleomycin, vincristine, mitomycin, ifosfamide, fluorouracil, etoposide, and methotrexate. Combination chemotherapy, such as cisplatin and ifosfamide with or without bleomycin, has been studied, yielding significantly higher response rates when compared with single-agent cisplatin. At present, the use of relatively more toxic of combination regimens is controversial because cisplatin alone may prolong survival equivalently. With recurrent squamous cancer, cisplatin produces a 20% to 30% response rate, 10% of cases being complete responses. No clear dose-response relation has been demonstrated, so cisplatin, 50 mg/m^2 i.v. every 3 weeks, is typically recommended.

d. **New approaches to advanced disease.** Use of neoadjuvant chemotherapy in certain clinical situations seems logical, and reports have been promising; but the result of five randomized trials comparing neoadjuvant chemotherapy followed by irradiation with irradiation alone have failed to show an improvement in outcome when neoadjuvant chemotherapy was added to radical radiotherapy. This is true despite the high response rates of locally advanced cancer to chemotherapy. Studies are continuing, however. Chemotherapy is being prospectively tested as a radiation sensitizer. Several small series suggested that better local control and survival are achieved using radiation concurrent with hydroxyurea, fluorouracil, cisplatin, or combinations of these agents. Although the absolute value of radiosensitizing chemotherapy is not proved, there appears to be reason for optimism based on a recent GOG study that found weekly cisplatin superior to hydroxyurea.

3. **Recurrent cervical cancer.** The recurrence rate for all cervical cancer is 35%. In contrast, only 10% to 20% of patients with stage IB disease have recurrence. This rate increases to 45% to 60%, however, when lymph nodes contain metastasis. Recurrences generally develop within 2 to 3 years of primary treatment, and most of these patients die from disease. Recurrent cervical cancer must be treated within the constraints presented by the site of the recurrence and the type of treatment originally rendered (i.e., surgery, radiation therapy, or both). Sites of recurrence are categorized as local/central (resectable, thus potentially curable), regional (in the pelvis but unresectable, extending to the sidewall or to lymph nodes (rarely curable), and distant.

A true central recurrence after primary surgery can be managed with radiation therapy (likely with sensitizing chemotherapy). Salvage rates as high as 25% to 50% are reported. A curative alternative for central recurrence, particularly in previously irradiated patients, is the select use of ultraradical surgery. Employed under ideal clinical circumstances, pelvic exenteration offers a 30% to 60% 5-year survival rate (i.e., if complete, negative-margin resection proves possible). Because of the high surgical complication rate and the risk of major long-term physical and psychological morbidity, exenterative surgery is indicated only with the intent of cure.

- **D. Survival.** The overall 5-year survival rate for cervical cancer is only 50%. Stage is the most significant predictor. The survival rate for stage IA is 98%; stage IB and IIA, 75% to 85%; stage IIB, 55%; stage III, 10% to 50%; and stage IVB, essentially none. Discouragingly, despite improvements in radiotherapy technology and better delineation of disease, survival rates have not improved in 30 years.

II. Endometrial cancer. Endometrial cancer is the most common gynecologic pelvic malignancy in developed nations. There will an estimated 36,100 new cases and 6,300 deaths from endometrial cancer in the United States this year. Because endometrial cancer usually presents as postmenopausal bleeding, any amount of postmenopausal bleeding is suspect. Epidemiologic risk factors for endometrial cancer include obesity, nulliparity, diet, advancing age, and unopposed estrogen use. The use of oral contraception and, surprisingly, smoking are negatively correlated. The diagnosis is established by simple, cost-effective, endometrial biopsy performed in the office. The physical examination and Pap smear are not usually contributory to diagnosis.

- **A. Pathology and patterns of spread**
  1. **Histology.** The dominant histologic type of endometrial cancer is endometrioid. Together with the other less common adenocarcinomas of the endometrium (adenosquamous, papillary serous, and clear cell cancers), they constitute 90% of cases of "uterine cancer." Differentiating among the adenocarcinoma subtypes is important because each has its own biologic behavior and outcome. For example, the patterns of spread and the 90% 5-year survival rate for early-stage endometrioid cancer differ greatly from those of papillary serous and clear cell carcinomas, which have 40% and 44% survival rates, respectively.
  2. **Patterns of spread.** Endometrioid carcinoma first invades the myometrium and then the vascular and lymphatic space. Metastases to the pelvic lymph nodes, and then to the periaortic

lymph nodes, follow. The vagina is another common site of lymphatic spread. Thus, metastases to the vagina usually represent only the "visible tip of the iceberg," rather than an innocuous, truly isolated lesion. The presence of simultaneous, but occult, lymphatic metastasis accounts for the high failure rate of treatment focused only on the obvious vaginal site. In another means of dissemination, malignant cells can exfoliate from endometrial primary tumor and implant throughout the peritoneal cavity, especially with serous or clear cell histologies. Hematogenous metastases to the lungs, liver, bone, and brain are usually late-occurring events. Concomitant endometrioid cancer found in both the endometrium and ovaries is surprisingly frequent, up to 15%. Distinguishing whether the simultaneous involvement of organs represents metastasis, one site to the other, or two separate stage I primary tumors has therapeutic relevance.

B. Pretreatment evaluation

1. Diagnostic tests. In clinically early-stage endometrial cancer, few preoperative tests are fruitful. Still, chest x-ray and CT studies are generally obtained to look for advanced disease. CA-125 levels are occasionally elevated in endometrial neoplasms and, if so, are useful in monitoring treatment response. Cystoscopy, sigmoidoscopy, and pelvic ultrasound invariably show negative results and hence should be avoided unless symptoms indicate otherwise. Magnetic resonance imaging (MRI) is sensitive in determining the extent and depth of myometrial invasion but is expensive and rarely alters current treatment.

2. Staging. Federation Internationale de Gynecologie et d'Obstetrique (FIGO) staging of endometrial cancer is surgical (Table 12-2). Stage according to disease distribution is further subcategorized by tumor grade. Because most endometrial cancers are heralded by abnormal bleeding, diagnosing the disease in a low stage is facilitated; consequently, 75% are stage I and 15% stage II at the time of diagnosis.

3. Risk stratification. Risk factors in stage I endometrial cancer are tumor grade (G1, G2, G3), depth of myometrial invasion, VSI, age, hormonal receptor status, tumor histology, DNA ploidy, and S-phase fraction. In a major GOG study of stage I endometrioid cancer, there was only a 3% risk of pelvic nodal involvement for G1 lesions, compared with 18% for G3 lesions. Without myometrial invasion, the risk of nodal metastases was 1%. This risk increased to 25%

Table 12-2.   FIGO staging for carcinoma of the corpus uteri

Stage	Definition
I	Tumor confined to the uterine fundus
IA G123	Tumor limited to endometrium
IB G123	Invasion to less than one half of the myometrium
IC G123	Invasion to more than one half of the myometrium
II	Tumor extends to the cervix
IIA G123	Endocervical glandular involvement only
IIB G123	Cervical stromal invasion
III	Regional tumor spread
IIIA G123	Tumor invades serosa and/or adnexa and/or has positive peritoneal cytology
IIIB G123	Vaginal metastases
IIIC G123	Metastases to pelvic and/or periaortic lymph nodes
IV	Bulky pelvic disease or distant spread
IVA G123	Tumor invasion of bladder and/or bowel mucosa
IVB	Distant metastases, including intraabdominal and/or inguinal lymph nodes

with myometrial penetration to the outer third. Among patients with cancer showing no VSI, 7% had pelvic nodal metastases, compared with 27% if there was VSI. The significance of finding malignant cells on cytology of abdominal and pelvic washings in the absence of other risk factors is controversial. Still, it appears that "positive" washings are an independent marker for aggressive disease, thus carrying a worse prognosis (e.g., risk of occult, current or later-developing extrapelvic disease). In recognition of this fact, FIGO has upstaged patients with malignant cytology to stage IIIA. (The best management for the situation is less clear, however.)

After surgery, the combined power of all the pathologically confirmed prognostic factors is used for risk stratification, and in that process, the need for adjuvant treatment is best determined.

C. **Management**
   1. **Surgery.** The standard and central treatment for endometrial cancer is surgery. Although historically, preoperative radiation therapy was widely used, for good reason, that practice has been abandoned.

   Surgery for endometrial cancer consists of exploratory laparotomy, cytologic washings, extrafascial total hysterectomy, bilateral salpingo-oophorectomy, and staging. A selective approach is often taken to decide on further staging. An intraoperative assessment is made of myometrial invasion and disease distribution; then, based on the presence or absence of those risk factors, lymph node sampling and other staging can be selectively performed. Specific adjustments in the operation are made according to histology, tumor grade, and intraoperative findings (e.g., if deep myometrial invasion exists).

2. For the rare patient deemed absolutely inoperable for medical reasons, **radiation therapy** (external-beam and intracavitary implants) as sole treatment becomes a not-so-unmorbid alternative. The cure rate achieved by radiation therapy alone, even with early-stage disease, is inferior to that of hysterectomy. Hormonal therapy as a medical alternative is rarely of sustained benefit.

3. **Postoperative management**
   a. **Adjuvant treatment.** Based on the surgical pathology, patients with a poor prognosis can be identified. Although proof of ultimate benefit is still lacking, pelvic irradiation is nevertheless the most common type of adjuvant treatment given patients considered at high risk of local recurrence. At Women and Infants Hospital/Brown University, adjuvant treatment protocols for stage I endometrioid cancer currently employ postoperative whole-pelvis irradiation if there is deep myometrial invasion, VSI, G3 lesions, or extension to the endocervix stroma—assuming the lymph nodes are negative for cancer. If the lymph nodes have metastasis, extrauterine disease is present, or abdominal or pelvic washings contain malignant cells, then the potential rationale of adjuvant radiation therapy is less obvious. Therefore, we view such patients as better candidates for advanced-disease treatment, preferably on protocols.
   b. **Advanced-disease treatment**
      (1) **Radiotherapy.** Effective treatment for advanced endometrial cancer remains elusive. Lacking other options, pelvic radiation therapy is often tried, even with high-risk or high-stage regional disease. The generally poor outcome is understandable because treating a simultaneously bulky and diffuse malignant process with necessarily constrained, nontumoricidal radiation doses is bound to fail.
      (2) **Systemic therapy.** Hormonal therapy, though logical and once highly touted, has thus far proved largely ineffective in controlled studies. Oc-

casionally, however, meaningful responses to high-dose progestins do occur, particularly with late-recurring grade 1 tumors, at sites outside the irradiated field. Similarly, there are individual responses to systemic chemotherapy, though larger studies have yet to identify a routine role for potentially toxic current drugs (especially administered to symptom-free patients). Despite a lack of compelling response data, doxorubicin (Adriamycin), considered the most active single agent, and other single agents with notable responses, including paclitaxel, cisplatin, cyclophosphamide, and combinations of these agents, may be given for their short-term benefit. Paclitaxel at higher doses (250 mg/m^2) has shown impressive response rates (36%), and paclitaxel in various dosages and schedules is being studied in drug combinations, as are other drugs.

What might be considered standard chemotherapy regimens for patients not wishing protocol treatment include the following:

Doxorubicin, 60 mg/m^2 i.v. every 3 weeks, *or*

Doxorubicin, 60 mg/m^2 i.v., *plus* cisplatin, 50 mg/m^2 i.v. every 3 weeks.

  c. **Recurrent disease.** In select patients with a presumably limited recurrence of endometrial cancer, surgical restaging can be helpful in the final decision-making process. When possible, complete resection of the recurrent tumor (e.g., upper vaginectomy) appears to enhance subsequent salvage therapy. In general, however, for advanced or recurrent endometrial cancer, surgery and radiation therapy are of limited local-control value, and systemic therapies are briefly palliative. Because individual good responses can occur, thoughtful chemotherapy, surgery, and radiation therapy, especially in the protocol setting, are justified for the informed patient wishing to try.

 4. **Special cases.** A variety of less common uterine neoplasms can also occur. These need to be managed according to their own unique biology, which differs from that of the endometrioid histology.

  a. **Papillary serous carcinoma** (PSC) of the endometrium behaves biologically more like the histologically identical PSC of the ovary. In an ovarian-like fashion, the endometrial PSC spreads and recurs diffusely on peritoneal serosal surfaces throughout the entire abdomen. Disappointingly, and unlike their ovarian counterpart, even the use of postsurgery cisplatin-based combination chemotherapy has had little impact in PSC of the endometrium. Nevertheless, systemic adjuvant therapy seems appropriate, given their biologic behavior.

b. **Other uterine malignancies.** About 5% of uterine malignancies are sarcomas, which can emanate from the myometrium or the endometrial stroma. The mixed müllerian mesodermal tumor (MMMT), formally called carcinosarcoma, is the most common type, followed by leiomyosarcoma and then endometrial stromal sarcomas.

In general, the primary treatment of MMMT and leiomyosarcomas is surgery: total abdominal hysterectomy and bilateral salpingo-oophorectomy and staging, followed by consideration of adjuvant treatment. Both lesions recur locoregionally and distally; thus, adjuvant pelvic irradiation may reduce local recurrence but has no overall survival benefit. Although there is a need, there is currently no proven role for adjuvant chemotherapy in the treatment of these malignancies. Ifosfamide as a single agent or in combination with other drugs is receiving the greatest interest for treating advanced disease.

Ifosfamide, 1.2 to 1.5 g/m^2 i.v. days 1 to 4 with mesna protection, *or*

Ifosfamide, 1.2 to 1.5 g/m^2 i.v. days 1 to 4 with mesna protection, *plus* cisplatin, 20 mg/m^2/day i.v. for 4 days every 3 weeks for eight cycles.

Other neoplasms (e.g., endometrial stromal tumors) occasionally develop in the uterine connective tissues as well. Most often, advanced or recurrent connective tissue tumors are of higher grade or are unresectable and thus must be treated systemically. Depending on hormonal receptor status and the type of histology, dramatic responses to hormonal ablation with high-dose progesterone, such as megestrol acetate (Megace) 240 to 360 mg p.o. daily, can occur. Others sometimes respond to chemotherapy, including etoposide, dactinomycin, doxorubicin combinations, ifosfamide alone or with cisplatin, or cisplatin. Unfortunately, most high-grade sarcomas that are not cured surgically do not have prolonged responses to systemic treatment.

    c. Preserving fertility. Infrequently, a young woman desirous of fertility will develop a well-differentiated endometrioid adenocarcinoma of the endometrium. Barring evidence of advanced disease or an MRI suggesting myometrial invasion, well informed patients can consider, as primary management, intensive hormonal therapy using high-dose progesterone (e.g., megestrol acetate, 240 mg p.o. daily × 3 months) instead of hysterectomy. A thorough dilation and curettage with or without hysteroscopy follows the limited trial of hormones. If the cancer is resolved, reproductive assistance with ovulation stimulation can be done in hope of completing fertility desires before a need for hysterectomy develops. Generally, however, the odds for achieving a successful pregnancy under these circumstances are considered poor, although successful full-term deliveries have occurred.

III. Fallopian tube cancer. Despite its direct physical and anatomic relation with the uterus, the rare tubal cancer is biologically and behaviorally more analogous to serous epithelial ovarian cancer. As a practical matter, fallopian tube cancer is staged and managed in a fashion similar to ovarian and not uterine malignancy. The diagnosis of a tubal cancer is usually fortuitous, or comes about retrospectively, after surgery is performed to address some other process. Preoperative symptoms are sometimes present, the classic being a profuse, intermittent, watery, vaginal discharge. Pelvic pain and an abnormal Pap smear suggesting adenocarcinoma that are not otherwise explained by routine testing, such as colposcopy, endocervical curettage, and dilation and curettage, can also lead to the diagnosis of fallopian tube cancer.

    Treatment is primarily surgery followed by postoperative chemotherapy for advanced disease, as in ovarian cancer.

IV. Ovarian cancer. Ovarian cancer is the leading killer among female pelvic malignancies in the United States. In 1998, there were an estimated 25,400 new cases and 14,500 deaths. Contrary to the common perception, ovarian cancer is a heterologous group of biologically diverse neoplasms, often having only their anatomic site, the ovary, in common. Thus, broad generalizations about ovarian cancer are difficult but are best made by subcategorizing it into three groups based on embryologic origin.

    A. Histologic types

        1. Germ cell ovarian cancers. These malignancies typically occur in young women and are curable. They often present as an asymptomatic pelvic mass and, in the past, were usually lethal (e.g., immature teratomas, endodermal sinus tumors, dysgerminomas), even though they were confined to the ovary. Today's therapeutic breakthrough is curative chemotherapy, which, as an added benefit, does not typically compromise future fertility. After surgery, which is done to remove the involved ovary, establish the diagnosis, and stage the disease, the same agents effective against male germ cell tumors (e.g., bleomycin, etoposide, and cisplatin [BEP]) also work well against their less common female counterparts (see Chapter 13.)

2. **Stromal tumors.** Stromal tumors of the ovary are rare anachronistic neoplasms occurring at any age but are stereotyped by their occasional sex hormone production. The uncommon but often discussed childhood granulosa cell tumor causing precocious puberty is a classic example. After surgical resection, the typical patient with a stromal tumor is observed without further intervention. This management strategy is chosen in part because most stromal tumors are benign or low grade (or of inscrutable malignant potential) and hence are resolved by simple removal. Recurrences can occur, sometimes many years later. If so, or with advanced or unresectable disease, chemotherapy (e.g., bleomycin, etoposide, and cisplatin; see Chapter 13) can be beneficial, even if not curative.

3. **Epithelial ovarian cancer.** Seventy percent of ovarian malignancies belong to the epithelial subgroup (e.g., serous, mucinous, endometrioid, clear cell). In contrast to germ cell tumors, epithelial ovarian cancer (EOC) generally occurs after menopause, is advanced at the time of diagnosis, and is rarely curable. The remainder of this section deals with the diagnosis and management of this common variety of ovarian cancer.

B. **Diagnosis and screening**

1. **Early diagnosis.** Diagnosing EOC at an early stage is a difficult, almost fortuitous occurrence because patients usually lack specific symptoms and findings. Little actual merit has come from attempts to screen healthy asymptomatic women for EOCs by using tumor markers with or without ultrasound. CA-125, alone or together with other tumor markers lacks sufficient sensitivity and specificity for general screening. By its nature, the normal ovary has a dynamic cyclic cyst-forming physiology. By comparison, the chance of developing an EOC—an estimated lifetime risk of 1 in 70 (1.4%) American women—is

rare. Although today's ultrasound technology can detect even the tiniest ovarian cysts, uncertainty in the true pathology and need for intervention persists in all but the small "simple" cysts. Consequently, the National Cancer Institute (NCI) and others have concluded that routine screening programs for EOC are inappropriate as a current standard of care.

In contrast, however, two classes of serum tumor markers, monoclonal antibodies (e.g., CA-125 with EOCs) and peptide markers (e.g., α-fetoprotein with endodermal sinus tumors, müllerian inhibiting factor, and inhibin with granulosa cell tumors) have proved useful in monitoring the treatment of, not the screening for, ovarian cancer. Additionally, preoperative evaluation of tumor markers and pelvic ultrasound may be useful in estimating risk of malignancy and aid in appropriate preoperative patient triage.

2. **Risk stratification for screening.** As mentioned, screening is not recommended for the general population. However, women deemed at high risk of developing EOC are still being advised to undergo extra surveillance and, at the extreme, prophylactic oophorectomy. Accepting for the moment the underlying premises of cancer prevention benefit, because the criteria defining high risk are not yet specific or proved, that designation can be subjectively extrapolated to encompass too many women.

Epidemiologically, low parity with a history of infertility correlates with an increased risk of EOC. In contrast, high parity, tubal ligation, and oral contraceptive use negatively correlate with the risk of EOC, with oral contraceptive use reducing the relative risk up to 50%. Ironically, in this era that clamors for cancer prevention, the use of safe, low-dose birth control pills (and possibly acetaminophen) stands out as a real but often ignored option that may be immediately advantageous.

Meanwhile, under present limitations, risk stratification for EOC relies largely on the family history. Fortunately, lacking multiple first-degree relatives with EOC, or repetitive generations (maternal or paternal) affected by the cancer, there is little (e.g., 5% to 7% lifetime risk) increase in risk. During the past several years, multiple genes have been identified that, when mutant, increase the risk of developing ovarian cancer. The breast and ovarian cancer syndrome associated with germline BRCA-1 and BRCA-2 mutations is inherited in an autosomal dominant fashion. BRCA-1 and BRCA-2 appear to function as tumor-suppressor genes, based on loss of heterozygosity at this locus in tumors from families with familial ovarian cancer. The precise increase in risk associated with a mutation of BRCA-1 ranges from about 26% to 44% to as high as 85% in a small subset of patients, and this is likely indicative of the specific mutation and penetrance. The risk of ovarian cancer in women harboring a mutation in the BRCA-2 gene is less, with a cumulative risk estimated to be less than 10% by 70 years of age. About 5% to 10% of ovarian cancer cases are likely attributable to such mutations. An increased risk of ovarian cancer is also associated with hereditary nonpolyposis colon cancer, with mutations documented in the mismatch repair genes MSH2, MLH1, PMS1, and PMS2. In this rare high-risk situation, prophylactic oophorectomy is being advocated and may have benefit. However, even after oophorectomy, serous carcinoma of the peritoneum, a disease similar to EOC, can still occur.

C. **Management**
   1. **The role of surgery.** After an initial work-up and assessment of tumor markers, the key first step in the evaluation of a pelvic or abdominal mass with or without ascites is surgery. Indeed, with surgery comes the primary intervention, almost without regard for patient age, clinically presumed diagnosis, or stage of disease. Preoperative diagnostic tests, such as needle biopsies and paracenteses, are generally meddlesome, risk disseminating disease, and do not alter the ultimate need for surgery. The surgery allows for accurate diagnosis, thorough staging of disease, and in abdominal disease, valuable tumor debulking.
      a. **Early disease and surgical staging** (Table 12-3). At laparotomy, the ovarian mass is resected intact if possible (i.e., without rupture), and diagnosis is established based on frozen-section evaluation. During surgery, 20% of EOCs appear visually or grossly confined to the ovary (i.e., stage I), but 30% to 50% of patients have extraovarian microscopic disease—thus, the stage of disease is more advanced. Surgical staging then permits postoperative treatment to be realistically directed at the true EOC distribution.
      b. **Advanced disease.** 80% of women have advanced disease (stage III or stage IV) at diagnosis. Most of the women have disease disseminating throughout the abdominal cavity with ascites. The finding of ad-

Table 12-3. FIGO staging system for ovarian cancer

Stage	Definition
I	Growth limited to the ovaries
IA	Growth limited to one ovary; no ascites, no tumor on the external surfaces, capsule intact
IB	Growth limited to both ovaries; no ascites; no tumor on the external surfaces, capsule intact
IC	Tumor either stage IA or IB but with tumor on the surface of one or both ovaries; or with capsule ruptured; or with ascites present containing malignant cells or with positive peritoneal washings
II	Growth involving one or both ovaries with pelvic extension
IIA	Extension and/or metastases to the uterus and/or tubes
IIB	Extension to other pelvic tissues
IIC	Tumor either stage IIA or IIB but with tumor on the surface of one or both ovaries; or with capsule ruptured; or with ascites present containing malignant cells or with positive peritoneal washings
III	Tumor involving one or both ovaries with peritoneal implants outside the pelvis and/or positive retroperitoneal or inguinal nodes; surface liver metastases equals stage III; tumor is limited to the true pelvis but with histologically verified malignant extension to small bowel, large bowel, or omentum
IIIA	Tumor grossly limited to the true pelvis with negative nodes but with histologically confirmed microscopic seeding of abdominal peritoneal surfaces
IIIB	Tumor of one or both ovaries; histologically confirmed implants of abdominal peritoneal surfaces, none exceeding 2 cm in diameter; nodes negative
IIIC	Abdominal implants greater than 2 cm in diameter and/or positive retroperitoneal or inguinal nodes
IV	Growth involving one or both ovaries with distant metastases; if pleural effusion is present, there must be positive cytologic test results to allot a case to stage IV; parenchymal liver metastases equals stage IV

vanced EOC often portrays a seemingly insurmountable picture of unresectable peritoneal and bulky pelvic and abdominal tumor. Fortunately, with the proper surgical approach, maximal tumor resection is possible in 80% of patients. Although the surgical risks of debulking are real and substantial, they seem justified by the improved survival experienced by patients whose tumor was optimally debulked relative to those in whom cytoreduction was suboptimal or not carried out. Therefore, if technically feasible, as is usual in experienced hands, optimal debulking remains the recommended surgical intervention for advanced EOC. The value of a focused expertise in managing EOC has been indirectly recognized by the NCI in their recommendation that where the potential for such cases exists, they be managed by fellowship-trained gynecologic oncologists.

2. **Chemotherapy.** The need for postsurgery chemotherapy is determined in the context of histology, grade, stage, amount of residual tumor, and other prognostic factors, such as DNA ploidy and proliferative index. With the exception of ovarian tumors of low adjuvant potential (borderline ovarian tumors) generally treated with bilateral salpingo-oophorectomy alone, or the occasional patient with stage I low-grade EOC, most patients benefit from postoperative therapy.

   a. **In early-stage, high-grade EOC,** adjuvant chemotherapy has proved to prolong disease-free survival and possibly survival itself. Various adjuvants have been used, among them intraperitoneal phosphorus 32 (^{32}P) and systemic treatment with melphalan and platinum-based chemotherapy. For the occasional patient with high-grade stage I EOC, judicious adjuvant platinum-based therapy for three to six cycles is a current recommendation. The GOG is formally addressing the issue of treatment duration in early-stage disease. Given the limited data on chemotherapy in early EOC, treatment regimens have been extrapolated from those used in advanced disease. Dosing and timing of treatment are identical to advanced disease as outlined next.

   b. **Patients with more advanced disease** are currently treated with a platinum and paclitaxel regimen after debulking surgery. Appropriate regimens include the following:

Carboplatin i.v. calculated with area under the curve (AUC) of 5 to 7.5 (using the Jeliffe formula to calculate the estimated creatinine clearance and the Calvert formula for determining the AUC), *plus* paclitaxel, 175 mg/m^2 i.v. over 3 hours.

Cisplatin, 75 mg/m^2 i.v., *plus* paclitaxel, 135 mg/m^2 i.v. over 3 hours.

Carboplatin i.v. calculated with an AUC of 5 to 7.5 *plus* cyclophosphamide, 500 to 600 mg/m^2 i.v.

Although paclitaxel and a platinum is the favored regimen, with improvement in response rate and in disease-free and overall survival rates when compared with cyclophosphamide and a platinum, the latter regimen may be favored in certain circumstances, such as the diabetic patient who has significant peripheral neuropathy. The regimen is typically administered every 3 weeks for six cycles. Overall, the response rate (complete response plus partial response) is 70% to 80%, of which 50% are complete clinical responses and 30% complete pathologic responses. Although paclitaxel administered over 3 hours plus carboplatin is the current favored regimen off protocol, given the ease of administration, the optimal duration of paclitaxel infusion (e.g., 3 versus 24 hours) and the equivalence of carboplatin to cisplatin are currently being evaluated.

Patients are carefully monitored to determine treatment efficacy. Before receiving each cycle, they undergo physical examination, including pelvic examination, CA-125 determination, and less frequently, other studies. If any parameter suggests treatment failure (i.e., progression of disease), the regimen is immediately curtailed, and strategic options that remain are presented to the patient. Patients opting for second-line treatment, on or off protocol, do so realistically and with a great concern for maintaining the best possible quality of life under difficult circumstances.

c. **Dose intensification** is also being looked at in an effort to improve disease-free and overall survival rates. Although results are mixed, most studies suggest that dose intensification within the conventional range offers no improvement in disease-free or overall survival rates but is clearly associated with greater toxicity. Several phase I and II studies have demonstrated the feasibility, initial high response rates, and impressive disease-free or overall survival with bone marrow or peripheral blood stem cell transplantation immediately after first-line chemotherapy. These studies, however, have significant selection bias and, therefore, need to be interpreted with extreme caution. It remains that transplantation as a component of initial therapy should only be done in the protocol setting and, at present, optimally as part of a phase III randomized trial. One such trial, GOG 164, is a prospective randomized intergroup trial using cyclophosphamide (Cytoxan), mitoxantrone, and carboplatin with stem cell support, compared with standard paclitaxel plus carboplatin in patients with chemosensitive, minimal residual disease at the time of second-look laparotomy.

The utility of transplantation in the relapsed setting also remains unclear, yet its feasibility for intensive therapy has been demonstrated. In patients who have chemosensitive disease in the relapsed setting, bone marrow transplantation is an appropriate alternative treatment modality if performed on protocol.

3. **Second-look laparotomy.** At the end of primary treatment, if there is a complete clinical response, a normal CA-125 level, and a normal-appearing CT scan, selected patients are offered a second-look laparotomy. Most typically, this is appropriate only in a protocol setting, in which the information gained from surgery is used to determine further protocol treatment. Despite a preoperative impression of no evidence of disease, about one third of second-look laparotomies reveal gross disease. Although controversial, under such circumstances, if optimal secondary debulking is technically feasible without undue morbidity, the effort seems prudent. Of the remaining second-look laparotomies, one third reveal microscopic residual disease, and one third are negative (i.e., all of the restaging biopsy and cytology studies are normal). Of patients with a pathologic complete response at second-look laparotomy, half are destined to recur.

4. **Intraperitoneal chemotherapy.** The risk of intraperitoneal (IP) chemotherapy is unclear in the current standard management of bulky EOC. Although most studies fail to show an advantage to intraperitoneal versus intravenous therapy, one study from the pre-paclitaxel era,

using intraperitoneal cisplatin in previously untreated, optimally debulked stage III EOC, noted
a survival benefit when compared will an all-
intravenous regimen. A follow-up intergroup
study including paclitaxel has recently been
completed and awaits maturity. An exception to
this, where IP chemotherapy may still have
value, is after a second-look laparotomy, when at
most only microscopic disease was found. In the
setting of exceedingly minimal disease, the limited but very-high-dose drug intensity IP chemotherapy delivers to the peritoneal surfaces at
risk of EOC is theoretically advantageous compared with intravenous administration. Samples
of regimens include the following:

^{32}P, *or*
Cisplatin, 100 mg/m^2 IP every 3 weeks × 6, *or*
Cisplatin, 200 mg/m^2 IP, *plus* etoposide (VP-16),
    350 mg/m^2 in 2 liters of normal saline every
    3 weeks × 6.

Thiosulfate should be used during high-dose
IP cisplatin to protect against nephrotoxicity.
Thiosulfate, 4 mg/m^2 i.v. bolus over 30 minutes
at the start of IP therapy and then 2 g/m^2/h continuous i.v. infusion for a total of 6 hours, has
been employed.
Access to the peritoneal cavity can be gained
before each IP infusion using a Veress needle
and employing local anesthesia. Fluoroscopic
confirmation of proper needle location and free
peritoneal cavity dispersion of contrast dye is established before installation of the IP drugs. If
IP chemotherapy is to be considered for a patient
seemingly ideal for the intervention, informed
entry into a proper protocol remains important.
D. **Follow-up.** Even the patients with negative findings
at second-look laparotomy may eventually develop recurrent disease. Recurrences are usually identified
using CA-125 levels, sometimes months before diagnosed disease. As with initial disease, recurrences are
most common within the abdomen. Current treatment
has greatly improved survival and quality of life, but
patients are not, in the strictest sense, cured. Time to
recurrence can range greatly, from a few months to
more than 15 years. Nevertheless, if patients are followed long enough, recurrences typically develop. It
may be that a recurrence many years later is actually
a new or second malignant process (e.g., *de novo* peritoneal disease) and not a treatment failure.
E. **Recurrent and persistent disease.** Various second-line chemotherapy regimens have yielded modest responses and some relative improvement in survival. Platinum-based agents can be retried if the
interval from complete response to recurrence is at
least 6 months. Paclitaxel, 135 to 175 mg/m^2 i.v., can

be given if it was not used upfront. Other agents with reported activity include the following (used as single agents, not in combinations):

- Liposomal doxorubicin (Doxil), 40 to 50 mg/m^2 every 3 weeks.
- Topotecan, 1.5 mg/m^2 on days 1 to 5 every 3 weeks.
- Oral etoposide, 50 mg/m^2 (30 mg/m^2 for prior radiotherapy), on days 1 to 21 every 28 days.
- Oral altretamine (Hexalen, hexamethylmelamine), 260 mg/m^2.
- Gemcitabine, 800 to 1,000/m^2 i.v. on days 1, 8, and 15 every 28 days.
- Paclitaxel, 80 mg/m^2 on days 1, 8, 15 every 28 days.
- Tamoxifen, 20 mg p.o. b.i.d.

Responses with second-line treatment range from 20% to 40%. Most are short, but responses can occasionally exceed 1 to 2 years, justifying the concept of second-line chemotherapy for the informed patient who still wishes to try.

V. Gestational trophoblastic neoplasm. Gestational trophoblastic disease encompasses a spectrum of neoplasms arising from fetal chorionic tissue. These tumors range from benign hydatidiform mole, to invasive or metastatic molar tissue, to malignant choriocarcinoma. All histologic classifications of this disease exhibit proliferation of cytotrophoblast and syncytiotrophoblast secreting human chorionic gonadotropin (β-hCG), which is a sensitive and specific tumor marker for gestational trophoblastic neoplasm (GTN). Historically, metastatic gestational choriocarcinoma was the first solid tumor to be cured with systemic chemotherapy. Today, most GTNs can be cured with systemic chemotherapy, even in the presence of widespread metastases.

A. Hydatidiform mole. By far the most common form of GTN is the hydatidiform mole. Cytogenetic techniques have established two distinct molar syndromes: complete moles and partial moles. The complete moles arise from a paternal diploid genotype (90% 46XX, 6% 46XY) and constitute 95% of GTNs overall. In contrast, partial moles are associated with triploidy incorporating an extra haploid paternal chromosome (69XXY or 69XYY). All hydatidiform moles have the potential for developing malignant sequelae. Indeed, malignant transformation occurs in 20% of complete moles, but only 4% to 6% overall develop metastasis. Only 10% of partial moles have malignant sequelae, and these usually take the form of nonmetastatic, postmolar GTN.

    1. Initial management. The evaluation and primary management of both complete and partial hydatidiform moles are similar: surgical evacuation of the uterus and then close monitoring of postevacuation β-hCG levels until proof of cure or malignant sequelae occur. Often, the diagnosis of hydatidiform mole is only established ret-

rospectively, following what was presumed to be
an otherwise unremarkable spontaneous or elective abortion. If, however, the actual diagnosis
is made before evacuating the uterus (typically
by antenatal ultrasound), a physical examination, complete blood cell count, chest x-ray, and
baseline β-hCG measurement should be done
preoperatively. Liver and thyroid function tests
should be considered. Hydatidiform moles can
present with a variety of severe medical syndromes; classic among them is early-gestational-
age preeclampsia. Occasionally, ultrasound
identifies a concomitant viable fetus with or
without large ovarian thecalutein cysts. Uncommonly, metastatic disease is found, requiring a
more extensive work-up and staging (to be discussed). Considering the complex array of problems associated with hydatidiform moles, if the
diagnosis is known preoperatively, clinical management is best rendered by physicians with extensive knowledge and experience with GTN.

2. **Monitoring.** After evacuation of a molar pregnancy, serum β-hCG levels are monitored weekly
until three consecutive measurements are normal, and then titers are followed monthly for
6 months. Resolution of the β-hCG to a normal
value typically occurs by 12 weeks. Throughout
the entire observation period, patients are recommended to practice effective birth control to
prevent pregnancy and its attendant β-hCG elevation, which confuses the situation.

3. **Malignant transformation.** Malignant transformation of a hydatidiform mole expresses itself as a prolonged plateau, or even a rise, in the
β-hCG titer during the follow-up period. Under
these circumstances, prompt referral to an oncologist is recommended to expedite further
evaluation and treatment. Such patients are
staged and managed in the manner described in
the next section. The risk of specific hydatidiform mole undergoing malignant transformation may be predicted by a number of factors
(e.g., signs of marked trophoblastic growth, including uterine size greater than dates, elevated
β-hCG titer, prominent ovarian thecauterine
cysts, toxemia, hyperthyroidism, age). At some
centers, patients deemed at high risk of developing malignant sequelae are recommended to
receive single-agent prophylactic chemotherapy
to reduce the transformation risk. However, because the accuracy of prognostic factors is less
than absolute and the transformation rate of hydatidiform mole overall is only 15%, most experts do not recommend or use prophylactic
chemotherapy, even in high-risk patients. In-

stead, all patients are observed, and treatment is reserved until actual malignant transformation is documented.

B. **Malignant GTN.** The FIGO staging system for GTN and that of the American College of Obstetricians and Gynecologists (ACOG) are shown in Tables 12-4 and 12-5. The latter means of classification has greater clinical utility because it facilitates treatment selection as well as classification. Prognostic factors including age, β-hCG titer, number and sites of metastases, antecedent pregnancy, interval between antecedent pregnancy and start of chemotherapy, and prior chemotherapy, are considered as part of the ACOG classification system for malignant GTN.

Unlike patients with hydatidiform moles, everyone with malignant GTN is ultimately treated with chemo-therapy. Before treatment is initiated, however, they undergo a more extensive metastatic survey. For example, chest x-ray studies and CT of the chest, abdomen, brain, and pelvis are usually done. Usually, however, in the setting of normal-appearing chest radiographs (and normal vaginal findings), metastases are rarely identified by any of the other more sophisticated tests. As such, clinicians experienced in GTN management often exercise cost-effective selectivity in the actual pretreatment evaluation of patients with malignant GTN.

The key treatment monitor for malignant GTN, as with all GTNs, is the serum β-hCG level. As a matter of further surveillance, the complete blood cell count, along with renal and liver functions, are also followed starting from their pretreatment baseline. As a further safeguard, a pretreatment ultrasound to exclude the possibility of an intrauterine pregnancy should be considered. Once the patient's malignant GTN data base is collected, permitting ACOG classification, those unlikely to be cured using single-agent chemotherapy can be identified. Such high-risk pa-

Table 12-4. FIGO staging for gestational trophoblastic neoplasia

Stage	Definition
I	Strictly confined to uterine corpus
II	Extends outside the uterus, but limited to genital structures
III	Extends to the lungs, with or without genital tract involvement
IV	All other metastatic sites

Modified from Pettersson F, et al. *Annual report on the results of treatment of gynecologic cancer.* Vol. 19. Stockholm: International Federation of Gynecology and Obstetrics, 1985.

Table 12-5.   Modified American College of Obstetricians and Gynecologists classification of gestational trophoblastic neoplasm

I. Nonmalignant gestational trophoblastic neoplasm (GTN)
   A. Hydatidiform mole
      1. Complete
      2. Incomplete
II. Malignant GTN
   A. Nonmetastatic GTN: no evidence of disease outside of uterus, not assigned to prognostic category
   B. Metastatic GTN: any metastases
      1. Good-prognosis metastatic GTN
         Short duration (<4 months)
         Low β-hCG level (<40,000 mIU/mL serum β-hCG)
         No metastases to brain or liver
         No antecedent term pregnancy
         No prior chemotherapy
      2. Poor-prognosis metastatic GTN: any high risk factor
         Long duration (>4 months since last pregnancy)
         High pretreatment β-hCG level (>40,000 mIU/mL serum β-hCG)
         Brain or liver metastases
         Antecedent term pregnancy
         Prior chemotherapy

tients are then treated with aggressive combination chemotherapy.

1. **Treatment of malignant nonmetastatic GTN.** Malignant GTN is divided into two subsets according to the presence or absence of metastatic disease. For the nonmetastatic group, most centers report almost 100% cure rates using single-agent treatment with either methotrexate or dactinomycin.

Methotrexate, 0.4 mg/kg i.m. for 5 days, with cycles repeated every 14 days has been standard, *but*

Methotrexate, 40 mg/m² i.m. weekly, has emerged as the preferred alternative because of its simplicity and relative lack of toxicity.

Alternative schedules for methotrexate with folinic acid rescue have been used, but with no obvious therapeutic advantage and possibly with greater toxicity.

Whichever primary treatment regimen is selected for nonmetastatic GTN, additional controversy exists regarding the number of cycles of therapy required for disease resolution. In the United States, nonmetastatic GTN has been treated using repeated doses, given at short intervals, until one or two negative β-hCG titers are achieved. This tact is in recognition of the subpopulation of trophoblastic cells that can theoretically persist even when the β-hCG titer is zero.

Fortunately, few patients with malignant nonmetastatic GTN fail primary therapy. Most patients who fail methotrexate, however, can still be salvaged using single-agent dactinomycin. Dactinomycin is given in i.v. doses of 9 to 13 μg/kg/day for 5 days, recycled at 14-day intervals, or as a single i.v. bolus of 40 μg/kg (1.5 mg/m^2) administered every 2 weeks. As mentioned, dactinomycin can also be used as an alternative to methotrexate as initial therapy of nonmetastatic disease. Patients prefer the latter, however, particularly because it does not cause alopecia.

For patients who do not desire continued fertility, hysterectomy is an alternative approach to the use of extended chemotherapy alone. The advantage is that performing hysterectomy concomitant with chemotherapy reduces the total number of chemotherapy cycles needed to produce remission. However, given the high effectiveness of chemotherapy in treating GTN and the uncertainty of most young patients regarding their future fertility, the hysterectomy option is rarely taken.

2. **Treatment of malignant metastatic GTN.** As defined by the ACOG criteria, patients with malignant metastatic GTN are further separated into low- and high-risk groups. This distinction is of major clinical relevance.

   a. **Low-risk (good-prognosis) metastatic GTN.** This is treated identically to nonmetastatic GTN discussed already. About two thirds of low-risk patients have complete remission after single-agent therapy. Similar to their nonmetastatic peers, nearly all low-risk patients with metastases who develop disease resistant to initial therapy are subsequently cured with either an alternative single-agent or with combination chemotherapy.

   b. **High-risk (poor-prognosis) metastatic GTN.** Not all patients with metastatic high-risk GTN survive. Most American centers treat patients with high-risk metastatic GTN using multiagent chemotherapy. The overall success rate in high-risk disease ranges between 63% and 80% for multiagent chemotherapy using methotrexate- and dactinomycin-based combinations. The two most commonly used combination regimens are outlined in Table 12-6. MAC chemotherapy (see Table 12-6) has been the combination regimen most often reported

Table 12-6. Multiagent chemotherapy for high-risk metastatic gestational trophoblastic disease (GTD)

MAC

Days 1–5: Methotrexate, 0.3 mg/kg i.m. (11.1 mg/m² i.v.)
Dactinomycin, 8–10 µg/kg i.v. (0.30–0.37 mg/m²)
Cyclophosphamide, 250 mg i.v.
Cycles repeated every 14–21 d

EMA-CO
Course A

Day 1: Dactinomycin, 0.5 mg i.v. bolus
Etoposide, 100 mg/m² i.v. infusion over 30 min
Methotrexate, 100 mg/m² i.v. bolus followed by 200 mg/m² i.v. infusion over 12 h
Day 2: Dactinomycin, 0.5 mg i.v. bolus
Etoposide, 100 mg/m² i.v. infusion over 30 min
Folinic acid, 15 mg, i.m./p.o. every 6 h for four doses; begin 12 h after methotrexate infusion is completed
In patients with central nervous system metastases, increase methotrexate to 1 g/m² as 24-h i.v. infusion.
Increase folinic acid to 15 mg i.m./p.o. every 8 h for nine doses, beginning 12 h after methotrexate infusion is completed.

Course B

Day 8: Vincristine, 1 mg/m² i.v. bolus
Cyclophosphamide, 600 mg/m² i.v. infusion
Day 15: Recycle course A
Patients with central nervous system metastases or with high-risk World Health Organization prognostic index sources receive 12.5 mg of methotrexate by intrathecal injection on day 8.

Modified from Newlands ES, et al. Developments in chemotherapy for medium- and high-risk patients with gestation trophoblastic tumors (1979–1984). *Br J Obstet Gynaecol* 1986; 93:63.

in American centers. MAC frequently produces significant toxic side effects, particularly when cycled at intervals of less than 21 days. Because of MAC's severe toxicity, this regimen has fallen out of favor in deference to less-toxic therapy. The alternative, increasingly preferred regimen is EMA-CO (see Table 12-6), given on an outpatient basis. This combination is attractive because its primary complete response rate appears to be slightly better than that of MAC.

3. **Special situations.** In general, high-risk metastatic and special-situation GTN should be managed by centers experienced with the disease.

a. **Central nervous system metastases.** Patients with metastases to the central nervous system (CNS) have a greater risk of failing primary therapy than do patients with disease limited to the lungs or vagina. Radiation therapy is often administered to patients with CNS metastasis in conjunction with their primary multiagent chemotherapy. Delivered in 10 equal fractions, 3,000 cGy has been safely administered with concurrent MAC chemotherapy. Survival rates approximate 70% to 89% for patients treated with primary brain metastasis; however, the survival rate falls to 30% for those who receive salvage treatment for brain metastasis. Patients with CNS metastasis are at risk of neurologic decompensation caused by cerebral edema and acute hemorrhage. Therefore, dexamethasone is frequently used throughout their course of whole-brain radiation to minimize cerebral edema. Surgical extirpation is generally reserved for patients who demonstrate neurologic decompensation or those who require salvage therapy for recurrent CNS disease.

b. **Metastases to the liver.** Liver metastases occur in 2% to 8% of patients presenting for primary therapy of metastatic GTN. Survival rates of 40% to 50% are reported for patients with primary involvement of the liver. Because these metastases tend to be highly vascular and death is frequently caused by intraabdominal hemorrhage, whole-liver radiation to 2,000 cGy in conjunction with combination chemotherapy is recommended.

c. **Drug-resistant disease.** Patients with high-risk metastatic GTN who have not responded to primary chemotherapy have a very poor prognosis. Surgical excision of drug-resistant foci of disease should be considered in patients with limited systemic metastases and has been curative when all else has failed. β-hCG–imaging techniques are available to identify small sites of drug-resistant disease. Regimens including cisplatin or etoposide (VP-16) and cisplatin plus ifosfamide plus etoposide in patients who did not respond to EMA-CO can be effective. Other experimental drugs can be considered as a last resort. Total parenteral nutrition and other systemic supports can be essential. In short, no therapeutic approach or support should be ignored on behalf of these compelling patients because they are young and salvage for cure is occasionally still possible.

4. **Posttreatment follow-up.** Most women with malignant gestational trophoblastic disease can be cured using chemotherapy alone, thus preserving the potential for future childbearing. During the first year after completion of therapy, pregnancy is deferred so that β-hCG surveillance is not disrupted by an intercurrent pregnancy. Several series of women treated with simple chemotherapy for nonmetastatic or low-risk metastatic GTN have shown normal reproductive capacity after treatment.

VI. **Vulvar cancer.** Vulvar cancer is relatively uncommon, accounting for only 4% to 5% of gynecologic malignancies. Squamous histology constitutes 85% of vulvar malignancies, but cancer of other cell types, including melanoma, Bartholin's gland adenocarcinoma, Paget's disease, and sarcoma, can occur as well. Because vulvar squamous cancers anatomically involve external skin and are slow growing, early diagnosis is possible and generally leads to high cure rates. Cancers of the other cell types can be more insidious and have variable prognoses.

A. **Pathology.** Squamous cancers of the vulva typically occur in older, often elderly, women and may be preceded by or associated with vulvar intraepithelial neoplasia. The risk factors correlating with disease include lower socioeconomic status, smoking, history of lower genital tract malignancies (particularly squamous neoplasia of the cervix), and immune-compromised states. Biologically, squamous cancers tend to be indolent, spread initially by direct extension to adjacent organs (e.g., to the vulva, vagina, urethra, anus), and at some point send tumor emboli to regional lymph nodes (inguinal and femoral nodes) and then to distant nodes. Hematogenous spread to the lungs and distant organs is usually a late finding.

B. **Diagnosis and work-up.** Diagnosing vulvar cancer, based simply on gross appearance, is generally not possible. To the contrary, clinical impression is notoriously incorrect, both overestimating and underestimating the degree of neoplasia present. Therefore, a biopsy of abnormal vulvar lesions is needed for definitive diagnosis. After malignancy is diagnosed, establishing the lesion size and location, as well as the regional lymph node status by clinical examination, is important. Further work-up includes a thorough examination (e.g., colposcopy) of the cervix and vagina looking for concomitant neoplasia, CT of the pelvis and abdomen to evaluate disease and nodes, and a chest x-ray.

C. **Treatment**

1. **Surgery.** Because of the biologic behavior and anatomic site, vulvar cancer is often ideal for surgical cure. Indeed, radiation therapy is a poorly tolerated alternative in that anatomic

area, leading to high morbidity with skin breakdown, infection, and pain. Currently, the extent of surgical resection (i.e., the radicalness of the vulvectomy) required to achieve cure is in the midst of reconsideration, but a trend toward less extensive, but still radical, surgery appears to be emerging. In addition to radical vulvectomy, inguinal lymphadenectomy is also part of the surgical management of vulvar cancer. Here too, the radicalness of the inguinal dissection is being reconsidered. Consideration is given to just superficial or superficial and deep node dissection, and whether ipsilateral or bilateral dissection is needed, based on lesion size, location, depth of invasion, and clinical status of the groin nodes.

2. **Staging, risk stratification, and management principles.** Staging of vulvar cancer has been changed from clinical to surgical (Table 12-7). Based on surgicopathologic findings (e.g., depth of invasion, nodal status), coupled with clinical prognostic factors (e.g., lesion size, location), risk stratification is possible and helps with further treatment planning. Most commonly after surgery, the lesion is found to be completely resected and the lymph nodes are negative. The good-prognosis patients are generally observed and do well. In contrast, if groin nodes are positive, the prognosis is significantly worse. In this circumstance, adjuvant radiation to the inguinal region as well as to the whole pelvis is usually recommended. In this poor-prognosis situation, the use of radiation therapy has increased survival relative to that of the former strategy (ultraradical surgery), including pelvic lymph node dissection.

3. **Candidates for chemotherapy.** Patients with distant metastasis and those with locally advanced disease who would otherwise require exenterative-type, ultraradical surgery for complete resection are candidates for chemotherapy. The latter group can receive, as an alternative, neoadjuvant chemotherapy with or without preoperative radiation therapy, followed by a less radical resection.

Experience with cytotoxic drugs in managing vulvar malignancy is largely restricted to treating squamous cell tumors. As would be expected, most agents effective against squamous neoplasms occurring at other sites also have an effect on the vulva. Cisplatin, bleomycin, fluorouracil, methotrexate, mitomycin, and doxorubicin have some reported activity, albeit brief. Various combinations of these agents have been used, particularly as neoadjuvant treatment or in conjunction with radiation therapy. The regimens are as follows:

Table 12-7.   1995 FIGO
staging for carcinoma of the vulva

Stage	Definition
Stage 0 Tis	Carcinoma *in situ;* intraepithelial carcinoma
Stage I T1, N0, M0	Tumor confined to the vulva and/or perineum, 2 cm or less in greatest dimension; nodes are negative
Stage IA	Lesions 2 cm or less in size confined to the vulva or perineum with stromal invasion no greater than 1 mm. No nodal metastases. The depth of invasion is defined as the measurement of the tumor from the epithelial–stromal junction of the adjacent most superficial derma papilla to the deepest point of invasion
Stage IB	Lesions 2 cm or less in size confined to the vulva or perineum with stromal invasion greater than 1 mm; no nodal metastases
Stage II T2,N0,M0	Tumor confined to the vulva and/or perineum, more than 2 cm in greatest dimension, nodes are negative
Stage III T3, N0, M0 T3, N1, M0 T1, N1, M0 T2, N1, M0.	Tumor of any size with (1) adjacent spread to the lower urethra and/or the vagina, or the anus; and/or (2) unilateral regional lymph node metastasis
Stage IVA T1, N2, M0 T2, N2, M0 T3, N2, M0 T4, any N, M0	Tumor invades any of the following: upper urethra, bladder mucosa, rectal mucosa, pelvic bone; and/or bilateral regional node metastasis
Stage IVB Any T Any N, M1	Any distant metastasis, including pelvic lymph nodes

TNM Classification
Primary tumor

Tis Preinvasive carcinoma (carcinoma *in situ*)
T1   Tumor confined to the vulva and/or perineum <2 cm in
     greatest dimension
T2   Tumor confined to the vulva and/or perineum >2 cm in
     greatest dimension
T3   Tumor of any size with adjacent spread to the urethra and/or
     vagina and/or to the anus
T4   Tumor of any size infiltrating the bladder mucosa and/or the
     rectal mucosa, including the upper part of the urethral
     mucosa and/or fixed to the bone

continued

Table 12-7.   (*Continued*)

Stage	Definition

Reginal lymph nodes

N0   No lymph node metastasis
N1   Unilateral regional lymph node metastasis
N2   Bilateral regional lymph node metastasis

Distant Metastasis

M0   No clinical metastasis
M1   Distant metastasis (including pelvic lymph node metastasis)

Cisplatin, 50 mg/m^2/day i.v. on day 1, *plus* fluorouracil, 1,000 mg/m^2 on days 1 to 4, continuous i.v. infusion every 3 weeks.

Mitomycin, 10 mg/m^2 i.v. on day 1, *plus* fluorouracil, 1,000 mg/m^2/day continuous i.v. infusion on days 1 to 4.

Cycles may be repeated in 3 or 4 weeks, depending on recovery of the blood cell counts and whether subsequent surgery is planned. When used together with radiation therapy, these regimens have been reported to shrink locally advanced lesions, making them amenable to a lesser surgical resection.

D.   Summary. At this time, it is impossible to determine the optimal combination or even the role of chemotherapy in the treatment of vulvar cancer. Studies are ongoing. Fortunately, most patients with vulvar cancers are cured surgically. Moreover, there is an optimistic trend toward more limited, less-disfiguring surgical management, at times creatively combined with chemotherapy with or without radiation therapy.

SELECTED READINGS

General

CME Journal of Gynecologic Oncology, Peter Bosze, Editor, Primed-X Press, Budapest, Vol. 1(1), December 1996.

Chemotherapy of Gynecologic Cancers, Society of Gynecologic Oncologist Handbook, Stephen C. Rubin, Editor, Lippincott-Raven, 1996.

Clinical Practice Guidelines, Management of Gynecologic Cancers, SGO Medical Practice and Ethics Committee, October 1996.

Surgical Oncology Clinics of North America, Cancers Unique to Women, C.O. Granai, Guest Editor, W.B. Saunders Co., Vol. 7(2), April 1998.

Carcinoma of the Cervix

Alberts DS, Garcia D, Mason-Liddil N. Cisplatin in advanced cancer of the cervix: an update. *Semin Oncol* 1991;18[Suppl 3]:11.

Ambros RA, Kurman RJ. Current concepts in the relationship of human papilloma virus infection to the pathogenesis and classification of precancerous lesions of the uterine cervix. *Semin Diagn Pathol* 1990;7:158.

American Cancer Society, Inc. *Cancer facts and figures—1998.* Reprinted by permission of the American Cancer Society, Inc.

Dottino PR, et al. Induction chemotherapy followed by radical surgery in cervical cancer. *Gynecol Oncol* 1991;40:7.

Killackey MA, Boardman L, Carroll DS. Adjuvant chemotherapy and radiation in patients with poor prognostic stage Ib/IIa cervical cancer. *Gynecol Oncol* 1993;49:377.

McGuire WP, et al. Paclitaxel has moderate activity in squamous cervix cancer: a Gynecologic Oncology Group study. *J Clin Oncol* 1996;14:792–795.

Park RC, Thigpen JT. Chemotherapy in advanced and recurrent cervical cancer: a review. *Cancer* 1993;71:1446.

van Nagell JR, et al. Surgical therapy for cervical cancer. In: Gershenson DM, DeCherney AH, Curry SL, eds. *Operative gynecology.* Philadelphia: WB Saunders, 1993:271.

Endometrial Carcinoma

American Cancer Society, Inc. *Cancer facts and figures–1998.* Reprinted by permission of the American Cancer Society, Inc.

Ball HG, et al. A phase II trial of Taxol in advanced and recurrent adenocarcinoma of the endometrium: a Gynecologic Oncology Group study. *Soc Gyn Oncol #42 in Gyn Oncol* 1995;56:120.

Burk TW, Morris M. Surgery for malignant tumors of the uterine corpus. In: Gershenson DM, DeCherney AH, Curry SL, eds. *Operative gynecology.* Philadelphia: WB Saunders, 1993:371–393.

Carcangiu ML, Chambers JT. Uterine papillary serous carcinoma: a study on 108 cases with emphasis on the prognostic significance of associated endometrioid carcinoma, absence of invasion, and concomitant ovarian carcinoma. *Gynecol Oncol* 1992;47:298.

Creasman WT, et al. Surgical pathologic spread patterns of endometrial cancer: a Gynecologic Oncology Group Study. *Cancer* 1987; 60:2035.

Davies JL, et al. A review of the risk factors for endometrial carcinoma. *Obstet Gynecol Surv* 1981;36:107.

Gurney H, Murphy D, Crowther D. The management of primary fallopian tube carcinoma. *Br J Obstet Gynaecol* 1990;97:822.

Morrow CP, et al. Relationship between surgical-pathological risk factors and outcome in clinical stage I and II carcinoma of the endometrium: a GOG study. *Gynecol Oncol* 1991;40:55.

Morris PJ, Malt RA, eds. *Oxford textbook of surgery.* Vol. 12. Oxford: Oxford Medical, 1994:1438–1443.

Muntz HG, et al. Primary adenocarcinoma of the fallopian tube. *Eur J Gynaecol Oncol* 1989;10:239.

Silverberg SG, et al. Carcinosarcoma (malignant mixed mesodermal tumor) of the uterus: a Gynecologic Oncology Group pathologic study of 203 cases. *Int J Gynecol Pathol* 1990;9:1.

Society of Gynecologic Oncologists Clinical Practice Guidelines. Practice guidelines: uterine corpus–sarcomas. *Oncology* 1998;12(2).

Thigpen JT, et al. A randomized comparison of doxorubicin alone versus doxorubicin plus cyclophosphamide in the management of advanced or recurrent endometrial carcinoma: a Gynecologic Oncology Group study. *J Clin Oncol* 1994;12:1408.

Fallopian Tube Cancer

Society of Gynecologic Oncologists Clinical Practice Guidelines. Practice guidelines: fallopian tube cancer. *Oncology* 1998;12(2).

Carcinoma of the Ovary

Advanced Ovarian Trialists Group. Chemotherapy in advanced ovarian cancer: an overview of randomized clinical trials. *Br Med J* 1991;303:884.

Alberts DS, Liu PY, Hannigan EV, et al. Intraperitoneal cisplatin plus intravenous cyclophosphamide versus intravenous cisplatin plus intravenous cyclophosphamide for stage III ovarian cancer. *N Engl J Med* 1996;335:1950–1955.

American Cancer Society, Inc. *Cancer facts and figures–1998*. Reprinted by permission of the American Cancer Society, Inc.

Arbuck SG. Paclitaxel: what schedule? what dose? *J Clin Oncol* 1994; 12:233.

Baker TR, Piver MS, Hempling RE. Long term survival by cytoreductive surgery to less than 1 cm, induction weekly cisplatin and monthly cisplatin, doxorubicin, and cyclophosphamide therapy in advanced ovarian adenocarcinoma. *Cancer* 1994;74:656.

Burke W, Daly M, Garber J, et al. Recommendations for follow-up care of individuals with an inherited predisposition to cancer. *JAMA* 1997;277:997–1003.

Cannistra S. Cancer of the ovary. *N Engl J Med* 1993;329:1550–1559.

Creemers GJ, Bolis G, Gore M, et al. Topotecan, and active drug in the second-line treatment of epithelial ovarian cancer: results of a large European phase II study. *J Clin Oncol* 1996;14:3056–3061.

Friedman JB, Weiss NS. Second thoughts about second look laparotomy in advanced ovarian cancer. *N Engl J Med* 1990;322:1079.

Gallion HH, et al. Molecular genetic changes in human epithelial ovarian malignancies. *Gynecol Oncol* 1992;47:137.

Gershenson DM. Chemotherapy of ovarian germ cell tumors and sex cord stromal tumors. *Semin Surg Oncol* 1994;10:290–298.

Granai CO, Gajewski WH, Arena B. Ovarian cancer: issues and management. *Cancer* 1994;7:1.

Kaye SB, Cassidy PJ, Lewis CR, et al. Mature results of a randomized trial of two doses of cisplatin for the treatment of ovarian cancer. *J Clin Oncol* 1996;14:2113–2119.

Kirmani S, et al. Intraperitoneal cisplatin/etoposide (IP/CDDP/VP-16) for consolidation of pathologic complete response (PCR) in ovarian carcinoma. *Proc Am Soc Clin Oncol* 1990;9:167.

Markman M. Intraperitoneal chemotherapy in the treatment of ovarian cancer. *Ann Med* 1996;28(4):293–296.

McGuire WP, Hoskins WJ, Brady MF, et al. Cyclophosphamide and cisplatin compared with paclitaxel and cisplatin in patients with stage III and stage IV ovarian cancer. *N Engl J Med* 1996;334(1):1–6.

McGuire WP, Hoskins WJ, Brady MF, et al. Assessment of dose-intensive therapy in suboptimally debulked ovarian cancer: a Gynecologic Oncology Group study. *J Clin Oncol* 1995;13:1589–1599.

Miki Y, Swenson J, Shattuck-Eidens D, et al. A strong candidate for the breast and ovarian cancer susceptibility gene BRCA1. *Science* 1994;266:66–71.

Muggia FM, Hainsworth JD, Jeffers S, et al. Phase II study of liposomal doxorubicin in refractory ovarian cancer: antitumor activity and toxicity modification by liposomal encapsulation, *J Clin Oncol* 1997;3:987–993.

NIH Consensus Conference. Ovarian cancer screening, treatment and follow-up. *JAMA* 1995;273:491.

Ozols RF, Schwartz PE, Eifel PJ. Ovarian cancer, fallopian tube carcinoma, and peritoneal carcinoma. *Cancer* 1997;X:1502–1534.

Ozols RF, et al. Update of the NCCN Ovarian Cancer Practice Guidelines. *Oncology* 1997;11(11A):95–105.

Piver MS, Jishi MF, Tsukada Y, Nava G. Primary peritoneal carcinoma after prophylactic oophorectomy in women with a family history of ovarian cancer. *Cancer* 1993;71:2651–2655.

Rose PG, Blessing JA, Mayer AR, Homesley HD. Prolonged oral etoposide as second-line therapy for platinum-resistant and platinum-sensitive ovarian carcinoma: a Gynecologic Oncology Group Study. *J Clin Oncol* 1998;16(2):405–410.

Stiff PJ, et al. High-dose chemotherapy with autologous transplantation for persistent/relapsed ovarian cancer: a multivariate analysis of survival for 100 consecutively treated patients. *J Clin Oncol* 1997;15:1309–1317.

Thigpen T, Vance RB, McGuire WP, Hoskins WJ. The role of paclitaxel in the management of coelomic epithelial carcinoma of the ovary: a review with emphasis on the Gynecologic Group experience, *Semin Oncol* 1995;22[6 Suppl 14]:23–31.

Wooster R, Bignell G, Lancaster J, et al. Identification of the breast cancer susceptibility gene BRCA2. *Nature* 1995;378:789–792.

Young RC, et al. Adjuvant therapy in stage I and stage II epithelial ovarian cancer: results of two prospective randomized trials. *N Engl J Med* 1990;322:1021.

Gestational Trophoblastic Neoplasms

Berkowitz RS. Gestational trophoblastic diseases: recent advances in the understanding of cytogenetics, histopathology, and natural history. *Curr Opin Obstet Gynecol* 1992;4:616–620.

Bolis G, et al. EMA/CO regimen in high-risk gestational trophoblastic tumor (GTT). *Gynecol Oncol* 1988;31:439.

Feldman S, et al. Low risk metastatic gestational trophoblastic tumors. *Semin Oncol* 1995;22:166–171.

Holmseley HD, et al. Weekly intramuscular methotrexate for nonmetastatic gestational trophoblastic disease. *Obstet Gynecol* 1988; 72:413.

Lurain JR. High-risk metastatic gestational trophoblastic tumors: current management. *J Reprod Med* 1994;39:217–222.

Mutch DG, et al. Recurrent gestational trophoblastic disease: experience of the Southeastern Regional Trophoblastic Disease Center. *Cancer* 1990;66:978.

Society of Gynecologic Oncologists Clinical Practice Guidelines. Practice guidelines: gestational trophoblastic disease. *Oncology* 1998; 12(3):XX.

Theodore C, et al. Treatment of high-risk gestational trophoblastic disease with chemotherapy combinations containing cisplatin and etoposide. *Cancer* 1989;64:1824.

Yordan EL, et al. Radiation therapy in the management of gestational choriocarcinoma metastatic to the central nervous system. *Obstet Gynecol* 1987;69:627–630.

Carcinoma of the Vulva

Berek JS, et al. Concurrent cisplatin and 5-fluorouracil chemotherapy. *Gynecol Oncol* 1991;42:197.

Figge DC, Tamimi HK, Greer BE. Lymphatic spread in carcinoma of the vulva. *Am J Obstet Gynecol* 1985;152:387.

Hacker NF, et al. Management of regional lymph nodes and their prognostic influence in vulvar cancer. *Obstet Gynecol* 1983;61:408.

Homesley HD, et al. Radiation therapy versus pelvic node resection for carcinoma of the vulva with positive groin nodes. *Obstet Gynecol* 1985;68:733.

Homesley HD, et al. Assessment of current International Federation of Gynecology and Obstetrics staging of vulvar carcinoma relative to prognostic factors for survival (a Gynecologic Oncology Group study). *Am J Obstet Gynecol* 1991;164:997.

Levin W, et al. The use of concomitant chemotherapy and radiotherapy prior to surgery in advanced stage carcinoma of the vulva. *Gynecol Oncol* 1986;25:20.

Podratz KC, et al. Carcinoma of the vulva: analysis of treatment and survival. *Obstet Gynecol* 1983;61:63.

Society of Gynecologic Oncologists Clinical Practice Guidelines. Practice guidelines: vulvar cancer. *Oncology* 1998;12:275–282.

Thomas G, et al. Concurrent radiation and chemotherapy in vulvar carcinoma. *Gynecol Oncol* 1989;34:263.

Urologic and Male Genital Malignancies

Scott B. Saxman and Craig R. Nichols

Malignancies that arise from the urinary and male genital tracts are highly diverse in their biologic behavior. They span a spectrum that includes one of the most chemotherapeutically curable of cancers (testicular germ cell tumors [GCTs]) and one of the most resistant (renal cell carcinoma [RCC]). The therapeutic approaches to these tumors are also diverse and should be multidisciplinary because chemotherapy, surgery, and radiation therapy all have important roles.

I. **Carcinoma of the kidney**
   A. **Background.** RCC, which is an adenocarcinoma that arises from the parenchyma of the kidney, accounts for 85% of primary renal neoplasms. Transitional cell carcinomas (TCCs) arise from the cells lining the collecting system. Their behavior and response to therapy are similar to those arising in the bladder (see Section II). Other rare malignancies of the kidney include oncocytomas (well-differentiated adenocarcinomas), undifferentiated carcinomas, and sarcomas. Wilms' tumor (nephroblastoma) is a cancer that is seen predominantly in childhood and is not covered here. The term *hypernephroma* is a misnomer and should no longer be used.
   B. **Staging.** Staging for RCC should include a computed tomography (CT) scan of the chest and abdomen, bone scan, and usually arteriography or venography if nephrectomy is being considered. The TNM staging system is as follows:

   Stage I: Tumor 2.5 cm or smaller confined to the kidney (T1, N0, M0)
   Stage II: Tumor larger than 2.5 cm confined to the kidney (T2, N0, M0)
   Stage III: Tumor extending into major veins, adrenal gland, or perinephric tissues but not beyond Gerota's fascia, or metastasis to single node smaller than 2 cm (T3, N0, M0; or T1-3, N1, M0)
   Stage IV: Tumor invading beyond Gerota's fascia, or multiple lymph node metastasis or distant metastatic disease (T4, any N, M0; any T, N2-3, M0; or any T, any N, M1)

   C. **General therapeutic approach.** The treatment of choice for RCC is radical nephrectomy, including removal of the perinephric fat and regional lymph nodes. Partial nephrectomy is an option in patients with bilateral RCC or a solitary kidney to prevent the need for dialysis or kidney transplantation. Rarely, patients with solitary metastatic lesions can be cured by surgical removal of the metastasis at the time of nephrectomy. RCC is relatively radioresistant; thus, adjuvant radiation therapy does not improve survival. Radiation therapy can be useful for palliation of painful metastasis. Although it is reasonable to consider patients with inoperable metastatic disease for treatment with biologic agents or chemotherapy, in most patients, these systemic therapies are of minimal benefit.

D. **Treatment regimens**

1. **Biologic response modifiers**

a. **Interleukin-2** (IL-2) mediates its antitumor effects through activation of the patient's immune system. IL-2 alone or in combination with lymphokine-activated killer (LAK) cells or interferon results in tumor regression in 15% of patients. Although some of these responses have been complete and long-lasting, it is not yet known whether this represents a therapeutic advance because patients in the reported studies were carefully selected. There is a wide dosage range in various protocols. Some generally accepted treatment regimens and schedules are shown in Table 13-1. Although the greatest experience has been with the high-dose bolus regimen, this regimen is not recommended for most patients because of its greater toxicity. Outpatient bolus therapy is probably equally efficacious and has less morbidity.

b. **Interferon** results in regression in 15% of treated patients. The optimal treatment regimen or duration of treatment is not known; it is most commonly used in an intermediate-dose regimen of 5 to 10 × 10^6 IU/m^2 s.c. three to five times per week. The average response duration is 6 to 10 months. Response correlates with prior nephrectomy, good performance status, long disease-free interval, and lung-predominant disease.

c. **Combination therapy.** Combinations of interferon and IL-2 have been tested but have not been shown to be superior to IL-2 or interferon alone.

2. **Cytotoxic chemotherapy.** The most commonly used regimen is vinblastine, 5 to 6 mg/m^2 i.v. weekly, which produces responses in 10% of patients. The major dose-limiting toxicity is hematologic, and therapy should be delayed when the white blood cell count is less than 3,000/µL or the platelet count is less than

Table 13-1.   Interleukin-2–based regimens for renal cell carcinoma

Regimen	Treatment plan[a]
High-dose bolus interleukin-2 (IL-2) (inpatient therapy; requires intensive care unit support)	IL-2: 600,000 or 720,000 IU/kg i.v. over 15 min every 8 h on days 1–5 and 15–19. Repeat the cycle in 6–12 weeks if stable or responding disease.
Low-dose bolus IL-2 (inpatient therapy, fewer complications, reduced use of vasopressor support and fewer admissions to the intensive care unit)	IL-2: 72,000 IU/kg i.v. bolus over 15 min every 8 h on days 1–5 and 15–19. Repeat cycle in 5–6 weeks if stable or responding disease.
Outpatient subcutaneous IL-2	IL-2: $9–18 \times 10^6$ IU/m²/d s.c. for 5 d/wk. Repeat weekly for 4–6 wk, then give a 2- to 3-wk rest period. For stable or responding disease, repeat for two or three cycles.

[a] **Daily premedication and additional symptomatic medication are required on all regimens.** Examples of medication for symptom control include ondansetron, 30 mg i.v. on each day of the IL-2; acetaminophen, 650 mg p.o. pretreatment and q4h PRN; cimetidine, 800 mg p.o. daily; diphenoxylate with atropine (Lomotil), one tablet up to six times daily for diarrhea; hydroxyzine, 25–50 mg q4–6h for itching. In any of the schedules, therapy may be stopped prematurely for constitutional symptoms or for cardiovascular, renal, hepatic, neurologic, pulmonary, or hematologic toxicity.

100,000/μL. Chemotherapy does not prolong survival in these patients; therefore, the minimal potential palliative benefit should be carefully weighed against the added toxicity.

3. **Hormonal therapy.** Hormonal therapy (medroxyprogesterone acetate or tamoxifen) has historically been the mainstay of treatment, initially used because of preclinical data suggesting activity. More recent studies do not support any beneficial effect of these agents. At best, these agents produce responses in fewer than 5% of patients and therefore cannot be recommended.

E. **Complications of therapy.** Complications of IL-2, particularly with higher doses, include fever, agitation, and a capillary leak syndrome that results in increased interstitial water in the lungs and respiratory insufficiency. This situation usually requires management in an intensive care unit. Interferon can cause nausea, anorexia, fatigue, myalgia, headache, and fever. Complications of cytotoxic therapy include nausea, mucositis, myalgia, and myelosuppression. Hormonal therapy is usually free of side effects other than fluid retention.

F. **Recommendations.** Most patients with metastatic RCC should be managed expectantly with the aggressive use of narcotics and radiation therapy for pain control or be placed in clinical trials. Well-informed patients with excellent performance status and cardiac and pulmonary function can be considered for treatment with one of the IL-2 or interferon regimens. More enthusiasm for the use of these agents will have to await the results of phase III trials.

II. **Bladder cancer**

A. **General considerations and staging.** Cancer arising in the bladder is usually TCC, although occasionally squamous cell carcinomas or adenocarcinoma is seen. TCC falls into two major groups: superficial and invasive. The biology and natural history of these two groups differ markedly. When planning treatment for bladder cancer, one must take into account the stage of the tumor (0 to IV), histologic grade (1 to 3), and location of the tumor within the bladder (related to surgical considerations of partial versus total cystectomy).

The standard evaluation of a patient with invasive bladder cancer should include a CT scan of the abdomen and pelvis, chest radiograph, complete blood cell count, and serum chemistry profile. The TNM staging system can be summarized as follows:

TX: Primary tumor cannot be assessed
T0: No evidence of primary tumor
Ta: Noninvasive papillary carcinoma
Tis: Carcinoma *in situ*
T1: Tumor invades subepithelial connective tissue
T2: Tumor invades superficial muscle (inner half)
  T3: Tumor invades deep muscle or perivesical fat
  T3a: Tumor invades deep muscle (outer half)
  T3b: Tumor invades perivesical fat
  T3bi: Microscopically
  T3bii: Macroscopically (extravesical mass)
T4: Tumor invades any of the following: prostate, uterus, vagina, pelvic wall, or abdominal wall
  T4a: Tumor invades the prostate, uterus, or vagina
  T4b: Tumor invades the pelvic wall or abdominal wall

Stage groupings are as follows:

Stage 0: Ta or Tis, N0, M0
Stage I: T1, N0, M0
Stage II: T2 or T3a, N0, M0
Stage III: T3b or T4a, N0, M0
Stage IV: T4b, N0, M0; any T, N1-3, M0-1

B. **General approach to therapy**

1. **Superficial-stage, low-grade tumors.** Patients with stage 0 or I tumors are usually treated with transurethral resection (TUR) and

fulguration, with a local control rate higher than 80%. However, TUR does not reduce the risk of recurrence at other sites in the bladder. This risk may be reduced by administration of intravesical therapy. Diffuse carcinoma *in situ* may also be treated with intravesical therapy.

2. **Deep-stage, high-grade tumors.** Patients with larger stage II lesions or with stage III disease are usually managed with partial or radical cystectomy (depending on the size and location of the tumor). Several trials have investigated the roles of preoperative radiation therapy and chemotherapy, with inconclusive results. The role of neoadjuvant therapy remains controversial, and it should not be considered standard care.

3. **Advanced and metastatic tumors.** Patients with locally advanced disease or local recurrences can be considered for radiation therapy. Patients with metastatic disease are candidates for systemic chemotherapy. There is evidence that chemotherapy can prolong survival and that combinations are superior to single agents.

C. **Treatment regimens and evaluation of response**
  1. **Intravesical chemotherapy**
      a. **Method of administration and follow-up.** Intravesical therapy is usually administered in a volume of 40 to 60 mL through a Foley catheter. The catheter is then clamped and the agent retained for 2 hours. This procedure delivers a high local concentration to the tumor area while usually avoiding systemic effects. Patients with superficial bladder cancers require lifelong surveillance with periodic cystoscopy (initially every 3 months, then every 6 months, then annually) because, even with intravesical therapy, an increased risk of new primary tumors persists. Patients being treated for diffuse carcinoma *in situ* should have biopsy confirmation of the return of normal mucosa after the installation therapy has been completed. These patients also require lifelong cystoscopic surveillance.
      b. **Selection of patients for intravesical therapy.** Only patients with superficial or small, minimally invasive tumors (T1) should be treated. The grade of the tumor is also a significant predictor of progression. Patients with grade 3 lesions should be considered for more aggressive treatment than intravesical therapy. Possible objectives for intravesical therapy are as follows:
          (1) Prevention of relapse in patients with Ta grades 2 and 3 and stage I lesions treated with TUR.

      (2) Prevention of occurrence of new bladder tumors. Patients with two or more previously resected bladder tumors should be treated in an effort to prevent development of *de novo* malignancies.

      (3) Carcinoma *in situ* may involve the bladder diffusely and thus not be amenable to TUR. A course of installation therapy is usually given, followed by repeat biopsies. Persistence of carcinoma *in situ* is an indication for radical cystectomy.

c. Specific intravesical therapeutic regimens

Bacillus Calmette-Guérin (BCG), 120 mg weekly for 6 to 8 weeks, *or*

Thiotepa, 30 to 60 mg weekly for 4 to 6 weeks, *or*

Mitomycin, 20 to 40 mg weekly for 6 to 8 weeks, *or*

Doxorubicin, 50 to 60 mg weekly for 6 to 8 weeks.

d. Selection of therapy. Although few controlled studies have been done, it appears that thiotepa, mitomycin, and doxorubicin are equally effective. Two separate studies have shown BCG to be superior to thiotepa and doxorubicin in preventing recurrence. Thus, BCG should be considered the agent of choice for intravesical therapy.

e. Response to therapy. About 40% to 70% of patients with existing or residual tumor after TUR respond to therapy. Whether adjuvant intravesical therapy prevents progression to invasive or metastatic bladder cancer or improves survival requires further study.

f. Complications of therapy. All of the agents mentioned can cause symptoms of bladder irritation (pain, urgency, hematuria) and allergic reactions. Thiotepa is systemically absorbed and can occasionally cause myelosuppression. This is rare with mitomycin and doxorubicin. Patients receiving thiotepa should have their blood cell counts monitored closely. Mitomycin can cause dermatitis in the perineal area and hands. BCG is occasionally associated with systemic symptoms, including fever, chills, malaise, arthralgias, and skin rash.

2. Adjuvant chemotherapy. Chemotherapy has been studied both preoperatively and postoperatively in patients with deeply invasive tumors or positive lymph nodes. To date, no randomized trial has demonstrated a clear-cut benefit. Although this question is still under study, neoadjuvant or adjuvant chemotherapy is not generally considered standard in this patient population.

3. **Systemic chemotherapy for advanced disease.**

   a. **Drugs** active against bladder cancer include cisplatin, doxorubicin, vinblastine, fluorouracil, cyclophosphamide, carboplatin, mitoxantrone, and methotrexate. Of these, cisplatin is probably the most active as a single agent. The combination of methotrexate, vinblastine, doxorubicin, and cisplatin (MVAC) is the most commonly used. A randomized trial showed MVAC to have a survival advantage over single-agent cisplatin.

   b. **Specific regimens** (Table 13-2). Combination chemotherapy that includes three or four agents should be considered standard first-line therapy. Single agents can be used for patients with congestive heart failure, renal dysfunction, or poor bone marrow reserve who are unable to tolerate more aggressive treatment.

   c. **Response to therapy.** MVAC may be expected to produce a complete response in 15% of patients and a partial response in

Table 13-2.   Combination chemotherapy and active single agents for cancer of the bladder

Regimen or single agent	Doses and schedules
MVAC	Methotrexate, 30 mg/m^2 i.v. on day 1 Vinblastine, 3 mg/m^2 i.v. on day 2 Doxorubicin, 30 mg/m^2 i.v. on day 2 Cisplatin, 70 mg/m^2 i.v. on day 2 (with vigorous diuresis) Repeat methotrexate and vinblastine on days 15 and 22 if white blood cell count >2,000/µL and platelet count >50,000/µL. Cycles should be repeated every 28 days.
CP	Paclitaxel, 200 mg/m^2 over 3 h, followed by: Carboplatin, AUC 5 Repeat cycle every 21 d.
Cisplatin	40–60 mg/m^2 i.v. every 3 wk
Doxorubicin	60, mg/m^2 i.v. every 3 wk
Cyclophosphamide	1 g/m^2 i.v. every 3 wk
Fluorouracil	500 mg/m^2 i.v. weekly

35%, for an overall response rate of about 50%. The median survival time is about 13 months. The toxicity of this regimen is substantial and must be weighed against the expected benefit when selecting therapy. Drug delivery can be enhanced by the coadministration of granulocyte colony-stimulating factor. However, there is no evidence that this improves survival. Response to any chemotherapy is monitored by periodic measurement of tumor masses with the expectation that most patients who will respond will do so within the first one to two cycles of treatment. Patients who relapse after or progress during MVAC occasionally respond to a second-line regimen. This should be undertaken for palliative reasons only because any survival benefit is minimal. Such patients should be considered for clinical trials.

    d. **Complications of systemic therapy.** The major dose-limiting toxicity of MVAC is myelosuppression, which often precludes the administration of chemotherapy on days 15 and 22. Cisplatin can cause renal damage, but this can usually be prevented by vigorous hydration and saline diure-sis. Mucositis, nausea and vomiting, and malaise are also commonly seen.

    e. **Follow-up.** Patients can be followed every few months for symptomatic progression. Serial x-ray studies or bone scans are costly and are of minimal value.

III. **Prostate cancer**

    A. **Background.** Carcinoma of the prostate is the most common cancer in the United States, with the exception of nonmelanoma skin cancers. Largely because of aggressive "screening" using prostatic specific antigen (PSA), the incidence of new cases increased 50% between 1980 and 1990, so that in 1998, about 185,000 new cases were diagnosed. Whether the earlier diagnosis and aggressive surgical or radiotherapeutic management of these patients will change the natural history of prostate cancer and decrease the mortality of this disease of older men remains unknown.

    B. **Staging.** Staging is usually done using a combination of clinical and pathologic indicators. Pathologic staging is necessary for completely accurate staging of low-stage disease but often is not needed once the disease has become metastatic to the bones or visceral organs. Accurate determination of extension beyond the prostate capsule and into lymph nodes requires pathologic evaluation in most circumstances. The modified Whitmore Jewett, or American Urologic Association, staging system is the most commonly used in the United States; the TNM system provides more detail about tumor extent and spread.

TX: Primary tumor cannot be assessed

T0: No evidence of primary tumor

T1: Clinically inapparent tumor not palpable or visible by imaging

T1a: Tumor incidental histologic finding in 5% or less of tissue resected.

T1b: Tumor incidental histologic finding in more than 5% of tissue resected.

T1c: Tumor identified by needle biopsy (e.g. because of elevated PSA)

T2: Tumor confined within prostate

T3: Tumor extends through the prostatic capsule

T4: Tumor is fixed or invades adjacent structures other than seminal vesicles

Stage groupings are as follows:

Stage I: T1a, N0, M0, G1
II: T1a, N0, M0, G2–4
   T1b, c, N0, M0, any G
   T2, N0, M0, any G
III: T3, N0, M0, any G
IV: T4, N0, M0, any G
   any T, N1–3, M0, any G
   any T, any N, M1, any G

In the American Urologic Association system, stages A, B, C, and D correspond closely to stages I, II, III, and IV in the TNM system. Additional prognostic information can be obtained by evaluating the differentiation of the tumor using the Gleason Grading System and the degree of elevation of the PSA.

Staging of prostate cancer should include abdominal and pelvic CT scans, chest radiographs, bone scans, liver function tests, and serum PSA and acid phosphatase measurements.

C. **General considerations and goals of therapy.** Selection of therapy for prostate cancer is complex and based on the extent of the disease as well as the age and general medical condition of the patient. Although many biases exist, there are no good randomized studies comparing treatment modalities in patients with organ-confined disease.

With the possible exception of young patients (less than 60 years of age), T1a (A1) prostate cancer should be followed without further therapy because survival is equal to that in age-matched controls. For other patients with organ-confined disease (T1b,c, T2), radical prostatectomy and high-dose radiation therapy are treatment options that probably have equal effectiveness. Observation alone may also be reasonable for patients with low-grade, organ-confined tumors. The choice between these three options must take into account the patient's performance status and the toxicities of each modality, which include anesthesia, blood loss, and incontinence for surgery versus tenesmus, rectal bleeding, and diarrhea for radiation. Stage III (c) tumors are usually treated with radiation therapy, although it is unclear whether this therapy prolongs survival. Very elderly patients or patients who have poor general health can be observed without therapy because the natural history is usually slow, with progression over years rather than months. Patients with metastatic disease are usually treated initially with hormonal therapy with or without radiation therapy to severely affected vertebral bodies or long bones. Patients asymptomatic metastatic disease can have treatment delayed until symptoms develop, with no decrease in likelihood of benefit from therapy.

D.   Treatment of symptomatic metastatic disease
1.   **Hormonal therapy.** Hormonal therapy results in a subjective response in nearly 75% of patients treated, lasting an average of 18 months. Most of these patients also have objective evidence of response, measured either radiographically or by a decreasing PSA level. In general, there is little evidence to suggest that one hormonal manipulation is superior to any other, so the choice can be based on patient preference, existing medical conditions, and cost. No good predictive markers for response currently exist in clinical practice.

   a.   **Orchiectomy** is often the treatment of choice because it is relatively inexpensive and obviates the need for injections or daily medications. This procedure can be done on an outpatient basis in all but the sickest of patients with minimal morbidity.

   b.   **Estrogens** are effective but less frequently used because of concern about potential cardiotoxicity and thrombophlebitis. Historically, 3 to 5 mg/day of diethylstilbestrol (DES) has been given; however, 1 mg/day produces fewer side effects without shortening survival. Painful gynecomastia can be prevented by superficial radiation (5 Gy) to the breast tissue before the start of therapy.

   c.   **Luteinizing hormone–releasing hormone** (LHRH) analogs are synthetic peptides administered by parenteral injection that occupy the receptors for LHRH in the pituitary gland. Initially, the release of luteinizing hormone is increased, causing a rise in the serum testosterone level. The continuous administration of therapeutic (super physiologic) doses of the LHRH analog blocks the physiologic pulsatile luteinizing hormone release from the pituitary, causing a fall in the serum testosterone to castrate levels. These agents can be administered either by s.c. injection daily, or monthly in a depot form. Currently used agents include the following:

Leuprolide, 7.5 mg i.m. depot monthly
Goserelin, 3.6 mg s.c. depot monthly or 10.8 mg s.c. every 3 months

Advantages of these agents are that they avoid the trauma of orchiectomy as well as the side effects of DES. Disadvantages include the potential for rapid worsening during the initial few weeks owing to a paradoxical transient increase in testosterone production. This flare can usually be avoided by the concurrent use of antiandrogens. Other disadvantages include the potential for poor patient compliance and the extremely high cost—more than $500 per month.

d. **LHRH analogs and antiandrogens** (total androgen blockade) have been used in combination. Synthetic antiandrogens (e.g., flutamide) act by competing with testosterone at the level of the cellular receptor. A recent randomized trial showed no improvement in survival when flutamide was given after orchiectomy. Because of the lack of benefit as well as added cost and toxicity, total androgen blockade should no longer be used in the treatment of patients with metastatic disease.

e. **Second-line hormonal therapies** that have been tried include orchiectomy (if not used as initial therapy), adrenalectomy, hypophysectomy, antiandrogens, progestins, and adrenal suppressants. The response rates to these therapies are low (less than 15%) and of brief duration. Patients who were initially treated with combined-modality therapy occasionally respond to withdrawal of the antiandrogen. This should be considered before proceeding to more toxic therapies.

2. **Cytotoxic chemotherapy.** Patients who relapse from or fail to respond to hormonal therapies can be considered for cytotoxic chemotherapy. In general, however, chemotherapy trials have been disappointing, with most agents having response rates lower than 10%.

Other most commonly used drugs are shown below. Except for the combination of estramustine and vinblastine, they are used as single agents.

There is no evidence that chemotherapy improves survival in these patients. A recent randomized trial demonstrated that patients treated with mitoxantrone (12 mg/m^2 every 3 weeks) and prednisone (5 mg b.i.d.) had improved pain control and reduced need for analgesic medications when compared with patients treated with prednisone alone. This is a reasonable option for patients with symptomatic hormone-refractory disease.

Doxorubicin, 60 mg/m^2 i.v. every 3 weeks
Cyclophosphamide, 1 g/m^2 every 3 weeks
Fluorouracil, 500 mg/m^2 i.v. weekly
Methotrexate, 40 mg/m^2 i.v. weekly
Cisplatin, 40 mg/m^2 i.v. every 3 weeks
Estramustine, 600 mg/m^2 p.o. on days 1 to 42, and **vinblastine,** 4 mg/m^2 i.v. weekly for 6 weeks. Courses of estramustine and vinblastine are repeated every 8 weeks

Patients who have received extensive radiation therapy should have their initial chemotherapy dose reduced by 20%. Patients who progress with hormonal therapy can still have severe symptomatic worsening if testosterone levels rise. Therefore, patients who have not undergone orchiectomy should continue with estrogen or LHRH therapy.

   3. **Evaluation of response.** Evaluating the response is often difficult because many patients do not have measurable disease. However, the serum PSA or alkaline phosphatase level is often elevated and can be serially measured as a marker for response. Bone scans are difficult to interpret because "hot spots" can reflect either the presence of disease or healing of bone in response to tumor regression.
   4. **Complications of therapy.** All hormonal therapies can cause sexual dysfunction, including impotence and decreased libido. Orchiectomy can rarely be complicated by local infection or hematoma. LHRH analogs can cause an initial flare of the disease and are frequently associated with hot flashes. Antiandrogens can cause diarrhea and hepatic dysfunction. Estrogens are associated with thromboembolic disease, fluid retention, and cardiac disease. Chemotherapy side effects include nausea and vomiting, mucositis, marrow suppression, and alopecia.
   E. **Follow-up.** Patients treated with radical prostatectomy can be followed with PSA measurements every 4 months. Patients with a rising PSA level, evidence of local recurrence, and no evidence of metastatic disease can be considered for radiation to the prostatic bed. Otherwise, there is no role for serial PSA measurements (except as a marker for response to hormonal therapy, noted in Section III.D.3) or bone

scans because patients are treated only for symptomatic progression.

IV. **Testicular cancer** (germ cell tumors [GCTs])

A. **Overview.** Although primary neoplasms of the testis can arise from Leydig's or Sertoli's cells, less than 95% of testicular cancers are of spermatogenic or germ cell origin. GCTs are rare, accounting for 1% of all malignancies in men. However, they are important malignancies because they represent the most common solid tumor in young men and because of their high degree of curability. With the advent of cisplatin-based chemotherapy, accurate tumor markers, and aggressive surgical approaches, overall cure rates for patients with disseminated disease approach 80%, and patients with early-stage disease are nearly always cured. GCTs are also one of the few solid tumors for which salvage chemotherapy can be curative.

B. **Histology.** GCTs are categorized as either *seminomatous* or *nonseminomatous* (which includes a variety of other histologies, such as embryonal cell carcinoma, choriocarcinoma, and yolk sac tumors). Pure seminoma accounts for 40% of patients with GCTs. Although mild elevations of the β-subunit of human chorionic gonadotropin (hCG) may be seen, pure seminoma is never associated with an elevation of α-fetoprotein (AFP). Nonseminomatous GCT can cause elevations of hCG, AFP, or both.

C. **Staging.** Pretreatment staging should include serum tumor markers (AFP, hCG) and CT of the abdomen and chest. Other radiographic procedures should be undertaken only if symptoms or physical examination dictate.

Stage I: Tumor confined to the testis with or without involvement of the spermatic cord or epididymis

Stage II: Tumor with metastasis limited to retroperitoneal lymph nodes

Stage III: Tumor spread beyond retroperitoneal lymph nodes

D. **Treatment strategies and management** of specific situations. The therapeutic approach to the patient with testicular cancer depends on the histology of the tumor and the clinical or pathologic stage of the disease.

1. **Seminoma.** Most patients with seminoma present with early-stage disease and are nearly always cured with radiation therapy. Patients with stage I disease are treated with 2,500 cGy given to abdominal nodes in daily fractions over 3 to 4 weeks. Patients with lymph node involvement on lymphangiogram or CT scans receive a slightly higher dose of 3,000 to 3,500 cGy. The contralateral testis should be shielded to maintain fertility. Radiation to the mediastinum is contraindicated and can compromise salvage chemotherapy. Residual radiographic abnormalities are most often scar tissue or necrosis and do not need to be surgically resected. Patients with bulky retroperitoneal disease larger than 5 cm or stage III disease should be treated with chemotherapy (see Section IV.D.2).

2. **Nonseminoma**
    a. **Stage I disease.** Historically, these patients have been pathologically staged and treated with a retroperitoneal lymph node dissection (RPLND). Patients with pathologically confirmed stage I disease do not need any further therapy because less than 10% show relapse. In about 25% of patients, clinical stage I disease is found to be stage II pathologically, and treatment for these patients is discussed in the following section. The major complication of RPLND is retrograde ejaculation with subsequent infertility, although this is rare with the currently used nerve-sparing procedure. The other option for selected patients is surveillance without RPLND. These patients should be chosen carefully and should not have any poor prognostic features for extratesticular involvement: microscopic evidence of lymphatic or vascular invasion, invasion of the tunica albuginea or epididymis, or embryonal cell carcinoma. Because 30% of these patients eventually experience relapse, they must be followed closely with monthly measurements of serum markers and chest radiographs for the first year and every other month the year after that. Abdominal CT scans should also be performed every 2 months the first year and every 4 months thereafter. If patients are selected and followed appropriately, overall survival is the same as for patients undergoing RPLND.
    b. **Stage II disease.** Patients with lymph nodes larger than 3 cm should be treated primarily with chemotherapy. If the lymph nodes measure less than 3 cm, a RPLND should be performed. Patients with pathologically confirmed and completely resected stage II disease have a relapse rate of about 30%. These patients either can be treated with two cycles of adjuvant chemotherapy after RPLND or can be followed closely and treated with standard chemotherapy if they show relapse. Patients who choose observation should receive monthly chest x-ray and serum marker evaluations and should be treated immediately if the disease recurs.

Patients with stage II disease who have elevated markers after RPLND or whose disease is not completely resected should be treated the same as patients with stage III disease.

c. **Stage III disease.** About 30% of patients present with stage III disease. The most common site of involvement is the lungs, but liver, bone, and brain can also be involved with metastatic disease. These patients are further categorized as good risk or poor risk based on the number, size, and sites of metastatic involvement. Poor-risk patients according to the Indiana Classification System include those with the following:

Advanced chest disease (mediastinal mass more than 50% of the intrathoracic diameter, or more than 10 pulmonary metastases per lung, or multiple pulmonary metastases larger than 3 cm), *or*

Palpable abdominal mass plus pulmonary metastases, *or*

Hepatic, osseous, or central nervous system metastasis.

An international germ cell prognostic classification has been developed based on a retrospective analysis of more than 5,000 patients with metastatic GCTs. This system will be the basis for future clinical trials.

d. **Recommended therapy.** All patients with stage II or III disease who require chemotherapy should receive cisplatin-based BEP chemotherapy, as follows:

Cisplatin, 20 mg/m^2 i.v. over 30 minutes on days 1 to 5, *and*

Etoposide, 100 mg/m^2 i.v. on days 1 to 5, *and*

Bleomycin, 30 U i.v. push weekly on days 1, 8, and 15.

Repeat cycle every 21 days regardless of blood cell counts for two (adjuvant therapy), three (good-risk patients), or four (poor-risk patients) cycles.

If the patient has fever associated with granulocytopenia, we would give the next cycle at the same doses, followed by daily subcutaneous injections of granulocyte colony-stimulating factor. Other chemotherapy regimens, such as VIP (etoposide, ifosfamide, cisplatin) have not improved outcome and are more toxic.

e. **Surgery for residual disease.** Patients who have a complete response with chemotherapy should be followed and do not require any further treatment. Patients whose marker levels normalize but who have not achieved a radiographic complete response should undergo complete surgical resection of residual disease. If the resected material reveals only teratoma, necrosis, or fibrosis, then no further therapy is necessary, and the patient should be followed. If there is carcinoma in the resected specimen, the patient should receive two more cycles of BEP chemotherapy.

   f. **Follow-up.** Most patients who experience relapse do so within the first 2 years, although late relapses do occur. In general, patients should be followed with monthly physical examination, chest x-ray studies, and serum marker measurements during the first year and every 2 months during the second year. Patients should then be followed about every 4 months for the third year, twice the fourth year, and yearly thereafter. Because tumors can arise in the contralateral testis, patients should be taught to do testicular self-examination.

E.   Salvage chemotherapy

   1. **Standard-dose therapy.** Patients who respond to first-line chemotherapy and then relapse are still curable with salvage regimens such as VIP.

   • Vinblastine, 0.11 mg/kg (4.1 mg/m^2) i.v. push on days 1 and 2, *and*
   • Ifosfamide, 1.2 g/m^2 i.v. over 30 minutes on days 1 to 5, *and*
   • Cisplatin, 20 mg/m^2 i.v. over 30 minutes on days 1 to 5.

   Repeat every 21 days for four cycles. Any radiographic abnormalities that persist after salvage chemotherapy should be surgically resected.

   2. **High-dose chemotherapy** with autologous bone marrow transplantation (ABMT). High-dose chemotherapy with carboplatin and etoposide with or without ifosfamide followed by ABMT should be considered for patients who show relapse after salvage chemotherapy or disease progression during first-line chemotherapy. Overall, about 15% of these patients are long-term survivors. The role of ABMT as first-line salvage therapy is being evaluated and should be considered experimental.

F.   Prognosis. With these strategies, the overall cure rate for patients with stage I disease is more than 98%; stage II disease, more than 95%; and stage III disease, more than 80%.

G. **Complications of therapy.** Because patients are cured, the short- and long-term toxicities are of considerable importance. The short-term toxicities of the described chemotherapy regimens include nausea and vomiting, myelosuppression, renal toxicity, and hemorrhagic cystitis. The major long-term morbidities include infertility, pulmonary fibrosis, and a small but definite risk of secondary leukemia.

H. **Mediastinal and other midline GCTs.** GCTs can arise in several midline structures, including the retroperitoneum, mediastinum, and pineal gland. All patients with GCTs at these sites should have a testicular ultrasound examination to exclude an occult primary tumor. Mediastinal nonseminomatous GCTs are associated with Klinefelter's syndrome and with rare hematologic malignancies (particularly acute megakaryocytic leukemia). Small mediastinal seminomas can be treated with radiation therapy alone. Widespread tumors or nonseminomatous tumors should be treated with four cycles of BEP chemotherapy. Salvage chemotherapy (including ABMT) in patients with nonseminomatous mediastinal GCT is ineffective.

V. **Cancer of the penis**

A. **General considerations.** Penile cancer is rare in North America but is a significant health problem in many developing countries. These tumors are nearly always squamous cell in origin and are associated with the presence of a foreskin and poor hygiene. Typically, these tumors present as a nonhealing ulcer or mass on the foreskin or glans. The most common treatment is wide surgical excision or penectomy, depending on the size and location of the lesion. Prophylactic inguinal lymph node dissection is indicated in certain subgroups of patients. Radiation therapy can also provide local control, although 15% to 20% of patients require surgical salvage.

B. **Chemotherapy for systemic disease.** Active single agents include bleomycin, cisplatin, and methotrexate, with response rates of 20% to 50%. Combination chemotherapy results in high response rates, but whether survival is improved over that with single agents is unknown. A reasonable regimen is cisplatin, 100 mg/m^2 on day 1, with fluorouracil, 1,000 mg/m^2/day given by continuous infusion on days 1 to 4. Cycles can be repeated every 21 days.

SELECTED READINGS

Kidney

Atkins MB, Sparano J, Fisher RI, et al. Randomized phase II trial of high-dose interleukin-2 either alone or in combination with interferon alfa-2b in advanced renal cell carcinoma. *J Clin Oncol* 1993; 11(4):661–670.

Bukowski RM. Natural history and therapy of metastatic renal cell carcinoma: the role of interleukin-2. *Cancer* 1997;80:1198–1220.

Fyfe G, Fisher RI, Rosenberg SA, et al. Results of treatment of 255 patients with metastatic renal cell carcinoma who received high-dose recombinant interleukin-2 therapy. *J Clin Oncol* 1995;13(3): 688–696.

Thrasher JB, Robertson JE, Paulson DF. Expanding indications for conservative renal surgery in renal cell carcinoma. *Urology* 1994; 43(2):160–168.

Yang JC, Topalian SL, Parkinson D, et al. Randomized comparison of high-dose and low-dose intravenous interleukin-2 for the therapy of metastatic renal cell carcinoma: an interim report. *J Clin Oncol* 1994;12:1572–1576.

Bladder

Herr HW, Schwalb DM, Zhang ZF, et al. Intravesical bacillus Calmette-Guerin therapy prevents tumor progression and death from superficial bladder cancer: ten-year follow-up of a prospective randomized trial. *J Clin Oncol* 1995;13(6):1404–1408.

Igawa M, Urakami S, Shiina H, et al. Long-term results with M-VAC for advanced urothelial cancer: high relapse rate and low survival in patients with a complete response. *Br J Urol* 1995;76:321–324.

Lacombe L, Dalbagni G, Zhang ZF, et al. Overexpression of p53 protein in a high-risk population of patients with superficial bladder cancer before and after bacillus Calmette-Guerin therapy: correlation to clinical outcome. *J Clin Oncol* 1996;14(10):2646–2652.

Lamm DL, Blumenstein BA, Crawford ED, et al. A randomized trial of intravesical doxorubicin and immunotherapy with bacille Calmette-Guerin for transitional-cell carcinoma of the bladder. *N Engl J Med* 1991;325:1205–1209.

Loehrer P, Elson P, Dreicer R, et al. Escalated dosages of methotrexate, vinblastine, doxorubicin, and cisplatin plus recombinant human granulocyte colony-stimulating factor in advanced urothelial carcinoma: an Eastern Cooperative Oncology Group trial. *J Clin Oncol* 1994;12:483–488.

Saxman SB, Propert K, Einhorn LH, et al. Long-term follow-up of a phase III intergroup study of cisplatin alone or in combination with methotrexate, vinblastine, a doxorubicin in patients with metastatic urothelial carcinoma: a cooperative group study. *J Clin Oncol* 1997;15:2564–2569.

Tester W, Caplan R, Heaney J, et al. Neoadjuvant combined modality program with selective organ preservation for invasive bladder cancer: results of Radiation Therapy Oncology Group phase II trial 8802. *J Clin Oncol* 1996;14(1):119–126.

Prostate

Chodak GW, Thisted RA, Gerber GS. Results of conservative management of clinically localized prostate cancer. *N Engl J Med* 1994; 330:242.

Eisenberger M, Crawford ED, McLeod D, et al. A comparison of bilateral orchiectomy with or without flutamide in stage D2 prostate cancer. *Proc Am Soc Clin Oncol* 1997;16:2a(abst 3).

Fowler FJ, Barry MJ, Lu-Yao G, et al. Outcomes of external-beam radiation therapy for prostate cancer: a study of Medicare beneficiaries in three Surveillance, Epidemiology, and End Results areas. *J Clin Oncol* 1996;14(8):2258–2265.

Pienta KJ, Esper PS. Risk factors for prostate cancer. *Ann Intern Med* 1993;118:793.

Pilepich MV, Caplan R, Byhardt RW, et al. Phase III trial of androgen suppression using goserelin in unfavorable-prognosis carcinoma of the prostate treated with definitive radiotherapy: report of Radiation Therapy Oncology Group protocol 85-31. *J Clin Oncol* 1997;15(3):1013–1021.

Prostate Cancer Trialists' Collaborative Group. Maximum androgen blockade in advanced prostate cancer: an overview of 22 randomised trials with 3283 deaths in 5710 patients. *Lancet* 1995;346(8970): 265–269.

Small EJ, Vogelzang NJ. Second-line hormonal therapy for advanced prostate cancer: a shifting paradigm. *J Clin Oncol* 1997;15(1): 382–388.

Tannock IF, Osoba D, Stockler MR, et al. Chemotherapy with mitoxantrone plus prednisone or prednisone alone for symptomatic hormone-resistant prostate cancer: a Canadian randomized trial with palliative end points. *J Clin Oncol* 1996;14(6):1756–1764.

Testis

Baniel J, Foster RS, Gonin R, et al.: Late relapse of testicular cancer. *J Clin Oncol* 1995;13(5):1170–1176.

Beyer J, Kramar A, Mandanas R, et al. High-dose chemotherapy as salvage treatment in germ cell tumors: a multivariate analysis of prognostic variables. *J Clin Oncol* 1996;14(10):2638–2645.

Einhorn LH. Treatment of testicular cancer: a new and improved model. *J Clin Oncol* 1990;8:1777.

Foster RS, McNulty A, Rubin LR, et al. The fertility of patients with clinical stage I testis cancer managed by nerve sparing retroperitoneal lymph node dissection. *J Urol* 1994;152(4):1139–1143.

International Germ Cell Cancer Collaborative Group. International Germ Cell Consensus Classification: a prognostic factor-based staging system for metastatic germ cell cancers. *J Clin Oncol* 1997;15(2): 594–603.

Loehrer PJ, Johnson D, Elson P, et al. Importance of bleomycin in favorable-prognosis disseminated germ cell tumors: an Eastern Cooperative Oncology Group Trial. *J Clin Oncol* 1995;13(2):470–476.

Nichols CR, Williams SD, Loehrer PJ, et al. Randomized study of cisplatin dose intensity in poor-risk germ cell tumors: a Southeastern Cancer Study group and Southwest Oncology Group protocol. *J Clin Oncol* 1991;9:1163–1172.

Read G, Stenning SP, Cullen MH, et al. Medical Research Council prospective study of surveillance for stage I testicular teratoma. *J Clin Oncol* 1992;10(11):1762–1768.

Saxman SB, Finch D, Gonin R, Einhorn LH. Long-term follow-up of a phase III study of 3 versus 4 cycles of bleomycin, etoposide and cisplatin in favorable-prognosis germ cell tumors: the Indiana University Experience. *J Clin Oncol* 1998;16(2):702–706.

Saxman S. Salvage therapy in recurrent testicular cancer. *Semin Oncol* 1992;19:143.

Williams SD, Stablein DM, Einhorn LH, et al. Immediate adjuvant chemotherapy versus observation with treatment at relapse in pathological stage II testicular cancer. *N Engl J Med* 1987;317:1433–1438.

Penis

Abi-Aad AS, deKemion JB. Controversies in ilioinguinal lymphadenectomy for cancer of the penis. *Urol Clin North Am* 1992;19:319.

Burgers JK, Badalament RA, Drago JR. Penile cancer: clinical presentation, diagnosis, and staging. *Urol Clin North Am* 1992;19:247.

Thyroid and Adrenal Carcinomas

Samir N. Khleif

Endocrine cancers account for 1.5% of all cancers diagnosed and for 0.4% of cancer deaths. Thyroid cancer is the most common endocrine malignancy, accounting for 90% of endocrine cancers and for 60% to 70% of the deaths from this group of diseases. Although the role of cytotoxic chemotherapy is limited in endocrine cancer, it is beneficial in selected patients. Pancreatic islet cell carcinomas and other pancreatic malignancies are discussed in Chapter 10. Here, thyroid and adrenal carcinomas are discussed. The pathology, presentation, and biologic behavior of thyroid and adrenal carcinomas are important determinants of therapy, and they are briefly considered.

I. **Thyroid carcinoma**
   A. **Background**
      1. **Incidence.** About 17,000 new cases of thyroid carcinoma are diagnosed each year, which result in about 1,200 deaths due to this cancer. The incidence of thyroid carcinoma is 5.9 per 100,000 women and 2.2 per 100,000 men. The prevalence at autopsy is 5 to 15 per 100,000 subjects. Thyroid carcinoma usually affects people between the ages of 25 and 65 years.
      2. **Etiology and prevention.** In most instances, the cause of thyroid carcinoma is unknown, although experimentally prolonged stimulation by thyroid-stimulating hormone (TSH) may lead to the development of thyroid carcinoma. Some cases appear to be related to a dose-dependent phenomenon involving radiation to the neck during childhood. Thyroid malignancy has been observed 20 to 25 years after radiation exposure in atomic bomb survivors and in children treated with radiation therapy for benign conditions of the head and neck. The frequency increases exponentially with doses up to 12 Gy and then decreases, so that with doses over 20 Gy, the risk of developing malignancy becomes relatively low because such high doses lead to the destruction and killing of cells rather than nonlethal damage of the DNA. Some cases of thyroid carcinoma (usually medullary carcinoma) are familial, as seen in the multiple endocrine neoplasia (MEN) syndrome, which was recently found to be associated with germline mutation of the RET protooncogene. Although ionizing radiation for benign conditions of the head and neck is no longer being used, thyroid carcinomas related to this

usage are still being seen. In cases of accidental nuclear exposure, it is thought that the use of potassium iodide to block the thyroid uptake of radioactive iodine (RAI) in children is helpful in reducing the incidence of subsequent thyroid cancer. This measure was used in eastern Europe after the Chernobyl accident.

3. **Histologic types.** The most common histologic types of thyroid carcinoma are as follows:

   a. **Well-differentiated adenocarcinoma** includes papillary carcinoma (40% to 50%), follicular carcinoma (25%), and mixed papillary and follicular adenocarcinoma (20%). Well-differentiated adenocarcinomas are derived from thyroglobulin-producing follicular cells.

   b. **Anaplastic or undifferentiated carcinoma** (15% to 20%).

   c. **Medullary carcinoma** (1% to 5%). Medullary carcinomas are derived from thyroid parafollicular or C cells. These cells produce both immunoreactive calcitonin and carcinoembryonic antigen (CEA).

   d. **Hürthle's cell carcinoma** (2% to 5%) used to be considered a variant of follicular carcinoma; recently, it was shown to be a separate pathologic entity.

   e. **Thyroid lymphoma** (5%).

4. **Prognosis**

   a. **Cell types.** Patients with papillary or mixed papillary and follicular histology (which have similar biologic and prognostic behaviors) have an excellent prognosis, with less than 15% mortality at 20 years. Patients with pure follicular carcinoma do not do as well as those with papillary elements, at least in part because there is a tendency for the follicular carcinoma to spread through the bloodstream, whereas the papillary carcinoma spreads more by lymphatic channels. Recent studies have shown that patients having follicular carcinoma with vascular invasion have a relatively bad prognosis, whereas patients with follicular carcinoma without vascular invasion do almost as well as those with papillary carcinoma. About half of medullary carcinomas are familial, as part of three clinical syndromes (MEN-IIa, MEN-IIb, and familial non-MEN medullary thyroid carcinoma). Regional lymph node and distant metastases are common in patients with medullary carcinomas and occur in early stages of the disease. The 10-year survival rate after surgical resection is 40% to

60%. Patients with anaplastic thyroid carcinoma have an abysmal prognosis, with a median survival time of 4 months, although occasional patients may be cured with combined radiotherapy and chemotherapy.

b. **Other factors.** In addition to the cell type, the prognosis of thyroid carcinoma is shown to be worse if the following factors are present:

- A large tumor size, especially more than 4 cm.
- Patient age more than 40 years.
- Distant metastases. Well-differentiated carcinoma tends to metastasize to the lung or bone. Patients with bone metastases have survival rates at 5, 10, and 15 years of 53%, 38%, and 30%, respectively.
- Abnormal DNA content in tumor cells in the papillary type; the more pronounced the aneuploidy, the more aggressively the cancer behaves.
- Male sex, which may be related to the fact that men tend to be older at the time of diagnosis and are more likely to have a worse histologic type.

In contrast to most other cancers, limited regional lymph node metastasis of well-differentiated thyroid carcinomas does not influence survival substantially, and radiation-induced thyroid carcinoma is not associated with a worse prognosis.

B. **Diagnosis and staging.** Any solitary nonfunctioning thyroid nodule ("cold" nodule) should be considered a possible malignant tumor until proved otherwise, especially in patients younger than 25 years and men older than 60 years. The overall incidence of cancer in a cold nodule is 25%. Although toxic goiters are less likely to contain carcinoma, a hyperfunctioning thyroid nodule does not automatically confer benignity. Because most thyroid tumors spread primarily by local extension and regional nodal metastasis, assessment of the extent of disease is concentrated on the neck. Presurgical studies include inspection and palpation, indirect laryngoscopy, radionuclide scanning, esophagogram, computed tomography (CT) scan of the neck, and needle aspiration cytology. The accuracy of needle aspiration biopsy ranges between 50% and 97%, depending on the pathologist and the institution. Whereas the best method for the diagnosis of well-differentiated thyroid and medullary carcinoma is surgical resection, large-needle biopsy is the method of choice for diagnosing thyroid lymphoma and anaplastic carcinoma. Chest radiography should be performed before surgery to rule out pulmonary metastasis. If there is any clinical or laboratory suggestion of bone metastases, a radionuclide bone scan should be performed. Patients with thyroid carcinoma are typically euthyroid. Thyroid carcinoma rarely destroys thyroid function to the point of frank hypothyroidism. However, elevated TSH levels with increased antimicrosomal antibodies may be seen with Hashimoto's thyroiditis, which may coexist in 20% of patients with papillary thyroid carcinoma.

C. **Treatment.** The therapeutic approach to patients with thyroid carcinoma depends considerably on the histologic type.

   1. **Well-differentiated thyroid carcinoma.** The management approach to the patient with well-differentiated thyroid carcinoma is illustrated in Table 14-1.

      a. **Surgery is the only definitive therapy.** Although the surgical approach may differ among surgeons and institutions, many surgeons prefer a bilateral near-total thyroidectomy, taking into consideration that with well-differentiated thyroid carcinoma, the incidence of the disease in the contralateral lobe is 20% to 87%. Limited lymph node involvement does not substantially influence the survival rate, but it is associated with an increase in local recurrence. Total thyroidectomy with modified neck dissection is often preferred for those who have cervical lymph node involvement. Mortality after thyroidectomy in well-differentiated thyroid carcinoma approaches 0%. Complications include permanent recurrent laryngeal nerve damage in 2% of patients and permanent hypoparathyroidism in 1% to 2%.

      b. **TSH suppression** is an essential component in the treatment of all of these tumors

Table 14-1.   Guidelines for the treatment of well-differentiated thyroid carcinoma

Patient Age (yr)	Extent of the Disease (cm)	Treatment
≤45	<2	Lobectomy or NTT + HS
	≥2	NTT + HS
	Metastasis	NTT + HS + RAI
>45	<2	NTT + HS
	≥2	NTT + HS + RAI
	Metastasis	NTT + HS + RAI

NTT, near-total thyroidectomy; HS, thyroid-stimulating hormone suppression; RAI, radioactive iodine.

(see Table 14-1) because there is good evidence that well-differentiated thyroid cancer cells are usually responsive to TSH. TSH suppresses the growth of malignant as well as normal thyroid tissue, and therefore, the recurrence rate is reduced; in a few patients, metastatic lesions are diminished markedly. This hormonal suppression can be achieved by the administration of exogenous thyroid hormone. Usually, 200 to 250 µg of levothyroxine (T_4) daily is necessary to obliterate the pituitary response to thyrotropin-releasing hormone (TRH) and thus to keep the TSH level below that detectable by standard assays. Not withstanding, the dose should be individualized to a maximum tolerable level. Side effects and dose-limiting factors include symptoms of thyrotoxicosis, angina, and cardiac arrhythmia. Other alternatives include liothyronine (triiodothyronine, or T_3) and desiccated thyroid preparations.

c. **Radiotherapy** depends to a large degree on the clinical practice of the institution. Treatment with RAI (^{131}I) is usually recommended for patients with well-differentiated thyroid carcinoma and known postoperative residual disease, patients with distant metastases, and patients with locally invasive lesions. It is also recommended in patients older than 45 years and in those with large lesions (see Table 14-1). When ablation of a thyroid remnant is carried out postoperatively, it is usually done 4 to 6 weeks after thyroidectomy. Although the effect of RAI on survival is not well determined, it is clear that the use of RAI and T_4 markedly decreases the recurrence rate. Effective use of RAI treatment requires the following:

(1) Tumor cells that are capable of receiving and concentrating iodide (i.e., well-differentiated papillary or follicular carcinoma), *and*

(2) Appropriate patient preparation by withholding thyroid hormone administration for 2 to 4 weeks to provide the iodine-concentrating cells with the highest endogenous TSH stimulation.

T_3 is cleared from the body much more rapidly than T_4. The shorter period of withdrawal minimizes the period of hypothyroidism. Accordingly, patients are switched from suppression therapy with T_4 to a corresponding dose of T_3 for 2 to 4 weeks to allow metabolic disposal of the T_4. This is followed by 2 weeks of T_3 withdrawal. Effective doses of thyroid ablation usually are 50 to 150 mCi, depending on the size and extent of the disease. Isolation of these patients is required by federal regulations until the total-body radiation activity decreases below 30 mCi. Postablation TSH follow-up should identify individuals who do not respond to the therapy. Ideally, serum levels should exceed 30 μm/mL. Potential side effects expected after radioiodine therapy include temporary bone marrow depression, nausea, sialoadenitis with possible permanent cessation of salivary flow (radiation mumps), skin reaction over the tissue concentrating the radioiodine, pulmonary fibrosis, and a small risk of later development of acute leukemia (2%). Once ablation is successful, patients are placed on suppressive therapy. Patients with lung metastases treated with RAI have a 20-year survival rate of 54%. In contrast, patients with bony involvement have a 10-year survival rate of 0%. Scintigraphy should be performed 4 to 6 weeks after therapy to detect any residual carcinoma. Most well-differentiated thyroid carcinomas grow very slowly. The rate of recurrence is 0.5% to 1.6% per year. Therefore, lifelong annual serum thyroglobulin assays are recommended. Scintigraphy is suggested if the thyroglobulin is found to be elevated (more than 23 ng/mL). The role of external radiation therapy in well-differentiated thyroid carcinoma is limited. It is considered for tumors that concentrate little or no iodine.

2. **Medullary thyroid carcinoma.** With familial medullary carcinoma, the disease is almost always bilateral. Regional lymph node involvement is common in early stages. Therefore, total thyroidectomy and central lymph node dissection are required. The overall 10-year survival rate after surgical resection is 40% to 60%. Postoperative annual evaluation is recommended by measuring levels of calcitonin and CEA, both of which are secreted by the medullary thyroid carcinoma cells, as a follow-up for residual disease or recurrence. Suppressive therapy is of no benefit because medullary cells do not have TSH receptors. RAI and cytotoxic chemotherapy are of little utility. Cisplatin, streptozocin, carmustine, methotrexate, and fluorouracil have shown little if any benefit. However, some studies have

shown doxorubicin chemotherapy to produce occasional responses of metastatic disease (see Section I.C.4.). Local radiation therapy is useful in some patients as palliative therapy.

3. **Anaplastic thyroid carcinoma.** Most anaplastic tumors are unresectable at the time of presentation. Combination chemotherapy or chemotherapy plus radiation therapy have shown encouraging results for local control, and some partial and complete remissions have been seen.

4. **Chemotherapy**

   a. **Single-agent chemotherapy.** The most widely applied cytotoxic agents are doxorubicin (Adriamycin), bleomycin, cisplatin, and etoposide. Each of these medications has demonstrated some activity against anaplastic and medullary thyroid carcinomas. Improved survival may be achieved in patients who respond to sequential exposure to these agents. Doxorubicin has proved to be the best single chemotherapeutic agent with the highest response rate. Doxorubicin in a dosage of 60 to 75 mg/m^2 i.v. every 3 weeks has resulted in objective responses in 20% to 45% (median, 34%) of patients with advanced refractory metastatic thyroid carcinoma. The response rate is probably highest for the medullary type and lowest for undifferentiated thyroid carcinoma. A high single dose of doxorubicin, which should be increased in patients with no response, appears to be essential for a therapeutic effect. Because of its apparently lower cardiotoxicity, epirubicin, although almost as effective as doxorubicin, may be given at higher doses and over longer periods and is therefore preferred by some investigators.

   b. **Combination chemotherapy usually includes doxorubicin.** Cisplatin, 40 mg/m^2 i.v., plus doxorubicin, 60 mg/m^2 i.v., given every 3 weeks has yielded a higher rate and quality of response than doxorubicin alone. These results included complete remission in 12% of patients, several of whom survived more than 2 years. Toxicity was no worse with the combination therapy. Other combination chemotherapy regimens are doxorubicin, bleomycin, vincristine, and melphalan, with a response rate of 36%; and doxorubicin, bleomycin, and vincristine, with an improved 64% response rate. Doxorubicin, 10 mg/m^2 i.v., has been used in combination with external radiotherapy 90 minutes before the first radiation treatment and weekly thereafter. In this combination, the radiotherapy was given at a dose of 1.6 Gy per treatment twice a day for 3 consecutive days weekly for 6 weeks. Patients with undifferentiated thyroid carcinoma treated in this fashion showed an improvement in the median survival compared with historical control subjects. In general, the highest response is observed in patients with pulmonary metastasis. If anaplastic thyroid carcinoma responds to chemotherapy, a prolongation of the median survival time from 3 to 5 months to 15 to 20 months can be achieved.

5. **Non-Hodgkin's lymphoma** is more thoroughly addressed in Chapter 23. The discussion here briefly highlights its significance concerning thyroid malignancies. By definition, lymphoma of the thyroid is, at the time of diagnosis, confined to the gland or to the gland and regional lymph nodes. The major histologic type is non-Hodgkin's lymphoma. Autoimmune thyroiditis is a predisposing factor. Lymphoma of the thyroid usually presents with rapid enlargement of the gland within a few weeks and is bilateral in 25% of patients. If the tumor is confined to the thyroid, surgical excision alone yields a 5-year survival rate of 70% to 90%. Once the lymphoma extends beyond the thyroid gland, however, surgical therapy does not improve survival, and radiation therapy and chemotherapy are indicated.

II. **Adrenal carcinoma**
  A. **Adrenocortical carcinoma**
    1. **Incidence and etiology.** Adrenocortical carcinoma is a rare tumor, with fewer than 200 new cases occurring yearly in the United States. It accounts for 0.05% to 0.20% of all cancers and for 0.2% of cancer deaths. It has a prevalence of 2 per 1,000,000 population worldwide. The peak incidence of adrenocortical carcinoma occurs during the fourth and fifth decades of life. The incidence in women in most reports is about 2.5 times higher than that in men, who tend to be older at diagnosis. Women have a tendency to develop a functional carcinoma, whereas men usually develop a nonfunctional malignancy. There is no family predilection, and no etiologic factors have been established. Sometimes, it occurs in the context of tumor-predisposing syndromes, such as Li-Fraumeni or Beckwith-Wiedemann syndrome.
    2. **Clinical picture.** Adrenal carcinoma may present in several modes.

    a. **A palpable abdominal mass** or an abdominal mass detected incidentally by abdominal imaging for some other purpose. About half of patients have a palpable abdominal mass at the time of diagnosis.

    b. **A functioning tumor** with or without endocrine signs and symptoms of Cushing's syndrome, virilization, or feminization. More than 60% of patients present with functioning tumor, depending on the age and sex of the patient. Such manifestations are due to an increase in the production of a wide variety of steroid hormones. Ten percent of adrenocortical carcinomas are associated with virilization and 12% with feminization. Adrenal carcinoma is the cause of 10% of all cases of Cushing's syndrome.

    c. **Other frequent presenting symptoms** include upper abdominal pain, weight loss, anorexia, and malaise. Usually, these symptoms are associated with advanced disease.

3. **Pathology and diagnosis.** Most malignant adrenal masses represent carcinomatous metastatic lesions, primarily from the lung and breast. Whether the coincidental finding of an adrenal mass requires complete screening of the patient for a hidden primary adrenal tumor depends on the clinical situation. There may be some difficulty distinguishing adenoma from carcinoma (Table 14-2). CT scan and magnetic resonance imaging (MRI) are helpful in diagnosing adrenocortical carcinoma. A CT finding of a large unilateral adrenal mass with irregular borders is almost always an indication of adrenal cancer. On MRI, adrenal cancer has intermediate to high signal intensity on T2-weighted images, in contrast to benign lesions, which have low signal intensity. In addition, MRI is a helpful tool in delineating adrenocortical carcinoma before surgery. Iodocholesterol scanning is rarely indicated. It shows poor uptake in carcinomas compared with adenomas. Adrenocortical carcinoma can be further divided into two categories according to the pathologic patterns of cellular arrangement and the cellular pleomorphism.

    a. **Well-differentiated adrenocortical carcinoma**, which occurs more commonly in women and usually presents with a functioning tumor, *and*

    b. **Anaplastic carcinoma**, which is more common in men and is often associated with a lack of hormone production.

Table 14-2. Diagnosis of malignancy in adrenocortical neoplasms

Reliability	Clinical Criteria	Pathologic Criteria
Diagnostic of malignancy	Weight loss, feminization, nodal or distant metastases	Tumor weight >100 g, tumor necrosis, fibrous bands, vascular invasion, mitoses
Consistent with malignancy	Virilism, Cushing's syndrome and virilism, no hormone production	Nuclear pleomorphism
Suggestive of malignancy	Elevated urinary 17-ketosteroid levels	Capsular invasion
Unreliable	Hypercortisolism, hyperaldosteronism	Tumor giant cells, cytoplasmic size variations, ratio between compact and clear cells

Adapted from Page DL, DeLellis RA, Hough AJ. Tumors of the adrenal. *In* Hartmann WH, Sobin LH, eds. *Atlas of tumor pathology.* Washington, DC: Armed Forces Institute of Pathology, 1986.

4. **Staging and prognosis.** Most patients (70%) present with stage III or IV disease. Adreno- cortical carcinoma is a highly malignant cancer with an overall 5-year mortality rate of 75% to 90%, depending on the stage and morphology of the disease. The most commonly used stag- ing system (derived from the TNM classifica- tion system) for adrenocortical carcinoma is as follows:

Stage	Size (CM)	Node or local inclusion	Metastasis
I	≤5	—	—
II	>5	—	—
III	Any	+	—
IV	Any	Both ±	+

Metastases of adrenocortical carcinoma most commonly occur in the lung (71%), lymph nodes (68%), liver (42%), and bone (26%). The median survival time of patients with well-differentiated carcinoma is 40 months, whereas patients with anaplastic carcinoma have a more dismal me- dian survival time of 5 months. The median sur- vival time of patients with stages I, II, or III dis- ease is 24 to 28 months, and for stage IV disease, 12 months.

5. **Treatment.** Because of the extremely low inci- dence of this disease, few medical centers have sufficient experience treating it, and an effort should be made to refer these patients to cen- ters that have clinical trials pertaining to this disease. This caveat notwithstanding, several guidelines regarding its treatment can be given.

   a. **Surgery.** In up to half of patients, adreno- cortical carcinomas can be resected, al- though incompletely in some patients; however, the remainder of patients have either local invasion that is too extensive or metastases to the abdomen, liver, lung, or other locations. Of the patients whose tumors are resected for cure, 40% remain disease free. The remainder die, usually with extensive metastatic disease, within an average of less than 1 year. Patients who undergo complete resection should initially be followed on a monthly basis (with measurements of steroid levels if they have a functioning tumor) to detect recurrence. Serial MRI may also be used to evaluate for recurrence.

   b. **Radiotherapy.** Radiation therapy pro- vides symptomatic relief from pain due to local or metastatic disease, especially bony metastases. It has also been used to pre- vent local recurrence after surgical resection (40 to 55 Gy over 4 weeks), but the benefit is uncertain, and there is no proof that it improves survival.

c. **Chemotherapy.** Indications for chemotherapy include recurrent, metastatic, and nonresectable adrenocortical carcinoma. Agents used are the following:

(1) **Adrenocortical suppressants**

(a) **Mitotane** (o,p'-DDD, Lysodren). An unconventional chemotherapy and a close chemical relative of the insecticide DDT, mitotane has been used to treat adrenocortical carcinoma since 1960. It inhibits corticosteroid biosynthesis and destroys adrenocortical cells secreting cortisol. The cytotoxic effect of mitotane has been considered transient and inconsistent. Included in its effects is the destruction of the adrenocortical cells. The part that is most affected by this action is the zona reticularis, and the least affected is the zona glomerulosa. Forty percent of the medication is absorbed from the gastrointestinal tract. The drug is highly lipid soluble and is subsequently concentrated in both normal and malignant adrenocortical cells. Reports of its plasma half-life range from 18 to 159 days.

(i) **Dosage and administration.** Treatment with mitotane is started at 2 to 6 g/day p.o. in three divided doses, then gradually increased monthly by 1 g/day until 9 to 10 g/day is reached or until the maximum tolerated dose is achieved with no side effects. Blood levels of o,p'-DDD should be maintained at more than 14 (g/mL to demonstrate a therapeutic response. Mitotane serum level was shown in a retrospective study to be the only significant prognostic factor for tumor response. Levels of more than 20 µg/mL have a higher incidence of toxicity.

(ii) **Response and follow-up.** Objective tumor regression usually occurs within 6 weeks after the initiation of therapy and is seen in 70% of patients as a decrease in excessive hormone production. However, the reduction in hormone production is not regularly accompanied by an objective tumor response. In about 30% to 40% of patients, the tumor size is reduced significantly, but complete remission is unlikely. The median duration of response is 10.5 months. If no clinical benefit is demonstrated at the maximum tolerated dose after 3 months, the case may be considered a clinical failure. Postoperative adjuvant therapy with mitotane has resulted in no improvement in survival. The combination of mitotane and radiation therapy has not conferred any additional benefit over mitotane alone.

(iii) **Side effects.** Nausea and vomiting occur in 80% of patients. Severe neurotoxicity, which may occur during long-term treatment, presents as somnolence, depression, ataxia, and weakness in 60% of patients. Reversible diffuse electroencephalographic changes may also occur. Adrenal insufficiency occurs in 50% of patients (without replacement), and dermatitis develops in 20% of patients. Because the maximal dosage is often limited by the severity of, and the patient's tolerance to, the side effects, the total dose may range widely from patient to patient.

(iv) **Glucocorticoid replacement.** During mitotane treatment, it is necessary to prevent hypoadrenalism. Replacement can be achieved by administering cortisone acetate, 25 mg p.o. in the morning and 12.5 mg p.o. in the evening, plus fludrocortisone acetate, 0.1 mg p.o. in the morning. Plasma cortisol rather than 17-hydroxycorticosteroid should be used to monitor adrenal function during mitotane use. If severe trauma or shock develops, mitotane should be discontinued immediately and larger doses of corticosteroids (e.g., hydrocortisone, 100 mg t.i.d.) should be administered.

(v) **Nonresponders to mitotane.** These patients can be treated with other adrenocortical suppressants, including metyrapone (75 mg p.o. every 4 hours) or aminoglutethimide (250 mg p.o. every 6 hours initially, with a stepwise increase in dosage to a total of 2 g/day or until limiting side effects that resemble those of mitotane appear). The latter drug inhibits conversion of cholesterol to pregnenolone. Metyrapone can induce hypertension and hypokalemic alkalosis. Neither of these medications has antitumor effects, but they are effective in relieving the signs and symptoms of excessive hormonal secretion. Another medication that can be used is ketoconazole, 200 to 600 mg/day. It is a potent adrenal inhibitor that produces clinical alleviation of the signs and symptoms within 4 to 6 weeks. In addition, it may cause regression of pulmonary and hepatic metastases, although the mechanism is not clear. Other drugs that might be of benefit in controlling symptoms include those that block the action of steroids in their target tissues, including antimineralocorticoid and antiandrogenic agents and, more recently, antiglucocorticoid agents, such as mifepristone (RU 486). None of these medications has an effect on tumor regression.

(2) Cytotoxic chemotherapy. Cytotoxic drugs are usually used in patients who show no response to mitotane. Because of the small number of patients who require such therapy, the experience with this treatment is limited despite many clinical trials. No cytotoxic drug has shown definite effectiveness in the treatment of adrenocortical carcinoma, although doxorubicin, cisplatin, and suramin have been reported to produce partial responses in patients with metastatic disease. Few combination chemotherapy regimens have been effective. Cyclophosphamide, 600 mg/m^2 i.v., plus doxorubicin, 40 mg/m^2 i.v., plus cisplatin, 50 mg/m^2 i.v., given in cycles every 3 weeks led to partial remission in 2 of 11 patients with adrenocortical carcinoma. The only combination that has induced complete remission is cisplatin 40 mg/m^2 i.v., plus etoposide, 100 mg/m^2 i.v., plus bleomycin, 30 U i.v. given every 4 weeks. Three of four patients responded, one with complete remission. Severe side effects occurred in patients in both of these studies.

Chemotherapy can also be given in combination with mitotane. Cisplatin, 75 to 100 mg/m^2, was combined with mitotane, 4 g p.o. daily. This resulted in a 30% objective response that lasted for 7.9 months. The survival duration in this study was 11.8 months. Other combinations of natural-product chemotherapy with mitotane are being tested; this may be pharmacologically advantageous because mitotane has been shown to be a multidrug resistance–blocking agent.

d. **Arterial embolization.** Another modality used for palliation of adrenocortical carcinoma is arterial embolization. It is used to decrease the bulk of the tumor, suppress tumor function, and relieve pain. Embolic agents used include polyvinyl alcohol foam and surgical gelatin.

B. **Pheochromocytoma**

1. **Description and diagnosis.** Pheochromocytoma is a tumor that arises from chromaffin cells mainly in the adrenal medulla (90% of cases) and in other sites (e.g., the urinary bladder, heart, and organ of Zuckerkandl). It is an uncommon tumor, with an estimated 800 cases diagnosed in the United States every year. It is found in up to 0.3% of autopsy subjects and is responsible for fewer than 0.1% to 0.5% of all cases of hypertension. Pheochromocytoma can be hereditary, as part of the MEN syndrome (MEN-IIa, MEN-IIb) or familial with no other manifestation of the MEN syndrome; when part of the MEN syndrome, it is never malignant. Also, it may be found as part of von Hippel-Lindau disease. The risk of developing a contralateral tumor in hereditary pheochromocytoma is more than 50%. The incidence of malignant pheochromocytoma ranges between 5% and 45%. The only definite proof of malignancy is the presence of tumor in secondary sites where chromaffin tissue is not normally present. The diagnosis of pheochromocytoma depends on a thorough history and physical examination, increased catecholamine levels in the plasma and the urine (including epinephrine, norepinephrine, dopamine, total metanephrines, and vanillylmandelic acid), an abnormal result on the clonidine suppression test, cross-sectional imaging such as with CT or MRI, and ^{131}I-metaiodobenzylguanidine ([131]-MIBG) scintigraphy. The overall 5-year survival rate for patients with malignant pheochromocytoma is 36% to 44%. Although pheochromocytoma is a rare tumor, early detection and treatment are crucial, owing to its high morbidity and potential mortality. Patients with pheochromocytoma can present with sustained or episodic hypertension. Hypertension does not usually correlate with the amount of

catecholamine production, and its severity varies widely among patients.

2. **Treatment**

   a. **Surgery.** Surgery is the only definitive therapy for pheochromocytoma. It is done for localized and regional unilateral or bilateral disease. Surgery requires careful preoperative preparation to achieve control of the blood pressure, blood volume, and heart rate. Phenoxybenzamine, an α-adrenergic receptor blocker, is started 1 to 2 weeks before surgery in a dose of 10 to 20 mg p.o. three or four times daily. Some patients require the addition of β-blockers (e.g., propranolol, 80 to 120 mg/day), which are indicated for persistent supraventricular tachycardia or the presence of angina. To prevent hypertensive crisis secondary to unopposed vasoconstriction, the β-blocker should never be given before the α-antagonist. Other α-adrenergic blockers are used for the same purpose, including prazocin, which is a selective $α_1$-antagonist that has also been used successfully for preoperative preparation of pheochromocytoma. Intraoperatively, blood pressure can be controlled by titration with nitroprusside. Postoperatively, blood pressure is best controlled with diuretics.

   Catecholamine levels should be measured 1 week after surgery to confirm total removal of the tumor. Operative mortality should be less than 2% to 3%. Patients whose localized disease is fully resected should have normal life expectancy. Close postoperative follow-up is mandatory because of the possibility of postoperative residual tumor and because 10% of patients have metastasis and another 10% have multiple primary tumors at the time of diagnosis.

   The follow-up should include a history and physical examination and catecholamine measurements every 3 months for a year, then every 6 months for another year, followed by a similar evaluation yearly for life. Redevelopment of any sign or symptom suggesting pheochromocytoma or a rising trend in catecholamine levels requires imaging, including ^{131}I-MIBG scintigraphy. Some groups recommend that ^{131}I-MIBG scintigraphy be done yearly regardless of the catecholamine levels or the clinical picture. The recurrence rate of pheochromocytoma postoperatively is 5% per year. Contralateral adrenalectomy of a normal gland is generally not recommended in patients with a high incidence of bilateral disease (e.g., MEN-II), despite the high risk of subsequent involvement. In patients with metastatic disease, there is no evidence to support improved survival after local debulking.

b. **Chemotherapy and radiation therapy.** These are reserved for locally invasive, metastatic, and inoperable lesions. Response to both of these treatments is evaluated by regression of tumor size and a decrease in the catecholamine levels. Owing to the small number of patients with pheochromocytoma, limited data are available regarding the effect of chemotherapy. Because of the functional and biologic similarities between pheochromocytoma and neuroblastoma, the combination of cyclophosphamide and dacarbazine, which induces an 80% response in neuroblastoma, was used in two series to treat pheochromocytoma. The chemotherapy regimen consisted of cyclophosphamide, 750 mg/m^2 i.v., plus vincristine, 1.4 mg/m^2 i.v. on day 1 and dacarbazine, 600 mg/m^2 i.v. on days 1 and 2; it was repeated in 21- to 28-day cycles. Analysis of 23 patients showed objective tumor size regression in 61% of patients, and the urinary catecholamine levels decreased in 74% of patients. The median response time averaged 28 months. Improvement of blood pressure control and performance status occurred with minimal toxicity. Because streptozocin has yielded favorable results in the treatment of neuroendocrine tumor in the gastrointestinal tract, it was used as a single agent in a patient with malignant pheochromocytoma. Streptozocin showed promising results, with a 73% reduction in urinary vanillylmandelic acid level and significant tumor size regression.

c. **Radiation therapy.** ^{131}I-MIBG is actively taken up and concentrated by pheochromocytoma cells with high sensitivity and specificity. Consequently, a high dose of ^{131}I-MIBG is used to treat pheochromocytoma. This treatment has shown some evidence of response in terms of tumor size regression and decreased catecholamine levels. The uptake of ^{131}I-MIBG by pheochromocytoma requires the presence of an active neuronal pump mechanism, which limits the use of this agent to patients with pheochromocytoma who have the ability to concentrate ^{131}I-MIBG in the cells. Therefore, initial screening of the ability of the pheochromocytoma to concentrate small doses of ^{131}I-MIBG is necessary to determine the probable efficacy of the treatment.

d. **Supportive pharmacologic therapy.** α-Blockers should be used to prevent severe hypertension-related morbidity and mortality, especially in untreated patients and those receiving chemotherapy. Another pharmacologic agent that can be used is α-methyl-L-tyrosine (metyrosine), which inhibits tyrosine hydroxylase, a rate-limiting step in catecholamine biosynthesis. Metyrosine allows the use of lower doses of α-blockers and has been shown to be effective in catecholamine-induced cardiomyopathy. Other medications include β-blockers, which are used to control arrhythmia; angiotensin-converting enzyme inhibitors; and calcium-channel blockers, which are also used for hypertension control.

SELECTED READINGS

Thyroid Carcinoma

Bucsky P, Parlowsky T. Epidemiology and therapy of thyroid cancer in childhood and adolescence. *Exp Clin Endocrinol Diabetes* 1997;105[Suppl]4:70–73.

Farid NR. Molecular pathogenesis of thyroid cancer: the significance of oncogenes, tumor suppressor genes, and genomic instability. *Exp Clin Endocrinol Diabetes* 1996;104[Suppl]4:1–12.

Galloway RJ, Smallridge RC. Imaging in thyroid cancer. *Endocrinol Metab Clin North Am* 1996;25(1):93–113.

Harmer CL. Radiotherapy in the management of thyroid cancer. *Ann Acad Med Singapore* 1996;25(3):413–419.

Moley JF. Medullary thyroid cancer. *Surg Clin North Am* 1995; 75(3):405–420.

Noguchi M, Katev N, Miwa K. Therapeutic strategies and long-term results in differentiated thyroid cancer. *J Surg Oncol* 1998; 67(1):52–59.

Robbins J. Prognostic factors in the management of thyroid cancer. *J Endocrinol Invest* 1995;18(2):159–160.

Soh EY, Clark OH. Surgical considerations and approach to thyroid cancer. *Endocrinol Metab Clin North Am* 1996;25(1):115–139.

Tezelman S, Clark OH. Current management of thyroid cancer. *Adv Surg* 1995;28:191–221.

Yeh SD, La Quaglia W. [131]I therapy for pediatric thyroid cancer. *Semin Pediatr Surg* 1997;6(3):128–133.

Adrenocortical Carcinoma

Boscaro M, Fallo F, Barzon L, Daniele O, Sonino N. Adrenocortical carcinoma: epidemiology and natural history. *Minerva Endocrinol* 1995;20(1):89–94.

Cook DM. Adrenal mass. *Endocrinol Metab Clin North Am* 1997; 26(4):829–852.

Dogliotti L, Berruti A, Pia A, et al. Cytotoxic chemotherapy for adrenocortical carcinoma. *Minerva Endocrinol* 1995;20(1):105–109.

Dunnick RN. Adrenal carcinoma. *Radiol Clin North Am* 1994;31:99.

Gicquel C, Baudin E, Lebouc Y, Schlumberger M. Adrenocortical carcinoma. *Ann Oncol* 1997;8(5):423–427.

Haak HR, Hermans J, Van deVelde CJ, et al. Optimal treatment of adrenocortical carcinoma with mitotane: results in a consecutive series of 96 patients. *Br J Cancer* 1994;69:947.

Kasperlik-Zaluska AA, Migdalska BM, Makowska AM. Impact of adjuvant mitotane on the clinical course of patients with adrenocortical cancer: two years later [letter]. *Cancer* 1996;78(7):1520–1521.

McGrath PC, Sloan DA, Schwartz RW, Kenady DE. Current advances in the diagnosis and therapy of adrenal tumors. *Curr Opin Oncol* 1998; 10(1):52–57.

Miller JA, Norton JA. Multiple endocrine neoplasia. *Cancer Treat Res* 1997;90:213–225.

Wooten MD, King DK. Adrenal cortical carcinoma: epidemiology and treatment with mitotane and review of the literature. *Cancer* 1993; 72:3145–3155.

Pheochromocytoma

Bravo EL. Pheochromocytoma. *Curr Ther Endocrinol Metab* 1997; 6:195–197.

Francis IR, Korobkin M. Pheochromocytoma. *Radiol Clin North Am* 1996;34(6):1101–1112.

Kenady DE, McGrath PC, Sloan DA, Schwartz RW. Diagnosis and management of pheochromocytoma. *Curr Opin Oncol* 1997;9(1):61–67.

Loh KC, Fitzgerald PA, Matthay KK, Yeo PP, Price DC. The treatment of malignant pheochromocytoma with iodine-131 metaiodobenzylguanidine (13 1 I-MIBG): a comprehensive review of 116 reported patients. *J Endocrinol Invest* 1997;20(11):648–658.

Neumann HP, Bender BU, Januszewicz A, Janetschek G, Eng C. Inherited pheochromocytoma. *Adv Nephrol Necker Hosp* 1997;27: 361–376.

O'Riordan JA. Pheochromocytomas and anesthesia. *Int Anesthesiol Clin* 1997;35(4):99–127.

Werbel SS, Ober KP. Pheochromocytoma: update on diagnosis, localization, and management. *Med Clin North Am* 1995;79(1):131–153.

Young WF Jr. Pheochromocytoma: issues in diagnosis & treatment. *Compr Ther* 1997;23(5):319–326.

15

Melanoma and Other Skin Malignancies

Larry Nathanson

Our skin is the organ which protects us from our environment, and against which both physical and chemical agents in the environment are first directed. It should be no surprise, therefore, that the incidence of skin cancer far exceeds that of any other body organ and approached 1 million cases in 1998 (ACS Statistics for 1998). About 95% of these cases will be basal and squamous carcinoma of the skin and the rest a variety of tumors, including melanoma, carcinomas of the skin appendages, Merkel's cell tumor, Kaposi's and other sarcomas, and cutaneous lymphomas (see Chap. 23). Because melanoma accounts for more than 70% of about 11,000 deaths cause by skin cancers annually in the United States, it is emphasized in this chapter.

I. **Melanoma**
  A. **Natural history**
      1. **Etiology, epidemiology, and prevention.** The normal precursor cell of malignant melanoma is the cutaneous pigment-producing melanocyte. During embryologic development, these cells differentiate in the neural crest and migrate to the skin and eye. About 10% of melanoma occurs in some extradermal site; primarily the eye and mucous membranes of the oropharynx, anal, and urogenital tracts. In the United States, melanoma occurs slightly more commonly in men than women, is rare in children, and has a peak age of incidence at 46 to 48 years. Because of the relative youth of many melanoma patients, melanoma ranks next to testicular cancer in the average number of years of life lost per patient among adult cancers in the United States. The incidence of the disease has tripled since the 1970s in the "developed" nations of the world, with a current lifetime risk of about 1%. Melanoma is now the seventh most common cancer and accounted for about 41,000 new cases and 7,300 deaths in the United States in 1998 (ACS Cancer Statistics, 1998). The striking increase in incidence, the greatest for any cancer in the United States, is presumably due to increased exposure to actinic (primarily ultraviolet [UV] radiation). Although UV-B appears to be the most carcinogenic part of the spectrum, UV-A also appears to have some carcinogenic potential. Diminution in the tropospheric ozone layer, increase in leisure time, and use of scanty leisure clothing have all probably

contributed to this increase. Epidemiologic studies suggest that the greatest risk of melanoma is from intermittent intense sun exposure, especially in children. A melanoma-susceptible phenotype characterized by fair, photosensitive skin also plays a role in defining the high-risk individual. Non-Caucasians have a lower incidence of melanoma than do Caucasians. African Americans have about 15% the incidence of melanoma, have a shorter survival owing to presentation at a more advanced stage of disease, and have a far higher proportion of lesions arising on the feet (especially plantar aspect) than do Caucasians. Sunny parts of the United States have the highest incidence of the disease, especially Hawaii, Southern California, Florida, and Arizona–New Mexico. Patient education in prevention, including use of sun-protective clothing, avoidance of the brightest sunlit hours of the day, use of topical sunscreens, refraining from use of sun-tan parlors, and use of skin self-examination, should be a responsibility of every clinical oncologist.

2. **Precursor lesions, genetics, and familial melanoma.** Benign, congenital, and dysplastic nevi may be precursor lesions for melanoma. Dysplastic nevi may be sporadic or familial and, along with large numbers of benign nevi, constitute markers for melanoma risk. Careful follow-up should be carried out in patients with these risk factors and in the 10% of patients with a family history of the disease. The familial atypical multiple mole/melanoma (FAMMM) syndrome is characterized by earlier age of diagnosis, thinner and often multiple lesions, and a higher cure rate. Mutations in the tumor-suppressor gene CDKN-2 (p16ink4a), CDK-4, and possibly p15ink4b, have been discovered in familial melanoma. This suggests that in the future, identification of susceptibility genes will be markers for, or provide an explanation of, genetic predisposition to this disease. In the meantime, early excision of suspicious lesions or congenital lesions, such as giant hairy nevi, may result in prevention of melanoma that might otherwise prove fatal. In xeroderma pigmentosa, a rare autosomal recessive condition in which the skin lacks means to repair UV-induced DNA damage, multiple nonmelanoma and melanoma malignancies occur.

3. **Types and appearance of primary lesions.** The four major clinical types of primary cutaneous melanoma, in order of increasing aggressiveness, are (a) lentigo maligna melanoma, often flat, large (1- to 5-cm) lesions found pri-

marily on the sun-exposed surfaces of the skin in the elderly; (b) superficial spreading melanoma, the most common type, seen on all areas of the skin; (c) nodular melanoma, usually fairly symmetric with early direct invasion into the skin (most mucosal melanomas seem to have this pattern); and (d) acral lentiginous melanoma (ALM), primarily on the subungual, palmar, and plantar surfaces (not all lesions in these locations are ALM). When primary melanoma becomes malignant, it usually presents with a history of recent growth, in addition to the following signs or symptoms: change in pigmentation, ulceration, itching, or bleeding. On examination, these lesions have a tendency to have absence of hair follicles, irregular margins, and variegated coloration, with hues of brown, red, white, blue, and gray. They often are larger than 6 mm in diameter, have an irregular or pebbled appearance on their surface, and may have satellites. None of these signs is pathognomonic, and they are frequently present in mild degree in atypical or dysplastic lesions; but they help to distinguish malignant from benign lesions. Although primary melanomas have a characteristic histopathologic appearance, some are relatively undifferentiated. In these lesions, the use of immunochemical stains (S-100, HMB-45) may be of great help.

4. **Patterns of metastases.** At initial presentation, up to 20% of patients have disease that has spread beyond the local lesion (about 15% regional lymph nodes and 5% distant metastases). Of the patients (80% of the total) who do not have diagnosed metastatic melanoma at presentation, about 15% develop metastasis. Of these patients, one fifth experience soft tissue metastases alone (lymph node, skin, subcutaneous) and the other four fifths visceral (especially lung, liver, brain, and bone), with or without soft tissue, metastases. Pregnancy during, before, or after diagnosis of primary melanoma does not appear to affect prognosis. About 5% of melanomas present with metastases (most often in regional nodes) without an identified primary melanoma. In these patients with unknown primary melanoma, either spontaneous primary regression, origin in an extracutaneous site, or some other mechanism is postulated to account for this pattern of presentation.

5. **Amelanotic melanoma** (about 1% to 2% of primaries) may have a somewhat worse prognosis; but this is controversial. Poorly pigmented primary or metastatic melanoma may present a

diagnostic challenge, and one should be suspicious of nonpigmented lesions that otherwise look or behave like melanoma.

6. **CNS metastasis.** One of the most vexing clinical problems in the treatment of this disease remains its predilection for development of central nervous system (CNS) metastases. Fully half of all cases that relapse, including those that have responded to systemic therapy in other sites, relapse in the CNS. Until this problem is solved, no attempt at systemic therapy will be successful.

7. **Ocular melanoma** arises predominantly in the uveal tract of the eye (choroid, ciliary body, iris) and is the most common malignancy of the eye in adults. Although enucleation was the standard treatment for this tumor in the past, sight preservation with local radiotherapy, surgery, or both is now being employed with promising, albeit preliminary, results. When metastatic (usually to the liver), this tumor appears to be less chemosensitive than its cutaneous counterpart.

B. **Staging.** Melanoma is staged based on the pathologically measured thickness of the primary tumor ("microstaging") and the extent of spread of metastatic tumor (see Table 15-1 for the current AJCC Staging system). The current AJCC Staging for melanoma (*AJCC Staging Manual,* 5th ed, 1997) has been widely criticized (Buzaid, 1997), and may soon be changed. Clinical staging is often unsatisfactory because of the poor resolution of available radiologic imaging modalities and the lack of a specific and sensitive blood test (serum S-100 is being studied as a marker). All patients should have a careful history and physical examination with special attention to the skin, mucous membranes, and regional lymph nodes. A chemistry profile (especially lactate dehydrogenase levels) may yield clues suggesting visceral metastases, and a chest x-ray may show pulmonary lesions. In addition, in primary melanomas thicker than 1.5 mm and in those with possible regional lymph node spread, the use of lymphoscintigraphy (lymphatic mapping) and blue dye or radionuclide probe studies (sentinel node identification) is indicated (for rationale for these tests, see Section I.C). Moreover, if abnormal signs, symptoms, or screening laboratory results are found, it may be cost-effective to consider ultrasonography, computed tomography, magnetic resonance imaging of the CNS, radionuclide bone scanning, or even positron emission tomography (if available). In follow-up of high-risk primary or node-positive patients, however, the history and physical examination yield the bulk of the useful diagnostic information, with chest x-rays occasionally being helpful (Table 15-2). Identification of circulating micrometastatic melanoma cells using reverse transcriptase polymerase chain reaction to detect

Table 15-1.   Staging and survival for melanoma

AJCC Stage	TNM classification	Site	Approximate 5-Yr survival rate (%)
		Primary Tumor Only—Thickness in Millimeters	
0	pTis	Carcinoma *in situ*	100
I	pT1	<0.75	97
	pT2	>0.75–1.5	90
II	pT3a	>1.5–3	85
	pT3b	>3–4	75
III	pT4a	>4	56
	pT4b	Local satellite metastasis (≤2 cm from primary)	48
	N1	Lymph nodes ≤3 cm	40
	N2a	Lymph nodes >3 cm	22
	N2b	"In transit" metastases	35
	N2c	Both N2a and N2b	22
IV	M1a	Distant metastasis in skin, subcutaneous tissue, or lymph nodes beyond regional nodes	10
	M1b	Distant visceral metastasis	5

From American Joint Committee on Cancer. *AJCC Cancer Staging Manual,* 5th ed. Philadelphia: Lippincott-Raven, 1997, pp 163–167.

melanoma-specific mRNA is now being studied as a method for finding patients whose disease is likely to recur.

C. **Prognosis and surgical treatment**. To microstage primary tumors optimally, the standard surgery for pigmented lesions suspected of being melanoma is excisional (not shave or incisional) biopsy. This is followed by reexcision: 1-cm tumor-free margin on all sides of the lesion for lentigo maligna melanoma and other melanomas of less than 1-mm thickness; 2-cm tumor-free margin for all other primary melanomas if technically possible. Survival of patients with an excised primary lesion varies inversely with the thickness of the lesion. Favorable factors also include female gender, extremity location (compared with trunk, head, or neck), and lack of ulceration of the primary (primary type is weak factor; see previo⌐ discussion, I.A.3). If elective lymph node dissecti⌐ primary melanoma is being considered, lym⌐ mapping (identification of the regional drair⌐ basin by use of lymphoscintography) m⌐

**Table 15-2.   Recommended staging
and follow-up tests for melanoma**

When	Tests	Follow-up interval
At presentation with and during follow-up of primary melanoma	Physical (including complete skin) examination History Chest radiograph CBC and chemistries (including LDH) Lymphatic mapping, sentinel node identification, and ELND may stage patients for adjuvant therapy Other studies as suggested by positive findings on above panel	Every 2 mo for six exams, then every 4 mo for three exams, then every 6 mo for six exams, then every year thereafter
At presentation with, and during follow-up of, nodal metastases	Physical examination CBC and chemistries (including LDH) Chest radiograph (or thoracic CT) Therapeutic node dissection Other studies as suggested by positive findings	Every 3 mo for four exams, then every 6 mo for eight exams, then every year thereafter
At presentation with, and during follow-up of, distant metastases	In treated patients, follow sites of measurable or active disease; otherwise limit to supportive care	Follow-up visits as indicated primarily by concern for quality of life

CBC, complete blood count; LDH, lactic dehydrogenase; CT, computed tomography; ELND, elective lymph node dissection.

cated for melanoma in skin regions where the node basin is ambiguous. It has been established that each lymph node basin possesses a sentinel node in which tumor cells first appear. When free of tumor, this node correctly predicts a tumor-free lymphatic basin and precludes the necessity of node basin dissection; if tumor is found, node dissection is mandated. Although elective lymph node dissection has not been shown to improve survival in patients with primary lesions of any thickness, sentinel lymph node identification (discussed earlier) and resection for staging, in anticipation of the use of adjuvant therapy, should be considered. Whether lymphatic mapping and sentinel node identification require two procedures or may be accomplished in a single step has yet to be determined. Surgery in carefully selected patients with metastatic disease may yield great benefit in the following circumstances: (a) for cytoreduction before systemic therapy (e.g., in patient with regional lymph node or visceral metastases); (b) for palliation in selected patients with one or two metastatic foci, in whom surgery may prolong survival and alleviate symptoms (e.g., in patients with CNS or pulmonary metastases); and (c) occasionally with curative intent (e.g., in patients with soft tissue or pulmonary metastases).

D. **Adjuvant therapy.** The report of a large randomized adjuvant trial of interferon-α_{2b} (IFN-α_{2b}) in patients with AJCC stages IIb (more than 4-mm thick primary tumor) and III (regional lymph node positive) melanoma, after elective or therapeutic lymph node dissection (ECOG trial 1684) has demonstrated that statistically significant prolongation of overall survival can be achieved in these patient subsets. The dose of IFN-α_{2b} is 20×10^6 IU/m^2 i.v. 5 days a week for 4 weeks followed by 10×10^6 IU/m^2 s.c. 3 days a week for 48 weeks (total duration of therapy, 1 year). Toxicity (influenza-like syndrome, hepatic and CNS abnormalities) is significant, but a careful quality-of-life analysis (Q-TWiST) demonstrated overall benefit. A subsequent ECOG trial (E 1690) also showed a disease-free survival benefit, but no overall survival benefit. Thus the role of adjuvant interferon is not certain. Adjuvant use of regional arteriovenous heated chemotherapy (usually melphalan) perfusion in patients with high-risk extremity melanoma has been reported to benefit this group of patients, but a larger repeat study (EORTC/WHO) has refuted this finding.

E. **Therapy of metastases**
   1. **Chemotherapy**
      a. **Patient selection.** Melanoma is relatively refractory to systemic therapy. Therefore, when patients are being considered as candidates for such therapy, factors predictive of favorable response must be kept in mind. These factors include good performance status (ECOG grades 0-2); Soft tissue or single visceral (pulmonary most sensitive) sites of metastases; young age (less than 65 years); no prior chemotherapy; normal hemogram and renal and hepatic function; and absence of CNS metastases.
      b. **Single-agent chemotherapy.** The response rates of the various agents to which melanoma has been reported to be sensi-

tive vary considerably as reported by different authors (Table 15-3): single institution studies tend to have higher response rates than cooperative groups. Doses are for single-agent treatment.

(1) Dacarbazine (DTIC), remains the standard single agent for the treatment of metastatic melanoma. Usually administered at a dose of 200 mg/m^2 i.v. on days 1 to 5 every 3 weeks, or 750 mg/m^2 i.v. on day 1 every 6 weeks. Response rate is 20% to 25%.

(2) Nitrosoureas have been used in melanoma and probably have about equal efficacy. Carmustine (BCNU), 150 mg/m^2 i.v. is given as a single dose every 6 weeks, *or* lomustine (CCNU), is given in a dosage of 100 to 130 mg/m^2 p.o. once every 3 to 6 weeks. Response rates are about 15% to 20%.

(3) Platinum-containing drugs. Cisplatin, 100 mg/m^2 i.v. every 3 weeks, *or* carboplatin, 400 mg/m^2 i.v. every 3 weeks, appears to have similar efficacy. The dose of the latter drug may be cautiously escalated. Response rates are 15% to 20%.

(4) Taxanes. Paclitaxel (Taxol), 135 to 215 mg/m^2 is given in 3-hour i.v. infusions every 3 weeks, *or* docetaxel (Taxotere), 60 to 100 mg/m^2 is given in 1-hour i.v. infusion every 3 weeks. Response rates are 10% to 15%.

Table 15-3.   Systemic chemotherapy for melanoma

Single agents	Estimated objective response rate (%)
Standard	
Dacarbazine	20
Nitrosoureas (BCNU, CCNU)	18
Cisplatin	16
Carboplatin	15 (?)
Paclitaxel	14
Vinca alkaloids (VCR, VLB)	14
Ifosfamide (with mesna)	10
Procarbazine	10–12
Dactinomycin	10–12
Biologic	
Interferon- α (2a or 2b)	15
Interleukin-2 (high dose)	15–20

(5) **Dactinomycin, ifosfamide (plus mesna), alkylating agents, vinca alkaloids, and procarbazine** at the appropriate doses all have been demonstrated to have response rates of 10% to 15%.

(6) **Experimental drugs** recently reported to have activity in melanoma include Temozolomide (an oral imidazole) and fotemustine (a nitrosourea). Both have substantial CNS penetration and possible anti-CNS metastases responses.

c. **Multiagent chemotherapy.** Two of the most commonly used regimens with data from a significant number of patients are shown in Table 15-4. However, even these chemotherapy combinations do not solve two problems that have plagued the oncologist. First, the median duration response is rarely greater than 6 months, and the median survival time is rarely greater than 10 months. Second, systemic polychemotherapy does not appear to effectively prevent or treat CNS metastases. Recent randomized studies of polychemotherapy versus single-agent regimens have not achieved significant differences in survival, even though somewhat higher response rates have been consistently re-

Table 15-4.   Multiagent systemic therapy for melanoma

Regimen	Drug dosages
DBD	DTIC (dacarbazine), 220 mg/m^2/d on days 1–3 every 3 wk BCNU (carmustine), 150 mg/m^2/d on day 1 every 6 wk DDP (cisplatin), 25 mg/m^2/d on days 1–3 every 3 wk
CVD	DDP (cisplatin) 20 mg/m^2/d on days 1–4 for 3 wks VLB (vinblastine) 1.6 mg/m^2/d on days 1–4 for 3 wks DTIC (dacarbazine) 800 mg/m^2 on day 1 only for 3 wks
Biochemo-therapy (see Legha, 1997)	CVD as above, together with: Interleukin-2, 9 MIU/m^2 qd by continuous i.v. infusion days 1–4 (96 h)* Interferon-α_{2b}, 5 MU/m^2 s.c. on days 1–5, 7, 9, 11, and 13 GCSF 5 µg/kg s.c. qd on days 7–16 Repeat cycle every 21 d for maximum of four cycles

*On day 1, begin IL-2 2 to 3 hours after chemotherapy.

ported for multiagent programs. We must conclude that no program has demonstrated consistent superiority to justify the label "standard regimen."

2. **Hormones.** Tamoxifen, 20 to 60 mg/day p.o. (see McClay, 1996) and megestrol, 40 to 80 mg q.i.d. p.o. (see Nathanson, 1994) appear to have no significant antitumor activity when used alone in patients with metastatic tumor; but when used concurrently with chemotherapeutic agents, these drugs may potentiate the activity of some cytotoxic agents. This finding, however, must still be considered controversial. In a preliminary small randomized study, now being repeated, megestrol was found to have benefit as an adjuvant treatment for high-risk AJCC stage II and III melanoma (Creagan et al., 1989).

3. **Biologic response modifiers**

   a. **Interferon-α$_{2a}$** (Intron A) and **interferon-α$_{2b}$** (Roferon), 3 to 50×10^6 IU/m^2 s.c, i.m., or i.v. administered three to five times per week, have been found to have an objective response rate of 10% to 15% in a variety of studies. Time to onset of response may be somewhat longer than that seen with chemotherapeutic agents.

   b. **Interleukin-2** (IL-2; Proleukin, aldesleukin) is an agent that, when used in high doses (600,000 IU/kg given in 15-minute i.v. infusions every 8 hours for a total of 14 doses) produces responses from 15% to 20%, some of long duration. This drug is associated with a capillary-leak syndrome and other severe toxic manifestations and usually requires inpatient care; it should only be used by those experienced in its administration. Low-dose, outpatient use of IL-2 is of questionable efficacy. The use of IL-2 and IFN-α together has also been reported; however, whether a truly additive clinical benefit is achieved is controversial.

4. **Biochemotherapy.** In one carefully implemented large study (see Legha, 1997 and Table 15-4) employing initial use of chemotherapy followed by biotherapy with both IFN and IL-2, 17% of patients achieved measurable complete responses that were durable (greater than 18 months). Moreover, 9% of patients experienced complete responses lasting longer than 3 years, leading to the conclusion that the regimen has curative potential. Substantial toxicity is encountered in such studies, and experience and strong medical support are required for their implementation. Moreover, a metaanalysis of small studies (some randomized) has reported

29% versus 41% objective response rates and 8.6 versus 9.8 month median survival durations for polychemotherapy regimens versus biochemotherapy, respectively—a modest gain indeed for a toxic and complex regimen.

F. Regional therapy

1. **Extremity perfusion.** Arteriovenous cannulation and perfusion with heated solution of chemotherapeutic agents (melphalan, nitrogen mustard [Mustargen], cisplatin, tumor necrosis factor-α [TNF-α, an experimental agent]) and other agents has consistently yielded higher tissue drug concentrations and objective response rates than has use of the same agents delivered by the intravenous route. In a randomized adjuvant study, however, this approach did not achieve superior survival, and when used (generally with soft tissue metastases) in patients with measurable regional disease, survival superiority is questionable. Because of the toxicity, cost, and technical expertise required, its usefulness has been questioned. One (nonrandomized) study suggested that the same results could be achieved with the same agents delivered with hyperthermia by intraarterial infusion. Hepatic arterial infusion therapy is uniquely suited to the metastatic pattern of ocular melanoma in the liver, where such infusion may encompass the critical mass of the tumor.

2. **Intralesional bacillus Calmette-Guérin** (BCG) has been primarily used in patients with extremity primary tumors with the in-transit (intradermal and subcutaneous) pattern of metastases (AJCC stage N2b). This pattern of metastases (2–3% of patients) is more common following regional lymph node dissection. It is more effective in patients with intradermal tumors and with fewer than 10 lesions, and it is associated with about an 80% overall response rate in injected lesions and with a 15% complete response rate. In both injected and uninjected lesions IFN-α, granulocyte-macrophage colony-stimulating factor, and other reagents have also been used intralesionally with varying degrees of success.

3. **Treatment of CNS metastases** should start with dexamethasone, 10 mg i.v. bolus, followed by 4 mg every 6 hours p.o. This should be accompanied as soon as possible by radiotherapy given by stereotactic or three-dimensional conformal techniques, if available, usually with whole-brain boost. In patients with solitary lesions, neurosurgical extirpation followed by radiotherapy may yield a significant group of survivors over one year who experience good quality of life.

4. **Intracavitary therapy** with thiotepa, bleomycin, or doxycycline may be of benefit in reducing the volume and rate of accumulation of intraperitoneal or intrapleural effusions. Each of these drugs must be administered (usually in multiple doses) through an indwelling thoracotomy tube.

5. **Radiotherapy** is of variable efficacy in the treatment of the regional or bony metastases but sometimes may yield gratifying symptomatic benefit. One group (Ang, 1994) has employed radiotherapy as an adjuvant in the treatment of high-risk regional lymph node positive head and neck melanoma in a nonrandomized trial, and reported an apparent significant survival benefit. This approach is being restudied in a randomized format by the Eastern Cooperative Oncology Group (E 3697). Trials on the use of radioprotectants, or radiopotentiators, are ongoing.

G. **Experimental and future therapies**

1. **Immunotherapy.** Active immunotherapeutic whole-cell vaccines have undergone extensive trials in patients with measurable disease. At least two, polyvalent melanoma cell vaccine (PMCV) and Melacine, have achieved objective responses as well as a suggestion of prolongation of survival in patients with nonbulky metastatic tumor. They are both being tested in large multiinstitutional adjuvant studies (John Wayne Cancer Institute and Southwest Oncology Group [SWOG 9035] respectively). A purified ganglioside, GM-2KLH/QS-21 (Livingston et al., 1994), has demonstrated prolongation of survival of patients in whom the vaccine is optimally immunogenic and is now being tested in an adjuvant setting (ECOG E1694). Other studies of a partially purified polyvalent vaccine and vaccinia-infected melanoma cell lysates are underway. Within a few years, the efficacy of such vaccines will be known; in the meantime, many clinical oncologists may wish to enroll their patients in such on-going trials.

2. **Gene therapy** is directed at an *ex vivo* adoptive cellular approach in which tumor or immunocompetent cells are transfected with genes coding for immunogenic elements (such as B-7 or CD-80/86) or antitumor cytokines (such as IL-2 or TNF-α) and then reinfused into the patient. Such clinical studies are underway in melanoma patients.

3. **Antiangiogenic factors** are being studied in melanoma because of its rich tumor vasculature (and subsequent tendency to demonstrate clinical bleeding in the skin or gastrointestinal tract). A new variation on this theme is the finding that certain peptides, to which cytotoxic

drugs can be bound, may selectively adhere to tumor vascular endothelial cells, allowing selective targeting of the respective chemotherapeutic agents.

II.   Nonmelanoma skin cancer

A.   Etiology and epidemiology. Cancer arising in the basal (BCC) and squamous (SCC) cells of the skin is the most common type of human malignancy, with an estimated 1,000,000 cases and 2,300 deaths in the United States in 1998 (ACS Statistics, 1998). About 80% of these are BCC and 20% SCC. Both are more common in men than in women, and although they are seen predominantly in the elderly, they are becoming more common in younger individuals. Whereas BCC occurs almost exclusively in those with fair photosensitive complexions, SCC is frequently present in individuals with darker skin as well. Both occur primarily in sun-exposed areas of the skin, have increased in incidence rapidly in the past few decades, and are primarily caused by cumulative UV-B and UV-A exposure. Consequently, unlike melanoma, people with outdoor occupations have a higher risk of SCC and BCC; although risk of developing BCC is more closely related to childhood exposure. UV damage to epidermal keratinocytes may produce inactivating mutations in the p53 gene (responsible for apoptosis and cell growth control), which in turn leads to skin cancer. Multiple cancers are common in predisposed patients. Other etiologic factors include chronic scarring and burns (especially SCC), chronic inflammation, irradiation to the skin, and arsenic exposure. Treatment with psoralen UV light (PUVA) and immunosuppressive agents, are risk factors for both SCC and BCC. Preventive measures (see Section I.A.1) should be employed, especially in high-risk individuals. Diagnosis of all of the malignant dermatoses is made by biopsy, which may be shave, incisional, or excisional, depending on the clinical setting.

B.   Premalignant lesions

   1.   Actinic (solar) keratosis

   a.   Natural history. These lesions are common, are found primarily on the exposed surfaces of the skin in photosensitive people, are usually multiple, and present as a reddish patch of about 3 to 10 mm, sometimes with scales, arising from "within" the skin. They give rise predominantly to SCC, and in high-risk individuals, prevention (see Section I.A.1) is particularly important. The differential diagnosis includes seborrheic keratoses, which are often dark, verrucous lesions that appear "stuck on" the skin.

   b.   Topical chemotherapy. Fluorouracil is used as a 1% solution or cream (Efudex) on the face and as an up to 5% solution on the hands or arms. It is applied daily for 2 to 4 weeks by the patient, rubbing it in with the fingertips of a gloved hand (if gloves are not used, the hand should be immediately washed). Care should be taken with periorbital application. It should be applied smoothly to avoid accumulation in the skin folds. Erythema followed by desquamation, erosion (with tenderness), and reepithelialization begin 3 to 7 days after treatment. The drug should be stopped as soon as erosion is observed. The reaction resolves rapidly, and lesions on the face heal within 2 to 6 weeks (this takes somewhat longer on the arms). Repeat courses may be used. An overly brisk reaction to EFUDEX may be treated with topical steroids. Mechanism of action of the drug may include both cytotoxic effects and possibly delayed-type hypersensitivity to the drug (causing slough of the lesion).

2. **Leukoplakia.** Leukoplakia presents as white plaques on the oral, genital, or anal mucous membranes. It progresses to dysplasia and carcinoma *in situ* in about 2% of patients. Because of its association with smoking, alcohol ingestion, and poor dental hygiene, avoidance of these behaviors is necessary for effective treatment. Standard treatment is surgery, with conventional, laser, or cryogenic techniques. Fluorouracil cream (Efudex) or adherent paste can be applied to the lesions as described previously. Use of oral systemic 13-*cis*-retinoic acid (isotretinoin) has been effective in some studies but remains controversial.

C. **Basal cell carcinoma**
1. **Natural history.** Histologically, this tumor consists of basaloid cells that arise from the basal layer of the epidermis and infiltrate into the dermis. The most common type of BCC is the nodular-ulcerative type ("rodent ulcer"). It presents as a well-defined nodule that has rolled, pearly, or translucent edges traversed by telangiectasis and a central concave area that is often ulcerated. Histologic subtypes of this tumor include solid, keratotic, cystic, and adenoid. A pigmented type exists that is often nodular and may resemble malignant melanoma; the pigmented basal cell epithelioma. The differential diagnosis of BCC and SCC includes keratoacanthoma, a rapidly growing, reddish, hyperkeratotic, papule. It has a rolled border like BCC and a central keratin plug and usually undergoes spontaneous regression within about 6 months. BCC may also have superficial, scle-

rosing, cystic, and multicentric forms. BCC has a low metastatic potential, and 85% of these tumors occur on the skin of the head and neck. In patients with neglected disease (0.1% to 0.2%), metastases may occur an average of 11 years after the lesion was first noted. Lymph nodes, lung, and bone are involved, in decreasing order of frequency.

2. **Treatment.** Superficial surgery, electrodesiccation, chemosurgery (Mohs' procedure), or irradiation (often electron beam), are equally effective (about 95% cure rate) and may be chosen based on the individual needs of the patient, anatomic area to be treated, or facilities available. Chemosurgery involves use of zinc chloride fixative paste in two stages, with biopsies at each stage to determine the margins of the lesion. Use of fluorouracil solution or ointment (see Section II.B.1.b) is restricted to multiple widespread or resistant lesions and is not effective in thick (more than 2 to 3 mm) or invasive lesions.

D. **Squamous cell carcinoma**
1. **Natural history.** On histopathologic examination, the primary lesion is in the epidermis, with cells penetrating into the dermis. Keratinization and epidermal pearl formation are often present. The degree of cellular differentiation, atypicality of cells, and depth of penetration of the tumor are prognostic indicators. SCC may occur on any site on the skin as well as on the mucous membranes of the lips, vulva, penis, and anus. The area from which SCC arises rarely appears normal but usually has the changes associated with actinic damage or keratosis. The latter process sometimes constitutes an *in situ* state of SCC. The exceptional lesions that arise in normal-appearing skin or in other preexisting conditions (scars of chemical, thermal, or radiation injury) tend to be more aggressive than those that arise in actinically damaged skin. A rough, scaly surface with thickening of the skin and often well-circumscribed macular changes is frequently present. Crusting, thickening, ulceration, or induration of the border strongly suggests malignant change. About 0.2% of patients develop metastatic tumors, and 90% of these metastases are only to lymph nodes. About half of the patients with spread to lymph nodes and 60% of those with distant metastases die of the disease.

2. **Treatment.** After histopathologic diagnosis, surgery employing a variety of techniques, as in BCC, is the conventional treatment for SCC. The choices include curettage and desiccation.

Chemosurgery, cryotherapy, and radiotherapy are all used in appropriate circumstances, and all are associated with cure rates in excess of 94%. Because of the tendency to infiltrate through adjacent tissue, therapeutic results in recurrent lesions may be less satisfactory, and prompt and adequate surgery, or other therapy, is important. Superficial SCC may be effectively controlled with 1% to 5% topical fluorouracil (see Section II.B.1.b) when used for 3 to 12 weeks. With more invasive lesions, when infiltrative disease may be present, 20% fluorouracil under occlusive dressing may be tried. More often, if not contraindicated, surgery or another modality is the treatment of choice in these patients.

E. **Skin appendage (adnexal) carcinomas**
   1. **Natural history.** These are a heterogenous group of tumors arising in the hair follicles, eccrine and apocrine sweat, and sebaceous glands. Many may present a histopathologic diagnostic puzzle, and most are slow growing and only locally invasive. They are rarely metastatic.
   2. **Treatment.** After histologic diagnosis, adequate surgical therapy with generous tumor-free margins should be carried out. Local radiotherapy may be helpful with local recurrence. The tumors are too rare to have a standard chemotherapeutic regimen for metastatic lesions.

F. **Merkel's carcinoma**
   1. **Natural history.** These uncommon tumors arise from the small, round undifferentiated neuroendocrine Merkel's cells in the basal layer of the epidermis and the hair follicles. Cells may be distributed in solid, trabecular, or diffuse patterns. Merkel's carcinoma occurs largely in elderly Caucasians, equally in men and women, and often on the sun-exposed area of the head and neck. It presents as a rapidly enlarging, nontender, firm, bluish-red, shiny nodule. Its progression is aggressive with a tendency to recur locally as well as spreading to lymph node and distant sites. Dermatofibrosarcoma protuberans is a locally aggressive tumor that should be considered in the differential diagnosis of Merkel's carcinoma.
   2. **Treatment.** Early wide local surgical excision with elective lymph node dissection and postoperative radiotherapy is recommended. The 3-year cure rates is about 50%, with women doing significantly better than men. Chemotherapy with cisplatin and etoposide with or without cyclophosphamide yields a modest objective response rate.

G.   Kaposi's sarcoma
1. **Natural history.** This tumor originates in cells of the vascular system, frequently of the skin, and presents as macular, painless, violaceous or red lesions of variable size. The disease was first described as occurring predominantly in elderly men of Mediterranean origin, often in the lower extremities. A new herpes virus (KSHV) appears to be etiologic. An indolent process, it does have the potential for spread to distant skin, lung, or gastrointestinal sites. Other types of the disease, found in Bantu men, African children, immunosuppressed graft recipients, and patients with human immunodeficiency virus infection (see Chap. 26), may have a more aggressive clinical course.
2. **Treatment.** Radiotherapy (usually electron beam) may be successful in controlling the cutaneous stage of the disease. With systemic manifestations of the disease, either metastatic or paraneoplastic therapy with vinca alkaloids, etoposide, or anthracyclines (including liposomal preparations), often in low doses, may be useful.

H.   Cutaneous T-cell lymphoma
1. **Natural history.** These rare neoplasms of T-cell derivation include cutaneous lymphoma, Sézary syndrome, and mycosis fungoides. They all appear to be epidermatotropic, or of dermal origin. The clinical presentation is with erythematous, sometimes scaling, macular, plaquelike, or tumorous lesions, often on the non–sun-exposed surfaces. The differential diagnosis includes adult T-cell leukemia or lymphoma and Ki-1 large cell anaplastic lymphoma.
2. **Treatment.** In the cutaneous phase of the disease, local therapy, including radiotherapy (electron beam), topical nitrogen mustard (or other cytotoxic), PUVA, and *ex vivo* photopheresis, may be curative. However, when systemic, the disease is rarely curable and is treated like systemic T-cell lymphoma.

SELECTED READINGS

Melanoma

Ang KK, Peters LJ, Weber RS, et al. Postoperative radiotherapy for cutaneous melanoma of the head and neck region. *Int J Radiat Oncolo Biol Phys* 1994;30:795–798.

Balch CM, Urist MM, Karakousis CP, et al. Efficacy of 2 cm. surgical margins for intermediate thickness cutaneous melanoma (1-4 mm.): results of a multi-institutional randomized surgical trial. *Ann Surg* 1993;218:262.

Balch CM, Houghton AN, Milton GW, et al., eds. *Cutaneous melanoma,* 3rd ed. Philadelphia: Lippincott-Raven, 1998:1.

Bedikian AY, Legha SS, Mavligit G, et al. Treatment of uveal melanoma metastatic to the liver. *Cancer* 1995;76:1665.

Bedikian AY, Weiss GR, Legha SS, et al. Phase II trial of docetaxel in patients with advanced melanoma previously untreated with chemotherapy. *J Clin Oncol* 1995;13:2895.

Buzaid AC, Tinoco L, Ross MI, et al. Role of computed tomography in the staging of patients with local-regional metastases of melanoma. *J Clin Oncol* 1995;13:2104.

Buzaid AC, Ross MI, Balch CM, et al. Critical analysis of the current AJC Committee on Cancer Staging system for cutaneous melanoma and proposal of a new staging system. *J Clin Oncol* 1997;15:1039.

Dalgleish A. The case for therapeutic vaccines. *Melanoma Res* 1996;6:5.

Creagan ET, Ingle JN, Schutt AJ, et al. A prospective randomized controlled trial of megestrol acetate among high-risk patients with resected melanoma. *Am J Clin Oncol* 1989;12:152.

Hwu P. The gene therapy of cancer. *PPO Updates* 1995;9(4):1–13.

Garrison M, Nathanson L. Prognosis and staging in melanoma. *Semin Oncol* 1996;23:725.

Haluska FG, Hodi FS. Molecular genetics of familial melanoma. *J Clin Oncol* 1998;16:670.

Kirkwood JM, Strawderman MH, Ernstoff MS, et al. Interferon alfa 2b adjuvant therapy of high-risk resected cutaneous melanoma: the Eastern Cooperative Oncology Group trial EST 1684. *J Clin Oncol* 1996;14:7.

Legha SS. Durable complete responses in melanoma treated with interleukin 2 in combination with interferon alfa and chemotherapy. *Semin Oncol* 1997;24:S4–39.

Legha SS, Ring S, Eton O, et al. Development of a biochemotherapy regimen with concurrent administration of cisplatin, vinblastine, darcarbazine, interferon alfa, and interleukin-2 for patients with metastatic melanoma. *J Clin Oncol* 1998;16:1752–1759.

Livingston PO, Wong GYC, Adluri S, et al. Improved survival in stage III melanoma patients with GM-2 antibodies: a randomized trial of adjuvant vaccination with GM-2 ganglioside. *J Clin Oncol* 1994;12:1036.

Margolin K, Liu P-Y, Flaherty L, et al. Phase II study of BCNU, DTIC, cisplatin (DDP) and tamoxifen (Tam) in advanced melanoma: a Southwest Oncology Group study. *J Clin Oncol* 1998;16:664–669.

McClay EF, guest ed. Melanoma. *Semin Oncol* 1996;23:649–783.

Miller K, Abeles G, Oratz R, et al. Improved survival of patient with melanoma with an antibody response to immunization to a polyvalent melanoma vaccine. *Cancer* 1995;75:495.

Mitchell MS, Jakowatz J, Harel W, et al. Increased effectiveness of interferon alfa-2b following active specific immunotherapy for melanoma. *J Clin Oncol* 1994;12:402.

Morton DL, Wen DR, Wong JH, et al. Technical details of intraoperative lymphatic mapping for early stage melanoma. *Arch Surg* 1992;127:392.

Morton DL, Foshag LJ, Hoon DSB, et al. Prolongation of survival in metastatic melanoma after active specific immunotherapy with a new polyvalent melanoma vaccine. *Ann Surg* 1992;216:463.

Nathanson L, ed. *Current research and clinical management of melanoma.* Boston: Kluwer Academic, 1993:1–388.

Nathanson L, Meelu MA, Losada R. Chemohormonal therapy of metastatic melanoma with megestrol plus dacarbazine, carmustine, and cisplatin. *Cancer* 1994;73:98.

Nathanson L. Interferon adjuvant therapy of melanoma. *Cancer* 1996;78:944.

Rosenberg SA. Cancer vaccines based on the identification of genes encoding cancer regression antigens. *Immunol Today* 1997;18:175.

Nonmelanoma Skin Cancer

Preston DS, Stern RS. Non-melanoma cancers of the skin. *N Engl J Med* 1992;327:1649.

Safai B. Management of skin cancer. In: DeVita VT, Hellman S, Rosenberg SA, eds. *Cancer: principles and practice of oncology,* 5th ed. Philadelphia: Lippincott-Raven, 1997:1879.

Fleming ID, Amonette R, Monaghan T, et al. Principles of management of basal and squamous carcinoma of the skin. *Cancer* 1995;75:699.

16

Primary and Metastatic Brain Tumors

Jane B. Alavi

I. **Occurrence and tumor characteristics**
   A. **Primary brain tumors**
      1. **Incidence.** Primary tumors of the brain result in 2% to 3% of all deaths caused by cancer. The overall incidence in the United States is about 5 per 100,000 population, but in children under the age of 14 years, the incidence is 6.5 per 100,000. These tumors account for about 20% of all cancers in children.
      2. **Histology.** Most intracranial neoplasms arise from meningeal or neuroectodermal tissue. Meningiomas (which arise from the meninges) are generally benign and encapsulated and can be removed surgically. They are rarely malignant (sarcomatous), and chemotherapy has no role in their treatment. Gliomas account for two thirds of primary brain tumors. They arise from astrocytes (astrocytoma and glioblastoma), oligodendroglia (oligodendroglioma), and the ependymal cells that line the ventricles (ependymoma). Medulloblastomas and primitive neuroectodermal tumors (pineoblastoma and cerebral neuroblastoma) arise from unknown precursor cells, are highly malignant, and have a propensity to spread by the cerebrospinal fluid (CSF) to the surface of the spinal cord. The astrocytomas occur within a broad range of histologic differentiation. The well-differentiated tumors can be cured by surgery. The more highly malignant types—anaplastic astrocytoma and glioblastoma—are not curable. Primitive ectodermal tumors (medulloblastoma, pineoblastoma, and cerebral neuroblastoma) tend to be more sensitive to the effects of radiation therapy and chemotherapy than the gliomas, and the prognosis is therefore better despite their aggressive nature. During childhood, two thirds of the neoplasms are found in the cerebellum or brainstem, and the common histologic types are medulloblastoma, ependymoma, and low-grade astrocytoma. Fewer than 20% are glioblastoma. In contrast, primary tumors in adults are nearly always supratentorial, more than 50% are glioblastomas, and about 18% are meningiomas.
      3. **Staging.** The astrocytomas remain localized to the brain throughout the disease course. Thus,

staging is not necessary. The prognosis depends on the degree of histologic malignancy. For medulloblastomas, staging should include magnetic resonance imaging (MRI) of the spine and cytology examination of the CSF.

B. Metastatic (secondary) brain tumors. The overall incidence of metastatic tumors to the brain is higher than the incidence of primary brain tumors in adults. About 20% of patients with cancer are found to have brain metastases at autopsy. The most common primary sites are the lung (all cell types) and breast. Metastases from melanoma, colorectal carcinoma, unknown primary tumors, and renal carcinoma occur less frequently. Some rare tumors, such as choriocarcinomas, give rise to brain metastases with unusual frequency. Most brain metastases are found in the cerebral hemispheres, few are found in the cerebellum or midbrain, and most are multiple at the time of diagnosis. Meningeal metastases are seen less frequently, and the primary tumors are usually breast or lung cancers, lymphoma, or melanoma.

II. Approach to therapy: primary and metastatic brain tumors

A. Primary tumors

1. **Surgery.** Surgical removal depends on the location of the lesion, its size, and its propensity to infiltrate surrounding areas of the brain. Because gliomas tend to infiltrate normal brain tissue surrounding the obvious tumor mass, it is unusual to cure patients with surgery alone without resultant unacceptable neurologic deficits. Patients with small, low-grade astrocytomas, however, are often curable.

2. **Radiation therapy.** This form of therapy has a major role in the treatment of gliomas. The radiation dose to the tumor must exceed 5,000 cGy to achieve control. Partial brain irradiation is usually adequate. In the case of medulloblastomas, radiotherapy is applied to the entire neuraxis at lower doses after surgical extirpation of the primary lesion because these tumors tend to metastasize by shedding cells into the CSF.

3. **Chemotherapy.** Chemotherapy is used to treat patients with the more malignant gliomas, including the anaplastic astrocytomas, anaplastic oligodendrogliomas, and glioblastoma multiforme. Because of the highly malignant features of medulloblastoma, chemotherapy is often used to treat this tumor.

4. **Supportive care.** Because of their location in the central nervous system (CNS), intracranial tumors can cause serious neurologic symptoms, including seizures, headaches, and impairment of mental, motor, and sensory function. This dysfunction is the result of the combined effects

of the tumor and a variable degree of surrounding cerebral edema. Therapy is therefore directed toward reducing the edema as well as reducing the size of the malignant tumor mass. Nearly all patients should be evaluated by a physical therapist and may achieve considerable benefit.

B. **Metastatic tumors**
1. **Surgery.** Because metastatic cancers often do not extensively infiltrate the surrounding normal brain parenchyma, they can sometimes be easily resected. This measure should be attempted only when the metastasis is solitary, as revealed by computed tomography (CT) or MRI and when the patient's cancer is under good control systemically. In these circumstances, surgery followed by radiotherapy results in a longer survival period than is produced by radiotherapy alone (40 versus 15 weeks for lung cancers).
2. **Radiation therapy.** Whole-brain irradiation is employed for metastatic cancers. Small tumors (generally less than 4 cm in diameter) that are solitary or persistent after whole-brain irradiation can be treated with stereotactic radiosurgery. This technique uses a stereotactic frame and specialized external-beam focusing and is noninvasive. It permits a high dose of radiation to be delivered to a small region in a single fraction. It has also been applied to small gliomas.
3. **Chemotherapy.** Chemotherapy probably has a limited role in the treatment of cerebral metastases. The exception to this is that metastases from breast cancer sometimes respond well to the usual regimens for breast tumors. On the other hand, malignant meningeal infiltrates, also called *carcinomatous meningitis,* may respond to a combination of radiation therapy and intrathecal chemotherapy.
4. **Evaluation for a primary tumor.** Occasionally, a patient presents with brain metastases as the first manifestation of cancer. In most cases, there is little benefit gained by an extensive search for the primary site, if the history, physical examination, chest radiograph, blood cell count, and chemistry profile do not give a clue because the prognosis for patients with brain metastases is generally poor. An exception to this rule should be made if the patient is a young male in whom metastatic testicular cancer (and occasionally other germ cell tumors) can be cured despite brain metastases. In these patients, measuring α-fetoprotein and β-human chorionic gonadotropin levels is warranted. In

addition, small cell lung cancer sometimes responds well to chemotherapy and radiation therapy. Therefore, it is reasonable to perform a chest CT scan and biopsy of any lung tumor if the patient has a good performance status.

III. Chemotherapy

A. General considerations

1. **Special characteristics of primary brain tumors.** The blood supply to brain tumors is not homogeneous owing to poorly vascularized areas of central necrosis. The tumor vessels lack the normal blood-brain barrier, but at the more rapidly growing outer edge of the tumor, the blood-brain barrier is mostly intact. Therefore, it has usually been assumed that the most effective chemotherapeutic agents are those that are lipid soluble or of relatively low molecular weight, such that they are able to cross the normal blood-brain barrier and achieve an adequate intracerebral concentration. Another requirement for the use of brain tumor chemotherapy is that it be able to achieve cell kill in a heterogeneous population of tumor cells, such as is found in malignant gliomas. An additional consideration is that a large percentage of the cells in gliomas appear to be in a resting state (G_0 phase) and thus are relatively insensitive to cell cycle–active agents.

2. **The two major aims of therapy for glioma** are to reduce the neurologic deficit and to prolong useful and comfortable life by reducing the tumor mass and associated edema. Surgical decompression, when possible, and radiation therapy are standard treatments. Adjuvant chemotherapy has been shown to prolong the survival of patients with anaplastic astrocytoma. Either carmustine (BCNU) or the PCV regimen (procarbazine, lomustine [CCNU], and vincristine) is commonly used, starting simultaneously with or immediately after radiation therapy and continuing for about 1 year. Anaplastic oligodendrogliomas are much more sensitive to chemotherapy than other types of gliomas. As many as 75% of patients may respond, some with complete disappearance of enhancing tumor. The PCV regimen is used, although there is interest in higher-dose regimens, including intensive therapy with stem cell rescue. All patients with this histologic type should receive adjuvant chemotherapy.

There is little evidence that adjuvant chemotherapy improves the survival time (median of less than 1 year) for glioblastoma. Survival has been shown to depend more on certain prognostic factors, such as patient age, performance status at diagnosis, and the extent of surgical resection. Therefore, adjuvant chemotherapy is usually offered only to glioblastoma patients who are younger than 50 years and in good general health. It is started during radiation therapy.

3. **Quality of life.** Quality of life is a complex issue with neurologic tumors because it depends largely on the type of deficit induced by the tumor (e.g., hemiparesis, aphasia, and inability to read or write). Treatment has been shown to improve quality of life somewhat.

4. **Response evaluation.** Responses are sometimes difficult to analyze because of symptoms due to edema, seizures, steroid therapy, and a fixed neurologic deficit from surgery. Nonetheless, regular neurologic examination with a scoring of the neurologic deficit and computed tomography (CT) or MRI scans of the brain usually enable the physician to make an objective determination of response. Scans are repeated every 2 to 3 months for the first year and less frequently thereafter.

B. **Specific chemotherapy agents**

1. **Nitrosoureas.** Nitrosoureas have been the most effective drugs against malignant gliomas and medulloblastomas. As first-line agents, these drugs result in responses in 30% to 50% of patients, with a median duration of about 6 months. When administered to patients with glioma as an adjuvant to radiation therapy, carmustine or lomustine appears to prolong survival minimally, compared with radiation therapy alone. The major benefit may be to young and middle-aged adults or to those with anaplastic astrocytoma rather than glioblastoma.

   a. **Carmustine (BCNU).** This is given usually at a dose of 80 mg/m^2 i.v. daily for 3 days every 6 to 8 weeks.

   b. **Lomustine (CCNU).** Lomustine may be given at a dose of 130 mg/m^2 p.o. once every 6 to 8 weeks.

   c. **Duration.** Two cycles are usually administered to patients with recurrent tumors. If a response is observed clinically or by CT, the drug is continued until progression is noted or a total dose of 1,200 mg/m^2 (of either drug) has been reached. Six cycles are given for adjuvant therapy.

   d. **Precautions.** These drugs may produce severe and delayed myelotoxicity. Some investigators decrease the dose by 25% in patients over the age of 60 years. All patients should have frequent blood cell counts during treatment, and subsequent doses should be lowered if there is a significant nadir: white blood cell (WBC) count less than 2,000/µL or platelet count less than 75,000/µL. Treatment to cumulative doses in excess of 1,200 mg/m^2 may be associated with pulmonary fibrosis that is usually irreversible and sometimes fatal. Less common toxicities are hepatotoxicity, renal toxicity, and phlebitis or pain in the arm used for treatment.

    2. **Combinations.** Vincristine and procarbazine are sometimes given together with a nitrosourea. The PCV regimen is a combination of procarbazine (60 mg/m^2 orally on days 8 to 21), lomustine (110 mg/m^2 orally on day 1), and vincristine (2 mg i.v. on days 8 and 29), repeated every 6 to 8 weeks. Other combinations or schedules have been used without clear advantage. Vincristine can be used at a dose of 1 to 2 mg/m^2 (maximum, 2 mg) i.v. weekly for up to 4 weeks; procarbazine can be given at a dose of 100 mg/m^2 p.o. daily for 2 weeks followed by a 2-week rest. Doses of the latter should be reduced if given with a nitrosourea.

C. **Primitive neuroectodermal tumors, including medulloblastoma: special considerations.** There is some evidence that adjuvant chemotherapy benefits high-risk patients (those with incomplete tumor resection, brainstem involvement, seeding to the subarachnoid space, or positive CSF cytology). One successful regimen consists of vincristine, 1.5 mg/m^2 (maximum, 2 mg) weekly during radiation therapy, followed by a 6-week break. This is then followed by lomustine 75 mg/m^2 p.o. on day 1; cisplatin, 68 mg/m^2 i.v. on day 1; and vincristine, 1.5 mg/m^2 (maximum, 2 mg) weekly for weeks 1 to 3 (days 1, 8, and 15). Cycles of the three-drug combination are repeated every 6 weeks for a total of eight cycles. This treatment results in considerable toxicity, especially pancytopenia and peripheral neuropathy. Patients must be followed very closely.

D. **Investigational therapy**

    1. **Recurrent gliomas.** In most patients with recurrent tumor after radiation therapy and primary chemotherapy with a nitrosourea, second-line chemotherapy offers little benefit. However, if the patient is young and has a good performance status, phase II trials of several available agents can be considered. Partial objective and symptomatic response rates to salvage chemotherapy are usually 15% to 25%, but complete responses are almost never observed. The drugs with activity include cisplatin (60 to 90 mg/m^2), carboplatin (350 to 500 mg/m^2 every 3 to 4 weeks), and etoposide (100 to 120 mg/m^2/day for 3 days). Tamoxifen in high doses (100 mg per day) is said to produce some responses. Interfer-

ons have not been very successful. Radiolabeled monoclonal antibodies or targeted toxins are being investigated at several centers. High-dose chemotherapy with stem cell rescue offers benefit to children and young adults with recurrent primitive neuroectodermal tumors, but not to those with gliomas. In adults, this approach has met with little success. The investigational drug temozolomide, an alkylating agent that is related to DTIC, has been successful in some clinical trials.

2. **Newer approaches.** Newer modalities for brain tumors include administration of drugs into the internal carotid artery to achieve higher-level doses. Intracarotid carmustine has been associated with severe ophthalmic and cerebral toxicity and cannot be recommended. Cisplatin by the intraarterial route does produce a large number of responses, but there is not yet evidence that this prolongs survival. Very-high-dose systemic chemotherapy with autologous bone marrow rescue is another investigational approach. Interferons do not appear to be effective. Interleukins and lymphokine-activated killer cells are being evaluated, but thus far there is little to suggest that biologic treatments are useful. Second surgical resection or brachytherapy may be used for localized recurrences. Surgically resectable recurrences may also be treated with implantation of BCNU-containing wafers, which supply the drug directly to the tumor bed, with delivery persisting for several weeks postoperatively. A low-dose wafer is commercially available, and higher doses are being evaluated. Gene therapy using direct injection of a virus vector into the tumor is another research approach. Although several different genes and vectors are under study, a commonly used technique is introduction of the herpes simplex thymidine kinase gene, which in theory would render the induced cells susceptible to cell kill by ganciclovir. The latter can be administered intravenously. Antiangiogenesis drugs and metalloproteinase inhibitors are in clinical trial.

E. **Meningeal carcinomatosis.** This is treated with radiation therapy to the symptomatic areas of the CNS (e.g., to the brain for cranial nerve dysfunction) together with intrathecal chemotherapy.

1. **Methotrexate.** The most commonly used agent is methotrexate, 12 mg/m^2 (maximum, 15 mg) per dose once or twice a week until the cytologic examination shows clearing of the CSF, then once a month as maintenance.

2. **Alternative agents.** Thiotepa, 2 to 10 mg/m^2, and cytosine arabinoside, 30 mg/m^2, are alternatives.

3. **Administration.** Each of these chemotherapy agents should be freshly prepared in preservative-free diluent. Because drugs administered into the lumbar intrathecal space do not always reach the upper region of the spinal cord, it is preferable to give the agents in an Ommaya reservoir, which may be implanted under the scalp and connected by a catheter, through a burr hole, to the frontal horn of the lateral ventricle. This method permits easy access to the CSF and achieves good drug levels throughout the CSF pathways. If the lumbar intrathecal route is used, it is recommended that the volume injected be larger than the volume withdrawn (e.g., withdraw 5 mL for analysis, and inject 10 mL).

4. **Complications.** Complications of intrathecal chemotherapy include painful arachnoiditis and leukoencephalopathy. The latter is more likely to occur if the Ommaya catheter tip becomes lodged in the brain tissue rather than the lateral ventricle. Bone marrow suppression is not usually severe unless the patient undergoes spinal irradiation or systemic chemotherapy as well. Oral leucovorin can be given after the intrathecal methotrexate (10 mg leucovorin p.o. every 6 hours for six to eight doses, starting 24 hours after the methotrexate) to prevent marrow toxicity.

IV. Treatment of cerebral edema

A. Corticosteroids. These are usually started soon after the diagnosis of a brain tumor is established. Dexamethasone, 10 mg i.v., followed by 4 to 10 mg every 6 hours p.o. or i.v., reduces or eliminates the lethargy, headaches, visual blurring, and nausea caused by cerebral edema and also often reduces some of the focal neurologic signs and symptoms, such as hemiparesis and dysphagia.

The corticosteroid dose may be tapered and stopped after radiation therapy is complete and resumed if symptoms recur. The dose should be held at a level that maximizes therapeutic benefit and minimizes unwanted side effects (e.g., gastric irritation, sleeplessness, mood swings, cushingoid body features, increased appetite, and proximal myopathy). It is also advisable to suggest that patients take an antacid with the steroid and that they watch for the occurrence of oral and vaginal thrush, which can be effectively treated with nystatin (suspension or suppositories) or clotrimazole (lozenges or suppositories).

B. Treatment of refractory cerebral edema

1. **When moderate doses of dexamethasone** do not effectively control cerebral edema, the dose may be increased transiently to 40 mg i.v. every 4 to 6 hours. This dose should usually not be maintained longer than 48 to 72 hours.

    2. **An osmotic diuretic** in an urgent situation acts more rapidly than a corticosteroid.

      a. **Mannitol,** 75 to 100 g (as a 15% to 25% solution) is given by rapid infusion over 20 to 30 minutes and repeated at 6- to 8-hour intervals as needed.

      b. **Cautions and duration.** Careful monitoring of electrolytes, fluid intake and output, and body weight is essential to avoid dehydration. The osmotic diuresis may be discontinued when there is improvement in the signs and symptoms of the cerebral edema and when the corticosteroids or other measures to reduce cerebral edema have taken effect.

V. **Seizure control.** Because the occurrence of seizures is common in patients with cerebral neoplasms, many physicians recommend starting all such patients on anticonvulsant therapy with phenytoin, 300 mg/day, regardless of whether the patient has already experienced a seizure. Other oncologists treat only if the patient has had seizures or has undergone craniotomy. Anticonvulsants are used for every patient who has had a craniotomy, regardless of the seizure history. For those on long-term anticonvulsant therapy, it is important to check drug levels at intervals, especially after dosages of other medications are changed or new medications are added, because interaction between drugs occurs, and the therapeutic range is narrow.

Seizures are a particular problem after cisplatin therapy. They result from falling phenytoin levels and hypomagnesemia. The blood level of phenytoin should be checked daily for several days, and magnesium should be replaced. If a patient cannot tolerate phenytoin or has poor seizure control, the best alternative is carbamazepine. The usual dose is 200 mg p.o. q.i.d., but higher doses may be necessary, and the dose should be adjusted according to the anticonvulsant blood level. Phenobarbital, 30 mg p.o. q.i.d., is another alternative.

SELECTED READINGS

Boogard W, Hart AA, van der Sande JJ, Engelsman E. Meningeal carcinomatosis in breast cancer. Prognostic factors and influence of treatment. *Cancer* 1991;67:1685–1695.

Brem H, Piantadosi S, Burger PC, et al. Placebo-controlled trial of safety and efficacy of intraoperative controlled delivery by biodegradable polymers of chemotherapy for recurrent gliomas. The Polymer-brain Tumor Treatment Group. *Lancet* 1995;345:1008–1012.

Burger PC, Vogel FS, Green SB, Strike TA. Glioblastoma multiforme and anaplastic astrocytoma. Pathologic criteria and prognostic implications. *Cancer* 1985;56:1106–1111.

Cairncross G, Macdonald D, Ludwin S, et al. Chemotherapy for anaplastic oligodendroglioma. National Cancer Institute of Canada Clinical Trials Group. *J Clin Oncol* 1994;12:2013–2021.

Duffner PK, Cohen ME, Heffner RR, Freeman AI. Primitive neuroectodermal tumors of childhood. An approach to therapy *J Neurosurg* 1981;55:376–381.

Grossman SA, Sheidler VR, Gilbert MR. Decreased phenytoin levels in patients receiving chemotherapy. *Am J Med* 1989;87:505–510.

Hubbard JL, Scheithauer BW, Kispert DB, et al. Adult cerebellar medulloblastomas: the pathological, radiographic, and clinical disease spectrum. *J Neurosurg* 1989;70:536–544.

Kornblith PL, Walker M. Chemotherapy for malignant gliomas. *J Neurosurg* 1988;68:1.

Kovnar EH, Kellie SJ, Horowitz ME, et al. Preirradiation cisplatin and etoposide in the treatment of high-risk medulloblastoma and other malignant embryonal tumors of the central nervous system: a phase II study. *J Clin Oncol* 1990;8:330–336.

Levin VA, Silver P, Hannigan J, et al. Superiority of post-radiotherapy adjuvant chemotherapy with CCNU, procarbazine, and vincristine (PCV) over BCNU for anaplastic gliomas: NCOG 6G61 final report. *Int J Radiat Oncol Biol Phys* 1990;18:321–324.

Mellet LB. Physicochemical consideration and pharmacokinetic behavior in delivery of drugs to the central nervous system. *Cancer Treat Rep* 1977;61:527.

Packer RJ, Sutton LN, Elterman R, et al. Outcome for children with medulloblastoma treated with radiation and cisplatin, CCNU, and vincristine chemotherapy. *J Neurosurg* 1994;81:690–698.

Patchell RA, Tibbs PA, Walsh JW, et al. A randomized trial of surgery in the treatment of single metastases to the brain. *N Engl J Med* 1990;322:494–500.

Shapiro WR, Green SB, Burger PC, et al. Randomized trial of three chemotherapy regimens and two radiotherapy regimens in postoperative treatment of malignant glioma. Brain Tumor Cooperative Group Trial 8001. *J Neurosurg* 1989;71:1–9.

Shapiro WR, Shapiro JR. Principles of brain tumor chemotherapy. *Semin Oncol* 1986;13:56.

Sposto R, Ertel IJ, Jenkin RD, et al. The effectiveness of chemotherapy for treatment of high grade astrocytoma in children: results of a randomized trial. A report from the Childrens Cancer Study Group. *J Neurooncol* 1989;7:165–177.

Tirelli U, D'Incalci M, Canetta R, et al. Etoposide (VP-16-213) in malignant brain tumors: a phase II study. *J Clin Oncol* 1984;2:432–437.

Trojanowski T, Peszynski J, Turowski K, et al. Quality of survival of patients with brain gliomas treated with postoperative CCNU and radiation therapy. *J Neurosurg* 1989;70:18–23.

Walker MD, Green SB, Byar DP, et al. Randomized comparisons of radiotherapy and nitrosoureas for the treatment of malignant glioma after surgery. *N Engl J Med* 1980;303:1323–1329.

Wasserstrom WR, Glass JP, Posner JB. Diagnosis and treatment of leptomeningeal metastasis from solid tumors: experience with 90 patients. *Cancer* 1982;49:759.

Weiss RB, Poster DS, Penta JS. The nitrosoureas and pulmonary toxicity. *Cancer Treat Rev* 1981;8:111–125.

Zimm S, Wampler GL, Stablein D, Hazra T, Young HF. Intracerebral metastasis in solid-tumor patients: natural history and results of treatment. *Cancer* 1981;48:384–394.

Soft Tissue Sarcomas

Robert S. Benjamin

I. Classification and approach to treatment

A. Types of soft tissue sarcomas. The soft tissue sarcomas are a group of diseases characterized by neoplastic proliferation of tissue of mesenchymal origin. Thus, they differ from the more common carcinomas, which arise from epithelial tissue. Sarcomas can arise in any area of the body and from any origin; however, they most commonly arise in the soft tissue of the extremities, trunk, retroperitoneum, or head and neck area. There are more than 20 different types of sarcomas, classified according to lines of differentiation toward normal tissue. For example, rhabdomyosarcoma shows evidence of skeletal muscle fibers with cross striations, liposarcoma shows fat production, and angiosarcoma shows vessel formation. Precise characterization of the type of sarcoma is often impossible, and these tumors are called *unclassified sarcomas*. All of the primary bone sarcomas may arise in soft tissue, leading to such diagnoses as extraskeletal osteosarcoma, extraskeletal Ewing's sarcoma, and extraskeletal chondrosarcoma. A common diagnosis at present is malignant fibrous histiocytoma (MFH). This tumor is characterized by a mixture of spindle (or fibrous) cells and round (or histiocytic) cells arranged in a storiform pattern with frequent areas of pleomorphic appearance and frequent giant cells. There is no evidence of differentiation toward any particular tissue type. Many tumors previously called pleomorphic fibrosarcoma, pleomorphic rhabdomyosarcoma, and so forth are now classified as MFH. As immunohistochemistry and molecular diagnostic techniques improve, it is possible that some of the tumors currently classified as MFH will again become pleomorphic something else.

B. Metastases. Metastatic spread of all sarcomas tends to be through the blood rather than through the lymphatic system. The lungs are by far the most frequent site of metastatic disease. Local sites of metastasis by direct invasion are the second most common area of involvement, followed by bone and liver. (Liver metastases are common with leiomyosarcomas of gastrointestinal origin, however, and metastases to soft tissue are common with myxoid liposarcomas.) Central nervous system (CNS) metastases are extraordinarily rare except in alveolar soft part sarcoma.

C. Staging. Staging of sarcomas is complex and demands an expert sarcoma pathologist. Tumors have been staged according to two systems, the American Joint Committee for Cancer (AJCC) staging system and the Musculoskeletal Tumor Society staging system. The new International Union Against Cancer UICC/AJC staging system with international acceptance takes portions from each of the older systems and more appropriately identifies patients at increased risk of metastatic disease. Since current and older publications still refer to the older systems, however, all will be included.

1. **The old AJCC staging system**
   a. **Tumor grade.** The primary determinant of stage is tumor grade.
      Grade 1 tumors are stage I.
      Grade 2 tumors are stage II.
      Grade 3 tumors are stage III.
      Any tumor with lymph node metastases is automatically stage III.
      Any tumor with gross invasion of bone, major vessel, or major nerve is stage IV.
   b. **Stage.** Further division of stages I to III into A and B are based on tumor size.
      A = tumor smaller than 5 cm.
      B = tumor size 5 cm or larger.
      In stage III, lymph node metastases are classified as IIIC; in stage IV, local invasion is called IVA; and IVB represents distant metastases.

2. **The Musculoskeletal Tumor Society staging system.** The Musculoskeletal Tumor Society stages sarcomas according to grade and compartmental localization. The Roman numeral reflects the tumor grade.
   Stage I: low grade
   Stage II: high grade
   Stage III: any grade tumor with distant metastasis
   The letter reflects compartmental localization. Compartments are defined by fascial planes.
      Stage A: intracompartmental (i.e., confined to the same soft tissue compartment as the initial tumor)
      Stage B: extracompartmental (i.e., extending outside of the initial soft tissue compartment into the adjacent soft tissue compartment or bone)
   A stage IA tumor is a low-grade tumor confined to its initial compartment, a stage IB tumor is a low-grade tumor extending outside the initial compartment, and so forth.

3. **The new AJCC staging system**. The stage is determined by tumor grade, tumor size, and tumor location relative to the muscular fascia.
   There are now four tumor grades:
   Grade 1: Well differentiated
   Grade 2: Moderately differentiated
   Grade 3: Poorly differentiated
   Grade 4: Undifferentiated

Tumor size is now divided at less than or equal to 5 cm or more than 5 cm (in the old AJCC system, it was less than 5 cm, or more than equal to 5 cm).

T1 = ≤5 cm

T2 = >5 cm

Tumor status is subdivided by location relative to the muscular fascia.

Ta = superficial to the muscular fascia

Tb = deep to the muscular fascia

The staging is as follows:

Stage I:

Stage IA—G1, 2; T1a, b; N0; M0

Stage IB—G1, 2; T2a; N0; M0

Stage II:

Stage IIA—G1, 2; T2b; N0; M0

Stage IIB—G3, 4; T1; N0; M0

Stage IIC—G3, 4; T2a; N0; M0

Stage III—G3, 4; T2b; N0; M0

Stage IV:

IVA—any G; any T; N1; M0

IVB—any G; any T; any N; M1

The new staging system divides patients according to necessary therapy:

Stage I patients are adequately treated by surgery alone.

Stage II patients require adjuvant radiation therapy.

Stage III patients require adjuvant chemotherapy.

Stage IV patients are managed primarily with chemotherapy, with or without other modalities.

D. **Evaluation.** Patients are evaluated and followed according to the plan in Table 17-1.

E. **Primary treatment**

1. **Surgery and radiotherapy.** Treatment of the primary tumor involves surgery with or without radiation therapy. If radiation therapy is not used, surgery must be radical. Although this may often involve amputation or complete excision of the involved muscle group from origin to insertion, more and more frequently, wide local resection is performed, with or without adjuvant radiation, depending on stage and extent of negative margins.

2. **Adjuvant chemotherapy.** The role of adjuvant chemotherapy remains controversial, with both positive and negative results reported. A recent metaanalysis indicated a highly significant decrease in the risk of disease recurrence (either local or distant) and death in patients treated with adjuvant chemotherapy; thus, *some investigators believe that adjuvant therapy is clearly indicated for patients whose his-*

Table 17-1. Soft tissue sarcoma evaluation

Tests[a]	Initial	During treatment	Follow-up (if no evidence of disease)
History and physical examination	X	Before each treatment	Yr 1: q2mo; yr 2, 3: q3mo; yr 4: q4mo; yr 5: q6mo; then yearly
CBC, differential, and platelet counts[b]	X	Twice weekly	Yearly
Electrolytes[b]	X	Before each treatment	—
Chemistry profile[b]	X	Before each treatment	q4mo
Urinalysis	If giving ifosfamide	Before each treatment	—
PT, APTT, fibrinogen	X	—	—
Chest radiograph	X	Before each treatment	Same as for history and physical examination
CT scan chest	If chest radiograph appears normal	To confirm chest radiograph findings (if initially abnormal) or for surgical planning	If chest radiograph becomes equivocal
MRI primary (if not intraabdominal), or	X	Preoperatively	—
Ultrasound primary	—	—	—
CT of the abdomen and pelvis	If myxoid liposarcoma or retroperitoneal or pelvic primary tumor	If baseline, every third cycle	Yr 1: q4mo; yr 2, 3: q6mo If baseline, yr 1: q4mo; yr 2, 3: q6mo
ECG	If cardiac history	—	—
Cardiac nuclear scan (for ejection fraction)	If cardiac history	If doxorubicin dose is to exceed standard limits for schedule	Yearly for 2 yr, then as clinically indicated
Central venous catheter	X	—	—
Bone marrow	If small cell tumor	—	—
Bone scan	If indicated by history	—	—
Plain film	If indicated by history	—	—

[a] Tests may be ordered more frequently based on clinical indications.
[b] Required more frequently if patient is on a medical treatment program. CBC, complete blood cell count; PT, prothrombin time; APTT, activated partial thromboplastin time; CT, computed tomography; MRI, magnetic resonance imaging; ECG, electrocardiography.

tologic type, grade, or location is known to convey a poor prognosis. A metaanalysis of individual patient data confirms a survival benefit for patients with primary sarcomas of the extremities as well as increased local or distant disease-free interval for all patients treated with doxorubicin (Adriamycin)-based adjuvant chemotherapy. A recent Italian cooperative group study using epirubicin and ifosfamide for patients with current stage III disease also demonstrated survival and disease-free survival advantage for patients treated with chemotherapy.

F. **Prognosis.** Prognosis is related to stage, with a 5-year survival rate of 75% for old AJCC stage I, 55% for stage II, and 29% for stage III. The survival rate for stage IV disease is less than 10%; however, a definite fraction of patients in this category can be cured. Most patients with stage IV disease, if left untreated, die within 6 to 12 months; however, there is great variation in actual survival, and patients may go on with slowly progressive disease for many years.

G. **Treatment response.** Response to treatment is measured in the standard fashion for solid tumors with the addition of tumor necrosis, both radiologically and pathologically.

  1. **Complete remission.** This implies complete disappearance of all signs and symptoms of disease.

  2. **Partial remission.** There is a 50% or greater decrease in measurable disease, calculated by comparing the sum of the products of perpendicular diameters of all lesions before and after therapy. When disease is not measurable in two dimensions but can be followed objectively by magnetic resonance imaging (MRI), x-ray, ultrasound, or computed tomography (CT), a definite decrease in the amount of metastatic disease confirmed by two independent investigators or marked tumor necrosis attributable to chemotherapy demonstrated by imaging or pathology is the equivalent of a partial response, as calculated by a 50% decrease in measurable tumor.

  3. **Stable disease or improvement.** Lesser degrees of tumor shrinkage are categorized by some physicians as stable disease and by others as improvement or minor response. Stable disease implies a smaller than 25% increase in disease for at least 8 weeks. For all response categories, no new disease must appear during response.

  4. **Progression.** New disease in any area or a 25% or more increase in measurable disease constitutes progressive disease.

5. **Survival.** All patients whose disease responds objectively to chemotherapy survive longer than do patients with progressive disease, and the degree of prolongation of survival is directly proportional to the degree of antitumor response that can be measured.

II. **Chemotherapy**

A. **General considerations and aims of therapy.** Although there are numerous types of soft tissue sarcomas, there are few differences among them regarding responsiveness to a standard soft tissue sarcoma regimen. Leiomyosarcomas of gastrointestinal origin and alveolar soft-part sarcomas, and to a lesser extent, clear cell sarcomas and epithelioid sarcomas respond less frequently than do the other soft tissue sarcomas. Leiomyosarcomas of gastrointestinal origin, in particular, should not be treated with doxorubicin- and ifosfamide-based chemotherapy. In contrast, in a fraction of patients, two tumors—Ewing's sarcoma and rhabdomyosarcoma—particularly in children, are responsive to dactinomycin, vincristine, or etoposide. The other tumors are not. The goal of therapy for patients with advanced disease is primarily palliative, although a small fraction (about 20%) of patients who achieve complete remission are, in fact, cured. The first aim, therefore, is to achieve complete remission. Several investigators, including the author, have shown that the prognosis is the same whether complete remission is obtained by chemotherapy alone or by chemotherapy with adjuvant surgery, that is, surgical removal of all residual disease. Short of complete remission, partial remission causes some palliation, with relief of symptoms and prolongation of survival by about 1 year. Any degree of improvement or stabilization of previously advancing disease likewise increases survival.

B. **Effective drugs.** The most important chemotherapeutic agent is doxorubicin, which forms the backbone of all combination chemotherapy regimens. Ifosfamide, an analog of cyclophosphamide that has documented activity even in patients who are refractory to combinations containing cyclophosphamide, is usually included in front-line chemotherapy combinations. It is always given together with the uroprotective agent mesna to prevent hemorrhagic cystitis. Dacarbazine (DTIC), a marginal agent by itself, adds significantly to doxorubicin in prolonging remission duration and survival as well as increasing the response rate. Cyclophosphamide adds marginally, if at all, but is included in some effective regimens.

The key to effective sarcoma chemotherapy is the steep dose-response curve for doxorubicin. At a dose of 45 mg/m^2, the response rate is lower than 20%, compared with a 37% response rate at a dose of 75 mg/m^2. A similar dose-response relationship

exists for ifosfamide and for combination chemotherapy, and the regimens with the best reported results
are those using the highest doses.

C. **Primary chemotherapy regimen (Adjuvant or
Advanced).** The most effective primary chemotherapy regimens include doxorubicin and ifosfamide
(high-dose AI); or doxorubicin and dacarbazine
(ADIC), with or without the addition of cyclophosphamide (CyADIC) or ifosfamide and mesna (MAID).
The CyADIC regimen is a modification of the standard CyVADIC regimen, which includes vincristine.
Because analysis has shown that vincristine makes
no significant contribution and produces neurotoxicity, its addition at a dose of 2 mg maximum or 1.4
mg/m^2 weekly for 6 weeks and then once every 3 to 4
weeks is recommended only for treatment of rhabdomyosarcoma and Ewing's sarcoma.

By giving doxorubicin and dacarbazine by continuous 72- or 96-hour infusion, with the two drugs
mixed in the same infusion pump, nausea and vomiting are markedly reduced, and the chemotherapy
can be continued until a cumulative doxorubicin dose
of 800 mg/m^2 is reached, with less cardiac toxicity
than with standard doxorubicin administration and
a cumulative dose of 450 mg/m^2.

1. **The high-dose AI regimen** is as follows:
   Doxorubicin, by continuous 72-hour infusion,
   75 mg/m^2 i.v. (25 mg/m^2/day for 3 days), *and*
   Ifosfamide, 2.5 g/m^2 over 2 to 3 hours daily for
   4 days.
   Mesna, 500 mg/m^2, is mixed with the first ifosfamide dose, and 1,500 mg/m^2 is given as a
   continuous infusion over 24 hours for 4 days
   in 2 liters of alkaline fluid.
   Granulocyte colony-stimulating factor, 5 µg/kg
   s.c., is given on days 5 to 15 or until granulocyte recovery to 1,500/µL.
   Repeat cycle every 3 weeks.

2. **The continuous-infusion CyADIC regimen**
   is as follows:
   Cyclophosphamide, 600 mg/m^2 i.v. on day 1,
   and
   Doxorubicin, by continuous 96-hour infusion,
   60 mg/m^2 i.v. (15 mg/m^2/day for 4 days), *and*
   Dacarbazine, by continuous 96-hour infusion,
   1,000 mg/m^2 i.v. (250 mg/m^2/day for 4 days)
   mixed in the same bag or pump as the doxorubicin. Doses should be divided into four
   consecutive 24-hour infusions.
   Repeat cycle every 3-4 weeks.

3. **The continuous-infusion ADIC regimen** is
   as follows:
   Doxorubicin, by continuous 96-hour infusion,
   90 mg/m^2 i.v. (22.5 mg/m^2/day for 4 days), *and*

Dacarbazine, by continuous 96-hour infusion, 900 mg/m^2 i.v. (225 mg/m^2/day for 4 days) mixed in the same bag or pump as the doxorubicin. Doses should be divided into four consecutive 24-hour infusions.

Repeat cycle every 3 to 4 weeks.

4. **The MAID regimen** is as follows:

Mesna, by continuous 96-hour infusion, 8,000 mg/m^2 i.v. (2,000 mg/m^2/day for 4 days).

Doxorubicin, by continuous 72-hour infusion, 60 mg/m^2 i.v. (20 mg/m^2/day for 3 days).

Ifosfamide, by continuous 72-hour infusion, 6,000 mg/m^2 i.v. (2,000 mg/m^2/day for 3 days). Doses should be divided into three consecutive 24-hour infusions. (Some investigators prefer to infuse ifosfamide over 2 hours rather than 24 hours because of higher single-agent activity with the shorter infusions.)

Dacarbazine, by continuous 72-hour infusion, 900 mg/m^2 i.v. (300 mg/m^2/day for 3 days) mixed in the same bag or pump as the doxorubicin. Doses should be divided into three consecutive 24-hour infusions.

Repeat cycle every 3 to 4 weeks.

5. **Dose modification.** Doses of doxorubicin, cyclophosphamide, ifosfamide, and mesna should be increased by 25% and may be decreased by 20% for each course of therapy to achieve a lowest absolute granulocyte count of about 500/μL if growth factors are not used. *The maximum doxorubicin dose is limited to 600 to 800 mg/m^2, depending on the duration (48 to 96 hours) of infusion, at which point therapy should be discontinued unless cardiac biopsy specimens indicate that it is safe to continue.* With Ewing's sarcoma and rhabdomyosarcoma, therapy may be continued, and dactinomycin, 2 mg/m^2 in a single dose or 0.5 mg/m^2 daily for 5 days, may be substituted for the doxorubicin, with continuation of the regimen for a total of 18 months.

6. **An alternative regimen for children with rhabdomyosarcoma** is an alternating regimen, using ifosfamide and etoposide alternating with the so-called VAdriaC regimen. Vincristine, 1.5 mg/m^2 is given weekly for the first two cycles of VAdriaC and then on day 1 only. Doxorubicin is given at a dose of 60 to 75 mg/m^2 as a 48-hour continuous infusion, and cyclophosphamide, 600 mg/m^2, is given daily for 2 days (with mesna). After 3 weeks, ifosfamide is given at a dose of 1,800 mg/m^2 daily for 5 days (with mesna), and etoposide is given at a dose of 100 mg/m^2 daily for 5 days. Chemotherapy cycles are alternated for 39 weeks.

7. **A less-intensive, older but still effective regimen for children with good-prognosis**

rhabdomyosarcoma is the so-called pulse VAC regimen. Dactinomycin is given at a total dose of 2 to 2.5 mg/m^2 by divided daily injection over 5 to 7 days (e.g., 0.5 mg/m^2 daily for 5 days) repeated every 3 months for a total of 5 courses. Cyclophosphamide pulses of 275 to 330 mg/m^2 daily for 7 days are begun at the same time but are given every 6 weeks with vincristine, 2 mg/m^2 on days 1 and 8 of each cyclophosphamide cycle. Cyclophosphamide cycles are terminated prematurely if the white blood cell counts fall below 1,500/μL. Chemotherapy continues for 2 years. (The necessity of the 2-year duration of the chemotherapy program is not certain.)

D. **Secondary chemotherapy.** Secondary chemotherapy for patients with sarcoma is relatively unrewarding, with response rates lower than 10% for almost all conventional drugs or regimens tested. The best commercially available drug is ifosfamide, which if not used in primary treatment, produces a response in about 20% of patients. High-dose ifosfamide (12 g/m^2 or higher) may produce responses in patients resistant to lower doses in combination. Methotrexate, with a response rate of about 15% regardless of schedule, is the only other active agent. Patients who do not respond to primary chemotherapy and ifosfamide should be entered in a phase II study of a new agent to see if some activity can be established because other reasonably good alternatives do not exist.

E. **Complications of chemotherapy.** Side effects of sarcoma chemotherapy can be classified into three categories: life-threatening, potentially dangerous, and unpleasant.

1. **Life-threatening complications of chemotherapy are infection or bleeding.** Thrombocytopenia lower than 20,000/μL occurs with this type of chemotherapy when growth factors are used to maintain dose intensity, but bleeding is rare and can be minimized by transfusing platelets at 10,000/μL. About 20% to 40% of patients have documented or suspected infection related to drug-induced neutropenia at some time during their treatment course. These infections are rarely fatal if treated promptly with broad-spectrum, bactericidal antibiotics at the onset of the febrile neutropenia episode.

2. **Potentially dangerous side effects of chemotherapy** include the following:

    a. **Mucositis**, which occurs in fewer than 25% of patients, may interfere with oral intake or may act as a source of infection.

    b. **Granulocytopenia** predisposes the patient to infection but, because of its brevity, rarely causes infection.

      c. **Cardiac damage** from doxorubicin rarely causes clinical problems at the doses recommended, with usually reversible congestive heart failure occurring in fewer than 5% of patients.

      d. **Renal insufficiency** is a rare complication of ifosfamide. Fanconi's syndrome, particularly manifested by a significant loss of bicarbonate, is a dose-related complication of ifosfamide, occurring in 10% to 30% of patients at standard ifosfamide doses and in close to 100% with high-dose regimens.

      e. **CNS toxicity** of ifosfamide is rarely a serious complication. Patients frequently demonstrate minor confusion, disorientation, or difficulty with fine movements. Somnolence and coma are rarely seen in patients without hypoalbuminemia and/or acidosis.

      f. **Hemorrhagic cystitis**, a rare complication of cyclophosphamide therapy, used to be the dose-limiting toxicity of ifosfamide. It can be prevented in most cases by administration of another agent, mesna, before and after each ifosfamide dose, allowing higher doses of ifosfamide to be used.

   3. **Unpleasant but rarely serious problems** include nausea and vomiting (primarily from dacarbazine and ifosfamide) and alopecia (from doxorubicin, cyclophosphamide, and ifosfamide).

F. Special precautions

   1. **Ifosfamide.** Patients must be kept well hydrated with an alkaline pH to prevent CNS toxicity and minimize nephrotoxicity. Sodium bicarbonate or sodium acetate should be added to intravenous fluids at an initial concentration of 100 to 150 mEq/L, and fluid administration should be adjusted to produce a urine output of at least 2 L/day and to maintain the serum bicarbonate concentration at 25 mEq/L or higher.

   2. **Doxorubicin.** Avoid extravasation. Continuous infusions must (and short infusions should) be administered through a central venous catheter. Attention to cumulative dose administered (varying according to the schedule of administration) is critical to minimize the risk of cardiac toxicity.

SELECTED READINGS

Adjuvant chemotherapy for localised resectable soft-tissue sarcoma of adults: meta-analysis of individual data. *Lancet* 1997;350:1647–1654.

Antman KH, Montella D, Rosenbaum C, Schwen M. Phase II trial of ifosfamide with mesna in previously treated metastatic sarcoma. *Cancer Treat Rep* 1985;69:499.

Antman KH, Crowley J, Balcerzak SP, et al. An intergroup phase III randomized study of doxorubicin and dacarbazine with or without ifosfamide and mesna in advanced soft tissue and bone sarcomas. *J Clin Oncol* 1993;11:1276.

Benjamin RS, Baker LH, Rodriquez V, et al. The chemotherapy of soft tissue sarcomas in adults. In: Martin RG, Ayala AG, eds. *Management of primary bone and soft tissue tumors.* Chicago: Year Book, 1977:309–316.

Benjamin RS, Legha SS, Patel RS, Nicaise C. Single agent ifosfamide studies in sarcomas of soft tissue and bone: the M. D. Anderson experience. *Cancer Chemother Pharmacol* 1993;31:S174–S179.

Elias A, Ryan L, Sulkes A, Collins J, Aisner J, Antman KH. Response to mesna, doxorubicin, ifosfamide, and dacarbazine in 108 patients with metastatic or unresectable sarcoma and no prior chemotherapy. *J Clin Oncol* 1989;7:1208.

Lindberg RD, Martin RG, Romsdahl MM, Barkley HT. Conservative surgery and radiation therapy for soft tissue sarcomas. In: Martin RG, Ayala AG, eds. *Management of primary bone and soft tissue tumors.* Chicago: Year Book, 1977:289–298.

Patel SR, Vadhan-Raj S, Papadopoulos N, et al. High-dose ifosfamide in bone and soft-tissue sarcomas: results of phase II and pilot studies. Dose response and schedule dependence. *J Clin Oncol* 1997; 15:2378–2384.

Patel SR, Vadhan-Raj S, Burgess MA, et al. Results of two consecutive trials of dose-intensive chemotherapy with doxorubicin and ifosfamide is highly active in patients with soft-tissue sarcomas. *Am J Clin Oncol* 1998;21:317–321.

Patel SR, Benjamin RS, eds. Sarcomas: part I and II. *Hematol Oncol Clin North Am* 1995;9:513–942.

Russell WO, et al. A clinical and pathological staging system for soft tissue sarcomas. *Cancer* 1977;40:1562.

Zalupski MM, Ryan J, Hussein M, Baker L. Defining the role of adjuvant chemotherapy for patients with soft tissue sarcoma of the extremities. In: Salmon SE, ed. *Adjuvant therapy of cancer VII.* Philadelphia: JB Lippincott, 1993:385–392.

Bone Sarcomas

Robert S. Benjamin

There are four major sarcomas of bone, each differing somewhat in clinical behavior, chemotherapy responsiveness, and prognosis. All present as painful bony lesions, and all metastasize preferentially to lung and then to other bones. The prognosis of untreated sarcomas of the bone is inversely proportional to their chemotherapy responsiveness. The sarcomas are considered in order of greatest to least chemotherapeutic responsiveness: Ewing's sarcoma, osteosarcoma, malignant fibrous histiocytoma of bone, and chondrosarcoma.

Response to treatment is evaluated according to the usual criteria used for solid tumors and identical to that reported in Chapter 17 for soft tissue sarcomas. Angiography is particularly helpful in defining the response of primary bone tumors to chemotherapy, and the angiographic response correlates well with pathologic tumor destruction. Complete resection and examination of the total specimen often are required to determine response to therapy in a primary lesion and to confirm complete remission.

I. **Staging.** Bone tumors are staged exclusively according to the criteria of the Musculoskeletal Tumor Society.
   A. The Roman numeral reflects the **tumor grade.**
   Stage I: Low grade
   Stage II: High grade
   Stage III: Any grade tumor with distant metastasis
   B. The companion letter reflects **tumor compartmentalization.**
   Stage A: Confined to bone
   Stage B: Extending into adjacent soft tissue
   C. Thus, a stage IA tumor is a low-grade tumor confined to bone, and a stage IB tumor is a low-grade tumor extending into soft tissue, and so forth. Patients are evaluated and followed according to the plan in Table 18-1.

II. **Ewing's sarcoma**
   A. **General considerations and aims of therapy**
      1. **Tumor characteristics.** Ewing's sarcoma is a highly malignant, small round-cell tumor of bone. It occurs most commonly in the second decade of life, and 90% of patients are younger than 30 years. There is a slight male predominance. The most common locations are the pelvis or the diaphysis of long tubular bones of the extremities. Often, systemic symptoms of fever and leukocytosis suggest infection. Radiographically, the predominant feature is osteolysis, although sclerosis does occur. Frequently,

Table 18-1.   Primary bone sarcoma evaluation

Tests[a]	Before therapy	On initial treatment	Preoperative	On subsequent treatment	Follow-up
History and physical examination	X	Before each treatment	X	Before each treatment	Yr 1: q2 mo; yr 2, q3–4 mo; yr 4: q4 mo; yr 5: q6 mo; then yearly
CBC, differential, and platelet counts[b]	X	Twice weekly	X	Twice weekly	Yearly
Chemistry profile[b]	X	Before each treatment	X	Before each treatment	Yr 1: q4–6 mo; then yearly
Creatinine clearance	X	For methotrexate	—	For methotrexate	—
Electrolytes, Mg[b]	X	Before each treatment	X	Before each treatment	—
Urinalysis	If ifosfamide is given	Before each treatment	X	Before each treatment	—
PT, APTT, fibrinogen	X	Before each intra-arterial (IA) treatment and qd while on IA treatment	X	—	—
Plain films of primary tumor	X	q2 cycles	X	q3mo	Yr 1: q 4–6 mo; then yearly
CT of primary tumor	X	After two to four cycles	X	—	At end of treatment for head and neck or pelvic primaries
MRI of primary tumor	—	For surgical planning only	—	—	—
Bone scan	X				

		After two to four cycles	If needed to assess response		
Sestamibi scan[c]	X	X	X	—	—
Chest radiograph	X	Before each treatment	X	Before each treatment	Yr 1: q2 mo; yr 2, 3: q3–4 mo; yr 4: q4 mo; yr 5: q6 mo; then yearly
Chest CT	If chest radiograph appears normal	If chest radiograph is equivocal or for surgical planning	—	If chest radiograph is equivocal or for surgical planning	If chest radiograph is equivocal or for surgical planning
Angiogram	—	Before each preoperative treatment	—	—	—
Bone marrow	Only for small cell tumors with metastases	—	—	—	—
ECG	If cardiac history	—	If cardiac history	—	—
Cardiac scan	If cardiac history	—	—	If doxorubicin dose exceeds standard limits for schedule	—
Central venous catheter	X	—	—	—	—
Bone tumor conference	X	—	—	—	If further multidisciplinary decisions are required

[a] Tests may be ordered more frequently based on clinical indications.

[b] Required more frequently if patient is on a medical treatment program.

[c] Name of the thallium-technetium isotope used for scanning. Trade name is Cardiolyte. Procedure is suggested but optional.

CBC, complete blood cell count; PT, prothrombin time; APTT, activated partial thromboplastin time; CT, computed tomography; MRI, magnetic resonance imaging; ECG, electrocardiogram.

the periosteal reaction has the so-called onion skin pattern with layering of subperiosteal new bone, frequently with spicules radiating out from the cortex. Prognosis, until recently, was extremely poor, with a 5-year survival rate lower than 10% and almost half of patients dying within 1 year of diagnosis. Because Ewing's sarcoma is a high-grade tumor by definition is almost always accompanied by a soft tissue mass, it usually is staged as IIB or IIIB depending on the demonstration of metastatic disease in lung, bone, or both.

   2. **Primary treatment.** For this reason and because of the mutilative surgery involved in resection of the primary lesion, radiotherapy has been the primary modality for local tumor control. As techniques for limb salvage surgery have become more widely practiced, attempts to use surgery rather than radiation therapy are again increasing.

B. **Chemotherapy**
   1. **CyVADIC regimen.** Perhaps the best chemotherapeutic regimen for Ewing's sarcoma is the continuous-infusion CyVADIC regimen, which is mentioned in Chapter 17 (see Section II.C).
   Cyclophosphamide, 600 mg/m^2 i.v. on day 1
   Vincristine, 1.4 mg/m^2 (2 mg maximum) i.v. weekly for 6 weeks, then on day 1 of each cycle
   Doxorubicin (Adriamycin), 60 mg/m^2 i.v. by 96-hour continuous infusion through a central venous catheter (15 mg/m^2/day for 4 days)
   Dacarbazine (DTIC), 1,000 mg/m^2 i.v. by 96-hour continuous infusion (250 mg/m^2/day for 4 days) mixed in the same bag or pump as the doxorubicin. Doses should be divided into four consecutive 24-hour infusions
   Repeat cycle every 3 to 4 weeks.
   2. **Dose modifications.** Courses are repeated with a 25% increase or decrease in the doses of cyclophosphamide and doxorubicin depending on morbidity. Courses are repeated in 3 to 4 weeks as soon as recovery to 1,500 granulocytes and 100,000 platelets occurs. Complications are as described in Chapter 17 (see Section II.E), with the addition of peripheral neuropathy from vincristine. When the cumulative dose of doxorubicin has reached 800 mg/m^2, therapy is discontinued.
   3. **Alternative regimens.** Alternative regimens omit dacarbazine; vary doses of cyclophosphamide up to 4,200 mg/m^2; give dactinomycin with, or in place of, doxorubicin; and in some patients, add other drugs. A common regimen at present alternates two regimens every 3 weeks: ifosfamide plus etoposide; and vincristine, doxo-

rubicin plus cyclophosphamide, with dactino-mycin substituted for doxorubicin after a cumulative (bolus) dose of 375 mg/m^2 (VAdCA). In a recent intergroup study, this regimen was superior to VAdCA alone. The schedule of drug administration is as follows:

  a. Initial combination
     Ifosfamide, 1,800 mg/m^2 i.v. daily × 5 (with mesna), *and*
     Etoposide 100 mg/m^2 daily i.v. × 5.

  b. Three weeks later, start
     Vincristine, 1.5 mg/m^2 i.v. on day 1, *and*
     Doxorubicin, 75 mg/m^2 i.v. on day 1, *and*
     Cyclophosphamide, 1,200 mg/m^2 i.v. on day 1.

  c. Three weeks later, return to the first regimen, and so forth. At a cumulative doxorubicin dose of 375 mg/m^2, substitute dactinomycin 1.25 mg/m^2. Chemotherapy continues for a total of 1 year.

  d. Another version of the alternating regimen starts with an intensive VAC regimen with the doxorubicin and vincristine given by 72-hour continuous infusion and the cyclophosphamide dose increased to 4,200 mg/m^2 divided into two equal doses on days 1 and 2.

4. Responses. Most patients with metastatic disease obtain complete remission; however, almost all patients experience relapse and ultimately die of disease. When chemotherapy is used in the therapy of primary disease with surgery or radiation therapy, prognosis depends on the size and location of the primary tumor. Patients with large flat-bone lesions have a lower than 30% cure rate compared with a 60% to 70% cure rate for those patients with long-bone lesions, which are generally smaller. An alarming complication of the chemotherapy and radiation therapy combination is a high frequency of second malignancies in cured patients, with 4 of 10 patients in one series developing secondary sarcomas within the radiated fields. This complication is another reason for considering surgical intervention rather than radiation because chemotherapy is required for cure whether or not the primary lesion can be controlled with radiation.

5. Secondary chemotherapy. Occasional responses have been seen with etoposide (VP-16), other alkylating agents (especially ifosfamide), the nitrosoureas, and cisplatin. A combination of etoposide and ifosfamide is now frequently used in patients for whom those drugs were not used in initial therapy. High-dose ifosfamide

(14 g/m² divided over 3 to 7 days, either as a 2-hour infusion with each dose or as a continuous infusion) with mesna or high-dose doxorubicin (90 mg/m²) plus dacarbazine (900 mg/m²) as a 96-hour continuous infusion is occasionally effective in producing brief remissions in patients for whom these agents were not used or were used at substantially lower doses during initial therapy. Nonetheless, secondary responses are extremely poor, and the survival of a relapsed patient with Ewing's sarcoma is measured in weeks.

6. **High-dose chemotherapy.** The standard chemotherapy used for Ewing's sarcoma is accompanied by severe but transient myelosuppression. The availability of hematopoietic growth factors to reduce infectious complications provides an added measure of safety but is not routinely required. Our policy has been to use growth factors only in patients who have had febrile-neutropenic episodes during a previous course of chemotherapy rather than to reduce the doses of the myelosuppressive drugs.

Bone marrow transplantation or peripheral stem cell rescue programs are being investigated in patients presenting with poor prognostic features (large pelvic primary tumors, metastatic disease) but have not yet been demonstrated to improve prognosis. Such regimens have been tried with negative results in patients relapsing after standard chemotherapy and have been demonstrated to have no significant benefit. Clearly, this approach should not be used in patients with relapse.

III. Osteosarcoma

A. **General considerations.** Osteosarcoma is a tumor with a poor prognosis in the absence of effective chemotherapy. It is the most common primary bone sarcoma. Frequently, it affects patients 10 to 25 years old and tends to be located around the knee in about two thirds of patients, with two thirds of those tumors involving the distal aspect of the femur. As with other sarcomas of bone, pulmonary metastases are most common, followed by bone metastases. Because conventional osteosarcoma is a high-grade tumor by definition and is accompanied by a soft tissue mass in 90% or more of patients, it is usually staged as IIB or IIIB, depending on the demonstration of metastatic disease in lung or bone.

B. **Role of chemotherapy.** Chemotherapy is usually employed in the adjuvant situation, and its value preoperatively has been conclusively demonstrated. Patients who show a complete response to preoperative chemotherapy with tumor destruction of at least 90% have significantly improved survival. Response rates in evaluable tumors range from 30% to 80%. Cure of primary disease with adjuvant chemotherapy is 50% to 80%.

C. **Effective agents.** The four major standard single agents in the treatment of osteosarcoma are cisplatin, doxorubicin, ifosfamide, and high-dose methotrexate. In addition, the combination of bleomycin, cyclophosphamide, and dactinomycin (BCD) has been effective.

D. **Recommended regimen.** A variety of regimens may be recommended based on preliminary, or more extensive, evaluation.

    1. **Doxorubicin and cisplatin**

        Doxorubicin, 90 mg/m^2 i.v. by 96-hour continuous infusion through a central venous catheter, *and*

        Cisplatin, 120 mg/m^2 intraarterially (for primary tumor) or i.v. on day 6.

        Repeat every 4 weeks.

        Three to four courses of therapy should be administered preoperatively. Postoperative therapy depends on the response of the primary tumor. Patients with tumor necrosis of 90% or more should continue on the same regimen for six postoperative courses or until a cumulative doxorubicin dose of 800 mg/m^2 is reached. If cisplatin must be discontinued earlier, substitute dacarbazine, 750 mg/m^2 i.v. over 96 hours (ADIC).

    2. **After primary chemotherapy,** if there is less than 90% tumor necrosis at surgery, **switch to the alternative regimen** as follows:

        a. High-dose methotrexate, 12 g/m^2 i.v. every 2 weeks for 8 weeks with leucovorin rescue (see Section III.E.2).

        b. Three weeks later, administer ifosfamide, 2 g/m^2 i.v. over 2 hours for 5 consecutive days, with mesna, 1,200 mg/m^2 i.v. in three divided doses each day (i.e., 400 mg/m^2 i.v. every 4 hours × 3) or by continuous infusion after a loading dose of 400 mg/m^2 mixed with the first ifosfamide dose. Three weeks later, repeat the course.

        c. Three weeks later, administer a 96-hour continuous infusion of doxorubicin, 75 mg/m^2, plus dacarbazine, 750 mg/m^2 (ADIC). Three to 4 weeks later, repeat the course.

        d. Three to 4 weeks later, repeat the entire cycle of 4 courses of methotrexate, two courses of ifosfamide, and two courses of ADIC. End with 4 more courses of high-dose methotrexate.

    3. **An alternative approach to alternating-cycle chemotherapy** is as follows:

a. High-dose methotrexate, 12 g/m² i.v. weekly for 4 weeks with leucovorin rescue (see Section III.E.2).

b. Three weeks later, administer BCD for 2 consecutive days.

Bleomycin, 12 U/m² i.v. daily on days 1 and 2, *and*

Cyclophosphamide, 600 mg/m² i.v. daily on days 1 and 2, *and*

Dactinomycin, 450 µg/m² i.v. daily on days 1 and 2.

c. Three weeks later, repeat high-dose methotrexate weekly for 2 weeks.

d. One week later, give doxorubicin, 45 mg/m² i.v. daily for 2 consecutive days.

e. Three weeks later, repeat high-dose methotrexate weekly for 2 weeks.

f. Repeat the cycles using the sequence of BCD, high-dose methotrexate, doxorubicin, and high-dose methotrexate for 5 courses.

E. **Special precautions in administration**

1. **Cisplatin.** Prehydration is necessary, with overnight infusion of i.v. fluids at 150 mL/h or 1 liter of fluid over 2 hours (for adults), followed by at least 6 liters of fluid containing potassium chloride (KCl), at least 20 mEq/L, and magnesium sulfate (MgSO₄), at least 4 mEq/L, for the first 1 or 2 days or after cisplatin administration. The addition of mannitol, 50 mL of a 20% solution, before cisplatin, followed by 200 mL of a 20% solution mixed with normal saline in a total volume of 1 liter to run simultaneously with the cisplatin over 2 to 3 hours, is preferred by many investigators. Particular care in electrolyte balance, including frequent determinations of magnesium levels, is necessary. In the presence of severe hypomagnesemia, magnesium sulfate, up to 1 to 2 mEq/kg, may be infused over 4 hours.

2. **High-dose methotrexate.** The pretreatment creatinine clearance rate should be at least 70 mL/min.

a. **Methotrexate administration and alkalization of urine.** Before administration of high-dose methotrexate, 0.5 mEq/kg of sodium bicarbonate is infused i.v. over 15 to 30 minutes in an attempt to create an alkaline urine. Allopurinol, 300 mg/day for 3 days, is given starting 1 day before the methotrexate infusion. Methotrexate is dissolved in no more than 1,000 mL of 5% dextrose in water, with a final concentration of about 1 g/100 mL. The total dose ranges from 8 g/m² for patients over 40 years old to

12 g/m^2 for children and young adults. The dose should be increased on subsequent courses if an immediate postinfusion methotrexate level is less than 10^{-3} M. Sodium bicarbonate, 50 mEq, is added per liter of methotrexate solution, which is infused over 4 hours. After completion of the methotrexate infusion, 10 mL/kg of an i.v. infusion of 5% dextrose in water with 50 mEq/L of bicarbonate is given over 2 hours if the patient is unable to drink or if the 24-hour methotrexate levels of the previous high-dose methotrexate treatment have been higher than 1.5×10^{-5} M. The intravenous infusion is then discontinued, and the patient is encouraged to drink sufficient fluid to produce about 1,600 mL/m^2 of alkaline urine for the first 24 hours, and 1,900 mL/m^2 daily for the next 3 days. Sodium bicarbonate, 14 to 28 mEq every 6 hours p.o., is administered to ensure alkaline urine. The pH of the urine is measured, and if it is less than 7, an extra dose of bicarbonate is administered.

   b. **Leucovorin rescue.** Twenty-four hours after the start of the methotrexate infusion, leucovorin, 15 to 25 mg, is administered p.o. every 6 hours for at least 10 doses, or intramuscularly if the oral medication is not tolerated.

   c. **Serum methotrexate levels.** These levels should be followed and should fall about 1 log/day. When methotrexate concentration falls below 1×10^{-7} M, leucovorin may be safely discontinued. Intravenous hydration is required whenever oral intake is inadequate to produce sufficient urine output as previously defined, for abnormal serum methotrexate concentration, for persistent vomiting, or for early toxicity.

3. **Ifosfamide.** Patients must be kept well hydrated with an alkaline pH to prevent central nervous system (CNS) toxicity and minimize nephrotoxicity. Sodium bicarbonate or sodium acetate should be added to intravenous fluids at an initial concentration of 100 to 150 mEq/liter and fluid administration adjusted to produce a urine output of at least 2 L/day and to maintain the serum bicarbonate concentration at 25 mEq/L or higher.

F. **Complications.** Complications of chemotherapy depend on the drugs. For doxorubicin and cyclophosphamide, the major complication is infection owing to neutropenia. Other complications include stomatitis, nausea and vomiting, and delayed cardiac toxicity, as discussed in the management of soft tissue sarcomas (see Chap. 17, Section II.E). Ifosfamide produces myelosuppression, nausea and vomiting, and alopecia, similar to doxorubicin. Hemorrhagic cystitis, once the dose-limiting toxicity, is rarely seen because the use of mesna has become routine. The most serious toxicities of ifosfamide are nephrotoxicity and CNS toxicity. Nephrotoxicity in the form of Fanconi's syndrome is a frequent problem, the morbidity of which can be minimized by the routine use of alkaline infusions and correction of electrolyte levels with oral replacement therapy. Only rarely does the nephrotoxicity progress to renal failure. Correction of acid–base balance and hypoalbuminemia can essentially prevent the CNS toxicity (see Chap. 17, Section II.E). Dactinomycin causes similar side effects to those of doxorubicin, but not cardiac toxicity. Methotrexate predominantly causes stomatitis, but it may cause myelosuppression and renal, hepatic, and CNS abnormalities. Cisplatin and dacarbazine cause severe nausea and vomiting. In addition, cisplatin nephrotoxicity is primarily a tubular defect, with hypomagnesemia as the most prominent manifestation, but hypocalcemia, hypokalemia, and hyponatremia also occur. Delayed cumulative nephrotoxicity can cause impaired glomerular function as well. Ototoxicity may occur but is less common. Delayed neurotoxicity also occurs. Both cisplatin and methotrexate can, by causing renal toxicity, exacerbate their other side effects.

G. **Recurrence and treatment of refractory disease.** Patients with osteosarcoma who are refractory to a combination of doxorubicin and cisplatin may respond to high-dose methotrexate; patients refractory to high-dose methotrexate may respond to doxorubicin plus cisplatin; and patients refractory to both may respond to ifosfamide or, rarely, to BCD. However, treatment of refractory disease is usually disappointing, and participation in studies of new agents is indicated for patients whose disease cannot be resected. Surgical resection of pulmonary metastases remains the only viable secondary therapy for most patients. For this reason, careful follow-up for detection of metastases while they are still at the stage of resectability is indicated.

H. **High-dose chemotherapy.** The standard chemotherapy used for osteosarcoma is accompanied by severe but transient myelosuppression. The availability of hematopoietic growth factors to reduce infectious complications provides an added measure of safety but is not routinely required. Our policy has been to use growth factors only in patients who have had febrile-neutropenic episodes during a previous course of chemotherapy rather than to reduce the doses of the myelosuppressive drugs.

Bone marrow transplantation or peripheral stem cell rescue programs are being investigated in patients presenting with poor prognostic features (e.g., poor-prognosis histologic subtypes, pelvic primary tumors, metastatic disease) but are not yet demonstrated to improve prognosis.

IV. **Malignant fibrous histiocytoma of bone.** This recently reported entity, characterized by a purely lytic lesion in bone, has an exceptionally poor prognosis when treated with surgery alone, although the number of reported patients is small. It may be extremely difficult to distinguish from fibroblastic osteosarcoma and may be best considered as a fibroblastic osteosarcoma with minimal (i.e., no detectable) osteoid production. The tumor responds well to the CyADIC regimen for soft tissue sarcomas, with more than half of patients obtaining at least partial remission. In addition, cisplatin at a dose of 120 mg/m^2 every 4 weeks has caused remissions, even in patients who did not respond to primary therapy. A particularly attractive approach for patients with large, unresectable primary tumors is the administration of cisplatin by the intraarterial route. Complete tumor destruction in one patient and a good partial remission in a second patient are the reported results among three patients so treated. Systemic doxorubicin may be added, as for osteosarcomas (see Section III.D.1). Alternatively, responses have been seen after high-dose methotrexate-based regimens for osteosarcomas (see Section III.D.2). After local tumor destruction, surgery may be employed to remove residual disease. Because of the poor prognosis, adjuvant chemotherapy with the continuous-infusion CyADIC regimen is recommended until an 800 mg/m^2 cumulative doxorubicin dose has been reached.

V. **Chondrosarcoma.** The chemotherapy for chondrosarcoma is totally inadequate, and no regimen can be recommended except for the rare patients with mesenchymal chondrosarcoma, a subtype that may respond to CyADIC chemotherapy or cisplatin, or with dedifferentiated chondrosarcoma, which should be treated the same way as osteosarcoma. Most patients have conventional chondrosarcoma and are candidates only for surgical management. Metastatic disease should be treated with phase II protocols in an attempt to determine some effective type of chemotherapy that may be recommended in the future.

SELECTED READINGS

Benjamin RS, Baker LH, O'Bryan RM, Moon TE, Gottlieb JA. Chemotherapy for metastatic osteosarcoma: studies by the M.D. Anderson Hospital and the Southwest Oncology Group. *Cancer Treat Rep* 1978;62:237.

Benjamin RS, Murray JA, Carrasco CH, et al. Preoperative chemotherapy for osteosarcoma: a treatment approach facilitating limb salvage with major prognostic implications. In: Jones SE, Salmon SE, eds. *Adjuvant therapy of cancer*, Vol IV. New York: Grune & Stratton, 1984:601–610.

Chawla SP, Benjamin RS, Abdul-Karim FW, et al. Adjuvant chemotherapy of primary malignant fibrous histiocytoma of bone: prolongation of disease free and overall survival. In: Jones SE, Salmon SE, eds. *Adjuvant therapy of cancer,* Vol IV. New York: Grune & Stratton, 1984:621–629.

Gehan EA, Sutow WW, Uribe-Botero G, Romsdahl M, Smith TL. Osteosarcoma: the M. D. Anderson experience, 1950–1974. In: Terry WD, Windhorst D, eds. *Immunotherapy of cancer: present status of trials in man.* New York: Raven, 1978.

Grier H, Krailo M, Link M, et al. Improved outcome in non-metastatic Ewing's sarcoma (EWS) and PNET of bone with the addition of ifosfamide (D) and etoposide (E) to vincristine (W), Adriamycin (Ad), cyclophosphamide (C), and actinomycin (A): a Children's Cancer Group (CCG) and Pediatric Oncology Group (POG) report. *Proc Am Soc Clin Oncol* 1994;13:A1443.

Kushner BH, Meyers PA, Gerald WL, et al. Very-high-dose short-term chemotherapy for poor-risk peripheral primitive neuroectodermal tumors, including Ewing's sarcoma in children and young adults. *J Clin Oncol* 1995;13:2796–2804.

Rosen G, et al. The successful management of metastatic osteogenic sarcoma: a model for the treatment of primary osteogenic sarcoma. In: van Oosterom AT, Muggia FM, Cleton FJ, eds. *Therapeutic progress in ovarian cancer, testicular cancer and the sarcomas.* Hingham: Leiden University Press, 1990:244–265.

Acute Leukemias

Chatchada Karanes and Neil A. Lachant

The acute leukemias are a heterogeneous group of disorders characterized by the abnormal proliferation and accumulation of hematopoietic progenitor cells. The appellation *acute* is now a historical anachronism because it refers to the short natural history of the disease before the modern chemotherapeutic era. Great therapeutic advances have been made since the early 1960s, so that many patients can now be cured of these otherwise fatal illnesses. Unfortunately, however, an unacceptably high proportion of affected patients still die. Many questions remain unanswered about the optimum way to treat these disorders. Therefore, all patients with acute leukemia should be considered candidates for well-designed randomized, prospective studies and should be cared for in centers where appropriate supportive care can be provided.

I. **Diagnosis and classification.** Acute leukemia is a clonal disorder that arises in an early hematopoietic progenitor and ultimately gives rise to a state of functional bone marrow failure. The acute leukemias are arbitrarily divided into acute myeloid (AML) and acute lymphoblastic (ALL) forms based on the stem cell of origin. Although the peripheral smear may be highly suggestive of acute leukemia, the diagnosis is made by examining the bone marrow. Classification into the AML and ALL categories is usually based on the morphologic, histochemical, enzymatic, and immunologic (antigenic) characteristics of the blast cells. Occasionally, electron microscopy, cytogenetics, and molecular biologic techniques aid in establishing the diagnosis. The principles used to diagnose and classify acute leukemia are briefly presented below.

    A. **Acute myeloid leukemia.** The French-American-British (FAB) system is the most widely used for the diagnosis and morphologic subclassification of AML. Normally, myeloblasts and promyelocytes constitute fewer than 5% of the nucleated cells in the marrow. In general, the diagnosis of AML is established by demonstrating that leukemic cells (myeloblasts, promyelocytes, monoblasts, promonocytes, megakaryoblasts) constitute more than 30% of the nucleated marrow cells (or more than 30% of the nonerythroid nucleated cells in the case of erythroleukemia). Classically, histochemical stains have been used to demonstrate that cells are of nonlymphoid origin. Common histochemical stains that are positive in nonlymphoid cells are Sudan black B and peroxidase (myeloblasts, promyelocytes), nonspecific esterases that are inhibited by sodium fluoride (monoblasts), and block-positive periodic acid–Schiff stains (pronormoblasts in erythroleukemia). Antigens commonly demonstrated by immunologic techniques include CD13 and CD33 on myeloblasts and monoblasts; CD14 on monoblasts; and von Willebrand factor, GPIIb (CD41), and GPIIIa (CD61) on megakaryoblasts. Electron microscopy is useful for demonstrating the presence of myeloperoxidase and platelet peroxidase in the FAB M0 and M7 variants, respectively. A simplified version of the FAB classification system is as follows:

M0: Myelocytic leukemia without maturation
M1: Myelocytic leukemia with minimal differentiation
M2: Myelocytic leukemia with maturation
M3: Promyelocytic leukemia
M4: Myelomonocytic leukemia
M5: Monocytic leukemia
M6: Erythroleukemia
M7: Megakaryoblastic leukemia

B. **Acute lymphoblastic leukemia.** Whereas mature lymphocytes may account for up to 25% of the nucleated cells in the adult bone marrow, recognizable lymphoblasts are not a component of normal marrow. In general, the diagnosis of ALL is established by demonstrating that leukemic lymphoblasts constitute more than 25% of the nucleated marrow cells. Because of its lack of reproducibility, the morphologic subclassification of ALL by the FAB system has been abandoned. In general, ALL is subclassified according to B-cell or T-cell lineage based on immunophenotyping. Immunologic markers classically suggesting B-cell lineage are the common ALL antigen (CALLA, CD10; common or pre-pre–B-cell ALL), intracytoplasmic heavy chains (pre–B-cell ALL), and surface membrane immunoglobulin (B-cell ALL). Ia, CD19, and CD22 are common generic markers for cells of B lineage, whereas CD20 is seen in more mature B-lineage cells. T-cell ALL arises from stage I (prothymocyte) and stage II thymocytes. Immunologic markers classically suggesting T-cell lineage are CD2 (sheep red blood cell [RBC] receptor), CD3, CD7, CD38 (panthymocyte), and CD71 (transferrin receptor). The enzyme terminal deoxynucleotidal transferase (TdT) can be demonstrated in cells of early B-cell (before pre–B-cell) and T-cell (through thymocyte) lineage.

C. **Acute mixed-lineage and stem cell leukemias.** With the expansion of immunophenotyping panels and the increased use of electron microscopy and gene rearrangement studies for the characterization of acute leukemia, increasing degrees of infidelity of myeloid and lymphoid markers can be demonstrated. Minimal deviation from the expected markers is not uncommon and may produce well-defined syndromes that do not alter the basic cellular lineage (e.g., CD13/CD33-ALL, CD7-AML, TdT-AML). There are no consensus guidelines for the diagnosis of true acute mixed-lineage leukemia, which is probably a rare disorder. In stem cell leukemia, the cells express only rudimentary hematopoietic markers (e.g., Ia antigen, TdT, CD34). The identification of entities such as CD13/CD33-ALL and stem cell leukemia may be of prognostic importance and have therapeutic implications.

II. **Initial support.** Once the diagnosis of acute leukemia has been established, the next 24 to 48 hours are usually spent preparing the patient for the initiation of cytotoxic chemotherapy. The following issues need to be addressed in almost all individuals facing induction chemotherapy because those who are in the best overall shape are best able to tolerate the rigors of induction chemotherapy.

A. **Hydration and correction of electrolyte imbalance.** Dehydration needs to be corrected and adequate urine output maintained to prevent renal failure due to the deposition of cellular breakdown products. In the absence of cardiac disease, normal saline with or without 5% dextrose is infused to maintain the urine output at more than 100 mL/h. The concomitant use of loop diuretics may be necessary in patients with congestive heart failure. Although a variety of electrolyte problems may occur in patients with acute leukemia, hypokalemia is the most troublesome, particularly in patients with AML. Serum potassium levels should be monitored closely because a normal serum potassium level does not reflect the diminished potassium stores of most of these patients.

B. **Prevention of uric acid nephropathy.** Hyperuricemia is common at presentation and may also occur with the tumor lysis caused by chemotherapy. Allopurinol is the mainstay of prevention of uric acid nephropathy. The usual initial adult dose is 300 mg (150 mg/m^2) b.i.d. for 2 to 3 days, which is then decreased to 300 mg once a day. Allopurinol should be stopped after 10 to 14 days to lessen the risk of rash and hepatic dysfunction. If chemotherapy needs to be initiated urgently, allopurinol at a dose of 600 mg b.i.d. is well tolerated for 1 to 2 days. With the advent of allopurinol, the role of urine alkalinization has become less clear. Although urine alkalinization increases uric acid solubility, it decreases the solubility of urinary phosphates and may promote phosphate deposition in patients susceptible to the tumor lysis syndrome (e.g., B-cell ALL and T-cell lymphoblastic leukemia). A commonly employed method of urine alkalinization is to hydrate the patient with 0.5 N saline to which two syringes of sodium bicarbonate (44 mEq NaHCO$_3$ per syringe) have been added per liter.

C. **Blood product support.** Most patients with acute leukemia present with bone marrow failure, so symptomatic anemia and thrombocytopenia must be corrected (see Chap. 29). It is recommended that HLA typing be obtained before initiating therapy because patients who are severely myelosuppressed during chemotherapy do not have enough lymphocytes for HLA typing. HLA-matched platelet transfusions may need to be administered to patients who become refractory to pooled or single-donor platelets.

D. **Fever or infection.** Patients frequently have a fever or an infection at initial diagnosis. The approach to fever and infection is discussed in Chap. 28. The cardinal rule is that all patients with acute leukemia and fever have an infection until proved otherwise. Given the additional myelosuppressive and immunosuppressive effects of chemotherapy, severe infections should be treated aggressively before initiating chemotherapy. However, the antibiotic treatment frequently needs to be administered concurrently with induction chemotherapy. Patients with acute leukemia need a careful physical examination daily. Close attention needs to be played to potential sites of infection, including the fundi, sinuses, oral cavity, intertrigenous areas, perineum (do not do internal rectal examination during neutropenia), and catheter sites. A dental consultation at the time of diagnosis is often useful.

E. **Vascular access.** Because of the need for several sites of venous access for at least 1 month, a multiple-lumen implantable catheter (e.g., Hickman catheter, PICC line) must be placed as soon as possible. An implantable port is not recommended for leukemic patients because there is higher risk of infection and hematoma at the access site.

F. **Suppression of menses.** A serum human chorionic gonadotropin (β-hCG) assay (pregnancy test) should be done in all premenopausal women before initiating chemotherapy. Because menorrhagia may occur owing to the severe thrombocytopenia that is seen during induction chemotherapy, preventing menses becomes desirable. Medroxyprogesterone (Provera) may be used for hormonal support of the progestational endometrium. Medroxyprogesterone, 10 mg b.i.d. p.o., should be started 5 to 7 days before the presumed starting time of the next menstrual period. It may be increased to 10 mg t.i.d. or higher if breakthrough bleeding occurs. Depo-Provera is contraindicated in the thrombocytopenic and neutropenic patient.

G. **Birth control.** Given the potential teratogenic effects of cytotoxic chemotherapy, appropriate measures for preventing conception must be addressed with women who are undergoing postinduction therapy and who may still be in their reproductive years. Although there are no clear data linking postinduction chemotherapy in the male partner to teratogenic effects in the fetus, it appears prudent to suggest that appropriate birth control measures be undertaken in this situation as well.

H. **Psychosocial support.** Patients with acute leukemia are usually previously healthy individuals who have suddenly had to accept their own imminent mortality. Intensive psychological support by the health care team, family, and religious leaders is critical for maintaining the patient's sense of well-being (see Chap. 33).

I. **Optimization of comorbid disease.** Patients with good performance status are best able to tolerate chemotherapy. Comorbid disease (e.g., heart failure, diabetes, chronic lung disease) should be aggressively treated before initiating induction chemotherapy.

III. **Therapeutic principles of and approach to therapy for acute leukemia**

A. **Therapeutic aim.** The goals of chemotherapy are to eradicate the leukemic clone and reestablish normal hematopoiesis in the bone marrow. Two important principles need to be remembered: (1) long-term survival is seen only in patients in whom a complete response (CR) is attained, and (2) with the exception of bone marrow transplantation (BMT) as salvage therapy, the response to initial therapy predicts the fate of the patient with acute leukemia. Although leukemia therapy is toxic and infection is the major cause of death during therapy, the median survival time of untreated (or unresponsive) acute leukemia is 2 to 3 months, and most untreated patients die of bone marrow failure. The doses of chemotherapy are never reduced because of cytopenia, since lowered doses still produce the unwanted side effects (further marrow suppression) without having as great a potential for eradicating the leukemic clone and ultimately improving marrow function.

B. **Forms of chemotherapy**

1. **Induction chemotherapy** is initial intensive chemotherapy given in an attempt to eradicate the leukemic clone and to induce a remission (CR).

2. **Postinduction (postremission) chemotherapy** is additional chemotherapy given after a CR has been obtained in a further attempt to eradicate the residual, but undetectable, leukemic cells. Given the generally high induction rate for acute leukemia, future advances are likely to be made through improved postinduction chemotherapy. Therefore, all patients should be candidates for experimental protocols evaluating options for postinduction therapy.

   a. **Consolidation.** This involves repeated courses of the same drugs at the same or similar doses as those used to induce the remission, which are given soon after the remission has been achieved. Consolidation often requires further acute hospitalization.

   b. **Intensification.** Intensive courses of drugs are given at increased dosages to take advantage of steep dose-response relationships (e.g., high-dose cytarabine) or of putatively non–cross-resistant drugs. Intensification is given soon after the remission has been achieved and requires further acute hospitalization.

   c. **Maintenance.** Low doses of drugs designed for outpatient use are given for months to years.

C. **Definition of response.** The criteria are based on the peripheral blood counts and the status of the bone marrow at the time of marrow recovery, not at the time of marrow aplasia.

   1. **Complete response** (complete remission) is the return of the complete blood count to a "normal" absolute neutrophil count (ANC) of more than 1,500/μL and to a platelet count of more than 100,000/μL in conjunction with a normal bone marrow [i.e., normal cellularity, less than 5% blasts or promyelocytes and promonocytes, and an absence of obvious leukemic cells (e.g., containing Auer's rods)].

   2. **Partial response** is the persistence of gross residual leukemia (5% to 25% leukemic cells in the bone marrow).

IV. **Therapy for adult acute myelogenous leukemia**

A. **General plan of therapy.** The day that induction chemotherapy is started is arbitrarily called day 1. Bone marrow aspiration and biopsy are repeated on about days 12 to 14. If the bone marrow is severely hypoplastic with fewer than 5% residual blasts or if the bone marrow is aplastic, no further chemotherapy is given, and the patient is supported until bone marrow recovery occurs (usually 1 to 3 weeks). If there is residual leukemia at day 14, a second course of chemotherapy is given. A bone marrow examination is repeated 2 weeks later (about days 26 to 28). Patients who have residual disease at day 28 should be considered primary treatment failures and switched to alternative therapy. Once a CR has been documented, the potential benefit of further post-induction therapy should be determined on an individual basis.

B. **Induction.** With the exception of acute promyelocytic leukemia (M3), the same chemotherapeutic regimens are used to treat the various subtypes of AML (M0 to M2, M4 to M7). Factors that influence the choice of the chemotherapeutic program to be employed include the patient's cardiac function, age, and performance status. The initial drug doses outlined below are based on the presence of normal hepatic function. They are not modified based on peripheral blood counts. The overall approach to induction therapy used at Wayne State University is shown in Table 19-1.

1. **_De novo_ AML.** Patients who develop AML _de novo_ have the best response to chemotherapy. Therapeutic options vary depending on the clinical situation. Cytarabine (ara-C) is the most active agent against AML and is the agent around which most active regimens are built.

   a. **Normal cardiac function.** The most commonly used program is "7 + 3". The addition of 6-thioguanine to this regimen (DAT), which was commonly used in the 1970s and 1980s, has not been shown to improve the response rate. Both regimens produce overall remission rates of 65% to 70%. The use of high-dose cytarabine (HDAC) as induction therapy when combined with daunorubicin or etoposide does not show an improved CR rate.

      (1) **"7 + 3"** is the combination of a 7-day infusion of cytarabine and 3 days of an anthracycline or anthracenedione. Idarubicin, a newer anthracycline, and mitoxantrone have been compared with daunorubicin in randomized trials in newly diagnosed patients. Idarubicin may offer a modest advantage over daunorubicin based on a slightly higher CR rate and a higher percentage of patients achieving CR after a single cycle of therapy. Thus, although many investigators have strong personal biases about the choice for induction therapy, we would consider daunorubicin, idarubicin, and mitoxantrone as essentially equivalent choices based on current data. All three should be considered potentially cardiotoxic.

      Cytarabine, 100 to 200 mg/m^2/24 hours continuous i.v. infusion on days 1 to 7, _and_

      Daunorubicin, 45 mg/m^2 i.v. bolus on days 1 to 3, _or_

      Idarubicin, 12 mg/m^2 i.v. bolus on days 1 to 3, _or_

      Mitoxantrone, 12 mg/m^2 i.v. bolus on days 1 to 3.

      If there is residual leukemia (more than 5% blasts and more than 15% cellularity) in the bone marrow spec-

Table 19-1. Initial therapeutic options for acute myelogenous leukemia outside of the experimental setting[a]

Prior chemotherapy or myelodysplastic syndrome	Age (yr)	Cardiac function	Induction chemotherapy	Postremission therapy
No, or Yes (favorable cytogenetics)	<60	Normal	7 + 3	HDAC (CALGB), or −2', or HDAC ± DNR +2', HDAC × 2
		Abnormal	HDAC	HDAC × 2
Yes (favorable cytogenetics)	>60	Normal	7 + 3 ± G-CSF, or VP-16 + mitoxantrone, or Supportive care	HDAC + G-CSF, or Maintenance
		Abnormal	Modified HDAC, or Supportive care	HDAC + G-CSF, or Maintenance
Yes (abnormal cytogenetics)	<60	Normal	HDAC + DNR, or 7 + 3	Allogeneic BMT, or HDAC (CALGB), or Autologous BMT HDAC × 2
		Abnormal	HDAC	
	>60	Normal	Supportive care, or 7 + 3 + G-CSF	Modified HDAC + G-CSF, or Autologous BMT
		Abnormal	Supportive care, or Modified HDAC + G-CSF	Modified HDAC + G-CSF

[a] Acute promyelocytic leukemia is excluded. All individuals with acute leukemia should be treated in clinical trials.
7+3, cytarabine days 1-7 and anthracycline or anthracenedione days 1-3; BMT, bone marrow transplantation; CALGB, Cancer and Acute Leukemia

imen obtained on day 14, the second course of chemotherapy is attenuated to a 5-day infusion of cytarabine and 2 days of the anthracycline or anthracenedione ("5 + 2"). There is no dose modification for the second course based on blood cell counts. The doses of both drugs may be decreased for the second cycle if hepatic dysfunction develops and is believed to be due to drug toxicity. If there has been little cytoreduction in the day 14 bone marrow specimen, 2 to 4 days of HDAC (see Section IV.B.1.b) would be a reasonable alternative to "5 + 2."

   (2) **Other agents.** HDAC (see Section IV.B.1.b) with or without an anthracycline has been shown to be active for the induction of AML. In the Southwest Oncology Group (SWOG) study 8600, HDAC plus daunorubicin was compared with "7 + 3" for induction and consolidation. There was no difference in the CR rate or survival, but there was more neurologic toxicity and a higher death rate in the HDAC arm. Although etoposide is active in relapsed and refractory AML, its addition to the "7 + 3" regimen at a dose of 75 mg/m^2/day on days 1 to 7 ("7 + 3 + 7") does not improve the CR rate compared with "7 + 3," but it may improve the response duration. However, the risk of secondary acute leukemia from topoisomerase inhibitors needs to be considered in patients who are potentially long-term survivors.

b. **Impaired cardiac function.** The use of an anthracycline or an anthracenedione is contraindicated for induction therapy in patients with severe underlying cardiac disease, particularly if the patient has had a recent myocardial infarction or has an ejection fraction of less than 50%. The choice of therapy in this situation is HDAC. Unique complications of HDAC include ulcerative keratitis and neurotoxicity. Because cytarabine is secreted in tears, ulcerative keratitis can be prevented by instilling eye drops (saline, methylcellulose, or steroid) every 4 hours while awake and Lacri-Lube ophthalmic ointment (Allergan Pharmaceuticals) at bedtime starting at the time HDAC is initiated and continuing for 2 to 3 days after the last dose of HDAC. The optimum form of HDAC therapy is not known (i.e., number of doses, dosage, infusion rate). Neurotoxicity (e.g., cerebellar dysfunction, somnolence) occurs more frequently in older patients and as the number of doses of HDAC increases. Renal and hepatic dysfunction contribute to the development of neurotoxicity. Because neurotoxicity appears to be decreased with shorter infusion times, 1- to 2-hour infusions are generally recommended as opposed to the original infusion rate over 2 to 3 hours. A commonly employed regimen is as follows:

- Cytarabine, 2 to 3 g/m^2 i.v. infusion over 1 to 2 hours every 12 hours for 12 doses.

The risk of neurotoxicity may be decreased by reducing the dose of cytarabine in face of renal dysfunction. The following schema has been suggested to decrease neurotoxicity in the face of renal dysfunction. For a baseline serum creatinine of 1.5 to 1.9 mg/dL or an increase in serum creatinine of 0.5 to 1.2 mg/dL from baseline, reduce the cytarabine to 1 g/m^2 per dose. For a baseline serum creatinine of more than 2 mg/dL or an increase of serum creatinine of 1.2 mg/dL from baseline, reduce the cytarabine dose to 100 mg/m²/day.

2. **AML in the elderly.** Given that the median age at presentation is about 60 years, AML in older patients is a common problem. Owing to the effects of comorbid disease and age on normal physiology, elderly people are less able to withstand the inherent toxicity of induction chemotherapy compared with young adults. There are also intrinsic differences in the biology of elderly AML (e.g., a higher percentage of the leukemic cells express P-glycoprotein at diagnosis, elderly patients have an increased background of myelodysplasia) that predispose to drug resistance. In addition, AML in the elderly is associated with high-risk cytogenetic abnormalities (including those of chromosomes 5 and 7, and trisomy 8). These poor prognostic features result in a lower CR rate and shortened survival. The decision to forgo therapy in an elderly patient with AML should not be made *a priori* based solely on age; rather, the decision to treat or not to treat should be based on more substantive factors, such as the presence of comorbid disease, performance status before diagnosis, quality of life before diagnosis, and projected long-term survival. In general, 40% to

50% of elderly patients can achieve a CR with chemotherapy. Although attenuated doses of "7 + 3" have been recommended in the past, full-dose therapy is now generally recommended owing to improvements in supportive care. The role of growth factors (granulocyte-macrophage colony-stimulating factor [GM-CSF] or granulocyte colony-stimulating factor [G-CSF]) to stimulate earlier marrow recovery in order to allow elderly patients to tolerate better full doses of induction is unclear. Although growth factors have been shown to decrease the neutropenic period by 2 to 5 days, there has been no change in CR rate or overall survival. Variable effects on the duration of hospitalization and antibiotic use have been reported. Good cost-benefit analyses have not been performed. Options include the following:

a. **Standard "7 + 3"** (see Section IV.B.1.a.1)

b. **"7 + 3" using idarubicin**. A recent French randomized trial has shown a higher CR rate with idarubicin compared with daunorubicin for patients aged 55 to 75 years.

Cytarabine, 100 mg/m^2/day i.v. continuous infusion on days 1 to 7, *and*

Idarubicin, 8 mg/m^2/day i.v. bolus on days 1 to 5.

c. **"7 + 3" plus growth factors**. G-CSF, 250 μg/m^2 s.c. beginning on day 8 until absolute granulocytes reach more than 500 for 2 or 3 successive days.

d. **Etoposide**, 100 mg/m^2/day i.v. on days 1 to 5, **and mitoxantrone**, 10 mg/m^2/day i.v. on days 1 to 5, represent an active and well-tolerated combination.

e. **Modified HDAC** decreases the cytarabine dose to try to diminish the neurotoxicity that is dose-limiting in the elderly. Modified HDAC is generally believed to be more toxic than the "7 + 3" regimen. We do not routinely recommend the use of HDAC for induction in elderly patients given the lack of data to support a higher CR rate and the significantly increased morbidity and mortality associated with HDAC during the induction period. In selected elderly patients with excellent performance status and a decreased ejection fraction, one can consider using modified HDAC. Although the optimum dose and schedule are not known, 1.5 to 2 g/m^2 every 12 hours for 8 to 12 doses is commonly used. The once-a-day regimen of

HDAC, 2 to 3 g/m²/day i.v. infusion over 3 hours for 5 days, as used by SWOG is also well tolerated in elderly patients (see Section IV.B.1.b).

3. **Secondary AML.** In general, secondary AML (e.g., arising after prior irradiation or chemotherapy with alkylating agents or topoisomerase inhibitors, or evolving from a myelodysplastic syndrome or myeloproliferative disorder) has been thought not to respond as well to standard induction chemotherapy as does *de novo* AML. The advisability of chemotherapy needs to be assessed in each individual situation. Recent data suggest that secondary AML with favorable cytogenetics [e.g., t(8:21), t(15:17), inv (16)] has a response rate similar to that of *de novo* AML with the same cytogenetic features. Therapeutic options include supportive care, "7 + 3," and HDAC ([1] standard HDAC [see Section IV.B.1.b.] and daunorubicin, 45 mg/m² i.v. on days 1 to 3; or [2] HDAC, 2 to 3 g/m²/day infusion over 3 hours on days 1 to 5, and daunorubicin, 45 mg/m² i.v. on days 6 to 8). In addition, younger patients with secondary AML should be considered for allogeneic BMT in first remission.

4. **AML during pregnancy.** The fortunes of both the mother and the fetus must be considered when discussing the therapeutic options for a pregnant woman who develops AML. Therapeutic abortion must be considered if AML develops during the first trimester. If therapeutic abortion is not an option or if AML develops during the second or third trimester, induction chemotherapy may be undertaken. Except for a modest increase in fetal deaths and an increased risk of premature labor, "7 + 3" appears to be well tolerated by both the patient and the fetus. However, the long-term effects of *in utero* exposure are not yet known because these exposed individuals are now just in the midst of their third decade of life.

C. **Postremission therapy.** The fact that most patients with AML relapse despite attaining a CR suggests that further postinduction therapy is indicated to attempt to eradicate the residual but undetected leukemic clone. Depending on the intensity, several types of postremission therapy have been studied, including consolidation, early intensification, and maintenance. Although the optimum form remains to be defined, almost all patients with AML benefit from further therapy. The type of postremission therapy should be determined based on age and prognostic factors. A high relapse-free survival rate is predicted by M3 morphology, a favorable karyotype [t(8;21), t(15;17), inv (16)], and the absence of dys-myelopoiesis. In contrast, the presence of myelo-dysplasia, age greater than 60 years, persistent leukemia after one course of induction therapy, or an unfavorable karyotype (abnormalities of chromosomes 5 or 7, trisomy 8, changes at position 11q23, and complex abnormalities), all predict a low relapse-free survival rate. Relative contraindications to postinduction therapy include complications during induction (e.g., posttransfusion hepatitis with persistent hepatic dysfunction, persistent systemic fungal infection), poor tolerance of induction by the elderly, and pregnancy. Patients with AML in first remission should be considered candidates for experimental protocols examining postinduction therapy options. For patients who are not able to be enrolled in protocol studies, the approach to postinduction therapy used at Wayne State University is shown in Table 19-1.

1. **Consolidation.** The current published data suggest that high-dose cytarabine intensification offers a distinct advantage over standard-dose cytarabine consolidation in patients under 60 years of age. Although consolidation with one to three cycles of "7 + 3" without maintenance has been empirically recommended as standard consolidation treatment in the past, patients younger than 60 years old or those who do not have favorable prognostic factors should be considered for early intensification with HDAC or BMT.

2. **Early intensification.** Early intensification represents the best strategy devised thus far for postremission chemotherapy. Uncontrolled series suggest that 40% to 50% of patients will be in a continuous CR 5 years after intensification with HDAC (with or without daunorubicin), whereas randomized Cancer and Leukemia Group B (CALGB) studies suggest that this rate may be closer to 40% to 50% at 4 years. There is about a 5% mortality rate with HDAC and with HDAC plus daunorubicin. Amsacrine appears to increase the toxicity of HDAC without a significant increase in benefit. Intensification is the best postinduction chemotherapeutic option currently available for patients under the age of 50 years who are standard risk or for those who are poor risk but do not have an HLA-identical sibling. Intensification should be strongly considered in patients between the ages of 50 and 60 years. Because of the significant morbidity and mortality, intensification is not recommended outside of the experimental

setting for patients older than 60 years. Intensification should be initiated when the peripheral blood counts have returned to normal (ANC more than 1,500/μL and platelet count more than 100,000/μL), marrow cellularity is normal, infections have cleared, and mucositis has resolved. The most tolerable intensification programs are based on HDAC. The optimum regimen is not known. Options include the following:

a. HDAC

Cytarabine, 3 g/m² i.v. infusion over 3 hours every 12 hours on days 1, 3, and 5 (CALGB HDAC) for four monthly courses (better tolerated), *or*

Cytarabine, 3 g/m² i.v. infusion over 2 hours every 12 hours on days 1 to 6 for one to three monthly courses (most patients cannot tolerate more than one or two courses of standard HDAC).

b. HDAC plus daunorubicin has been used in two different programs:

(1) Cytarabine, 3 g/m² i.v. infusion over 1 to 2 hours every 12 hours on days 1 to 6, *and* daunorubicin, 30 mg/m² i.v. on days 7 to 9, are given for 1 to 3 cycles, *or*

(2) Alternative program

Month 1: Cytarabine, 3 g/m² i.v. infusion over 2 hours every 12 hours on days 1 to 4, *and* daunorubicin, 45 mg/m² i.v. on days 1 to 3.

Month 2: Cytarabine, 200 mg/m²/24 hours continuous i.v. infusion on days 1 to 5, *and* daunorubicin, 45 mg/m² i.v. on days 1 to 3.

c. HDAC plus multiple agents

Month 1: Cytarabine 3 g/m² i.v. infusion over 2 hours every 12 hours on days 1 to 4, *and* mitoxantrone, 10 mg/m² i.v. on days 1 to 3.

Month 2: Etoposide 200 mg/m²/day on days 1 to 5, *and* mitoxantrone, 10 mg/m² i.v. on days 1 to 3.

Month 3: Cytarabine, 2 g/m² i.v. infusion over 2 hours every 12 hours on days 1 to 4, *and* daunorubicin, 45 mg/m² i.v. on days 1 to 3.

3. Maintenance. Previous trials from CALGB have shown that low doses of postremission maintenance therapy do not prolong the remission duration when given after more intensive postinduction therapy. Therefore, no further therapy is recommended after the completion of consolidation or early intensification.

Given the rigors of further intensive, cytoreductive chemotherapy, however, maintenance may be the postremission treatment of choice for elderly (older than 60 years) patients as well as for younger patients who did not tolerate induction well. In general, remission duration is 12 to 15 months and overall survival time is 18 to 24 months with maintenance chemotherapy. About 15% to 20% of patients treated with maintenance therapy remain long-term disease-free survivors. Maintenance may be initiated when the peripheral blood counts have returned to normal, marrow cellularity is normal, infections have cleared, and mucositis has resolved. Maintenance may be alternating blocks of drugs or repetitive courses of the same drugs.

a. **Alternating courses.** A commonly used program of alternating blocks of drugs has been devised by CALGB. Each of the four courses is given on a monthly basis during the cycle. Two cycles are given for a total of 8 months of therapy. If a bone marrow examination shows that the patient is still in a CR at the end of the second cycle, no further therapy is given. Minimal blood counts for initiating maintenance are an ANC of more than 2,000/µL and a platelet count of more than 100,000/µL. Each cycle consists of the following four courses:

Course 1: Cytarabine, 100 mg/m^2 s.c. b.i.d. on days 1–5, *and* 6-thioguanine, 100 mg/m^2 p.o. b.i.d. on days 1–5.

Courses 2 and 4: Cytarabine, 100 mg/ m^2 s.c. b.i.d. on days 1 to 5, *and* vincristine, 2 mg i.v. on days 1 and 8, *and* prednisone, 40 mg/m^2 p.o. on days 1 to 5 (100 mg maximum).

Course 3: Cytarabine, 100 mg/m^2 s.c. b.i.d. on days 1 to 5, *and* daunorubicin, 45 mg/m^2 i.v. on days 1 and 2. This course may require support for pancytopenia.

Once maintenance has been started, the next course may be given in 4 weeks, provided that infection and mucositis from the previous course have cleared, the ANC is more than 2,000/µL, and the platelet count is more than 100,000/µL. If the ANC and platelet count are below the minimum, repeat them in 1 week and use the following criteria:

Dose (%)	ANC (/µL)	Platelets (/µL)
100	≥2,000	≥100,000
50	1,000–1,999	50,000–99,999
0	<1,000	<50,000

Dose adjustments for hematologic toxicity should also be based on nadir blood counts or the development of grade 4 bleeding or infection during the previous course.

Dose (%)	Nadir ANC (/µL)	Nadir platelets (/µL)
100	≥1,000	≥50,000
50	<1,000	<50,000

   b. **Cytarabine and daunorubicin** produce similar results according to recent data from CALGB.

Cytarabine, 100 mg/m²/24 hours continuous i.v. infusion on days 1 to 5 monthly for 4 months, *then*

Cytarabine, 100 mg/m² s.c. b.i.d. on days 1 to 5, *and*

Daunorubicin, 45 mg/m² i.v. on day 1, both monthly for 4 months.

D. **Relapsed AML.** Cytotoxic chemotherapy offers little chance for long-term survival for patients with relapsed AML. Given the palliative nature of further chemotherapy at this point, a realistic appraisal of the situation should be offered to the patient to enable development of a plan that can optimize both the quantity and quality of meaningful life. A long first remission portends a better chance of attaining a substantial second remission. Unfortunately, second remissions tend to be short, with median durations in the range of 4 to 6 months. Patients with relapsed AML should be considered prime candidates for experimental protocols or stem cell transplantation. Depending on prior therapy, age, and perceived ability to tolerate another induction, chemotherapeutic options using commercially available drugs would include the following:

   1. **"7 + 3."** Up to half of patients who undergo induction with the "7 + 3" regimen followed by maintenance respond to a repeat course of "7 + 3." Patients who relapse within 6 months of the last chemotherapy are unlikely to respond to the same regimen again. Thus, a different regimen should be considered.

   2. **HDAC**. Fifty to 70% of patients respond to a form of HDAC. Although HDAC combination regimens may have a slightly higher response rate, their increased toxicity may not make them significantly better than single-agent HDAC. Patients who relapse within 6 months of HDAC intensification are unlikely to have a significant response to further HDAC. The doses given for the

HDAC are those originally described for each regimen. Options include the following:

  a. **HDAC**, *or*
  b. **HDAC plus anthracycline** (see Section IV.B.3), *or* HDAC, 3 g/m² i.v. infusion over 2 hours every 12 hours on days 1 to 4, *plus* mitoxantrone, 10 mg/m²/day i.v. on days 2 to 5 or 2 to 6, *or*
  c. **FLAG-Ida**
      Fludarabine, 30 mg/m²/day i.v. infusion over 30 minutes on days 1 to 5, *and*
      HDAC, 2 g/m²/day i.v. infusion over 4 hours starting 3.5 hours after the fludarabine is finished on days 1 to 5, *and*
      Idarubicin, 10 mg/m² iv on days 1 to 3, *and*
      G-CSF, 300 g/m²/day i.v. over 2 hours on days −1 to +5, *then*
      G-CSF, 300 g/m²/day s.c. on day 12 (i.e., 7 after *end* of chemotherapy) until neutrophil recovery (ANC more than 500/µL), *or*
  d. **MEC.** This regimen produces significant gastrointestinal and cardiac toxicity. It is not recommended for patients over 60 years of age or those with borderline cardiac function. A variation of MEC currently used by the ECO is:
      Etoposide, 40 mg/m²/day i.v. infusion over 1 hour on days 1 to 5, *followed immediately by*
      Cytarabine, 1 g/m²/day i.v. infusion over 1 hour on days 1 to 5, *and*
      Mitoxantrone, 4 mg/m²/day i.v. side arm push on days 1 to 5, given after completion of HDAC each day.

  3. **Etoposide**, 100 mg/m²/day i.v. on days 1 to 5, **and mitoxantrone**, 10 mg/m²/day i.v. on days 1 to 5, represents an active and well-tolerated combination that is commonly used for relapsed or refractory leukemia.

  4. **High-dose etoposide**, 70 mg/m²/hour continuous i.v. infusion for 60 hours, **and high-dose cyclophosphamide**, 50 mg/kg (1,850 mg/m²)/day i.v. infusion over 2 hours on days 1 to 4, is a highly toxic but active regimen that does not require bone marrow support. It is active against HDAC-resistant AML (30% CR). (For details, see Brown et al., 1990.) This regimen may be useful for young patients who are good candidates for allogeneic BMT while waiting for an unrelated donor search to be completed.

E. **Role of BMT in AML.** The role and timing of BMT in the management of adult AML, especially in first remission, have been the subject of much speculation and controversy because of the reporting of uncontrolled results (see Chap. 6). With the prolongation of first remission after the use of increasingly aggressive postinduction therapy, the role of allogeneic BMT is less well defined. The results of recently available randomized prospective trials that compare the outcome of BMT with that of less intensive postinduction therapies than are now used may not be applicable to patients receiving multiple courses of HDAC as postremission intensification. The benefit of BMT needs to be carefully considered on an individual basis. Factors to be considered include the risk of transplant-related mortality, age, and other prognostic factors. Patients with good prognostic factors at diagnosis [i.e., t(8;21), t(15;17), inv (16)] should receive standard postinduction therapy regardless of age. Those without good risk factors may benefit from either autologous or allogeneic BMT in first remission, especially those who have unfavorable bone marrow cytogenetics. An unrelated donor allogeneic BMT in first remission is still considered investigational unless one is dealing with therapy-related AML or AML following myelodysplastic syndromes. Potential candidates for BMT should be enrolled in prospective, randomized studies to define further its use.

1. **Allogeneic transplantation.** Although allogeneic BMT receives much fanfare in the medical literature and the lay press, it has been estimated that in reality at most 10% of patients with AML are candidates for a BMT from an HLA-compatible sibling. Although allogeneic BMT has been considered an option for patients younger than 40 to 45 years, many centers now take patients up to 60 years old. For patients with AML in second remission, allogeneic BMT is the treatment of choice because it offers a 20% to 30% chance of long-term survival. Recent randomized studies have suggested that the use of BMT in patients in their first remission does not improve the overall survival rate compared with patients treated with postinduction chemotherapy followed by BMT during the second remission should they experience relapse. As the "community standard," BMT should be considered as the optimum form of salvage therapy to be used for patients in second remission. It should also be considered for primary induction failures, early relapse, or high-risk patients. However, eligible patients should continue to be entered into randomized prospective clinical trials that examine the use of allogeneic BMT.

2. **Autologous transplantation** uses the recipient's own stem cells obtained from bone marrow or peripheral blood. The potential benefits of using the person's own stem cells are the absence of graft-versus-host disease, a readily

available donor, and better tolerance by older patients. The obvious disadvantage is the potential to reinfuse leukemic cells. Although still experimental, as methods of purging improve and new technology (e.g., polymerase chain reaction) allows for the better detection of residual leukemia, autologous BMT may become the best form of early intensification.

3. **Relapse.** Relapse after BMT performed during first remission occurs in about 20% of allogeneic transplantations and 40% of autologous transplantations. Salvage of these patients is difficult, especially if relapse occurs within 3 months of transplantation. Although 35% of patients may achieve a remission with subsequent "7 + 3" reinduction, long-term leukemia-free survival is rare. A second allogeneic BMT can be considered in highly selected patients who have achieved a second remission after reinduction chemotherapy and whose disease has relapsed at least 6 months after the initial BMT and who have no residual organ damage. The use of donor lymphocyte infusions has been reported to be successful in a small number of patients who are not candidates for a second BMT. The addition of interleukin-2 or interferon to the donor lymphocyte infusion to improve the antileukemic effect requires further investigation. Preliminary data have also suggested that G-CSF (μ 5 g/kg/day s.c.) can stimulate the normal hematopoietic clone in posttransplantation chimeras.

V. **Therapy for adult ALL**

A. **Overview.** All adults have high-risk ALL compared with children. Although 75% to 85% of adults with ALL can attain a CR, only 20% to 35% remain disease free. The emphasis in recent years has been on the development of therapeutic regimens that contain more intensive induction and postremission therapies. These regimens have usually been developed as complete programs without testing the contributions of the individual components. With the advent of these more aggressive regimens, long-term disease-free survival has improved. Whether this is due to a true improvement in chemotherapy as opposed to the biases of patient selection and better supportive care is not clear. Given the lessons learned from the "evolution" of therapy for diffuse large cell lymphoma in the 1980s and 1990s, these improved regimens (and the components thereof) need to be tested in rigorous, randomized prospective trials. All patients with ALL should be considered as candidates for chemotherapy in well-designed, randomized, prospective trials.

B. **Prognostic features.** As opposed to AML, in which chemotherapy is the same regardless of FAB classification, prognostic features are now being used to determine the intensity of induction and postremission therapy for adult ALL. The most important risk factor influencing the type of induction therapy is based on immunophenotypic subclassification of the leukemic cells at diagnosis (B-lineage ALL, T-cell ALL, or B-cell ALL). Other factors to consider when planning therapy include age, cytogenetic abnormalities, and the presence of extramedullary disease (i.e., testicular or central nervous system [CNS] involvement).

C. **General plan.** The general plan of therapy for adult ALL is somewhat different from that of AML. Adults with ALL should be stratified according to known risk factors at the time of diagnosis and started on a regimen appropriate for the perceived risk of failure. As opposed to AML, the bone marrow in adult ALL has usually been checked for residual leukemia only at the time of marrow recovery. Some newer, more aggressive protocols do base therapeutic decisions on the status of the day-14 bone marrow. Once a CR has been attained, the form of CNS prophylaxis and postinduction therapy should be determined on an individual basis. The overall approach to the treatment of ALL used at Wayne State University is shown in Table 19-2.

D. **B-cell–lineage ALL.** Standard-risk ALL consists of disease that is CD10 positive, does not express myeloid antigens, and does not have the Philadelphia chromosome (Ph^1). With the use of more intensive regimens (e.g., CALGB 8811), the presence of myeloid antigens loses its prognostic significance. Complete programs are described next.

1. **Normal cardiac function.** In the presence of normal cardiac function, adults with ALL are usually treated with an anthracycline-containing program.

a. **VPD with L-asparaginase.** Historically, regimens for the induction of adult ALL have been built around vincristine, prednisone, and daunorubicin (VPD). L-Asparaginase is commonly added. The overall response rate is 75-85%. Although L-asparaginase proved to be of value in the pre-anthracycline era, its role in anthracycline-based adult programs is unclear. Given the significant toxicity of L-asparaginase, many investigators no longer recommend its use, especially in elderly patients. The newer pegalated form of L-asparaginase (peg-L-asparaginase) offers a more prolonged half-life and has been shown to be effective in children who had a prior hypersensitivity reaction to other forms of L-asparaginase.

Table 19-2. Initial therapeutic options for acute lymphoblastic leukemia outside of the experimental setting[a]

Immunophenotype	Risk	Age (yr)	Cardiac function	Therapy
B-cell lineage	Standard	<60	Normal	CALGB 8811, or
				VPD ± A → maintenenance
			Abnormal	MOAD
		>60	Normal	VPD → maintenenance, or
				CALGB 8811
			Abnormal	MOAD
	High (Ph1+,	<60	Normal	CALGB 8811 ± BMT, or
	CD11/CD33+)			VPD ± A → allogeneic BMT or
				autologous BMT
T cell			Normal	Linker protocol, or
				CALGB 8811
B cell		<50	Normal	B-NHL 86
		>50	Normal	Modified B-NHL 86

[a] All patients with acute leukemia should be treated in clinical trials.
CALGB, Cancer and Acute Leukemia Group B; VPD, vineristine, prednisone, daunorubicin; A, asparaginase; BMT, bone marrow transplantation; BNHL, (see Section V.F.).

Preliminary data have shown that the combination of VPD with peg-L-asparaginase is well tolerated and produces a high CR rate in adult patients with ALL. The dose schedule and frequency of treatment requires further study. A number of variations on the basic VPD program are described below. VPD should be used for patients who are thought not to be able to tolerate a more intensive chemotherapy program. Some options are shown in parentheses.

(1) **Induction**

> Vincristine, 2 mg i.v. on days 1, 8, 15, (22), *and*

> Prednisone, 40 or 60 mg/m^2 p.o. on days 1 to 28 or days 1 to 35, followed by rapid taper over 7 days, *and*

> Daunorubicin, 45 mg/m^2 i.v. on days 1 to 3, *and*

> L-Asparaginase, 500 IU/kg (18,500 IU/m^2) i.v. on days 22 to 32.

(2) **CNS prophylaxis** is given as six doses of intrathecal methotrexate and whole-brain irradiation starting on about day 36 (see Section V.J.).

(3) **Maintenance for adult ALL** usually consists of methotrexate and 6-mercaptopurine. Pulses of vincristine and prednisone are given as "reinforcement" because they have relatively little toxicity. Maintenance is usually started once the marrow suppression and the oral toxicity of the CNS prophylaxis have cleared. Maintenance may be given in a pulse or a continuous manner. Although allopurinol is usually not needed after remission is achieved, the dose of 6-mercaptopurine should be decreased by 75% when given concomitantly with allopurinol.

(a) **Pulse maintenance** is an 8-week cycle consisting of three courses of methotrexate and 6-mercaptopurine given every 2 weeks, followed by a 2-week pulse of vincristine and prednisone.

> Methotrexate, 7.5 mg/m^2 p.o. on days 1 to 5, weeks 1, 3, and 5, *and*

> 6-Mercaptopurine, 200 mg/m^2 p.o. on days 1 to 5, weeks 1, 3, and 5, *and*

Vincristine 2 mg, i.v. on day 1, weeks 7 and 8, *and*

Prednisone 40, mg/m² p.o. on days 1 to 7, weeks 7 and 8.

Oral methotrexate should be taken in a single daily dose because splitting the daily dose significantly increases the mucositis. About three doses of intrathecal methotrexate are needed once maintenance has started. The schedule should be coordinated so that the intrathecal methotrexate is given on day 1 of the 5 scheduled days of oral methotrexate. On those days when intrathecal methotrexate is given, the oral methotrexate is not given. Pulse maintenance is given for 3 years.

Dose adjustments for hematologic toxicity from the methotrexate and 6-mercaptopurine should be made based on blood cell counts obtained before the start of each course.

Dose	ANC (/μL)	Platelets (/μL)
100%	≥2,000	≥100,000
75%	1,500–1,999	75,000–99,999
50%	1,000–1,499	50,000–74,999
0%	<1,000	<50,000

   (4) Intensification with cytarabine and daunorubicin given as "7 + 3" and "5 + 2" does not improve remission duration or overall survival compared with pulse maintenance in randomized prospective trials.

b.   CALGB 8811 consists of a five-drug combination devised to achieve more rapid cytoreduction during the induction phase. For B-cell–lineage ALL, it produced an 82% CR rate with 41% disease-free survival at 36 months. Patients in remission receive multiagent consolidation treatment, CNS prophylaxis, late intensification, and maintenance chemotherapy for a total of 24 months. CALGB 8811 should be considered for patients regardless of age who are thought to be able to withstand the rigors of an intensive program.

   (1) Induction

Cyclophosphamide, 1,200 mg/m² i.v. on day 1, *and*

Daunorubicin, 45 mg/m² i.v. on days 1, 2, 3, *and*

Vincristine, 2 mg i.v. on days 1, 8, 15, 22, *and*

Prednisone, 60 mg/m²/day p.o. on days 1 to 21, *and*

L-Asparaginase, 6,000 IU/m² s.c. on days 5, 8, 11, 15, 18, and 22.
For patients older than 60 years:
Cyclophosphamide, 800 mg/m² on day 1, *and*

Daunorubicin, 30 mg/m² on days 1, 2, 3, *and*

Prednisone, 60 mg/m²/day on days 1 to 7.

(2) **Early intensification** (two cycles)
Intrathecal methotrexate, 15 mg on day 1, *and*

Cyclophosphamide 1,000 mg/m² i.v. on day 1, *and*

6-Mercaptopurine, 60 mg/m²/day p.o. on days 1 to 14, *and*

Cytarabine, 75 mg/m²/day s.c. on days 1 to 4, 8 to 11, *and*

Vincristine, 2 mg i.v. on days 15 and 22, *and*

L-Asparaginase, 6,000 IU/m² s.c. on days 15, 18, 22, and 25.

(3) **CNS prophylaxis and interim maintenance**
Cranial irradiation, 2,400 cGy on days 1 to 12, *and*

Intrathecal methotrexate, 15 mg on days 1, 8, 15, 22, 29, *and*

6-Mercaptopurine, 60 mg/m²/day p.o. on days 1 to 70, *and*

Methotrexate, 20 mg/m² p.o. on days 36, 43, 50, 57, and 64.

(4) **Late intensification**
Doxorubicin, 30 mg/m² i.v. on days 1, 8, 15, *and*

Vincristine, 2 mg i.v. on days 1, 8, 15, *and*

Dexamethasone, 10 mg/m²/day p.o. on days 1 to 14, *and*

Cyclophosphamide, 1,000 mg/m² i.v. on day 29, *and*

6-Thioguanine, 60 mg/m²/day p.o. on days 29 to 42, *and*

Cytarabine, 75 mg/m²/day s.c. on days 29 to 32 and 36 to 39.

(5) **Prolonged maintenance** (monthly until 24 months from diagnosis)
Vincristine, 2 mg i.v. on day 1, *and*

Prednisone, 60 mg/m²/day p.o. on days 1 to 5, *and*

Methotrexate, 20 mg/m^2 p.o. on days 1, 8, 15, and 22, *and*

6-Mercaptopurine, 60 mg/m^2/day p.o. on days 1 to 28.

2. **ALL in the elderly.** Although elderly patients are often considered a poor risk because of their comorbid disease and the increased incidence of the Ph^1 chromosome, they cannot tolerate more intensive therapy. Thus, they are usually treated in the manner described above. In general, full doses of VPD induction therapy are used in elderly patients with ALL. Some investigators decrease the dose of vincristine by 50%. CALGB 8811 should also be considered for those who are thought to be able to tolerate more intensive therapy.

3. **Impaired cardiac function**

   a. **Induction.** Underlying cardiac disease may preclude the use of an anthracycline for induction therapy. Vincristine, prednisone, and asparaginase in the doses described above represents suboptimal therapy. An active program is MOAD, which is given in sequential 10-day courses (minimum 3, maximum 5) until remission is achieved. Once a CR has been attained, two additional courses of MOAD are given.

   Methotrexate, 100 mg/m^2 i.v. on day 1 (increase by 50% courses 2 and 3, and by 25% each additional course until mild toxicity is achieved), *and*

   Vincristine, 2 mg i.v. on day 2, *and*

   L-Asparaginase, 500 IU/kg (18,500 IU/m^2) i.v. infusion on day 2, *and*

   Dexamethasone, 6 mg/m^2/day p.o. on days 1 to 10.

   b. **Consolidation therapy** is repeated every 10 days for six courses.

   Methotrexate, (final dose from induction) i.v. on day 1, *and*

   L-Asparaginase, 500 IU/kg (18,500 IU/m^2) i.v. infusion on day 2.

   c. **Cytoreduction** begins on day 30 of the last consolidation cycle of methotrexate and L-asparaginase. Cytoreduction is given monthly for 12 months.

   Vincristine, 2 mg i.v. on day 1, 30 minutes, before methotrexate, *and*

   Methotrexate, 100 mg/kg (3.7 g/m^2) i.v. infusion over 6 hours on day 1, *and*

   Leucovorin, 5 mg/kg (185 mg/m^2) divided into 12 doses starting 2 hours after the methotrexate infusion over days 1 to 3, *and*

Dexamethasone, 6 mg/m²/day p.o. on days 2 to 6.

d. Maintenance begins on day 30 of the last course of cytoreduction. It is repeated monthly until relapse.

Vincristine, 2 mg i.v. on day 1, *and*

Dexamethasone, 6 mg/m²/day p.o. on days 1 to 5, *and*

Methotrexate, 15 mg/m² p.o. weekly, *and*

6-Mercaptopurine, 100 mg/m² p.o. daily.

E. T-cell lymphoblastic leukemia. This form of leukemia constitutes 20% to 25% of cases of adult ALL. Although it previously had a poor prognosis with standard induction and maintenance chemotherapy, with the advent of more intensive chemotherapy regimens, T-cell ALL has become a potentially curable malignancy. There was a 100% response rate, with 59% of responders projected to have long-term disease-free survival, with the regimen devised by Linker and colleagues (1991). CALGB 8811 produced a 100% CR rate with a 63% relapse-free survival rate at 3 years. The Linker regimen is as follows:

1. Induction

Daunorubicin, 60 mg/m² i.v. on days 1 to 3, *and*

Vincristine, 2 mg i.v. on days 1, 8, 15, and 22, *and*

Prednisone, 60 mg/m² p.o. on days 1 to 28, *and*

L-Asparaginase, 6,000 IU/m² i.m. on days 17 to 28.

If a bone marrow examination on day 14 shows residual leukemia, a single dose of daunorubicin, 50 mg/m², is given. If a bone marrow examination on day 28 shows residual leukemia, additional induction therapy is given:

Daunorubicin, 50 mg/m² i.v. on days 29 and 30, *and*

Vincristine, 2 mg i.v. on days 29 and 36, *and*

Prednisone, 60 mg/m² p.o. on days 29-42, *and*

L-Asparaginase, 6,000 IU/m² i.m. on days 29 to 35.

2. CNS prophylaxis consists of cranial radiation (1,800 cGy) and six weekly doses of intrathecal methotrexate.

3. Consolidation therapy is given monthly for 9 months if the ANC is higher than 1,000/μL and the platelet count is higher than 100,000/μL.

a. Treatment A is given in months 1, 3, 5, and 7.

Daunorubicin, 50 mg/m² i.v. on days 1 and 2, *and*

Vincristine, 2 mg i.v. on days 1 and 8, *and*

Prednisone, 60 mg/m² p.o. on days 1 to 14, *and*

L-Asparaginase, 12,000 IU/m² i.m. on days 2, 4, 7, 9, 11, and 14.

      b. **Treatment B** is given in months 2, 4, 6, and 8.
  Teniposide, 165 mg/m² i.v. on days 1, 4, 8, and 11, *and*
  Cytarabine, 300 mg/m² i.v. on days 1, 4, 8, and 11.

      c. **Treatment C** is given in month 9.
  Methotrexate, 690 mg/m² continuous i.v. infusion over 42 hours, *and*
  Leucovorin, 15 mg/m² every 6 hours for 12 doses starting at hour 42.

   4. **Maintenance** is continued for 30 months.
  Methotrexate, 20 mg/m² p.o. weekly, *and*
  Mercaptopurine, 75 mg/m² p.o. daily.

F. B-cell acute lymphoblastic leukemia is a rare ALL subtype constituting only 2% to 4% of cases of adult ALL. The leukemic cells are characterized by L3 morphology, by expression of monoclonal surface immunoglobulin (sIg), and by specific nonrandom chromosomal translocations [t(8;14) (q24;q32), t(2;8) (9q24:q11)]. In the past, the results of the treatment of B-cell ALL in both children and adults had been poor, with a CR rate of about 35% and leukemia-free survival (LFS) of 0% to 33%. The current pediatric studies designed specifically for B-cell ALL by the French and German study group have substantially improved the CR rate to about 90% and the LFS to 50% to 87%. The changes involve the use of higher doses and fractionation of the cyclophosphamide to expose the rapidly dividing B cells to the active alkylating metabolites of cyclophosphamide over a longer period as well as the use of high-dose methotrexate. These regimens are of brief duration and require no maintenance. Hoelzer and colleagues (1996) recently reported their experience in adapting these treatments to adults with B-cell ALL. The CR rate increased from 44% to 74%, the probability of LFS increased from 0% to 71%, and the overall survival rate increased from 0% to 51% when the intensive treatment was compared with a standard ALL regimen.

   Study B-NHL 86 consists of six alternating courses of regimens A and B.

   1. **Prephase therapy** is given to avoid tumor lysis syndrome and to correct possible metabolic abnormalities.
  Cyclophosphamide, 200 mg/m² i.v. infusion over 1 hour on days 1 to 5, *and*
  Prednisone, 60 mg/m²/day p.o. in three divided doses days 1 to 5.

   2. **Regimen A** begins 1 week after the first dose of cytoxan
  Methotrexate, 15 mg, *plus* cytarabine, 40 mg, *plus* dexamethasone, 4 mg intrathecally on day 1, *and*
  Vincristine, 2 mg i.v. on day 1, *and*
  Ifosfamide, 800 mg/m² i.v. on days 1 to 5, *and*

Teniposide, 100 mg/m^2 i.v. on days 4 and 5, *and*

Cytarabine, 150 mg/m^2 i.v. every 12 hours on days 4 and 5, *and*

Dexamethasone, 10 mg/m^2 p.o. on days 1 to 5, *and*

Methotrexate, 150 mg/m^2 IVPB bolus over 30 minutes on day 1, *immediately followed by* methotrexate, 1,350 mg/m^2 i.v. infusion over 23.5 hours (total methotrexate dose is 1,500 mg/m^2 i.v. in 24 hours), *and*

Leucovorin rescue, 30 mg/m^2 i.v. 36 hours after the beginning of high-dose methotrexate infusion, *followed by* oral leucovorin, 30 mg/m^2, 15 mg/m^2, and three doses of 5 mg/m^2 given at 42, 48, 54, 68, and 78 hours, respectively, for an appropriate decrease in methotrexate levels. If the methotrexate level at 42 hours is more than 0.5 μmol/L, give leucovorin, 50 mg/m^2 i.v. every 6 hours through 60 hours. If the methotrexate level at 68 hours is more than or equal to 0.1 μmol/L, give leucovorin, 30 mg/m^2 i.v. every 6 hours for four more doses.

3. **Regimen B**

Methotrexate, 15 mg, *plus* cytarabine, 40 mg, *plus* dexamethasone, 4 mg intrathecally on day 1, *and*

Vincristine, 2 mg i.v. on day 1, *and*

Methotrexate, 150 mg/m^2 IVPB bolus over 30 minutes on day 1, *then* methotrexate, 1,350 mg/m^2 i.v. infusion over 23.5 hours (total methotrexate 1,500 mg/m^2 i.v. in 24 hours). This is followed by leucovorin rescue as per cycle A, *and*

Cyclophosphamide, 200 mg/m^2 IVPB over 1 hour on days 1 to 5, *and*

Doxorubicin, 25 mg/m^2 IVP over 15 minutes on days 4 and 5, *and*

Dexamethasone, 10 mg/m^2 p.o. on days 1 to 5.

4. **For patients older than 50 years**, an intermediate dose of methotrexate (see below) is used instead of high-dose methotrexate owing to prolonged hematologic toxicity and mucositis.

On day 1, give methotrexate, 50 mg/m^2 loading dose by IVPB over 30 minutes, followed by methotrexate, 450 mg/m^2 i.v. infusion over the next 23.5 hours (total methotrexate dose, 500 mg/m^2/day). This is followed by leucovorin rescue, 12 mg/m^2 i.v. starting 32 hours after the beginning of methotrexate infusion; then repeat the same dose every 6 hours for a total of four doses. Thereafter, oral leucovorin (12 mg/m^2) is given until the methotrexate level is less than 0.01 μM (1×10^{-8} M).

5. **CNS prophylaxis.** Patients in CR after the first two cycles of chemotherapy (A and B) receive

prophylactic cranial irradiation of 2,400 cGy in addition to the triple intrathecal therapy as described above.

G. **Ph¹-positive ALL**. Ph¹-positive ALL accounts for 25% to 30% of cases of adult ALL and for about 50% of CD10-positive ALL in adults. Overall, Ph¹-positive ALL has the worst prognosis. Although Ph¹-positive ALL has a 50% to 70% induction rate, long-term responses are rare even with aggressive regimens (e.g., CALGB 8811, Linker protocol). Because cytogenetic analysis is not usually available in a timely manner and not all institutions can examine for bcr-abl rearrangement on site, patients with Ph¹-positive ALL are usually treated with standard induction therapy or with an appropriate experimental protocol. Patients who can tolerate a more aggressive approach should be treated with the CALGB 8811 regimen (see Section V.D.1.b). Those who attain a CR should be offered allogeneic BMT if possible. If not, they should be viewed as candidates for aggressive or novel postinduction experimental protocols.

H. **Relapsed ALL.** Although a second remission can usually be achieved in adults with ALL, it tends to be short lived. This is particularly true in patients treated with the contemporary intensive regimens described above. If a second remission can be attained, suitable patients with relapsed ALL should be considered as candidates for BMT. None of the regimens used for relapse is distinctly superior to the others, and any perceived differences are likely attributable to the usual biases of study selection. Chemotherapeutic options using commercially available agents are shown.

1. **"7 + 3"** (cytarabine and daunorubicin) as used for the induction of AML is active in ALL. Vincristine and prednisone may be added.

2. **HDAC as a single agent** has modest activity in ALL, with a CR rate of about 34% and a median remission duration of 3.6 months in data from combined studies. The addition of idarubicin or mitoxantrone increases the response rate to 60%, but the median response time remains 3.4 months.

3. **Cytarabine and fludarabine** comprise an active noncardiotoxic combination. The median response duration is 5.5 months. Neurotoxicity is low. A second course can be given in 3 weeks if needed.

   a. **Induction**
       Cytarabine, 1 g/m²/day i.v. over 2 hours on days 1 to 6, *and*
       Fludarabine, 30 mg/m²/day i.v. over 30 minutes 4 hours before cytarabine on days 2 to 6.

   b.   Consolidation is given monthly for two
        or three courses.
        Cytarabine, 1 g/m^2/day i.v. over 2 hours on
           days 1 to 4, *and*
        Fludarabine, 30 mg/m^2/day i.v. over 30 min-
           utes 4 hours before cytarabine on days
           1 to 4.
   c.   Maintenance
        6-Mercaptopurine 50 mg p.o. t.i.d., *and*
        Methotrexate, 20 mg/m^2 p.o. per week.
**4.   Sequential methotrexate and L-asparagi-
     nase** is another option. Stomatitis was dose
     limiting. Twenty-three percent of treated pa-
     tients had allergic reactions to L-asparaginase.
   a.   Induction
        Methotrexate, 50 to 80 mg/m^2 i.v. on day 1,
           and
        L-asparaginase, 20,000 IU/m^2 i.v. 3 hours
           after methotrexate on day 1, *followed by*
        Methotrexate, 120 mg/m^2 i.v. on day 8, *and*
        L-asparaginase 20,000 IU/m^2 i.v. on day 9.
           Repeat day 8 and 9 doses for methotrex-
           ate and L-asparaginase every 7 to 14 days
           until remission is attained.
   b.   Maintenance is repeated every 2 weeks.
        Methotrexate, 10 to 40 mg/m^2 i.v. on day 1,
           and
        L-asparaginase, 10,000 IU/m^2 i.v. on day 1.
5.   Etoposide and cytarabine are given every
     3 weeks for up to 3 courses until marrow
     hypoplasia and remission are achieved. They
     are then repeated monthly until relapse.
     Etoposide, 60 mg/m^2 i.v. every 12 hours on days
        1 to 5, *and*
     Cytarabine, 100 mg/m^2 i.v. bolus every 12 hours
        on days 1 to 5.
6.   Hyper CVAD consists of eight courses of alter-
     nating intensive chemotherapy with growth
     factor support, followed by oral maintenance
     chemotherapy.
   a.   Courses 1, 3, 5, and 7:
        Cyclophosphamide, 300 mg/m^2 i.v. every
           12 hours on days 1 to 3, *and*
        Vincristine, 2 mg i.v. on days 4 and 11, *and*
        Doxorubicin, 50 mg/m^2 i.v. on day 4, *and*
        Dexamethasone, 40 mg/day on days 1 to 4
           and days 11 to 14.
   b.   Courses 2, 4, 6 and 8:
        Methotrexate, 1 g/m^2 i.v. over 24 hours on
           day 1, *and*
        Cytarabine, 3 g/m^2 i.v. infusion over 1 hour
           every 12 hours × four doses on days 2
           and 3 (reduce cytarabine dose to 1 g/m^2
           for patients over 60 years old), *and*

Leucovorin rescue (see Section V.F.2) starting 12 hours after the completion of methotrexate, *and*

G-CSF is started 24 hours after chemotherapy is completed and is continued until the white blood cell (WBC) count is more than 3,000/μL and the platelet count is more than 30,000/μL.

   c. **Maintenance therapy** for 2 years
6-Mercaptopurine, 50 mg p.o. t.i.d., *and*
Methotrexate, 20 mg/m^2 p.o. per week.

I. **BMT.** As with adult AML, the role of BMT in the management of adult ALL is constantly in evolution (see Chap. 6). Eligible candidates should be entered into randomized prospective trials to define further the use of BMT in adult ALL.

   1. **Allogeneic BMT.** Allogeneic transplantation has been compared with chemotherapy in randomized prospective trials. For standard-risk patients, the outcome is similar. Thus, for standard-risk patients, BMT should be considered as salvage therapy in second remission. BMT should be considered the postremission treatment of choice in Ph^1-positive ALL and strongly considered for other high-risk patients.

   2. **Autologous BMT.** Autologous stem cell transplantation in patients in first remission appears to offer no advantage over chemotherapy in the prospective trials reported to date. Autologous transplantation in second remission can lead to a significant prolongation of leukemia-free survival.

   3. **Relapse after BMT.** Although up to 50% of patients can attain another remission with reinduction chemotherapy (vincristine and prednisone plus daunorubicin and/or L-asparaginase), fewer than 10% are leukemia free after 3 years. If a second remission can be attained with chemotherapy, a second BMT may improve survival, especially in those who have relapsed more than 1 year after the initial transplantation. Donor lymphocyte infusion is usually ineffective owing to lack of graft-versus-leukemia effect in ALL.

J. **CNS prophylaxis.** In the era before prophylaxis of the CNS, more than half of children and adults experienced relapse solely in the CNS. Treatment of the CNS sanctuary after a CR has been attained has dramatically decreased the risk of CNS relapse. The timing of CNS prophylaxis depends on the intensity of postremission therapy and the perceived risk of developing CNS leukemia. Two equivalent options exist.

   1. **Cranial irradiation and intrathecal methotrexate.** Cranial irradiation with intrathecal methotrexate has been the classic method of

CNS prophylaxis. It has usually been initiated within 2 weeks of attaining a CR when classic maintenance is given.

a. **Cranial irradiation** is usually given to the cranial vault (anteriorly to the posterior pole of the eye and posteriorly to C2) in 0.2-Gy fractions for a total of 18 to 24 Gy. The spine is not irradiated because marrow toxicity significantly limits the ability to give further chemotherapy. Common acute complications of radiation include stomatitis, parotitis, alopecia, marrow suppression, and headaches. Long-term complications include dental caries. Like children, young adults may develop learning disorders, impaired growth, and leukoencephalopathy.

b. **Intrathecal methotrexate.** Methotrexate is used instead of radiation therapy for prophylaxis of the spinal cord. A commonly used program is 12 mg/m^2 (maximum, 15 mg) of preservative-free methotrexate diluted in preservative-free saline or Elliot's B solution given intrathecally once a week for 6 weeks. Some investigators also give 10 mg of hydrocortisone succinate intrathecally to try to prevent lumbar arachnoiditis because the latter may limit the ability to give all six of the planned doses of intrathecal methotrexate. After cerebrospinal fluid (CSF) is obtained for appropriate studies, 5 mL of CSF is withdrawn into a syringe containing methotrexate diluted in 10 mL of vehicle. This produces a final methotrexate concentration of 1 mg/mL or less (higher concentrations increase the risk of arachnoiditis). The intrathecal methotrexate is then given in an "in-and-out" manner. One to 2 mL of the methotrexate solution is injected into the spinal canal. Then, 0.5 to 1 mL of spinal fluid is withdrawn back into the syringe. This in-and-out process is repeated until all of the methotrexate has been given. This method is used to ensure that the methotrexate is actually given into the subarachnoid space. Leucovorin, 5 to 10 mg, may be given orally every 6 hours for four to eight doses to ameliorate the mucositis, although this usually is not needed unless the patient is receiving concurrent systemic methotrexate. Complications of methotrexate include chemical arachnoiditis and leukoencephalopathy.

2. **Chemoprophylaxis.** Given the toxicity of
    whole-brain irradiation in patients younger
    than 25 years, other strategies of CNS prophy-
    laxis have been developed. The combination of
    systemic intermediate- to high-dose methotrex-
    ate with intrathecal methotrexate is considered
    to be as effective as cranial irradiation with in-
    trathecal methotrexate. HDAC used for inten-
    sification is also an active adjunct to intrathecal
    methotrexate.

VI. **Management problems.** Although patients receiving
therapy for acute leukemia often have a "predictable"
course, certain clinical manifestations require further individualization of the therapeutic approach.

A. **CNS leukemia.** Leukemic involvement of the CNS
bodes poorly for the adult with acute leukemia given
the morbidity of the associated neurologic dysfunction,
the inability to control CNS leukemia on a long-term
basis, and the common association with active marrow
disease. CNS involvement occurs most frequently
with hyperleukocytosis and with the monoblastic,
B-cell, and T-cell lymphoblastic leukemias.

1. **Diagnosis.** The occurrence of CNS involve-
    ment in ALL at diagnosis is well recognized.
    In patients with ALL, high peripheral blast
    counts, and no CNS symptoms, it is usually
    prudent to perform the lumbar puncture after
    chemotherapy has decreased the blast count. In
    this way, contamination of the CSF specimen in
    the event of a traumatic lumbar puncture is
    prevented. Common clinical features of CNS
    leukemia (in ALL and AML) include headache,
    altered sensorium, and cranial nerve palsy (es-
    pecially cranial nerve VI). Features suggestive
    of CNS involvement indicate the need for an im-
    mediate lumbar puncture because neurologic
    dysfunction is most amenable to therapy within
    the first 24 hours and infectious meningitis
    must be excluded in the immunocompromised
    host. The diagnosis of CNS leukemia is made by
    finding five or more blast cells on a cytospin
    preparation of 1 mL of CSF. Essentially all pa-
    tients with CNS leukemia have an elevated
    CSF protein level as well; however, in the ab-
    sence of infection, elevated protein by itself is
    suggestive but not diagnostic of CNS leukemia.

2. **Treatment.** Although the therapy for CNS
    leukemia is usually only palliative, it should be
    initiated as soon as possible. The rapid initiation
    of therapy may reverse or prevent cranial nerve
    palsies, which are a morbid complication for both
    patients and care takers. Treatment of CNS
    leukemia is usually concomitant cranial irra-
    diation and intrathecal chemotherapy. Cranial

irradiation is usually given to a total of 30 Gy in 1.5 to 2 Gy fractions. Intrathecal chemotherapy is given in the manner described under CNS prophylaxis (see Section V.J.). Intrathecal chemotherapy is repeated every 3 to 4 days, with appropriate laboratory studies being done with each lumbar puncture. When blast cells are no longer seen on the cytospin preparation, two more doses of intrathecal drug are given, usually followed by a monthly "maintenance" intrathecal injection. Intrathecal methotrexate, 12 mg/m² (maximum, 15 mg), is most commonly used for ALL. Oral leucovorin, 5 to 10 mg p.o. every 6 hours for four to eight doses starting at the time of the lumbar puncture, may be added to decrease systemic toxicity. Cytarabine, 50 mg given intrathecally, is most commonly used for AML. The addition of 10 mg of intrathecal hydrocortisone succinate may ameliorate chemical arachnoiditis and have some antileukemic effect as well. Some investigators advocate instilling intrathecal cytarabine and methotrexate at the same time or alternating doses of cytarabine and methotrexate. Some investigators advocate the routine use of an intraventricular reservoir for treating patients with CNS leukemia.

The use of systemic therapy with high-dose cytarabine, 1 to 3 g/m² i.v. infusion over 2 hours every 12 hours, is also effective for the treatment of CNS leukemia. A practical approach is to initiate intrathecal chemotherapy until the time that the HDAC is started. Further intrathecal therapy can then be given based on the results of subsequent CSF analysis after the HDAC is completed.

B. **Hyperleukocytosis** (blast counts of more than 100,000/µL) predisposes to rheologic problems.

　1. **Leukostasis** (vascular plugging) occurs almost exclusively with AML. Cerebral and cardiopulmonary dysfunction due to vascular obstruction, vessel wall necrosis with hemorrhage, or both are the most common clinical manifestations. Hyperleukocytosis is an oncologic emergency. Given the increased risk of early death with hyperleukocytosis, therapy should be rapidly initiated as soon as the diagnosis is made. If the patient is hemodynamically stable, leukapheresis is the most rapid way to lower the blast count. The goal of the leukapheresis session is to lower the blast count to less than 100,000/µL if possible. With very high blast counts (more than 200,000/µL), decreasing the blast count by 50% may have to be the initial goal because mathematic modeling suggests

that prolonged leukapheresis after a "3-liter exchange" does not significantly decrease the blast count further. Leukapheresis may be repeated daily. Systemic chemotherapy should be initiated immediately after emergent leukapheresis or if leukapheresis cannot be performed. Hydroxyurea, 3 to 5 g/m^2/day split into three doses daily, is most commonly used. Hydroxyurea is stopped at the time more specific induction chemotherapy is initiated. In patients presenting with hyperleukocytosis, an allopurinol dose of 600 mg b.i.d. is well tolerated for the first 2 days, followed by 300 mg b.i.d. for 2 to 3 days.

2. **Hyperviscosity.** Blood viscosity increases as the blast count rises. Fortunately, concomitant anemia produces a decrease in viscosity. Aggressive red blood cell (RBC) transfusion in patients with hyperleukocytosis may precipitate symptoms of hyperviscosity. RBC transfusions should be used judiciously (e.g., 1 U at a time until symptoms of anemia resolve), with a blast count of more than 200,000/μL, especially in patients with AML. Unless the patient has symptoms due to anemia, a packed cell volume (hematocrit) of 20% to 25% is a reasonable goal.

C. **Acute promyelocytic leukemia** (APL) is an uncommon (about 10%) form of AML that presents unique management challenges.

1. **Promyelocytic coagulopathy.** Hypergranular promyelocytic leukemia predisposes to the development of a devastating coagulopathy that is due to a combination of disseminated intravascular coagulation (DIC) and primary hyperfibrinolysis. Pooled data through the late 1980s suggest that under the best of circumstances with cytotoxic induction chemotherapy, 5% of these patients would die of CNS hemorrhage within the first 24 hours of hospitalization and another 20% to 25% would die of CNS hemorrhage during induction chemotherapy. With intensive supportive care, the most recent studies suggest that about 10% of patients will die of hemorrhage during induction chemotherapy. If looked for carefully, essentially all patients with APL have clinical or laboratory features of DIC. Even with severe thrombocytopenia, in most patients, the bleeding usually stops quickly at the site of bone marrow examination. Prolonged oozing (1 to 2 hours) at the bone marrow site is a telltale sign of DIC. Subtle laboratory signs suggestive of an underlying consumptive coagulopathy in APL include a prolongation of the prothrombin time (more than 0.1 second) or a normal rather than increased

fibrinogen titer (fibrinogen is an acute phase reactant that is normally elevated in acute leukemia at presentation).

a. **Therapy for promyelocytic coagulopathy.** The first rule of managing DIC is to treat the underlying cause. Thus, once the patient has been stabilized, the rapid initiation of induction therapy is the cornerstone of the management of APL (ideally within 24 hours of diagnosis). If anthracycline-based chemotherapy, as opposed to all-*trans*-retinoic acid (ATRA), is used for induction, lysis of the leukemic promyelocytes transiently exacerbates the clinical and laboratory manifestations of DIC. Intensive blood product support is usually necessary. Reasonable transfusion goals would be to keep the platelet counts above 50,000/μL (especially if heparin is used or there is a significant elevation of the fibrin degradation products, which may impair platelet function) and the fibrinogen concentration higher than 150 mg/dL. Platelet and cryoprecipitate transfusions may be needed as often as every 4 hours to maintain hemostasis. The most controversial aspect of the management of APL is the role of heparin in controlling the DIC. Given that APL is an uncommon form of AML, it is not possible to assess the efficacy of heparin in the usual randomized prospective manner. Thus, all of the available data are based on retrospective analyses.

(1) **Supportive care.** Retrospective single institution data suggest that aggressive replacement with coagulation factors and platelets can control the coagulopathy in APL with an acute hemorrhagic death rate of 10% to 15%.

(2) **Heparin.** The goal of therapy with heparin is to slow the rate of consumption of coagulation factors and platelets and thus prevent the development of microvascular thromboses and an uncontrolled hemorrhagic state. Even if heparin does not decrease the risk of initial fatal hemorrhage, control of the consumptive coagulopathy should translate into a decreased need for replacement with coagulation factors and platelets and hence a decreased risk from the morbidity and long-term mortality associated with multiple transfusions (e.g., viral infection, alloimmunization). If

heparin is to be used, it should be initiated immediately if the patient has clinical or laboratory evidence of DIC. If even subtle laboratory signs of DIC are absent, then heparinization probably can be delayed until the time when chemotherapy is to be initiated. Because the goal of heparin therapy is to control the clinical manifestations of DIC, the heparin dose should be adjusted by monitoring the platelet count and the fibrinogen titer every 4 to 6 hours initially depending on the severity of the DIC, and not by aiming for an arbitrary partial thromboplastin time, as is done with thromboembolic disease. A reasonable initial heparin dose is 500 U/h (7 U/kg) by constant infusion given without an initial heparin bolus. The duration of heparin therapy is empiric. The heparin can usually be tapered and stopped within 7 to 10 days as the manifestations of DIC subside.

(3) **Antifibrinolytic therapy.** Patients who have uncontrolled bleeding despite aggressive transfusion therapy and heparin and those with disproportionate fibrinolysis may benefit from epsilon-aminocaproic acid (EACA) given as either 1 g p.o. every 2 hours or as a 3 to 4 g i.v. bolus *followed by* continuous i.v. infusion at 1 g/h. Tranexamic acid, 6 g/24 hours by continuous i.v. infusion for up to 6 days, has also been suggested. Given that an underlying consumptive coagulopathy is present, concomitant heparin may be needed to prevent life-threatening thrombosis.

2. **Chemotherapy.** Therapy for APL has represented the most exciting recent advancement in the treatment of acute leukemia. ATRA is a unique chemotherapeutic agent that is able to induce a high rate of clinical remission by promoting cell maturation without producing marrow hypoplasia. Induction therapy consists of either ATRA-based or anthracycline-based chemotherapy. ATRA-based therapy is preferred for induction because it carries less morbidity from hemorrhage and improved overall survival.

a. **Anthracycline-based chemotherapy** can induce a remission in 70% to 90% of patients with APL. Using high-dose daunorubicin (70 mg/m^2/day on days 1 to 3) and cytarabine (100 mg/m^2/day for 7 days),

SWOG reported 70% leukemia-free survival at 10 years. The European APL 91 Group using daunorubicin (60 mg/m²/day on days 1 to 3) and cytarabine (200 mg/m²/day on days 1 to 7) had a 91% CR rate and a 28% relapse-free survival rate at 4 years. The recently completed Intergroup APL study used daunorubicin and cytarabine in the standard "7 + 3" regimen. The CR rate was 69%, with a 14% mortality rate. Unexplainedly, the projected 3-year relapse-free survival rate was only 18%. Death during induction is usually due to bleeding or infection. Drug resistance is rare.

   b. **ATRA, as a single agent**, induced a remission in 72% to 81% of patients with APL in large randomized trials. ATRA is usually continued for an additional 30 days after complete remission is documented. In nonresponders, it is continued for a maximum of 90 days. If the WBC is more than 10,000/μL, hydroxyurea should be started before the ATRA to prevent the retinoic acid syndrome (RAS). The hemorrhagic death rate, which was reported to be lower in earlier studies with the use of ATRA, has been found to be similar to that seen with induction chemotherapy in the APL 91 and Intergroup APL studies. RAS and infection are the other major causes of death during induction. Induction and maintenance with ATRA alone results in a short remission duration. Given that APL is the form of AML with the highest rate of long-term survivorship, the current trend has been to use ATRA during induction to decrease the risk of early hemorrhagic death, followed by intensification with an anthracycline-based combination to maximize leukemic cell kill once the risk of hemorrhage has returned to normal. The Intergroup APL study showed significantly better event-free survival in patients receiving ATRA as maintenance therapy for 1 year after completing two courses of consolidation chemotherapy. Given the rarity of APL, it is imperative that all eligible patients be entered into the available cooperative trials. The Intergroup APL regimen has a projected 75% 3-year disease-free survival rate.

      (1) **Induction**. ATRA, 45 mg/m²/day p.o., is divided into two doses with food every day until 30 days after complete remission.

(2) Consolidation

Course 1: Daunorubicin, 45 mg/m² i.v. on days 1 to 3, *and* cytarabine, 100 mg/m²/24 hours continuous i.v. infusion on days 1 to 7.

Course 2: Cytarabine, 2 g/m² as a 1-hour i.v. infusion every 12 hours on days 1 to 4, *and* daunorubicin, 45 mg/m²/day on days 1 and 2.

(3) Maintenance

ATRA, 45 mg/m²/day p.o., divided into two doses with food for 1 year

RAS occurs in 15% to 25% of patients, most commonly 7 to 14 days after starting ATRA. It has rarely been observed during recovery from chemotherapy-induced aplasia as well as during ATRA maintenance. RAS is a "capillary leak" syndrome that is mediated in part by interleukin-2. The cardinal clinical manifestations are fever, respiratory distress, and pulmonary infiltrates, which are seen in 80% to 90% of cases. Weight gain, plural or pericardial effusion, and renal failure occur in half of patients. Prevention is the best therapy for RAS. Although a rising WBC count is a risk factor for RAS, it may occur with a WBC count below 5,000/μL. If the WBC count is greater than 5,000 to 10,000/μL before initiating treatment with single-agent ATRA, hydroxyurea (see Section VI.B.I) should be used to lower the WBC count to the target range. If the WBC count rises to more than 10,000/μL during ATRA monotherapy, hydroxyurea (see Section VI.B.1), cytarabine (100 mg/m²/24 hours continuous i.v. infusion on days 1 to 5), or induction chemotherapy should be started. Regardless of the WBC count or the risk of neutropenic sepsis, at the first sign of dyspnea or pulmonary infiltrates with or without fever, dexamethasone (10 mg i.v. b.i.d.) should be initiated, and ATRA should be discontinued until RAS resolves.

c. **ATRA plus idarubicin** may represent the best approach for the initial treatment of APL. ATRA is given concomitantly with idarubicin. The best prospective results come from GIMEMA-AIEOP using the AIDA regimen. Although the data are not randomized and the median follow-up is short (12 months), 95% of patients achieved hematologic CR and 98% achieved molecular remission by polymerase chain reaction at the end of consolidation. Only 5% died of complications during induction, and 7% had RAS. The projected event-free survival rate is 79% at 2 years. We would recommend the concomitant use of ATRA plus idarubicin for induction, if cardiac function permits, in all patients with APL and especially those at high risk of developing RAS. If there is concern about the leukemogenic potential of etoposide for consolidation during first remission, or if there is concern about not using ATRA maintenance, using the Intergroup consolidation and maintenance regimens would be a reasonable alternative to the consolidation portion of AIDA. AIDA is as follows:

(1) Induction

ATRA, 45 mg/m^2/day p.o., divided into 2 doses with food until complete remission, *and*

Idarubicin, 12 mg/m^2/day i.v. on days 2, 4, 6 and 8.

(2) Consolidation

Course 1: Cytarabine, 1 g/m^2/day as a 6-hour i.v. infusion on days 1 to 4, *and* idarubicin, 5 mg/m^2 rapid i.v. infusion given 3 hours after completion of cytarabine on days 1 to 4.

Course 2: Mitoxantrone, 10 mg/m^2 i.v. rapid infusion on days 1 to 5, *and* etoposide, 100 mg/m^2 i.v. infusion over 60 minutes given 12 hours after the mitoxantrone on days 1 to 5.

Course 3: Idarubicin, 12 mg/m^2 i.v. on day 1, *and* cytarabine, 150 mg/m^2 s.c. every 8 hours on days 1 to 5, *and* 6-thioguanine, 70 mg/m^2 p.o. every 8 hours on days 1 to 5.

(3) Maintenance. There is no maintenance in the AIDA regimen. An intuitive approach based on the Intergroup APL study would be to add ATRA, 45 mg/m^2/day for 1 year.

3. **Residual disease.** Residual promyelocytes are not uncommonly found in the bone marrow after the second attempt at induction with anthracycline-based chemotherapy. Primary disease resistance is unusual in APL. Although residual disease in other forms of AML needs further vigorous treatment if long-term survivorship is to be attained, data suggest that "promyelocytic maturation" and bone marrow recovery may occur in patients with residual APL. The use of bone marrow cytogenetics and molecular monitoring of the PML/RARA fusion gene may also be useful in documenting a remission.

4. **Relapsed APL.** Despite an excellent response rate and a high relapse-free survival rate with

the use of the current regimens, patients with a high WBC at presentation and elderly patients are at the highest risk of relapse. Attempts to reinduce remission are successful in patients with a long duration of first CR, but the second CR is usually short. The chemotherapy options for relapsed APL are the same as those for other forms of relapsed AML. Liposomal ATRA and arsenic trioxide are under investigation for relapsed APL.

D. **Extramedullary leukemia.** Infiltration of organs outside the marrow may occur with acute leukemia. Diffuse organ infiltration (e.g., multiple skin nodules and gum infiltration with acute monoblastic leukemia) is best treated with systemic chemotherapy. Testicular involvement can occur in <5% of adults with acute leukemia and is most commonly seen with Ph[1]-positive ALL. Isolated accumulations of leukemic cells may occur with AML (granulocyte sarcoma, chloroma) and less often with ALL (lymphoblastoma). These foci are best treated with local irradiation at curative doses (30 Gy). Although most commonly associated with active marrow disease, chloromas and lymphoblastomas may occur as a sole site of relapse or as an initial presentation in association with a normal bone marrow. In either case, they universally herald the subsequent development of leukemic infiltration of the bone marrow. An intuitive approach is to treat these patients with "adjuvant" induction chemotherapy.

VII. **Growth factors.** Several randomized trials have recently been completed evaluating the effect of hematopoietic growth factors (G-CSF, GM-CSF) as adjuncts to the treatment of patients with acute myeloid leukemia. Most studies have shown a 2- to 5-day reduction in the duration of severe neutropenia. There has been no evidence for a selective advantage for regrowth of the leukemia clone when growth factors are given before marrow hypoplasia is achieved. There has been no consistent benefit as measured by improvement in CR rate, CR duration, or overall survival. There appears to be no role at this time for the priming of leukemia cells by growth factors to enhance the effect of chemotherapy. No specific recommendation for the use of growth factors during induction chemotherapy can be made at this time. It is clear that growth factors administered after consolidation chemotherapy can shorten the duration of neutropenia, without a significant effect on treatment outcome. The use of growth factor can be cost-saving if patients are hospitalized only for chemotherapy administration or for serious complications during the neutropenic period. Consolidation chemotherapy followed by growth factor support can even be administered on an outpatient basis, with less than half of patients being readmitted to the hospital for neutropenic fever. The use of other growth factors, such as interleukin-11 and thrombopoietin, in AML are under investigation.

SELECTED READINGS

Appelbaum FR, Gilliland DG, Tallman MS. *The biology and treatment of acute myeloid leukemia.* In McArthur JR, Schecter GP, Schrier SL (eds.), Hematology 1998: The American Society of Hematology education program book. Washington DC: The American Society of Hematology 1988:63–88. (Available at **http://www.hematology.org**)

Ball ED, Rybka WB. Autologous bone marrow transplantation for adult acute leukemia. *Hematol Oncol Clin North Am* 1993; 7:201–231.

Boucheix C, David B, Sebban C, et al. Immunophenotype of adult acute lymphoblastic leukemia, clinical parameters, and outcome: an analysis of a prospective trial including 562 tested patients (LALA87). *Blood* 1994 1:84:1603–1612.

Brown RA, Wolff SN, Fay JW, et al. High-dose etoposide, cyclophosphamide and total body irradiation with allogeneic bone marrow transplantation for resistant acute myeloid leukemia: a study by the North American Marrow Transplant Group. *Leuk Lymphoma* 1996;22:271–277.

Bishop JF. The treatment of adult acute myeloid leukemia. *Semin Oncol* 1997;24:57–69.

Cassileth PA, Lynch E, Hines JD, et al. Varying intensity of postremission therapy in acute myeloid leukemia. *Blood* 1992;79:1924–30.

Christiansen NP. Allogeneic bone marrow transplantation for the treatment of adult acute leukemias. *Hematol Oncol Clin North Am* 1993;7:177–200.

Ellison RR, Mick R, Cuttner J, et al. The effects of postinduction intensification treatment with cytarabine and daunorubicin in adult acute lymphocytic leukemia: a prospective randomized clinical trial by Cancer and Leukemia Group B. *J Clin Oncol* 1991;9:2002–2015.

Hirsch-Ginsberg C, Huh YO, Kagan J, Liang JC, Stass SA. Advances in the diagnosis of acute leukemia. *Hematol Oncol Clin North Am* 1993;7:1–46.

Ho AD, Lipp T, Ehninger G, et al. Combination of mitoxantrone and etoposide in refractory acute myelogenous leukemia-an active and well tolerated regimen. *J Clin Oncol* 1988;6:213–217.

Hoelzer DF. Therapy of the newly diagnosed adult with acute lymphoblastic leukemia. *Hematol Oncol Clin North Am* 1993 Feb;7(1): 139–160.

Hoelzer D, Ludwig WD, Thiel E, et al. Improved outcome in adult B-cell acute lymphoblastic leukemia. *Blood* 1996;87:495–508.

Kantarjian HM. Adult acute lymphoblastic leukemia: critical review of current knowledge. *Am J Med* 1994;97:176–84.

Koller CA, Kantarjian HM, Thomas D, et al. The hyper-CVAD regimen improves outcome in relapsed acute lymphoblastic leukemia. *Leukemia* 1997;11:2039–2044.

Kumar L. Leukemia: management of relapse after allogeneic bone marrow transplantation. *J Clin Oncol* 1994;12:1710–7.

Laport GF, Larson RA. Treatment of adult acute lymphoblastic leukemia. *Semin Oncol* 1997;24:70–82.

Larson RA, Dodge RK, Burns CP, et al. A five-drug remission induction regimen with intensive consolidation for adults with acute lymphoblastic leukemia: cancer and leukemia group B study 8811. *Blood* 1995;85:2025–37.

Larson RA, Stock W, Hoelzer DF, and Kantarjian HM. Acute lymphoblastic leukemia in adults. Hematology 1998: The American

Society of Hematology education program book. Washington DC: The American Society of Hematology 1988:44–62. (Available at **http://www.hematology.org.**)

Linker CA, Levitt LJ, O'Donnell M, Foreman SJ, Ries CA. Treatment of adult acute lymphoblastic leukemia with intensive cyclical chemotherapy: a follow-up report. *Blood* 1991;78:2814–2822.

Mandelli F, Diverio D, Avvisati G, et al. Molecular remission in PML/RAR alpha-positive acute promyelocytic leukemia by combined all-trans retinoic acid and idarubicin (AIDA) therapy. Gruppo Italiano-Malattie Ematologiche Maligne dell'Adulto and Associazione Italiana di Ematologia ed Oncologia Pediatrica Cooperative Groups. *Blood* 1997;90:1014–1021.

Mayer RJ, Davis RB, Schiffer CA, et al. Intensive postremission chemotherapy in adults with acute myeloid leukemia. Cancer and Leukemia Group B. *N Engl J Med* 1994;331:896–903.

Parker JE, Pagliuca A, Mijovic A, et al. Fludarabine, cytarabine, G-CSF and idarubicin (FLAG-IDA) for the treatment of poor-risk myelodysplastic syndromes and acute myeloid leukemia. *Br J Haematol* 1997;99:939–944.

Schwartz BS, Williams EC, Conlan MG, Mosher DF. Epsilon-aminocaproic acid in the treatment of patients with acute promyelocytic leukemia and acquired alpha-2-plasmin inhibitor deficiency. *Ann Intern Med* 1986;105:873–7.

Schiffer CA. Hematopoietic growth factors as adjuncts to the treatment of acute myeloid leukemia. *Blood* 1996;88:3675–85.

Shen ZX, Chen GQ, Ni JH, et al. Use of arsenic trioxide (As2O3) in the treatment of acute promyelocytic leukemia (APL): II. Clinical efficacy and pharmacokinetics in relapsed patients. *Blood* 1997;89:3354–3360.

Smith GA, Damon LE, Rugo HS, Ries CA, Linker CA. High-dose cytarabine dose modification reduces the incidence of neurotoxicity in patients with renal insufficiency. *J Clin Oncol* 1997;15:833–839.

Stone, RM, Mayer RJ. The approach to the elderly patient with acute myeloid leukemia. *Hematol Oncol Clin North Am* 1993;7:65–79.

Stone RM, Mayer RJ. Treatment of the newly diagnosed adult with de novo acute myeloid leukemia. *Hematol Oncol Clin North Am* 1993;7:47–64.

Suki S, Kantarjian HM, Gandhi V, et al. Fludarabine and cytosine arabinoside in the treatment of refractory or relapsed acute lymphocytic leukemia. *Cancer* 1993;72:2155–2160.

Tallman MS, Andersen JW, Schiffer CA, et al. All-trans-retinoic acid in acute promyelocytic leukemia. *N Engl J Med* 1997;337:1021–1028. (Published erratum appears in *N Engl J Med* 1997;337:1639)

Uckun FM, Reaman G, Steinherez PG, et al. Improved clinical outcome for children with T-lineage acute lymphoblastic leukemia after contemporary chemotherapy: a Children's Cancer Group Study. *Leuk Lymphoma* 1996;24:57–70.

Welborn JL. Impact of reinduction regimens for relapsed refractory acute lymphoblastic leukemia in adults. *Am J Hematol* 1994;45:341–344.

Weick JK, Kopecky KJ, Appelbaum FR, et al. A randomized investigation of high-dose versus standard-dose cytosine arabinoside with daunorubicin in patients with previously untreated acute myeloid leukemia: a Southwest Oncology Group study. *Blood* 1996;88:2841–2851.

Chronic Leukemias

Carol S. Palackdharry

In the chronic leukemias, there is excessive proliferation of functionally mature, differentiated cells. This contrasts with the acute leukemias and myelodysplastic syndromes, in which there is abnormal proliferation of immature cells with impaired differentiation. Thus, the chronic leukemias are postulated to be diseases caused by impaired signal transduction and regulation of cell proliferation, rather than impaired differentiation. This chapter briefly covers four chronic leukemias: chronic myelogenous leukemia (CML), chronic lymphocytic leukemia (CLL), hairy-cell leukemia (HCL), and adult T-cell leukemia and lymphoma (ATLL).

I. **Chronic myelogenous leukemias (CML, chronic granulocytic leukemia)**

   A. **Diagnosis.** CML is a clonal myeloproliferative disorder of a hematopoietic stem cell. Its incidence peaks in the fifth and sixth decades of life and declines thereafter. The hallmark presentation is leukocytosis in which cells at all stages of myeloid differentiation are present. These myeloid cells typically have low or absent leukocyte alkaline phosphatase activity. At diagnosis, splenomegaly is common, and small numbers of peripheral blasts may be present. Patients commonly have anemia, thrombocytosis, and a white blood cell (WBC) count of more than $100 \times 10^3/\mu L$. Because molecular studies on peripheral blood can be performed, the bone marrow is examined for prognosis rather than for diagnosis.

   CML involves the marrow myeloid, erythroid, megakaryocytic, and rarely, lymphocytic cell lines. The disease is characterized by the presence of the Philadelphia chromosome (Ph), which is the result of a reciprocal translocation involving chromosomes 9 and 22 [t(9;22) (q34;q11)]. This translocation transposes the c-abl protooncogene on chromosome 9 to the breakpoint cluster region (bcr) on chromosome 22, creating a hybrid oncogene, BCR-ABL. This oncogene produces a fusion protein with tyrosine kinase activity, which is thought to be responsible for the transformation of normal cells into CML cells. In about 90% of patients, routine cytogenetics demonstrate this translocation. For patients with the morphologic picture of CML but negative findings on cytogenetic analysis, Southern blot analysis of bcr gene rearrangement can identify a subset of Ph-negative, rearrangement-positive patients (additional 5%). The natural history and treatment for the 5% of patients with myeloproliferative disorders without any evidence for a translocation are different from those for patients with the translocation.

B. **Natural history.** CML characteristically has a biphasic or triphasic course. The median survival time after diagnosis with conventional therapy and routine supportive care is 3 to 4 years. During the indolent, or chronic, phase, the disease is easily controllable with therapy. Even with standard treatment, it progresses to an accelerated phase, which can last up to 1.5 years. The exact definition of the accelerated phase remains controversial. However, standard criteria are being developed and include circulating blasts of more than 15%, circulating blasts plus promyelocytes of more than 30%, peripheral basophils of more than 20%, and cytogenetic evolution. Cytogenetic analysis during transformation may demonstrate clonal evolution with new DNA abnormalities, including more than one Philadelphia chromosome or loss of the original Philadelphia chromosome. About 25% of patients die of complications during the accelerated phase, whereas 25% progress into the blastic phase (blast transformation) without going through a definable accelerated phase. Blast transformation is the final phase and in most patients represents a terminal event either from complications of therapy or from complications of marrow failure. About 67% transform to an acute nonlymphocytic leukemia (ANLL, AML), which is usually refractory to standard antileukemic treatment. The remaining 33% transform to an acute lymphocytic leukemia (ALL), which may have a better prognosis because some remissions are obtained with appropriate treatment.

C. **Therapy.** Transplantation of allogeneic bone marrow (AlloBMT) from a sibling or of bone marrow from an unrelated donor is the only known potentially curative therapy for CML. Therapy with interferon-α (IFN-α) is providing encouraging results for patients unable to undergo transplantation. Standard chemotherapy with hydroxyurea prolongs survival of patients with CML but does not prevent disease evolution.

   1. **Bone marrow transplantation.** All patients in the accelerated or blastic phases of CML who are candidates for AlloBMT (age less than 55 years, related matched or one antigen–mismatched donor) should be offered this procedure. The overall disease-free survival rate may correlate with the patient's disease state at the time of AlloBMT, but is about 40% at 5 years. There continue to be late relapses, possibly because of the primitive stem cell involved. The timing of AlloBMT during the chronic phase is more controversial because of the risks of the procedure, with an average transplantation-related mortality of 30%.

   Unrelated donor transplantations are yielding encouraging results, especially in young patients (younger than 30 years) with complete human leukocyte antigen (HLA) matches. The overall 2-year disease-free survival rate is about 30% to 50%, depending on the patient's age and degree of HLA matching. However, this procedure is associated with significant transplant mortality (40% to 60%) and is still considered investigational. For most patients, a trial of interferon is warranted before consideration of unrelated donor transplantation unless disease progression has occurred and the patient is younger than 30 years with an HLA-identical donor.

The use of adoptive immunotherapy with donor lymphocyte infusions in patients with CML who relapse after AlloBMT produces a response rate of 70% to 80%. This is the treatment of choice in such cases. Refinements of the technique are under investigation.

Autologous stem cell transplantation remains investigational in CML. This procedure may prolong survival, although it does not appear curative. Follow-up of ongoing studies will help clarify the role of autologous transplantation. This approach should be considered in the context of a clinical trial for patients who did not respond to interferon and do not have matched related donors (or unrelated donors, if young).

2. **IFN-α**

a. **Responses.** A number of clinical trials have confirmed the high complete hematologic remission rate (55% to 80%), with a substantial rate of cytogenetic remissions (20% to 60%), with the use of high-dose IFN-α. Response rates appear to be dose dependent, with the highest responses seen at 5×10^6 U/m^2 s.c. daily. Maturing results from initial trials demonstrate a median survival time of 5 to 6 years, with 25% of patients maintaining durable cytogenetic remissions; with conventional hydroxyurea therapy, there are no major cytogenetic responses, and the median survival time is about 4 years. The combination of IFN-α and cytarabine may produce longer survival than IFN-α alone, but these preliminary results need to be confirmed before this approach is adopted as standard therapy.

b. **Side effects.** Most patients experience self-limited influenza-like symptoms (fever, chills, anorexia) during the first few weeks of therapy, which are not considered dose limiting. This can be minimized by starting at 50% dosage (2.5×10^6 U/m^2 s.c. daily) for the first week and by giving the dose at bedtime with acetaminophen. Using hydroxyurea to reduce initial WBC counts to 20,000/μL also decreases early side effects. However, there are a number of dose-limiting late side effects, including depression, fatigue, neurotoxicity, and hepatitis. Antidepressants may be required in some patients. Other dose-limiting complications include immune-mediated hemolysis or thrombocytopenia, collagen vascular syndromes, and immune-mediated nephrotic syndrome or hypothyroidism. Rare cases of cardiac toxicity are reported.

c. **Recommendations** (Kantarjian et al., 1996). For patients who are not marrow transplantation candidates, give an initial trial of IFN-α. If there is a cytogenetic response with some reduction in Ph-positive cells by 6 months, IFN-α is continued indefinitely until the cytogenetic response is lost. By 12 months, there should be less than 65% Ph-positive cells to qualify for a response. For those patients who have grade 3 or 4 toxicity, therapy is temporarily held, and when the toxicity abates, dose reductions of 50% are given. If there is persistent grade 2 toxicity that does not improve with supportive therapy, the dose is reduced by 25%. Other indications for dose reduction are a WBC count less than 2×10^3/μL or platelet count less than 60×10^3/μL.

Were it not for the significant side effects associated with IFN-α, this therapy would more widely be considered the treatment of choice for older patients and for younger patients who do not have a matched related donor for AlloBMT. Because of cost and the IFN-α–associated side effects, however, many clinicians (and patients) still opt for chemotherapy.

3. **Chemotherapy in the chronic phase.** Therapy should be initiated in patients at the time of diagnosis. The goal of palliative chemotherapy is to lower the WBC count into the normal range (less than 10,000/μL). Two agents are currently used. Recently, hydroxyurea was shown to provide a survival advantage when compared with busulfan and is currently considered the treatment of choice. In addition, busulfan therapy is associated with a higher transplantation-related mortality and should not be used in patients in whom bone marrow transplantation is a consideration.

a. **Hydroxyurea.** In patients with a WBC count higher than 100,000/μL at diagnosis, hydroxyurea, 3 to 5 g p.o. daily, is required until the WBC count falls to 30,000 to 50,000/μL. At this point, lower doses can be instituted. Maintenance doses of hydroxyurea range from 500 to 2,000 mg/day. It is not unusual to have to adjust the maintenance dose routinely. An increase in the required dose may herald evolution of the disease.

b. **Busulfan.** This drug inhibits stem cell proliferation. Given the therapeutic advantage of hydroxyurea, busulfan is now considered second-line chemotherapy. The time to response is long (3 to 4 weeks after initiation of therapy). The initial dose is usually 4 or 8 mg p.o. daily. The dose should be cut in half each time the WBC count decreases by 50%. Therapy should be stopped when the WBC count reaches 20,000/μL because counts will continue to fall 1 to 2 weeks after discontinuing therapy. Busulfan therapy is associated with a number of long-term side effects, including pulmonary fibrosis, skin pigmentation, and an Addisonian-like wasting syndrome.

4. **Therapy in aggressive phase.** Outside the setting of bone marrow transplantation, therapy during the aggressive phase produces few responses. Interferon therapy produces far fewer responses than when this therapy is used in the chronic phase. Eligible patients in the aggressive phase should be considered for AlloBMT or experimental therapies, such as autologous, unrelated donor transplantation or other interferons.

5. **Splenectomy.** Symptomatic splenomegaly usually responds to therapy. Splenectomy is reserved for patients with cytopenia due to sequestration not responsive to other therapies. Radiation therapy may also be used in this situation.

6. **Therapy in blast transformation.** In most patients, this represents a terminal event. Patients with AML transformation respond poorly to any conventional AML regimen. Even AlloBMT in this setting produces poor results, with disease in most patients relapsing. Some patients who undergo ALL transformation obtain remissions to standard ALL therapy (see Chap. 19).

7. **Leukapheresis.** Patients with CML may develop symptoms of leukostasis, including CNS changes, hypoxia, cardiac ischemia, and renal insufficiency, when the WBC count approaches 500,000/μL, even without increased numbers of blasts and promyelocytes. However, when the

blast and promyelocyte counts are 50,000 to 100,000/µL, leukostasis can develop even with lower total WBC counts. Symptoms of leukostasis are absolute indications for leukapheresis, which alleviates symptoms until hydroxyurea takes effect.

8. **CML and pregnancy.** All therapy for CML is potentially teratogenic and represents a significant risk to the fetus. Effective contraception should be discussed and offered to sexually active patients with childbearing potential. If pregnancy occurs while a female patient is taking hydroxyurea and therapeutic abortion is not an option, busulfan should be used because it appears to be less teratogenic than hydroxyurea.

II. **Chronic lymphocytic leukemia.** Lymphoid ontogeny results in the production of a variety of immunologically and morphologically different lymphocytes. As a result, chronic lymphoid leukemias include many types of mature clonal proliferations, including B-cell chronic lymphocytic leukemia (B-CLL), T-cell chronic lymphocytic leukemia (T-CLL), HCL, prolymphocytic leukemia (PLL), small cleaved cell leukemia, Sézary syndrome, ATLL, and large granular lymphocytic leukemia (LGL). This section discusses issues attendant to B-CLL, whereas HCL and ATLL are discussed separately.

A. **Diagnosis of B-CLL.** In North America and Western Europe, B-CLL is the most common chronic lymphoid malignancy, accounting for 30% of all adult leukemias. The median age at diagnosis is 64 years, after which the incidence continues to increase. There is a 2 : 1 male-to-female ratio, with only 10% of patients being diagnosed before the age of 50 years. Most patients do not have symptoms at the time of diagnosis, likely due to the increased use of automated cell counters and routine complete blood cell (CBC) counts.

In June 1996, National Cancer Institute–sponsored working group guidelines for the diagnosis and treatment of CLL were revised. The demonstration of B-cell monoclonality (CD5; CD19 or CD20; often CD23; and either monoclonal γ or κ) with an absolute lymphocyte count (ALC) of more than 5,000/µL is sufficient for diagnosis. Flow cytometric analysis of peripheral blood demonstrates clonal B-CLL cells that differ from normal B lymphocytes in their characteristic expression of the T-cell antigen CD5, the common CLL antigen (cCLLa), and mouse red blood cell receptors. Morphologically, the cells appear as mature or hypernature small lymphocytes, though varying amounts of atypical prolymphocytic-like cells may be present. Examination of the bone marrow is not necessary for diagnosis but may aid in prognosis. Cytogenetic analysis is currently considered a research tool.

B. **Staging.** Tumor burden is linked to survival. There are many proposed staging systems for CLL, of which the modified Rai (Table 20-1) and the Binet (Table 20-2) staging systems are the most widely used. Both of these systems correlate extent of disease with median survival. Autoimmune cytopenias are not considered part of the staging systems. Both staging systems are comparable and provide the same general guidelines for a staging work-up, which should include a thorough physical examination, a CBC count, and peripheral blood flow cytometry, usually with a bone marrow examination. Computed tomography (CT) of the chest, abdomen, and pelvis may also be done to assess adenopathy, hepatomegaly, or splenomegaly not clinically detectable.

C. **Prognostic factors.** The major prognostic factor in CLL is the clinical stage of disease. However, a number of laboratory parameters have prognostic significance. A diffuse pattern of lymphocyte infiltration in the bone marrow as shown by histology is associated with a poor prognosis. Patients with short lymphocyte-doubling times (less than 12 months) also have a poor prognosis.

About 55% of patients with B-CLL have clonal DNA changes, the most common of which is trisomy 12. The role of trisomy 12 in the pathogenesis of CLL remains unclear. Other abnormalities include structural changes of the long arms of chromosomes 13 and 14. In addition, translocations involving the regions of the bcl-1, -2, or -3 protooncogenes have been identified in subsets of patients with CLL. Which chromosomal changes portend a poor prognosis remains uncertain.

D. **Therapy.** Not all patients with CLL require therapy. Because no standard therapy is curative, the goal of therapy remains palliation. Patients with early-

Table 20-1. Modified Rai staging system for chronic lymphocytic leukemia

Stage	Distribution %	Criteria	Median survival time (yr)
Low risk	30	Lymphocytosis only (in blood and bone marrow)	10
Intermediate risk	60	Lymphocytosis plus adenopathy or lymphocytosis plus splenomegaly or hepatomegaly	6
High risk	10	Lymphocytosis plus anemia (hemoglobin <11 g/dL) or thrombocytopenia (platelets $<100 \times 10^3/\mu L$)	2

Table 20-2.   Binet staging system for chronic lymphocytic leukemia

Distribution		No. of lymphoid areas involved[a]	Anemia or thrombocytopenia[b]	Median survival time (yr)
Stage	(%)			
A	60	0–2	No	9
B	30	3–5	No	5
C	10	0–5	Yes	2

[a] Five areas are included: cervical, axillary, inguinal, spleen, and liver. Bilaterality does not increase the number of areas designated.
[b] Anemia is defined as hemoglobin <10 g/dL; thrombocytopenia as platelets <100 × 10³/μL.

stage, stable disease require no antineoplastic therapy. Standard therapy with oral alkylating agents in patients with early-stage, stable, asymptomatic disease does not prolong survival and actually may be associated with a shorter survival time. For this reason, the standard of care for patients with early-stage, stable disease remains observation.

1. **Treatment of autoimmune hemolytic anemia (AIHA) and immune thrombocytopenia.** About 20% to 35% of CLL patients have immune-mediated cytopenias. These disorders are thought to be due to the production of polyclonal immunoglobulin G antibodies by cells other than the malignant clone. The mainstay of therapy remains prednisone, 60 to 100 mg/day for 3 to 6 weeks or until hemolysis subsides, after which the prednisone is tapered. Unresponsive patients may benefit from splenectomy, intravenous immunoglobulin, danazol, or splenic irradiation. Cytotoxic therapy has no direct benefit, and therapy with adenosine deaminase inhibitors appears to increase the incidence of AIHA.

2. **Treatment of progressive or advanced-stage disease.** Indications for treatment include progressive early-stage disease, B symptoms (fever, night sweats, weight loss), bulky nodal disease or hepatosplenomegaly, and evidence of a compromised bone marrow (early disease with extensive diffuse marrow infiltrate, developing anemia, or thrombocytopenia). The optimal duration of therapy is unknown. In general, therapy is discontinued when the disease is controlled, and maintenance therapy is not indicated unless necessary for disease control.

   a. **Purine nucleoside analogs.** Three nucleoside analogs, fludarabine, cladribine (2-chlorodeoxyadenosine, 2-CdA), and pentostatin (2-deoxycoformycin), have demonstrated potent antitumor activity in CLL and related disorders and are currently considered either first- or second-line therapy of CLL. Of the three drugs, current studies indicate that fludarabine is the most effective against CLL, with 2-CdA and pentostatin being less effective at the currently recommended doses.

(1) **Fludarabine.** This is currently considered the first-line therapy of choice in CLL without AIHA. The estimated overall response rate in previously untreated patients is 80%, with a 70% complete response (CR) rate. In previously treated patients, the overall response rate is 57%, with a 29% CR rate. Prednisone does not improve response rates and may increase mortality due to infection; thus, it is not recommended.

  (a) **Recommended dose.** The recommended dose is 25 mg/m²/day i.v. on days 1 to 5, every 4 weeks for 6 to 10 months. The combination of fludarabine with other agents, such as chlorambucil and low-dose cytarabine (ara-C), is currently being investigated and is not considered standard practice.

  (b) **Toxicities.** Fludarabine is usually well tolerated, with its major side effects being myelosuppression, reversible neurologic dysfunction (peripheral neuropathy), muscle weakness, and hearing loss. Severe and prolonged CD4 lymphopenia is a long-term side effect, and these patients must be monitored closely for associated infections. Allergic pneumonitis may masquerade as a pulmonary infection in these immunocompromised hosts. Occasionally, severe and nonreversible central and peripheral neurologic toxicity is seen.

  (c) **Cross-resistance.** Fludarabine and 2-CdA have similar structures. Recently, cross-resistance was confirmed, with only 20% of fludarabine-refractory patients achieving a response to 2-CdA.

       (2) **Cladribine and pentostatin.** These appear to have less activity in CLL than fludarabine. Dosing information for these drugs can be found in Section III.D.

   b. **Single alkylating agents with or without prednisone.** Oral chlorambucil is the best tolerated and most active alkylating agent administered alone or in combination with prednisone. It can be administered on a daily or intermittent (pulse) schedule. Prednisone appears effective in reducing adenopathy and splenomegaly and in improving anemia and thrombocytopenia. However, whether prednisone improves response rates or survival remains unclear. Its use must be balanced against the greater risk for infection with corticosteroid therapy.

       (1) **Continuous chlorambucil.** Three to 6 mg/m^2 p.o. is given daily. Doses should be reduced for hematologic toxicity (absolute neutrophil count [ANC] less than 1,000/μL, or platelet count less than 75,000/μL); dose reductions are often required as the disease responds.

       (2) **Intermittent chlorambucil.** A single dose of chlorambucil, 20 to 30 mg/m^2 p.o., can be given every 2 to 4 weeks. An alternative approach is to give a single dose of chlorambucil, 75 mg p.o., plus prednisone, 30 mg/day for 7 days with each course of chlorambucil. This dose may be repeated in 4 weeks when the WBC count returns to pretreatment levels. This may be associated with a higher response rate and longer survival than daily dosing, but the toxicity is greater.

       (3) **Cyclophosphamide.** Cyclophosphamide is an acceptable alternative to chlorambucil. The recommended dose is 80 to 120 mg/m^2/day p.o. Because of the risk of hemorrhagic cystitis, it should always be taken in the morning, and oral hydration with 2 to 3 liters of fluid daily is encouraged.

   c. **Combination chemotherapy.** Combinations with a variety of regimens have been used to treat advanced-stage disease, although the advantage to this approach remains unclear, and many oncologists would consider these options inferior to the newer purine nucleoside analogs. Updated data from earlier promising reports with aggressive combination chemotherapy regimens fail to demonstrate a clear survival advantage when compared with chlorambucil and prednisone. Commonly employed regimens are as follows:

(1) **CVP**

Cyclophosphamide, 400 mg/m² p.o. on days 1 to 5 (or 750 mg/m² i.v. on day 1), *and*

Vincristine, 1.4 mg/m² i.v. on day 1, not to exceed 2.0 mg, *and*

Prednisone, 100 mg/m² p.o. on days 1 to 5.

Repeat every 3 to 4 weeks.

(2) **CHOP**

Cyclophosphamide, 750 mg/m² i.v. on day 1, *and*

Vincristine, 2 mg i.v. on day 1, *and*

Doxorubicin, 50 mg/m² i.v. on day 1, *and*

Prednisone, 100 mg p.o. daily for 5 days.

Repeat every 3 or 4 weeks,

(3) **Modified CHOP**

Cyclophosphamide, 300 mg/m² p.o. on days 1 to 5, *and*

Vincristine, 2 mg i.v. on day 1, *and*

Doxorubicin, 25 mg/m² on day 1, *and*

Prednisone, 40 mg/m² p.o. on days 1 to 5.

Repeat every 3 to 4 weeks.

3. **Alternative therapies.** Virtually all CLL patients become resistant to the above-described therapies. Experimental approaches include AlloBMT, biologic response modifiers (BRMs), and monoclonal antibody (MoAB) therapy.

a. **AlloBMT.** AlloBMT is considered investigational for the treatment of CLL. Current reports on limited numbers of patients suggest a 53% disease-free survival rate with a median follow-up of 26 months. Early studies reported a high transplantation-related mortality (50%) and late relapses. More recent studies with different preoperative regimens showed a reduced early mortality to 10% and clearly prolonged survival. Although still investigational, this therapy should be considered for young patients with poor-risk disease who are refractory to fludarabine.

b. **BRMs.** Very few of the many BRM agents have reached clinical trials in CLL. Interleukin-2 appears ineffective in CLL, and the response to IFN-α either for therapy or maintenance remains disappointing.

c. **MoABs.** There are a number of MoABs directed against CLL-associated antigens, including CD5, cCLLa, CD19, CD20, lym-1, lym-2, and CAMPATH-binding protein. Encouraging results are being seen, especially with the CAMPATH-binding protein MoAB. Additional data and results from the conjugated MoAB trials are needed before the usefulness of these antibodies in the treatment of CLL can be determined. These should be considered within the framework of a clinical trial for refractory patients who are not eligible for an Allo-BMT trial.

E. **Complications**

   1. **Infections.** Infections, particularly bacterial infections, account for up to 60% of deaths in patients with CLL. Hypogammaglobulinemia is the factor most responsible for the susceptibility to bacterial infections. Special attention to unusual upper respiratory tract pathogens, such as *Listeria* species or *Pneumocystis carinii,* should be given to patients with CD4 lymphopenia. All patients treated with fludarabine should receive *Pneumocystis pneumoniae* prophylaxis until CD4 lymphopenia resolves. Immunizations are ineffective in CLL patients. Antibiotic or immunoglobulin prophylaxis should be considered in patients with repeated severe infections. Immunoglobulin prophylaxis is expensive. If it is done, doses of 400 mg/kg every 3 weeks significantly reduce infections and increase infection-free intervals, but a survival advantage over routine antibiotics has not been demonstrated.

   2. **Richter's transformation.** This is transformation to an aggressive large cell non-Hodgkin's lymphoma (NHL) in patients with previously existing or coexisting CLL or other indolent lymphoproliferative disorders. The exact incidence is difficult to determine but is estimated at 3% to 15%. Fever, marked progression of adenopathy, and an elevated lactate dehydrogenase level herald transformation, with most patients dying within 6 to 8 months, despite treatment.

   3. **PLL transformation.** The diagnosis is heralded by the sudden appearance of prolymphocytes (more than 55% of the ALC) in the peripheral blood. It is usually refractory to therapy.

   4. **Second malignancies.** New reports confirm a higher incidence of second malignancies in patients with CLL, which does not appear to be influenced by stage of disease or treatment

modality. There appears to be a combined 28% increased risk of the following malignancies: NHL, intraocular melanomas, malignant melanoma, brain tumors, and lung cancers. The explanation for this increased risk is unclear at present.

III. **Hairy-cell leukemia**

A. **Diagnosis.** HCL was first identified in 1958, but because of the recent development of purine nucleoside analogs, which are very active in producing durable complete remissions, there has been a substantial body of new literature on this disease. This is now the most treatable type of chronic lymphoid malignancy.

HCL is an uncommon disorder that characteristically presents with infection due to pancytopenia, splenomegaly, and a bone marrow that is difficult or impossible to aspirate. HCL is most commonly seen in elderly men, with a male-to-female ratio of $5 : 1$. Diagnosis can be made by morphologic, biochemical, and flow cytometric examination of peripheral blood cells or bone marrow elements (if obtainable).

In most patients with typical HCL, the malignant cells are monoclonal B cells that are tartrate-resistant acid phosphatase (TRAP)-positive. These cells have hairlike projections, best seen on wet mounts with phase-contrast light microscopy. There is a small subset of patients with "atypical" HCL, some with atypical B-cell phenotypes (TRAP-negative), and isolated patients who may represent T-cell variants. Variant HCL is less responsive to therapy and is not discussed here. The following sections apply to typical B-cell HCL.

Flow cytometric analysis has become the mainstay in differentiating HCL from other chronic lymphoid malignancies. The most specific findings are coexpression of B-ly7 with CD19, coexpression of CD11c with CD19, and moderate staining for CD25 (interleukin-2 receptor) and CD19. Most HCL cells do not express CD5. The most specific marker appears to be B-ly7, which is positive in all patients with HCL and negative in all patients with CLL.

B. **Natural history.** Before the advent of the purine nucleoside analogs, the prognosis for patients with HCL was poor because there was no known curative therapy. The median survival time was only 53 months. Some patients had palliation of cytopenias with splenectomy, and most still required systemic therapy within the first year after splenectomy. Exciting new developments have made this a highly treatable and possibly curable disease.

C. **Staging.** There is no formal staging system for HCL because staging does not alter therapy or outcome.

D. **Treatment.** About 10% to 20% of patients with HCL never require therapy and have stable disease without complications. These patients are best managed by observation and are offered therapy if there is disease progression. Indications for treatment include significant cytopenias, repeated infections, massive splenomegaly, painful adenopathy, and vasculitis.

1. **Purine nucleoside analogs.** These are now considered first-line therapy for the treatment of HCL. They all produce high CR rates, which appear to be durable for years. Longer follow-up is needed to determine whether these therapies are curative. Responses appear to be independent of previous splenectomy or interferon therapy. The three drugs differ in their response rates, duration of remission, side effects, degree of immunosuppression, and cost of therapy.

   a. **Definition of response.** Because of the impressive activity seen with these drugs, a more rigorous definition of CR has been devised (Table 20-3). Documentation of response requires examination of both the bone marrow and peripheral blood.

   b. **Cladribine.** A single 7-day continuous infusion of 2-CdA consistently produced CR rates above 80% in multiple studies. The additional 20% of patients are partial responders. At this point, remissions appear durable, with a median follow-up time of 16 months. The recommended dose is 0.09 to 0.1 mg/kg/day as a continuous i.v. infusion for 7 days. Alternatively, 0.14 mg/kg i.v. bolus over 2 hours daily for 5 days or 0.14 mg/kg s.c. daily for 5 days may be used. An oral form of the drug shows promise.

   The major side effects are myelosuppression and associated fever. However, with longer follow-up of patients treated with 2-CdA, a lengthy period of profound CD4

Table 20-3. Definition of response in hairy-cell leukemia

Response	Physical examination	Bone marrow	Peripheral blood
Complete remission	Absence of all signs and symptoms of hairy-cell leukemia	Absence of hairy cells	Hemoglobin >12 g/dL ANC >1,500/µL Platelets >100 × 10³/µL
Partial remission	50% Reduction of all findings of hairy-cell leukemia	1% to 5% Hairy cells	Hemoglobin >12 g/dL ANC >1,500/µL Platelets >100 × 10³/µL

ANC, absolute neutrophil count.

and CD8 lymphopenia has been seen and can last years after treatment, rendering patients susceptible to a variety of opportunistic infections. CD4 counts should be monitored regularly. Rare side effects include late bone marrow failure, peripheral neuropathy, and disturbing isolated incidence of severe proximal myopathy.

c. **Pentostatin (2-deoxycoformycin).** Pentostatin is an inhibitor of adenosine deaminase. The overall response rate is about 80%, with a CR rate of more than 50%. As with 2-CdA, many remissions have been durable to date, with about a 15% relapse rate. The recommended dose is 4 mg/m^2 i.v. every 2 weeks for 6 months, or 2 cycles beyond CR. In many cases, this is given with intravenous hydration (1 liter) because of reports of a high frequency of renal toxicity in the higher-dose phase I studies.

As with all of the purine nucleoside analogs, pentostatin is a potent depressor of CD4 and CD8 cells, which may last for many months after discontinuation of therapy. The incidence of neurologic, renal, hepatic, and bone marrow toxicities has decreased with the above-recommended dose. Patients must be monitored closely for opportunistic infections for at least 1 year after therapy and should have CD4 counts monitored.

d. **Fludarabine.** Current clinical trials indicate that fludarabine may have activity in HCL similar to that of 2-CdA. Results of ongoing studies will help determine the exact response and remission rates of this drug as well as the extent and duration of long-term immunosuppression. Current data suggest that fludarabine is not as active in HCL as 2-CdA or pentostatin.

2. **Splenectomy.** This is no longer considered the treatment of choice for patients with HCL because most patients still require systemic treatment. It is reserved for patients with life-threatening thrombocytopenia due to splenic sequestration.

3. **Interferon.** Splenectomy followed by interferon therapy produces very low remission rates (less than 10%) that are not usually durable. Like splenectomy, this is also no longer considered first-line therapy.

4. **Treatment failures.** There are few data on salvage therapy after treatment failure with one of the above-mentioned purine analogs.

A few patients may benefit from crossover to another purine analog, but there is expected to be a relatively high degree of cross-resistance. As a palliative measure, therapy with granulocyte colony-stimulating factor (G-CSF) may increase the ANC into an acceptable range, thus decreasing infection complications. Sparse data suggest that HCL cells are not stimulated by G-CSF.

IV. Adult T-cell leukemia and lymphoma

    A. Diagnosis. ATLL is characterized by hypercalcemia and the presence of malignant helper T cells in the skin and blood. There can be involvement of the lungs, liver, and spleen; lymphadenopathy (sparing the mediastinum); and lytic bone lesions. The initial clinical course may be chronic but is usually followed by a rapidly progressive phase that is terminal. The disease is caused by human T-cell lymphotropic virus type I (HTLV-I). HTLV-I is endemic in southwest Japan, the Caribbean, and the southeastern United States. There appears to be a lengthy latency phase necessary before the development of ATLL, with infected patients having a 5% lifetime risk of developing ATLL. Those with the highest risk of developing ATLL were likely infected perinatally.

    Diagnosis is made by the classic appearance of the T cells, which have indented or lobulated nuclei; flow cytometric studies demonstrating the CD4 phenotype; hypercalcemia; and the clinical presentation.

    B. Natural history. In the early or pre-ATLL phase, the disease is usually asymptomatic. Leukemic cells can usually be identified in the peripheral blood. Studies of HTLV-I integration demonstrated these cells to be polyclonal. In 50% of patients, these cells disappear spontaneously. In others, smoldering ATLL occurs and is manifested by circulating leukemia cells (normal total WBC count) and skin involvement, without visceral involvement. In this phase, the malignant cells demonstrate clonality. This can progress to a chronic or acute phase.

    In the chronic phase, an elevated WBC count reflects an increase in circulating ATLL cells. There is visceral involvement with hepatosplenomegaly and adenopathy. There is no hypercalcemia, although the serum lactate dehydrogenase level may be elevated.

    The acute phase is the most common form of presentation. Up to 25% of acute-phase cases present as lymphoma (skin lesions, adenopathy, and hepatosplenomegaly) without circulating ATLL cells. Hypercalcemia is seen in 50% of patients, with or without bone lesions, and is thought to be a paraneoplastic syndrome with elaboration of parathyroid hormone-related protein.

    C. Treatment. Acute ATLL is usually resistant to standard leukemia therapy, and most patients die within weeks to months. These patients should be treated with experimental protocols. Currently, there are some responders to 2-CdA infusions. Larger studies and longer follow-up are needed to determine the extent of activity of 2-CdA. Compound 506U (an ara-g analog) appears to show promise. Scattered case reports in the Japanese literature suggest that some patients respond to topical tretinoin (all-*trans*-retinoic acid), including some CRs in patients with visceral disease. Studies to confirm this using oral and topical tretinoin are just beginning in the United States. It is too early to confirm these findings.

SELECTED READINGS

Cheson BD, Bennett Jm, Grever M, Kay N, Keating MJ, O'Brien S. National Cancer Institute Sponsored Working Group guidelines for chronic lymphocytic leukemia: revised guidelines for diagnosis and treatment. *Blood* 1996;87:4990–4997.

Cheson BD, Vena DA, Foss FM, Sorensen JM. Neurotoxicity of purine analogs: a review. *J Clin Oncol* 1994;12:2216–2228.

Doane LL, Ratain MJ, Golumb HM. Hairy cell leukemia: current management. *Hematol Oncol Clin North Am* 1990;4:489.

Johnson S, Smith AG, Loffler H, et al. Multicenter prospective randomized trial of fludarabine versus cytoxan, doxorubicin, and prednisone (CAP) for treatment of advanced stage chronic lymphocytic leukemia. *Lancet* 1996;347:1432–1438.

Kantarjian NM, O'Brien S, Anderlini P, Talpaz M. Treatment of chronic myelogenous leukemia and investigational options. *Blood* 1996;87:3036.

Kyle RA, Tefferi A. Multiple myeloma, chronic lymphocytic leukemia, and hairy cell leukemia. *Curr Opin Hematol* 1994;4:195.

Neely SM. Adult T-cell leukemia-lymphoma. *West J Med* 1989;150:557.

Palackdharry CS. Non-Hodgkins lymphoma: why the increasing incidence? *Oncology* 1994;8:67.

Piro LD, Carrera CJ, Carson DA, Beutler E. Lasting remissions in hairy-cell leukemia induced by a single infusion of 2-chlorodeoxyadenosine. *N Engl J Med* 1990;322:1117–1121.

Robbins BA, Ellison DJ, Spinosa JC, et al. Diagnostic application of two color flow cytometry in 161 cases of hairy cell leukemia. *Blood* 1993;82:1277–1287.

Saven A, Piro LD. Treatment of hairy cell leukemia. *Blood* 1992; 79:1111.

Myeloproliferative and Myelodysplastic Syndromes

Peter White and Carol S. Palackdharry

I. **Myeloproliferative syndromes.** The myeloproliferative syndromes are clonal disorders of the pluripotent hematopoietic stem cell or of lineage-committed progenitor cells. These syndromes are characterized by autonomous and sustained overproduction of morphologically and functionally mature granulocytes, erythrocytes, or platelets. The diagnostic label of the individual syndrome indicates the cellular element most strikingly increased, but it is not uncommon to have modest or even major elevations in other lineages (e.g., thrombocytosis and leukocytosis in polycythemia vera). Bone marrow aspirates and biopsy specimens show hyperplasia of megakaryocytes and of granulocytic and erythroid precursors, but maturation is normal. The progeny of the neoplastic lineages display essentially normal physiologic function in most respects, although it is not unusual for platelet dysfunction (reflected by prolonged bleeding time and abnormal aggregation studies) to contribute to bleeding. Chronic granulocytic leukemia is discussed in Chap. 20. The other myeloproliferative disorders are discussed here.

   A. **Polycythemia vera**
      1. **Diagnosis.** Polycythemia vera must be distinguished from relative or spurious polycythemia (normal red blood cell [RBC] mass, decreased plasma volume) and from secondary erythrocytosis (increased RBC mass due to hypoxia, carboxyhemoglobinemia, inappropriate erythropoietin syndromes with tumors or renal disease, etc.). The following diagnostic criteria adopted by the Polycythemia Vera Study Group have proved useful:

      Category A
      A1 Increased RBC mass (measured with ^{51}Cr-labeled RBCs): males $\geq$ 36 mL/kg; females $\geq$ 32 mL/kg
      A2 Normal arterial oxygen saturation: $\geq$92%
      A3 Splenomegaly

      Category B
      B1 Thrombocytosis: platelets $\geq$ 400,000/μL
      B2 Leukocytosis: white blood cell (WBC) count $\geq$ 12,000/μL (in absence of fever or infection)
      B3 Elevated leukocyte alkaline phosphatase score: > 100 in absence of fever or infection

B4 Elevated serum vitamin B_{12} or unbound vitamin B_{12}–binding capacity: $B_{12} > 900$ pg/mL; unbound $B_{12} > 2200$ pg/mL

Polycythemia vera is considered established if parameters A1, A2, and A3 are all present, or if A1 and A2 are present plus any two category B parameters. RBC mass and arterial oxygen saturation should be determined routinely. It is also advisable to perform bone marrow aspiration and biopsy, to assess iron stores and karyotype (abnormal in 10% to 15% of patients), presence of panmyelosis (hyperplasia of all non-lymphoid elements), and fibrosis. Measurements of serum B_{12} and unsaturated B_{12}-binding capacity levels and imaging studies for splenomegaly (detectable by physical examination alone in 70% of polycythemia vera patients) are helpful in questionable cases but are not needed routinely. Serum erythropoietin levels should be measured when the diagnosis is not straightforward: Patients with polycythemia vera should have a subnormal level; elevated values should prompt a search for occult tumor, renal disease, and other causes of secondary erythrocytosis.

2. **Aims of therapy.** Thrombosis is a major cause of morbidity in polycythemia vera, primarily due to increased blood viscosity and stasis, and leading to stroke, myocardial infarct, and venous thromboembolism. Lowering the hematocrit to 40% to 45% reduces the risk of thrombosis, and risk is best minimized by concomitant use of phlebotomy and hydroxyurea or other myelosuppressive agents, particularly if platelets are elevated. It is particularly important to maintain good control of hematocrit and platelets in the elderly and in others predisposed to thrombosis.

3. **Treatment regimens**

   a. **Phlebotomy.** Removal of 350 to 500 mL of blood every 2 to 4 days (less often in the elderly or in patients with cardiac disease) is the standard initial approach, with the aim of lowering the hematocrit to 40% to 45%. The blood cell count is then checked monthly, and phlebotomy is repeated as needed to maintain the hematocrit at less than 45%. Rapid lowering of the hematocrit may also be achieved in surgical or thrombotic emergencies by erythroapheresis. Elective surgery should be deferred for 2 to 4 months after stabilizing the hematocrit at 45%. Platelet function should be evaluated (using bleeding time, aggregation studies, or both) before surgery or invasive procedures.

b. **Myelosuppressive agents** are commonly
indicated in conjunction with phlebotomy,
particularly for persistent thrombocytosis,
recurrent thrombosis, enlarging spleen, or
similar problems. They may also reduce
the risk of progression to myelofibrosis
compared with phlebotomy alone. Alkylating agents, such as chlorambucil, carry a
high risk of producing leukemia and are no
longer recommended. Currently recommended choices are as follows:

(1) **Hydroxyurea**, 600 to 800 mg/m² p.o.
daily. This drug requires weekly blood
cell counts initially and dosage adjustments to maintain the hematocrit
at 40% to 45%, the platelet count at
100,000 to 500,000/μL, and the WBC
count at more than 3,000/μL. Side
effects are usually minimal, but long-
term use may cause painful leg
ulcers and aphthous stomatitis; risk
of leukemia is probably increased
as well.

For cases that are difficult to control with hydroxyurea, acceptable alternatives include the following:

(2) **Interferon-α** is usually effective in
controlling hematocrit, platelet count,
and splenomegaly, according to recent
reports. The starting dose is 1 to 3 million U/m² three times weekly. Side
effects include myalgia, fever, and asthenia, usually controlled with acetaminophen. Leukemogenic effects are
presumably absent, but high cost is a
deterrent to long-term use.

(3) **Radioactive phosphorus** (³²P), 2.3
mCi/m² i.v. (5 mCi maximum single
dose). Repeat in 12 weeks if the response is inadequate (25% dose escalation optional). Lack of response
after a third dose mandates a switch
to other forms of therapy. Use of ³²P
entails about a 10% risk of leukemia
by 10 years, and it is best reserved for
use in the elderly and in patients
refractory to other modalities. Supplemental phlebotomies may be required for patients with satisfactory
platelet and WBC counts but with
rising hematocrit levels.

(4) **Busulfan** appears to have less leukemogenic potential than other alkylating agents and is appropriate
in patients whose disease is not

controlled by other treatments, or in the elderly. It is best given in short courses over several weeks (to avoid prolonged marrow suppression) at 2 to 4 mg/day.

(5) **Anagrelide** selectively inhibits platelet production, and a decrease in the platelet count is seen after 7 to 14 days. The WBC count is unaffected, and the hemoglobin level may fall slightly. Responses to anagrelide have been reported in more than 80% of patients with all myeloproliferative syndromes. The recommended starting dose is 0.5 mg q.i.d. Side effects include headache (44%), palpitations, diarrhea, asthenia, and fluid retention. Anagrelide appears to reduce risk of thrombosis.

c. **Ancillary treatments.** Allopurinol, 300 mg/day, is commonly needed to control hyperuricemia. Pruritus is a frequent problem but usually abates with myelosuppressive therapy. Cyproheptadine, 5 to 20 mg/day, and cimetidine, 900 mg/day, may be helpful. Aspirin and similar antiplatelet agents are often helpful for erythromelalgia (hot, red, painful digits) and are commonly used to prevent thrombosis, although their efficacy is unclear.

4. **Evolution and outcome.** The median survival time for patients with polycythemia vera is about 10 years. One third of deaths are caused by thrombosis. The risk of leukemia is small in patients treated by phlebotomy alone. Many patients progress to a "spent phase," with increasing splenomegaly and stable or falling hematocrit. A substantial number show extensive myelofibrosis (see Section I.C). Splenectomy or splenic irradiation may be indicated for massive splenomegaly in such patients.

B. **Essential thrombocythemia**
1. **Diagnosis** of essential thrombocythemia requires (a) a persistent elevation of the platelet count above 600,000/μL, plus (b) the absence of other known causes of reactive or secondary thrombocytosis (e.g., iron deficiency, malignancy, or chronic inflammatory disease). The hematocrit level and RBC mass should not be elevated; differentiation from "bled-out" polycythemia vera may be difficult. Marrow aspiration and biopsy should be performed to assess hyperplasia of megakaryocytes, evaluate iron stores, and exclude myelofibrosis and myelodysplasia. Marrow chromosome studies

are desirable to exclude the Philadelphia chromosome, bcr/abl gene rearrangements, and myelodysplastic syndrome (MDS; notably, 5q–syndrome), but an abnormal karyotype is found in less than 10% of patients. Palpable splenomegaly is present in less than 50% of patients. Platelet function studies may show either spontaneous aggregation or impaired response to agonists. Microvascular occlusion may cause digital gangrene, transient ischemic attacks, visual complaints, and paresthesias. Large-vessel occlusion (myocardial infarct, cerebrovascular accident) and hemorrhagic manifestations due to platelet dysfunction are also seen.

2. **Treatment regimens.** Observation alone is considered a reasonable course in younger, symptom-free patients with fewer than 1×10^6 platelets/μL. Therapy for the lower platelet count should be undertaken in patients at increased risk for hemorrhagic or thrombotic complications and in the elderly. Options include the following:

   a. **Hydroxyurea**, 600 to 800 mg/m^2 p.o. daily, with dosage adjustments on the basis of the weekly complete blood cell count, should achieve satisfactory response in 2 to 6 weeks. Protection against thrombosis has been shown.

   b. **Anagrelide** can now be considered a reasonable alternative to hydroxyurea, with presumed protection against thrombosis (see Section I.A.3.b.[5]).

   c. **Interferon-α.** Most thrombocythemic patients respond to this agent, at an initial dose of 3 million U/day s.c. As noted in Section I.A.3.b.(2), side effects and expense are potential problems, and its effectiveness in reducing thrombotic and hemorrhagic complications remains uncertain.

   d. **Platelet apheresis** may be indicated in emergent situations (e.g., cerebral ischemia), but the effect is usually short-lived. On occasion, platelet transfusion may be indicated to control hemorrhage despite high platelet count.

   e. **^{32}P and alkylating agents** are effective but carry increased risk of secondary leukemia. Nitrogen mustard (mechlorethamine, 0.15 to 0.3 mg/kg [6 to 12 mg/m^2] i.v.) can be helpful when rapid reduction in platelet count is needed. Busulfan, 2 to 4 mg/day initial dose, is appropriate in selected patients resistant to other agents, particularly the elderly.

      f. Aspirin, 300 mg/day, may control erythromelalgia and similar vasoocclusive problems but is contraindicated in patients with a history of hemorrhagic symptoms or platelet dysfunction (e.g., prolonged bleeding time). Aspirin may be useful in the management of pregnant patients, in whom the preceding agents are contraindicated.

    3. Evolution and outcome. The course of essential thrombocytopenia is often indolent, particularly in young patients. The median survival time probably exceeds 10 years, and some patients appear to have normal life expectancy. In a few patients, the disease transforms to other myeloproliferative disorders or to acute leukemia.

C. Agnogenic myeloid metaplasia (AMM)

    1. Diagnosis. This disorder of the stem cell, also called *idiopathic myelofibrosis,* is marked by (a) an intense reactive fibrosis of the marrow; (b) splenomegaly (frequently massive), reflecting ectopic hematopoiesis in the spleen and portal hypertension; and (c) the presence of immature granulocytes, nucleated RBCs, and teardrop RBCs in the peripheral blood (leukoerythroblastic blood picture). An abnormal karyotype is demonstrable in 50% to 60% of patients. Causes of secondary marrow fibrosis, such as metastatic carcinoma, hairy-cell leukemia, and granulomatous infections, must be excluded. Postpolycythemic myelofibrosis is clinically indistinguishable but carries a poor prognosis, evolving to acute leukemia in 25% to 50% of patients (compared with 5% to 20% for *de novo* AMM). Acute myelofibrosis is also distinct from AMM and may be identical or closely related to acute megakaryoblastic leukemia.

    2. Treatment regimens. The median survival time is about 5 years, but symptom-free patients may do well without treatment for a number of years. Intervention is indicated in the following cases:

      a. Anemia. Androgens (e.g., testosterone enanthate, 600 mg i.m. weekly, or oxymetholone, 50 mg q.i.d. p.o., for men; danazol, 600 mg p.o. daily, for women) are recommended and frequently reduce transfusion requirements. Corticosteroids (e.g., prednisone, 40 mg/m^2 p.o. daily) should be tried if overt hemolysis is present. Erythropoietin is helpful in a small percentage of patients (4,000 to 10,000 units two or three times weekly).

    b. **Splenomegaly.** Massive splenomegaly may lead to cytopenias, portal hypertension, variceal bleeding, abdominal pain, or compression of adjacent organs. Anorexia, fatigue, and hypercatabolic complaints may be prominent. Options for control include myelosuppressive therapy with hydroxyurea as for polycythemia vera (see Section I.A.3.b.) or busulfan, 2 mg/day, in older patients. Interferon-α produces responses in a significant percentage of cases, but its role is not established in AMM.

        Radiation, 50 to 200 cGy, may improve splenomegaly and occasionally is indicated for extramedullary hemopoietic tumors causing compression syndromes or for bone pain. Splenectomy is indicated in carefully selected cases but carries significant perioperative mortality and morbidity from bleeding, sepsis, and postoperative thrombocytosis.

    c. **Curative intent.** Allogeneic marrow or stem cell transplantation from appropriately matched donors appears to be potentially curative, on the basis of limited experience. Marrow fibrosis does not prevent successful engraftment.

II. MDSs, also referred to as *preleukemia* or *oligoblastic leukemia,* represent clonal abnormalities of hematopoietic stem cells. In contrast to myeloproliferative syndromes, dysplastic morphologic features are prominent, reflecting impaired maturation and functional abnormalities. Even without transformation to acute leukemia, there are fatal disorders, with death resulting from the complications of bone marrow failure (infection, bleeding, or both).

    A. **Diagnosis.** The bone marrow is usually hypercellular, but hematopoiesis is ineffective, and anemia with or without other cytopenias is the rule. Occasionally, the bone marrow is hypocellular or normocellular. Reticulocyte counts are normal or low, despite erythroid hyperplasia. Diagnostic features include dysplasia, megaloblastoid changes, or both in RBC precursors; ring sideroblasts; bilobed neutrophils (i.e., pseudo–Pelger-Huet anomaly); hypogranulation of neutrophils; monolobular or hypolobular megakaryocytes; and agranular platelets. Small numbers of blast cells may be found in the peripheral blood, and up to 30% may be found in the marrow. Transformation to acute leukemia can be diagnosed when the bone marrow blast count is greater than 30%.

        The French-American-British (FAB) classification divides MDSs into five categories.

    1. Refractory anemia (RA) (<5% blasts in marrow).
    2. Refractory anemia with ring sideroblasts (RARS) (<5% blasts, >15% ringed sideroblasts).

3. Refractory anemia with excess blasts (RAEB) (5% to 20% blasts in marrow)
4. Refractory anemia with excess blasts "in transformation" (RAEB-T) (20% to 30% blasts in marrow)
5. Chronic myelomonocytic leukemia (CMML) (5% to 20% blasts in marrow, >1000 monocytes/μL)

B. Cytogenetics and prognostic variables

1. **Karyotypic abnormalities.** A number of chromosomal abnormalities have been associated with MDSs, especially on chromosomes 5 and 7. Patients with 5q–syndrome (female predominance, anemia with a normal or high platelet count, and monolobulated or bilobulated megakaryocytes) have a longer survival time and less frequent transformation to acute nonlymphocytic leukemia (ANNL) than do patients with other DNA abnormalities. Recent studies demonstrated the translocation of chromosome 11q21 in MDSs secondary to epipodophyllotoxins and chromosome 21q22 in MDSs secondary to anthracyclines.

2. **Prognostic factors.** Several prognostic factors have been postulated. The most consistent predictors of a poor prognosis include advanced age, very low peripheral blood counts, increased blasts in the bone marrow, increased cytogenetic abnormalities, and a high ALIP (abnormal localization of immature precursors) score in the bone marrow.

C. Clinical course. These are fatal disorders, even without transformation to acute leukemia. Patients die from complications of bone marrow failure or acute leukemia. The median survival time for patients without transformation is only 2 to 4 years for RA and RARS, and less than 1 year for RAEB and RAEB-T. The frequency of transformation to acute leukemia before death correlates with the FAB classification.

RA, RARS	10% to 20%
CMML	20% to 30%
RAEB	40% to 50%
RAEB-T	60% to 75%

Transformation into a secondary acute leukemia is usually fatal. Durable remissions are rare, and in most studies involving induction chemotherapy, the toxic death rate equals or exceeds the response rate.

D. Treatment regimens

1. **Allogeneic bone marrow transplantation (BMT).** This is the only known curative therapy for MDS. BMT should be considered the treatment of choice in young patients for whom a matched related donor is available. Improvements in supportive care have allowed some centers to perform allogeneic BMT safely in healthy patients up to the age of 70 years. Stud-

ies indicate that 30% to 50% of eligible patients may be cured.

2. **Supportive care.** Most patients diagnosed with MDS do not qualify for allogeneic BMT because of advanced age, poor health, or lack of an HLA-identical sibling donor. For these patients, supportive care with antibiotics and transfusions when the disease is symptomatic should be considered the standard of care.

3. **Growth factors**
    a. **Erythropoietin.** Only about 20% of patients with MDS have a meaningful increase in hemoglobin with high-dose erythropoietin. Response does not correlate well with baseline endogenous erythropoietin levels.

    b. **Granulocyte-macrophage colony-stimulating factor (GM-CSF) and granulocyte colony-stimulating factor (G-CSF).** Although these factors can transiently increase the number of functioning neutrophils, studies have not demonstrated an improved survival with these therapies. A recent large randomized trial demonstrated a decreased survival rate after G-CSF treatment compared with supportive care. Given these data and the concern regarding the possible stimulation of progression to ANNL, these factors remain experimental.

    c. **Other hematopoietic growth factors.** Other factors currently being investigated include interleukin-3 (IL-3), IL-6, IL-11, Pixy 321, and stem cell factor. Sufficient data regarding response rates are not yet available.

4. **Hormonal therapies.** Several studies using steroids have been performed but have found essentially no durable responses and an increase in infectious complications. For this reason, steroids are relatively contraindicated in MDS. Neither androgens nor danazol has been shown to prolong survival or produce meaningful responses.

5. **Cytotoxic chemotherapy.** Trials using acute leukemia induction regimens to treat MDS (without transformation to ANNL) have produced response rates of 15% to 50%; however, the toxic death rates have equaled or exceeded response rates in most trials. Similar results are seen when transformation to a secondary ANNL occurs, with a 20% to 40% complete response rate but a 20% to 60% mortality rate with induction chemotherapy. This approach could be considered for young patients without

a match for allogeneic BMT but may result in early death in elderly patients.

6. **Differentiating agents**

   a. **Retinoids.** Initial promising data reporting a 20% complete response rate with the use of isotretinoin (*cis*-retinoic acid) have not been confirmed by additional studies. Currently, neither isotretinoin nor tretinoin (all-*trans*-retinoic acid) has demonstrated a survival advantage.

   b. **Low-dose cytarabine (ara-C).** Studies demonstrate only a 16% complete response rate in MDS; however, patients with MDS appear ultrasensitive to ara-C, and toxicities are significant. Despite an increase in disease-free survival, overall survival has not been prolonged by this therapy.

   c. **Vitamin D analogs.** Thus far, early trials have failed to demonstrate a significant effect.

   d. **5-Azacitidine.** Limited experience has not demonstrated a superior response rate compared with cytarabine.

E. **Summary.** For most patients in whom allogeneic BMT is not feasible, MDSs represent fatal disorders. Even without transformation to ANNL, most patients die from complications of bone marrow failure. Allogeneic BMT is the only known curative modality. Supportive care is considered standard therapy outside the setting of a clinical trial for most patients.

SELECTED READINGS

Appelbaum FR, Barrall J, Storb R, et al. Bone marrow transplantation for patients with myelodysplasia: pretreatment variables and outcome. *Ann Intern Med* 1990;112:590–597.

Bennett JM, Catovsky D, Daniel MT, et al. Proposals for the classification of the myelodysplastic syndromes. *Br J Haematol* 1982;51:189–199.

Bilgrami S, Greenberg B. Polycythemia rubra vera. *Semin Oncol* 1995;22:307–326.

Cheson BD. The myelodysplastic syndromes: current approaches to therapy. *Ann Intern Med* 1990;112:932.

Murphy S. Therapeutic dilemmas: balancing the risks of bleeding, thrombosis, and leukemic transformation in myeloproliferative disorders (MPD). *Thromb Haemost* 1997;78(1):622–626.

Petitt RM, Silverstein MN, Petrone ME. Anagrelide for control of thrombocythemia in polycythemia and other myeloproliferative states. *Semin Hematol* 1997;34:51–54.

Tefferi A, Silverstein M. Agnogenic myeloid metaplasia. *Semin Oncol* 1995;22:327:333.

Zuckerman KS. Myelodysplasia. *Curr Opin Hematol* 1993;4:183.

22

Hodgkin's Disease

Richard S. Stein

Hodgkin's disease is a lymphoproliferative malignancy that accounts for about 1% of cancers in the United States. The disease generally presents as solitary or generalized lymphadenopathy and spreads in a contiguous fashion. Most patients present with disease limited to lymph nodes or to lymph nodes and the spleen. The average age at presentation is 32 years, with a bimodal incidence curve; one peak occurs at age 25 years, the other at age 55 years. Patients with limited disease can be cured by radiation therapy; patients with advanced disease can be cured by combination chemotherapy. Patients who relapse after initial treatment may be cured by salvage therapy. Salvage chemotherapy may produce cures in patients initially treated with radiation therapy. Readministration of standard-dose chemotherapy, or more commonly, the administration of high-dose chemotherapy in conjunction with autologous stem cell transplantation, may produce cures in patients initially treated with combination chemotherapy.

Paradoxically, this success in the therapy of Hodgkin's disease makes it difficult to make definitive recommendations regarding initial treatment because the treatment options associated with superior disease-free survival may not necessarily produce superior overall survival when the results of salvage therapy are considered. However, for each stage of Hodgkin's disease, a number of rational therapeutic options exist.

I. **Pathologic subtypes.** Diagnosis of Hodgkin's disease requires biopsy of an involved node and review of the material by a hematopathologist. Four major histologic subtypes of Hodgkin's disease exist: lymphocyte predominant (2% to 7%), nodular sclerosis (60% to 75%), mixed cellularity (17% to 26%), and lymphocyte depleted (1% to 6%). Nodular sclerosis Hodgkin's disease is commonly seen in young adults and is frequently associated with a large mediastinal mass. Lymphocyte-depleted Hodgkin's disease is usually associated with symptomatic disease (see Section II.A) and frequent involvement of the bone marrow and retroperitoneal nodes. Although Hodgkin's disease can present below the diaphragm and may occasionally present at an extranodal site, these presentations are infrequent enough that the pathologic diagnosis of Hodgkin's disease should be made with great care in these circumstances.

II. **Staging.** In determining therapy for the patient with Hodgkin's disease, the critical variable is the stage of the patient. However, it must be recognized that stage and histologic type co-vary in Hodgkin's disease. The average patient with lymphocyte-predominant disease has a lower stage than the average patient with nodular sclerosis

Hodgkin's disease, who, in turn, has a lesser stage than the average patient with mixed cellularity Hodgkin's disease.

A. Cotswold staging system. The Cotswold modification of the Ann Arbor staging system is used for patients with Hodgkin's disease. Clinically, patients are placed in one of four stages (I through IV) and are further classified as to the presence or absence of symptoms. The subscript A denotes that no symptoms are present. The subscript B denotes that any or all of the following are present: fever, night sweats, unexplained weight loss of 10% or more of body weight. In addition, the subscript E (e.g., II_E) may be used to denote involvement of an extralymphatic site primarily, or, more commonly, by direct extension, such as a large mediastinal mass extending into the lung. Stage III Hodgkin's disease is often subdivided into stages III_1 and III_2 based on the extent of intra-abdominal disease.

Stage I: Involvement of a single lymph node region

Stage II: Involvement of two or more lymph node regions on the same side of the diaphragm

Stage III_1: Involvement of lymph node regions on both sides of the diaphragm. Abdominal disease is limited to the upper abdomen, that is, the spleen, splenic hilar, celiac, and/or porta hepatis nodes

Stage III_2: Involvement of lymph node regions on both sides of the diaphragm. Abdominal disease includes paraaortic, mesenteric, iliac, or inguinal nodes, with or without disease in the upper abdomen.

Stage IV: Diffuse or disseminated involvement of one or more extralymphatic tissues or organs, with or without associated lymph node involvement.

B. Staging tests. Staging must be performed with consideration of therapeutic options and not just to complete a checklist. When performing staging tests, one should remember that Hodgkin's disease tends to spread in a contiguous manner. Considering that the thoracic duct makes the left supraclavicular area and the abdomen contiguous sites, it is not surprising that abdominal disease is found in 40% of patients with left supraclavicular presentation and in only 8% of patients with right supraclavicular presentation. Additionally, one should consider that staging tests are designed to establish a baseline extent of disease so that completeness of response can be evaluated after completion of therapy. Procedures used in the staging of Hodgkin's disease are as follows:

  1. History taking. In addition to noting symptoms that may suggest unusual sites of disease, such as bone pain, it is critically important to determine if the patient should be categorized as A or B. Therefore, fever, night sweats, and weight loss must be evaluated.

  2. Complete physical examination. Attention must be paid to all lymph node regions and the spleen.

3. **Laboratory tests.** Complete blood counts, erythrocyte sedimentation rate, serum alkaline phosphatase levels, and tests of liver and kidney function should be obtained. Hepatic enzymes may be elevated nonspecifically in patients with Hodgkin's disease and do not necessarily indicate hepatic involvement by Hodgkin's disease.

4. **Chest radiograph.** Computed tomography (CT) of the chest is useful in establishing the baseline dimensions of a mass when the chest radiograph demonstrates an abnormality. Although the chest CT is often obtained as part of routine staging, the clinical value of detecting minimal disease that might be missed by routine chest radiographs alone is not established.

5. **Lymphangiogram.** The lymphangiogram is useful in that it can detect normal-sized nodes in which the internal architecture has been obliterated by Hodgkin's disease. These nodes may be too small to be detected by CT of the abdomen. However, performance of lymphangiography is dependent on the availability of a radiologist who can perform the test and interpret the results. As a result, clinical staging of the abdomen is often limited to performance of an abdominal CT scan.

    Because lymphangiography can be associated with embolization of lipid dye to the lungs, the procedure should not be performed in patients with pulmonary Hodgkin's disease or a large mediastinal mass. Omission of the lymphangiogram is of no clinical consequence in these patients because they are candidates for chemotherapy anyway.

6. **CT of the abdomen.** This test is routinely obtained as part of staging and is helpful when results are positive. Use of the abdominal CT scan has eliminated the need for performing isotopic scans of the liver and spleen. As noted previously, CT is less sensitive than the lymphangiogram.

7. **Bone marrow biopsy.** This test is rarely positive except in patients who are found to have at least stage III disease by other tests. However, because of the potential use of autologous bone marrow transplantation (BMT) or stem cell transplantation as salvage therapy, a bone marrow biopsy is a reasonable baseline study in all patients with Hodgkin's disease.

8. **Staging laparotomy.** Staging laparotomy is the most accurate means of determining the extent of abdominal involvement with Hodgkin's disease. Criteria for performing staging laparotomy vary widely. Some physicians recommend laparotomy whenever the therapeutic plan is to

administer radiation therapy. Others favor laparotomy whenever clinical staging is equivocal. However, one can compensate for uncertain clinical staging by omitting laparotomy and proceeding with chemotherapy. Relative indications for staging laparotomy in patients who are candidates for radiation therapy include the presence of mixed-cellularity Hodgkin's disease, Hodgkin's disease involving the left supraclavicular lymph nodes, patients older than 28 years, and patients in whom a lymphangiogram has not been performed. Staging laparotomy should include inspection, liver biopsies (wedge biopsy of the left lobe plus needle biopsy of both lobes), and biopsies of the splenic hilar, celiac, porta hepatis, mesenteric, paraaortic, and iliac lymph nodes. Ovariopexy may be performed to move the ovaries out of the radiation port. However, this is relevant only if the radiation therapist is willing to shield the ovaries, and only if radiation therapy to pelvic ports is planned, such as total nodal radiation. Because total nodal radiation therapy has been employed less frequently in recent years, ovariopexy has been employed less frequently as well.

C. **Therapy for Hodgkin's disease**
   1. **General considerations.** Therapy for Hodgkin's disease must be considered on a stage-by-stage basis. The incidence of various stages of Hodgkin's disease is presented in Table 22-1, which also presents an estimated cure rate for each stage. In general, limited stages of Hodgkin's disease (stages IA and IIA) are generally treated with radiation therapy, whereas advanced stages (IIIB, IVA, and IVB) are generally treated with combination chemotherapy. Therapy of the intermediate stages (IIB, IIIA) remains somewhat controversial, and although

**Table 22-1. Hodgkin's disease:
incidence of stages and results of therapy**

Stage	Relative Incidence (%)	Potential Cure Rate (%)
IA	10	95
IIA	35	85
IB, IIB	13	70
III_1A	12	85
III_2A	8	65
IIIB	12	60
IVA, IVB	10	60

radiation therapy can be considered for these patients, the tendency of most oncologists is to treat these patients with combination chemotherapy.

Despite the success in the treatment of Hodgkin's disease, decisions regarding the optimal choice of therapy for all stages of Hodgkin's disease have become more complex.

Late complications of radiation therapy for Hodgkin's disease include breast cancer, lung cancer, hypothyroidism, thyroid cancer, coronary artery disease, and valvular heart disease. Although the incidence of each of these complications is fairly low, the cumulative risk of all of these complications may be as much as 15% at 15 years after treatment. It is therefore reasonable to consider chemotherapy or chemotherapy plus involved field radiation therapy as an approach to limited-stage Hodgkin's disease. Unfortunately, there are no data showing that the overall survival of patients with limited-stage Hodgkin's disease can be improved with this alteration of therapy. Thus, after decades of "knowing" that radiation therapy was the optimal approach to limited-stage Hodgkin's disease, there is now uncertainty as to whether this is the case.

Although chemotherapy has clearly been established as the optimal therapy for advanced-stage disease, clinical trials have not resolved the question of which regimen represents optimal treatment. Regardless of the chemotherapy regimen chosen, standard regimens should not be altered arbitrarily because dose reductions may decrease the possibility of cure. Although most patients receive six monthly cycles of chemotherapy, the data actually support the policy of administering a minimum of six cycles, with therapy being given until a complete remission has been achieved and then administered for an additional two cycles. Although the tumor lysis syndrome has not been reported in Hodgkin's disease, it is prudent to administer allopurinol during the first cycle of chemotherapy or during the first 2 weeks of radiation therapy.

2. **Radiation therapy.** Studies conducted in the 1960s established that the optimal dose for local control is 36 to 40 Gy given over 3.5 to 4.0 weeks. Standard radiation therapy ports are illustrated in Fig. 22-1.

   With modern equipment, adequate radiation can be administered to involved areas while shielding adjacent tissues. Nevertheless, radiation injury, such as radiation pneumonitis or radiation pericarditis, occurs rarely. Inappro-

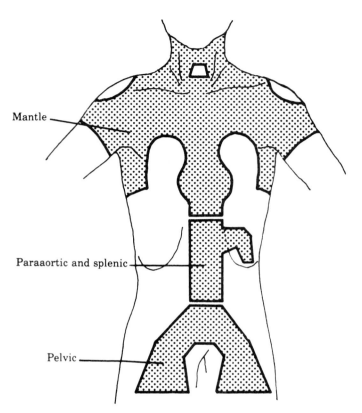

Fig. 22-1.   Standard radiation ports used for the treatment of Hodgkin's disease. For disease presenting above the diaphragm, the mantle plus paraaortic and splenic ports would be regarded as extended field radiation therapy. The use of all three ports would be considered total nodal irradiation. (Reprinted by permission from JR Salzman and HS Kaplan. Effect of prior splenectomy on hematologic tolerance during total lymphoid radiotherapy of patients with Hodgkin's disease. *Cancer* 27:472, 1972.)

priate overlapping of radiation ports can result in damage to the overtreated area. Because of the common occurrence of hypothyroidism and the less common occurrence of thyroid cancer in patients who receive radiation to the thyroid gland, thyroid-stimulating hormone (TSH) levels should be monitored yearly in these patients. Patients with elevated levels of TSH, even if clinically euthyroid, should be placed on thyroid hormone replacement to limit stimulation of the irradiated thyroid gland by elevated levels of TSH. Although radiation therapy alone has not been associated with an increased risk of acute leukemia, the use of radiation therapy in conjunction with combination chemotherapy has been associated with a risk of acute non-lymphocytic leukemia as high as 7% to 10% in the decade after therapy.

3. **Stages IA and IIA.** Patients with stage IA disease are most commonly treated with mantle irradiation when the disease occurs above the diaphragm (as it does in 90% of cases) or with pelvic radiation therapy when the disease presents in an inguinal node. Patients with stage IIA disease presenting above the diaphragm are most commonly treated with mantle plus paraaortic-splenic radiation therapy. There is no firm evidence that adding chemotherapy improves results in these patients. In attempts to limit long-term toxicity, investigators at Stanford have studied the use of involved-field radiation in conjunction with a combination regimen less toxic than usually employed, specifically VBM (vinblastine, bleomycin, and methotrexate.) Early results have been encouraging, but long-term follow-up is needed to determine if the risk of late toxicities is significantly decreased by this approach.

4. **Stage IIE disease with bulky mediastinal mass.** Patients with bulky mediastinal masses (disease diameter > 9 cm, or greater than one third of the chest diameter) present a special problem (Hancock et al., 1991). When treated with radiotherapy alone, these patients have a risk of relapse that approaches 50%. Combination chemotherapy, with or without radiation therapy, is most commonly employed in these patients. Because combined-modality therapy creates a risk of inducing acute leukemia, our approach is to treat these patients with combination chemotherapy and to give low-dose radiation therapy (20 Gy) only to patients with residual disease upon completion of chemotherapy and only to the area of residual disease. Unfortunately, there are no data showing that overall survival with this approach is superior to results achieved with other approaches, such as the initial use of radiation therapy followed by chemotherapy at the time of relapse.

5. **Stages IB and IIB.** In view of the limited number of patients with these stages of disease, available data do not allow firm treatment recommendations to be made. These patients are most commonly treated with extended-field radiation therapy or radiation therapy in conjunction with combination chemotherapy, such as MOPP, ABVD, or MOPP/ABV (Table 22-2). A discussion of the relative merits of the chemotherapy options for advanced-stage

Table 22-2. Chemotherapy regimens used in the treatment of Hodgkin's disease

Regimen	Drugs and Dosages
MOPP	Mechlorethamine, 6 mg/m^2 i.v. on days 1 and 8
	Vincristine (Oncovin), 1.4 mg/m^2 i.v. on days 1 and 8 (not to exceed 2.5 mg)
	Procarbazine, 100 mg/m^2 p.o. on days 1–14
	Prednisone, 40 mg/m^2 p.o. on days 1–14, cycles 1 and 4 only
	Repeat cycle every 28 days
ABVD	Doxorubicin (Adriamycin), 25 mg/m^2 i.v. on days 1 and 15
	Vinblastine, 6 mg/m^2 i.v. on days 1 and 15
	Bleomycin, 10 U/m^2 i.v. on days 1 and 15
	Dacarbazine, 375 mg/m^2 i.v. on days 1 and 15
	Repeat cycle every 28 days
MOPP/ABV	Mechlorethamine, 6 mg/m^2 i.v. on day 1
	Vincristine (Oncovin), 1.4 mg/m^2 i.v. on day 1 (not to exceed 2.5 mg)
	Procarbazine, 100 mg/m^2 p.o. on days 1–7
	Prednisone, 40 mg/m^2 p.o. on days 1–14
	Doxorubicin (Adriamycin), 25 mg/m^2 i.v. on day 8
	Vinblastine, 6 mg/m^2 i.v. on day 8
	Bleomycin, 10 U/m^2 i.v. on day 8
	Repeat cycle every 28 days
VBM	Vinblastine, 6 mg/m^2 i.v. on days 1 and 8
	Bleomycin, 10 U/m^2 i.v. on days 1 and 8
	Methotrexate, 30 mg/m^2 i.v. on days 1 and 8
	Repeat cycle every 28 days
EVA	Etoposide, 100 mg/m^2 p.o. days 1–3
	Vinblastine, 6 mg/m^2 i.v. day 1
	Doxorubicin (Adriamycin), 50 mg/m^2 i.v. day 1
	Repeat cycle every 3 weeks

Hodgkin's disease is found in the discussion of stages IIIB, IVA, and IVB disease.

6. **Stage IIIA.** Therapy for stage IIIA disease has become less controversial in the past 10 to 15 years, although consensus regarding the optimal therapy for these patients has not been achieved. Therapeutic options include total nodal radiation therapy alone, combination chemotherapy alone, or combined-modality therapy (i.e., radiation therapy plus chemotherapy).

With the demonstration that combined-modality therapy was associated with a high risk of acute leukemia, combined-modality therapy fell from favor. Additionally, studies in the early 1980s established that total nodal radiation therapy was adequate therapy only for patients with limited stage III disease (i.e., III_1 disease). For patients with stage III_2 disease, the use of radiation therapy alone was associated with a significant increase in mortality due to unacceptably high relapse rates and the inability of these patients to tolerate salvage chemotherapy at the time of relapse.

If one decides to use different approaches to stage III_1 disease and stage III_2 disease, a staging laparotomy is necessary to stage these patients definitively. As a result, the simplest approach to clinical stage III disease is to treat all stage III patients with combination chemotherapy.

7. **Stage IIIB, IVA, and IVB.** Combination chemotherapy is the standard approach to these stages of Hodgkin's disease, although there remains some controversy as to which chemotherapy approach is optimal.

In 1970, the demonstration by investigators at the National Cancer Institute (NCI) that MOPP chemotherapy could cure advanced Hodgkin's disease was one of the major milestones of the modern chemotherapy era because it was the first demonstration that a previously incurable advanced disease could be cured by combination chemotherapy. This has provided the rationale for the use of combination chemotherapy in medical oncology.

    a. **Dose and duration of therapy.** The optimal regimen for use in Hodgkin's disease has not been established, although several effective regimens exist. Arguments regarding selection of the "best" regimen should not obscure the following principles. Drugs should be administered in accordance with prescribed doses and schedules and not modified for toxicities, such as nausea and vomiting (which should be controlled symptomatically). Full doses should be given when cytopenias are due to bone marrow involvement with Hodgkin's disease. Vincristine should be decreased only in the presence of ileus, motor weakness, or numbness involving the whole fingers, not just the fingertips. Patients should be treated for a minimum of six cycles, but also until a complete remission is documented, and then for another two cycles. If tests are equivocal, it is better to treat with additional cycles rather than to discontinue therapy prematurely.

    b. **Classic MOPP therapy.** When MOPP was initially administered, 81% of patients achieved a complete remission. Of these patients, 66% (representing 53% of the total series) remained in complete remission for 5 years, and an identical percentage remained in complete remission for 10 years. Thus, although late relapses have been seen on occasion, 5-year disease-free survival probably represents cure for most patients. Because salvage therapy can cure patients who are not cured by initial chemotherapy, the figure of 53% represents a minimal estimate for the cure of advanced Hodgkin's disease.

c. **Alternatives to MOPP induction therapy.** Many efforts have been made to develop combination regimens that are more effective and less toxic than the standard MOPP regimen. Some regimens represent minimal modifications of MOPP, but the regimen that has attracted the most interest is ABVD, a regimen composed of agents not cross-resistant to MOPP. In a large randomized trial, ABVD was shown to be superior to MOPP with respect to remission rates and survival. Defenders of the MOPP regimen have noted that in the MOPP versus ABVD trial, MOPP was administered at doses less than those used in the initial NCI trial. Because the MOPP dose modifications were not arbitrary but rather reflect problems that clinicians and patients have with the classic MOPP regimen, this argument may be of limited value. In any case, ABVD has been established as an alternative to MOPP therapy.

An additional approach to advanced Hodgkin's disease is to integrate MOPP and ABVD into a single chemotherapy regimen. Based on kinetic models of tumor resistance, initial studies alternated 1 month of MOPP with 1 month of ABVD. That alternating regimen has been shown to produce results equivalent to those achieved with ABVD. However, for the past decade, one of the standard approaches to advanced Hodgkin's disease has been to integrate both effective regimens into a hybrid regimen, MOPP/ABV, in which all drugs are given during each cycle. Using the MOPP/ABV hybrid, a complete remission rate of 84% has been achieved. This complete remission rate was elevated to 97% by administration of radiation therapy to areas of residual adenopathy. At a median follow-up approaching 4 years, 90% of complete responders remained free of disease, for a projected disease-free survival rate of 88%.

In a randomized trial comparing hybrid MOPP/ABV with sequential MOPP and ABVD, the hybrid regimen was found to be superior to the sequential regimen. The MOPP/ABV hybrid produced complete remissions in 83% of patients, with a failure-free survival rate of 64%. Whether MOPP/ABV is superior to ABVD will not be known until ongoing trials are completed and analyzed.

Thus, standard MOPP, ABVD, MOPP-ABVD (alternating months), and the hybrid regimen MOPP/ABV are reasonable choices for the initial chemotherapy of patients with Hodgkin's disease. In patients who are concerned about fertility, ABVD is the treatment of choice.

Although some investigators have combined chemotherapy with radiation therapy as treatment of advanced disease, there is no evidence that the standard use of this approach can improve results enough to compensate for the leukemogenic risk of that practice. In selected patients with bulky disease, however, it is reasonable to consider supplementing combination chemotherapy with local radiation therapy to sites of bulky disease.

8. **Salvage therapy.** Salvage therapy may produce cures in patients with Hodgkin's disease who relapse after initial therapy. However, the chance of curing a patient with relapsed Hodgkin's disease is greater if the relapse is nodal than if the relapse is visceral. Additionally, the chance of cure is greater when the initial stage of disease was limited than when the initial stage was advanced.

For patients with limited nodal relapses after radiation therapy, additional radiation therapy may be considered. If the recurrence represents a marginal miss at the edge of a radiation field, this may be feasible. However, if the recurrence is within a treatment field, further irradiation of the area is usually contraindicated, and chemotherapy is needed.

For patients who relapse after chemotherapy, the variable that best predicts the chance of cure is the disease-free interval. Among patients initially treated with MOPP therapy, patients whose first complete remission lasted less than 1 year had a second complete remission rate of 29%, and only 14% of these second remissions lasted more than 4 years. Among patients whose first complete remission lasted

more than 1 year, 93% achieved a second remission, and 45% of these second remissions
were projected to last more than 20 years. Although the drugs used to obtain the first complete remission may be successful as salvage
therapy, the general trend is to use drugs to
which the patient has not been exposed. Thus,
for patients treated with MOPP, the ABVD
combination is the most commonly used salvage
therapy.

Although the use of combination chemotherapy, with drugs to which the patient has not
been exposed, is a rational therapeutic alternative, the widespread use of MOPP/ABV renders
this policy moot. The general approach to salvage therapy is, therefore, to use high-dose
chemotherapy in conjunction with autologous
BMT or peripheral blood stem cell transplantation (PBSCT).

High-dose therapy in conjunction with autologous BMT or PBSCT is based on the rationale
that bone marrow toxicity limits the dosages of
the drugs that are most effective in Hodgkin's
disease. When autologous marrow or stem cells
are stored, and reinfused after chemotherapy,
drug doses can be escalated to levels that would
ordinarily be fatal. A number of standard preparative regimens exist for use in conjunction
with autologous BMT and PBSCT, which are
presented in Table 22-3.

**Table 22-3.   Preparative regimens for
autologous transplantation in Hodgkin's disease**

Regimen	Drugs and Dosages
CBV	Cyclophosphamide, 1,800 mg/m^2 i.v. on days −7, −6, −5, −4
	BCNU, 600 mg/m^2 i.v. on day −3
	Etoposide (VP-16), 800 mg/m^2 i.v. on days −7, −6, −5
CBV	Cyclophosphamide, 1,500 mg/m^2 i.v. on days −5, −4, −3, −2
	BCNU, 300 mg/m^2 i.v. on day −5
	Etoposide (VP-16), 300 mg/m^2 i.v. on days −5, −4, −3
BEAM	BCNU, 300 mg/m^2 i.v. on day −6
	Etoposide (VP-16), 100–200 mg/m^2 i.v. on days −5, −4, −3, −2
	Cytosine arabinoside, 200–400 mg/m^2 i.v. on days −5, −4, −3, −2
	Melphalan, 140 mg/m^2 i.v. on day −1

Day 0 is the day of reinfusion of progenitor cells. Therefore, day −5
would be 5 days before reinfusion.

Controlled trials comparing preparative regimens for autologous BMT have not been conducted, and in view of the heterogeneity of relapsed patients with respect to prior therapy, sensitivity to therapy, site of relapse, and disease-free interval, it is impossible to compare regimens across studies. Nevertheless, because improvements in supportive care, such as the use of granulocyte or granulocyte-macrophage colony-stimulating factor, have lowered treatment-related mortality to about 5%, it appears that long-term disease-free survival may occur in about 50% of patients treated with autologous BMT or PBSCT. Patients who achieve long disease-free intervals with standard treatment, especially if they have good performance status and remain sensitive to standard chemotherapy, have an even better chance of long-term disease-free survival.

9. **Treatment of symptoms.** Fever, and occasionally pruritus, may be disabling for some patients with Hodgkin's disease. The basic approach to these problems is to treat the disease. However, if disease is drug resistant, that approach may be an oversimplification. Indomethacin. 25 to 50 mg t.i.d., may be helpful in these patients. Anecdotal experience also supports the use of other nonsteroidal antiinflammatory agents in these patients.

10. **Follow-up.** Hodgkin's disease patients who achieve a complete remission and who later relapse usually do so at a site of previous disease. Our policy for follow-up is to see the patient every 2 months for the first year, every 3 months for the second year, every 4 months during the third year, every 6 months during the fourth year, and every year thereafter. Follow-up evaluation for possible relapse is limited to physical examination (the most important tool for detecting relapse) and chest radiographs (for patients with mediastinal involvement at presentation). If the chest radiograph is indeterminate for relapse, a chest CT scan can be obtained. Some investigators have found gallium scanning to be useful in monitoring patients for relapse. However, it has not been proved that the routine use of gallium scanning is cost-effective in detecting relapses that would otherwise go undetected.

If a patient who presented with B symptoms develops recurrent symptoms while in apparent remission, an abdominal CT scan should be performed, even though the ability of CT scanning to detect retroperitoneal disease is limited. Areas suspicious for relapse should be biopsied to confirm the diagnosis of recurrent

Hodgkin's disease before proceeding with treatment.

Because of the risk of acute leukemia following therapy, we obtain complete blood counts at the time of each visit in patients who received combination chemotherapy. Monitoring for hypothyroidism was discussed in the section on radiation therapy. Although elevated sedimentation rates and lactic dehydrogenase levels may provide hints of relapse, we have not routinely used these tests for follow-up monitoring in our practice.

SELECTED READINGS

Andrieu JM, Ifrah N, Payen C, et al. Increased risk of secondary leukemia after extended field radiation combined with MOPP chemotherapy for Hodgkin's disease. *J Clin Oncol* 1990;8:1148–1154.

Canellos GP, Anderson JR, Propert KJ, et al. Chemotherapy of advanced Hodgkin's disease with MOPP, ABVD, or MOPP alternating with ABVD. *N Engl J Med* 1992;327:1478–1484.

Crnkovich MJ, Leopold K, Hoppe RT, Mauch PM. Stage I to IIB Hodgkin's disease: the combined experience at Stanford University and the Joint Center for Radiation Therapy. *J Clin Oncol* 1987; 5:1041–1049.

DeVita VT Jr, Serpick AA, Carbone PP. Combination chemotherapy in the treatment of advanced Hodgkin's disease. *Ann Intern Med* 1970;73:881–895.

Glick JH, Young ML, Harrington D, et al. MOPP/ABV hybrid chemotherapy for advanced Hodgkin's disease significantly improves failure-free and overall survival: the 8-year results of the intergroup trial. *J Clin Oncol* 1998;16:19–26.

Hancock SL, Cox RS, McDougall IR. Thyroid diseases after treatment of Hodgkin's disease. *N Engl J* Med 1991;325:599–605.

Horning SJ, Hoppe R, Hancock SL, Rosenberg SA. Vinblastine, bleomycin, and methotrexate: an effective regimen in favorable Hodgkin's disease. *J Clin Oncol* 1988;6:1822–1831.

Klimo P, Connors JM. An update on the Vancouver experience in the management of advanced Hodgkin's disease treated with MOPP/ABV hybrid regimen. *Semin Hematol* 1988;25[Suppl 2]:34–40.

Lister TA, Crowther D. Staging for Hodgkin's disease. *Semin Oncol* 1990;17:696–703.

Longo DL, Duffey PL, Young RC, et al. Conventional-dose salvage combination chemotherapy in patients relapsing with Hodgkin's disease after combination chemotherapy: the low probability of cure. *J Clin Oncol* 1992;10:210–218.

Mauch P, Larson D, Osteen R, et al. Prognostic factors for positive surgical staging in patients with Hodgkin's disease. *J Clin Oncol* 1990;8:257–265.

Mauch P, Tarbell N, Weinstein H, et al. Stage IA and IIA supradiaphragmatic Hodgkin's disease: prognostic factors in surgically staged patients treated with mantle and paraaortic irradiation. *J Clin Oncol* 1988;6:1576–1583.

Stein RS, Golomb HM, Wiernik PH, et al. Anatomic substages of stage IIIA Hodgkin's disease. *Cancer Treat Rep* 1982;66:733–741.

Vose JM, Bierman PJ, Armitage JO. Hodgkin's disease: the role of bone marrow transplantation. *Semin Oncol* 1990;17:749–757.

Non-Hodgkin's Lymphoma

Richard S. Stein and John P. Greer

Non-Hodgkin's lymphoma (NHL) is a term used to identify the diverse group of malignancies in which the cell of origin is a lymphocyte and for which the site of origin is outside the bone marrow. The disorders included in NHL differ in many basic characteristics. At the time of presentation, follicular small cleaved cell lymphomas are almost always disseminated, with a high incidence of bone marrow involvement. Diffuse large noncleaved cell lymphomas, on the other hand, may present with disease limited to one or two lymph node areas in up to 30% of cases; bone marrow involvement is seen at presentation less than 20% of the time. Some types of lymphoma, primarily follicular lymphomas, have a slow, indolent course; the disease continually responds and relapses, before having a fatal outcome after 4 to 12 years. By contrast, other types of lymphoma, such as diffuse large cell lymphomas, are fatal in 4 to 12 *months* in the absence of therapy but may be cured by combination chemotherapy in 40% to 50% of cases. In most NHLs, including the types previously discussed, the cell of origin is a B lymphocyte; in a minority of cases, the cell of origin is a T lymphocyte.

In this context of clinical diversity, accurate classification of NHL is essential for scientific and clinical purposes. Ideally, one would want a classification system to divide NHL into entities that were both scientifically and clinically meaningful; that is, a classification system should define entities that are relatively homogeneous from a morphologic, immunologic, and clinical point of view. One would also want a classification system that could be widely used by pathologists so that results could be compared from one institution to another. This would enable clinicians to apply the results of a study to individual patients secure in the knowledge that the pathologic terms used in the study meant the same thing to the academic pathologist writing the paper as to the local pathologist reviewing a specific case. Such an ideal classification system does not exist, and because confusion over pathology is a major limitation to the generation of meaningful clinical data regarding NHL, it is reasonable to start a discussion of NHL with a consideration of pathologic classification.

    I. Pathologic classification of NHL. The pathologic classification of NHL can best be appreciated from a historical perspective. In the 1960s, Rappaport proposed a classification of NHL that divided the disorders on the basis of whether the predominant cell was small (poorly differentiated lymphocytic lymphoma), large (histiocytic lymphoma), or a mixture of small and large cells (mixed-cell lymphoma). Lymphomas were also categorized as nodular or diffuse. This system was easy to use, and concordance among pathologists was high. Studies conducted using this system demonstrated that nodular lymphomas composed of small lymphocytes were generally indolent disorders, whereas so-called histiocytic lymphoma was curable with combination chemotherapy. However, the Rappaport system predated the understanding that lymphocytes were B cells or T cells and that many adult lymphomas were composed of the cells found in normal follicular centers. Rappaport's use of the term *nodular* was specifically chosen to emphasize the fact that it had not been proved that the nodules of nodular lymphoma were similar to the follicles normally seen in lymph nodes. The demonstration that the nodules of nodular lymphoma are composed of the same cells found in germinal follicles rendered this distinction a moot point. With the recognition that "histiocytic lymphoma" was composed of large B lymphocytes, rather than histiocytes, there was an obvious need for either better terminology or a more meaningful classification system.

In the 1970s, therefore, a large number of morphologically based classification systems were created, each trying to define immunologically homogeneous entities. In the United States, the most prominent of these systems was the Lukes-Collins classification system. Although the Lukes-Collins system represented a large scientific step forward, several problems limited its adoption. First, several systems considering immunologic features were simultaneously advocated by various hematopathologists, creating a chaos of competing terminologies. Second, while attempting to define lymphomas by immune origin, as many of 25% of lymphomas were unclassified in the Lukes-Collins system unless fresh tissue was available for the study of surface markers or until techniques to study gene rearrangements were developed. Third, as would be expected for any new system, concordance of diagnoses between pathologists was obtained less frequently than with the Rappaport system. As a result, there were major concerns regarding generalizability of data obtained using the Lukes-Collins classification. Fourth, although the Lukes-Collins system emphasized that "histiocytic lymphoma" was actually many disorders, (i.e., large noncleaved cell lymphoma, large cleaved cell lymphoma [LCCL], immunoblastic sarcoma of B cells, and peripheral T-cell lymphoma [PTCL]), it would not be until the middle to late 1980s that there would be evidence demonstrating which of these hematopathologic distinctions were of clinical significance. Thus, although the Lukes-Collins system was a scientific step forward, concerns over its practical applicability led to confusion.

In this context, the National Cancer Institute created a working panel of hematopathologists who created the New Working Formulation. This classification considered many of the concepts of the Lukes-Collins system (and other immunologically oriented systems). However, instead of defining entities based on their "cell of origin," the New Working Formulation (Table 23-1) defined broad cat-

**Table 23-1. New working
formulation for non-Hodgkin's lymphoma**

Low-grade lymphomas

Small lymphocytic consistent with chronic lymphocytic leukemia
(CLL) or plasmacytoid cell lymphoma
Follicular, predominantly small cleaved cell
    Diffuse areas
    Sclerosis
Follicular, mixed, small cleaved cell and large cell
    Diffuse areas
    Sclerosis

Intermediate-grade lymphomas

Follicular, predominantly large cell
    Diffuse areas
    Sclerosis
Diffuse small cleaved cell
Diffuse mixed, small cleaved cell and large cell
    Sclerosis
    Epitheliod cell component
Diffuse large cell
    Cleaved cell
    Noncleaved cell
    Sclerosis

High-grade lymphomas

Large cell, immunoblastic
    Plasmacytoid
    Clear cell
    Polymorphous
    Epitheliod cell component
Lymphoblastic
    Convoluted cell
    Nonconvoluted cell
Small noncleaved cell
    Burkitt's
    Follicular areas

Miscellaneous

Composite
Mycosis fungoides
Histiocytic
Extramedullary plasmacytoma
Unclassifiable
Other

Modified from the Non-Hodgkin's Lymphoma Pathologic Classification
Project. National Cancer Institute sponsored study of classification of non-
Hodgkin's lymphomas: summary and description of a working formulation for
clinical usage. *Cancer* 1982; 49:2112.

egories of lymphoma based on general clinical prognosis. Specifically, the New Working Formulation defined low-grade lymphoma, intermediate-grade lymphoma, and high-grade lymphoma.

Low-grade lymphomas are indolent lymphomas (such as chronic lymphocytic leukemia and follicular nodular small cleaved cell lymphoma). In patients with asymptomatic disease, even with widespread disease, watchful waiting (i.e., no initial treatment) may be appropriate management. These disorders are associated with a high response rate to single-agent or combination chemotherapy, but responses are eventually followed by relapses. Eventually, after a prolonged clinical course (4 to 12 years), and often after progression to a higher grade of lymphoma, these diseases are invariably fatal.

Intermediate-grade lymphomas are more aggressive lymphomas, associated with a fatal course within months to years in the age of single-agent chemotherapy, but curable 40% to 50% of the time in the era of combination chemotherapy. This category includes diffuse large non-cleaved cell lymphoma (the most common "histiocytic lymphoma") as well as diffuse forms of small cleaved cell lymphoma. Mixed-cell lymphomas are considered intermediate grade when diffuse and low grade when nodular, a policy that is compromised by the fact that more than 70% of mixed-cell lymphomas are both nodular and diffuse.

High-grade lymphomas are associated with a very high growth fraction and a rapidly lethal clinical course in the absence of effective therapy. This category includes small noncleaved cell lymphoma, a term that is equivalent to Burkitt's and Burkitt's-like NHL. At the time the New Working Formulation was designed, the complete remission rate in patients with high-grade lymphoma was only 20%. In the intervening years, however, as response rates in intermediate-grade NHL remained at a plateau of 40% to 50%, complete response rates in high-grade lymphoma rose from the 20% range to the 40% to 50% range with the use of more aggressive chemotherapy (Fig. 23-1).

Although the New Working Formulation provided a framework for clinical trials, at the time of its promulgation, it represented a scientific step backward. As additional information was discovered regarding the cell of origin of lymphomas, it became clear that grouping diverse entities together creates concordance among pathologists at the price of defining entities that are heterogeneous and potentially of limited biologic meaning. Based on the assumption that the scientific study of lymphomas requires the delineation of meaningful entities, the Revised European American Lymphoma (REAL) classification system has been developed to delineate the entities that hematopathologists, immunologists, and molecular biologists have defined in the past 15 years.

The REAL classification system (Table 23-2) has the advantage of recognizing lymphomas that can be defined at

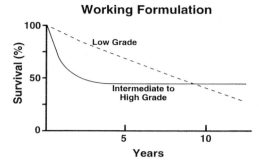

Fig. 23-1.   Survival related to classification by the New Working Formulation. With modern therapies, 40% to 50% of patients with intermediate- and high-grade lymphomas may experience long-term disease-free survival. Patients with low-grade lymphoma are, for the most part, incurable but have a median survival time of between 5 and 10 years. This leads to the paradox of lymphomas, the fact that low-grade lymphomas have better short-term survival but inferior long-term survival when compared with intermediate- and high-grade lymphomas.

the pathologic and molecular level but that are obscured by the use of the New Working Formulation. Entities such as mantle cell lymphoma, with its specific t(11;14) translocation, and large cell anaplastic lymphoma are recognized as distinct entities in this system. The impact of the REAL classification system on the delineation of prognostic subsets of low-grade lymphoma is shown in Fig. 23-2. In the REAL classification (see Table 23-2), however, the largest entity, diffuse large B-cell disease (31% of cases), is likely a heterogeneous disease, and the division of follicular lymphoma (22% of cases) into three grades does not clarify the classification of those entities. Thus, the REAL classification may run the risk of delineating uncommon lymphomas while neglecting the lymphomas most commonly encountered in clinical practice. Only time will tell if this approach leads to a more scientific clinical analysis of lymphoma or to a situation in which clinicians and hematopathologists "classify the frosting and neglect the cake."

II. **Staging**

A. **Limited versus advanced disease.** The Cotswold modification of the Ann Arbor classification is used for NHL as well as for Hodgkin's disease. However, the clinical applicability of the four-stage model to NHL is uncertain. For practical purposes, there may be only two stages of NHL, limited (stage I) and advanced (stages II, III, and IV). Additionally, in contrast to Hodgkin's disease, which arises at an extranodal site in less than 1% of cases, about 10% to 20% of NHLs have an extranodal presentation.

Table 23-2.   International study group classification (revised European American lymphoma classification)

B-cell lymphomas

  Precursor B-lymphoblastic
  Small lymphocytic chronic lymphocytic leukemia (CLL) (7%)
  Lymphoplasmacytic (1.2%)
  Mantle cell (6%)
  Follicle center, follicular (22.1%)
    Grade I (10%)
    Grade II (6%)
    Grade III (6%)
  Follicle center diffuse, small cell
  Marginal zone B-cell, MALT type (8%)
  Marginal zone B-cell, nodal
  Marginal zone B-cell, splenic (<1%)
  Hairy-cell leukemia
  Plasmacytoma
  Diffuse large B-cell (31%)
  Diffuse mediastinal large B-cell (2.4%)
  Burkitt's (<1%)
  High grade B-cell Burkitt's-like (2.1%)
  Unclassifiable low-grade
  Unclassifiable high-grade

T-cell and natural killer cell lymphomas

  Precursor T-lymphoblastic (1.7%)
  T-cell chronic lymphocytic leukemia
  Large granular lymphocyte leukemia
  Mycosis fungoides (<1%)
  Peripheral T-cell, unspecified (7%)
    Medium sized (3.7%)
    Mixed medium and large cell
    Large cell
    Lymphoepitheliod (<1%)
    Hepatosplenic (<1%)
    Subcutaneous panniculitic
  Angioimmunoblastic (1.2%)
  Angiocentric, nasal (1.4%)
  Intestinal (<1%)
  Adult T-cell lymphoma/leukemia (<1%)
Anaplastic large cell (including null phenotype) (2.4%)

Others

  Composite lymphoma
  Malignant lymphoma, unclassifiable low-grade
  Malignant lymphoma, unclassifiable high-grade
  Malignant lymphoma, unclassifiable
  Hodgkin's disease

Provisional categories are in italics; percentages represent the data presented after an international review of cases of non-Hodgkin's lymphoma; entities that represent ≥5% of cases are in boldface.

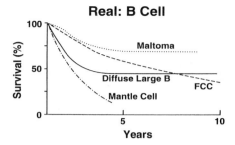

Fig. 23-2.   Survival of B-cell lymphomas as related to classification by the Revised European American Lymphoma classification system. Mantle cell lymphoma, MALToma, and FCC (follicle center cell, follicular lymphoma) were previously included in "low-grade lymphoma."

Radiation therapy plays less of a role in NHL than in Hodgkin's disease. In the case of stage I intermediate-grade lymphomas, radiation therapy has been supplanted by chemotherapy as the treatment modality of choice, although combined-modality therapy (radiation therapy and combination chemotherapy) is favored by some oncologists. With the possible exception of low-grade NHL, it has been established that radiation therapy alone has no role in the curative treatment of stage II NHL.

Perhaps as important as the staging of lymphoma in general is the International Prognostic Index (IPI) designed for use in patients with intermediate-grade lymphoma. This prognostic index (Table 23-3) predicts the probability of cure in intermediate-grade NHL based on age, stage, performance status, number of extranodal sites of disease, and lactate dehydrogenase (LDH) level (Fig. 23-3). For patients less than 60 years of age, a prognostic index based on stage, LDH, and performance status predicts the

Table 23-3.   International prognostic index for non-Hodgkin's lymphoma

Variable	0 points	1 point
Age	≤ 60	> 60
Stage	I or II	III or IV
Number of extranodal sites	≤ 1	> 1
Performance status	0 or 1	≥ 2
Lactate dehyrogenase level	normal	Elevated

Low risk, 0 or 1; low intermediate risk, 2; high intermediate risk, 3; high risk, 4 or 5.

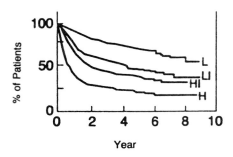

Fig. 23-3. Survival in intermediate-grade lymphoma as related to International Prognostic Index. L, low risk; LI, low intermediate risk; HI, high intermediate risk; H, high risk. (Reprinted with permission from the International Non-Hodgkin's Lymphoma Prognostic Factors Project. A predictive model for aggressive non-Hodgkin's lymphoma. N Engl J Med 1993;329:987–994.)

probability of cure. The IPI also correlates with overall prognosis in low-grade lymphoma.

  B. Special considerations in staging NHL. The tests used in the staging of Hodgkin's disease can be used in the staging of NHL, but because of differences in the two diseases, several important differences must be noted.

   1. History and physical examination. The history should consider prelymphomatous conditions, such as organ transplantation; acquired immunodeficiency syndrome (AIDS); and autoimmune disorders, such as Sjögren's syndrome, rheumatoid arthritis, and systemic lupus erythematosus. History of diphenylhydantoin or methotrexate therapy should be noted, as should a history of infection with Epstein-Barr virus, human T-cell leukemia/lymphoma virus type 1, *Helicobacter pylori,* or hepatitis C. When performing a physical examination, special attention should be given to Waldeyer's ring, epitrochlear nodes, femoral nodes, and popliteal nodes, sites that are almost never involved in Hodgkin's disease but that may be involved in a small percentage of cases of NHL. The association of specific sites of disease (e.g., Waldeyer's ring with gastrointestinal lymphoma, and CNS involvement in nasopharyngeal and testicular lymphoma) warrants special consideration.

   Although the designations A and B are used in NHL, treatment decisions are based on extent of disease. Unlike in Hodgkin's disease, there are no standard circumstances in which there are different treatments for stage IIA and stage IIB NHL (or for IIIA and IIIB disease).

2. **Bone marrow biopsy** is a key diagnostic procedure in the staging of NHL, owing to the high incidence of involvement, especially in small cleaved cell lymphoma. In other histologic types of NHL, the test is important as a baseline test because of the possible use of autologous bone marrow or stem cell transplantation at the time of relapse. Molecular genetics testing (bcl-2 and immunoglobulin gene rearrangement in follicular lymphomas, bcl-1 and immunoglobulin gene rearrangement in mantle cell lymphomas) may be of value in excluding lymphomatous involvement that may not be detected by routine pathologic studies.

3. **Lumbar puncture** should be considered in patients with small noncleaved cell lymphoma or lymphoblastic lymphoma as well as in patients with testicular or nasopharyngeal involvement and in patients with bone marrow involvement and intermediate-grade lymphoma.

4. **Computed tomography (CT) scans.** The abdominal CT and chest CT scans are routine parts of the staging of NHL. The abdominal CT scan is far more useful in NHL than in Hodgkin's disease. In Hodgkin's disease, involved nodes are often small and may be missed by CT scanning, whereas lymphangiography can detect small nodes in which the internal architecture is effaced. With NHL, retroperitoneal masses are often large and easily detected by CT scans. In addition, whereas mesenteric nodes are rarely involved in Hodgkin's disease, they are involved in most cases of follicular NHL.

5. **Gallium scans and positron emission tomography scans** may be helpful in identifying loci of disease and can be a sensitive marker for detecting residual disease.

6. **Gastrointestinal endoscopy** is indicated in patients with lymphoma involving Waldeyer's ring because of the association of gastrointestinal lymphoma with lymphoma involving Waldeyer's ring.

7. **Serum LDH and other prognostic markers.** The serum LDH is an important prognostic indicator and is one of the variables considered in the IPI. β_2-Microglobulin, interleukin-6, markers for multidrug resistance, and molecular markers, such as bcl-2, bcl-6, and p53, have been shown to have prognostic value but are not part of standard staging systems.

8. **Peripheral blood counts** are an insensitive measure of bone marrow involvement, but abnormal tests suggest marrow infiltration by

lymphoma. Because most patients with NHL receive chemotherapy, evaluation of the blood counts is a basic part of staging of NHL.

9. **Cytologic assessment** of pleural effusions or ascites should be performed if these fluid collections are present.

10. **Staging laparotomy** has no role in the evaluation of NHL because CT scans and biopsy of the bone marrow provide adequate staging information in nearly all patients.

III. **Radiation therapy of NHL: general considerations.** Because most patients with NHL have disseminated disease, radiation therapy plays a more limited role in NHL than in Hodgkin's disease. However, the value of radiation therapy should not be overlooked. With most histologic types of follicular lymphoma, doses of 44 Gy can achieve control of local disease. Because disease occurs outside of treatment fields (e.g., in bone marrow), radiation therapy is rarely curative. When patients with follicular lymphoma have large masses, however, local radiation therapy may be the most effective means of palliation. A dose-response curve for radiation therapy of large cell lymphoma is less well established, although radiation therapy may play a role in palliating patients with large cell lymphoma who have become refractory to chemotherapy.

Although 30% of patients with large cell lymphoma have stage I or II disease, the role of radiation therapy as the sole treatment in these patients has not been supported by clinical studies. Radiation therapy has been associated with cure rates exceeding 80% in stage I large cell lymphoma only when patients have been staged by laparotomy. Rather than subjecting these patients to laparotomy, the usual approach is to treat clinical stage I patients with either six cycles of a chemotherapy regimen such as CHOP (Table 23-4), or three cycles of CHOP in conjunction with involved-field radiation therapy. These approaches are associated with cure rates exceeding 90%. Stage II patients with large cell lymphoma are generally considered as having advanced disease and are treated the same as patients with stage III or IV disease.

IV. **Therapy of low-grade NHLs.** Follicular small cleaved cell lymphomas represent most cases of low-grade lymphoma, and the following discussion relates to the management of that disease entity. Although the terms *follicular small cleaved cell lymphoma* and *low-grade lymphoma* are used somewhat interchangeably in the following discussion (and in the medical literature), it must be recognized that other disorders are included in the latter category. Many of the studies of low-grade lymphoma involve patient populations in which follicular small cleaved cell lymphomas are a majority, but not the totality, of cases.

Follicular small cleaved cell lymphomas are associated with widespread disease at presentation. Bone marrow in-

Table 23-4. Combination chemotherapy regimens useful in treating low-grade lymphoma

Regimen	Drug and Dosage
CVP	Cyclophosphamide, 400–600 mg/m^2 i.v. on day 1 Vincristine (Oncovin), 1.4 mg/m^2 i.v. on day 1 (not to exceed 2 mg) Prednisone, 100 mg p.o. on days 1–5 Repeat every 21 days.
COPP	Cyclophosphamide, 600 mg/m^2 i.v. on days 1 and 8 Vincristine (Oncovin), 1.4 mg/m^2 i.v. on days 1 and 8 (not to exceed 2 mg) Procarbazine, 100 mg/m^2 p.o. on days 1–10 Prednisone, 100 mg p.o. on days 1–5 Repeat every 28 days.
CHOP	Cyclophosphamide, 750 mg/m^2 i.v. on day 1 Doxorubicin (Adriamycin), 50 mg/m^2 i.v. on day 1 Vincristine (Oncovin), 1.4 mg/m^2 i.v. on day 1 (not to exceed 2 mg) Prednisone, 100 mg p.o. on days 1–5 Repeat every 21 days.
CNOP	As above for CHOP, but substituting Mitoxantrone (Novantrone), 10 mg/m^2 i.v. on day 1 for the day 1 dose of doxorubicin

The alphabetic abbreviations used in these regimens consider doxorubicin (Adriamycin) as hydoxyldaunorubicin (H).

volvement is the most easily demonstrated site of advanced disease because it is found in 55% to 85% of cases on routine bone marrow biopsy. A higher incidence of marrow involvement has been noted when sensitive molecular techniques, such as bcl-2 and immunoglobulin gene rearrangement, have been employed. Nevertheless, despite the advanced stage of disease at presentation, median survival time in most series ranges from 5 to 10 years.

Combination chemotherapy regimens (see Table 23-4) have produced complete remissions in up to 80% of patients. However, such remissions are not durable, and the administration of combination chemotherapy may be associated with myelotoxicity, nausea, vomiting, and neurotoxicity. Because therapy is palliative, and because there is no proof that survival is improved by the early use of combination chemotherapy, many clinicians employ a policy of watchful waiting, as might be employed for chronic lymphocytic leukemia. In a large randomized trial, overall survival was similar for patients initially receiving aggressive combination chemotherapy and those receiving no initial treatment.

In patients not requiring initial treatment (i.e., patients with asymptomatic disease and minimal adenopathy), it is not uncommon for years to elapse before treatment is necessary. Patients with minimal symptoms or moderate lymphadenopathy are often treated with chlorambucil, either 2 to 4 mg p.o. daily or 30 to 60 mg p.o. every 2 weeks, with or without prednisone. In patients with enlarging nodes, progressive splenomegaly, cytopenia, fever, sweats, weight loss, or visceral involvement other than bone marrow or microscopic liver involvement, one would generally initiate therapy with CVP, CHOP, or, less frequently, one of the other regimens presented in Table 23-4. Although CHOP is effective in treating low-grade lymphomas, the initial use of anthracyclines in combination chemotherapy has not been proved to improve overall survival in these patients.

In patients who relapse after initial therapy, several options are available. If initial therapy has been low-dose chlorambucil, a regimen such as CHOP or CNOP would be reasonable. If a regimen such a CHOP or CNOP has been used initially, one can consider fludarabine, 25 mg/m^2/day i.v. for 5 days. Steroids are usually avoided in patients receiving nucleoside analogs such as fludarabine because of the risk of opportunistic infection. Interferon-α, 2 to 10 $\times$ 10^6 U/m^2 i.m. three times a week, has been shown to be effective in low-grade lymphoma. Although its inclusion in primary therapeutic regimens has not been consistently associated with improved survival, it is a reasonable option for salvage therapy. Preliminary evidence suggests that the monoclonal antibody rituximab may produce responses in 40% to 50% of patients with low-grade lymphoma; however, these are usually partial responses of less than 1 year's duration.

Another alternative for patients who relapse after initial treatment or fail to respond to initial therapy is one of the salvage regimens designed for use in intermediate-grade lymphoma, such as DHAP or MINE (Table 23-5). Because low-grade lymphomas are associated with prolonged survival despite multiple recurrences, there is no single clinical algorithm for all patients. Palliative treatments should be individualized based on extent of disease, clinical pace of disease, and age of the patient.

Another approach to low-grade NHL involves the use of high-dose chemotherapy, with or without total-body irradiation, in conjunction with autologous bone marrow or stem cell transplantation. This approach is limited by the fact that the bone marrow, and presumably the peripheral blood, is frequently involved in low-grade lymphoma. Even when genetic markers such as bcl-2 are used to confirm successful purging of tumor cells, lymphoma may not be completely removed from the reinfused stem cell product. Autologous transplantation has produced long-term disease-free survival in patients whose disease remains sensitive to chemotherapy at the time of transplantation. As with other therapies for low-grade lymphoma, however, there is no evidence that these results represent cures. Additionally, the optimal timing of such therapy (after one, two, or three chemotherapy regimens), the op-

Table 23-5.   Combination chemotherapy regimens useful as salvage regimens in lymphoma

Regimen	Drugs and Dosages
DHAP	Dexamethasone, 40 mg p.o. or i.v. days 1–4 Cytarabine (high-dose ara-C), 2g/m² over 3 hours, every 12 hours for two doses; on day 2, starting after completion of cisplatin infusion. If age >70 years, reduce to 1 g/m² Cisplatin 100 mg/m² continuous i.v. over 24 hours on day 1 Repeat every 3–4 weeks.
ESHAP	Etoposide, 60 mg/m² i.v. on days 1–4 Methylprednisolone, 500 mg i.v. on days 1–4 Cytarabine, 2 g/m² over 2 hours on day 5 after completion of cisplatin Cisplatin, 25 mg/m²/day continuous i.v. on days 1–4 Repeat every 3–4 weeks.
EPOCH	Etoposide, 50 mg/m²/24 hours continuous i.v. on days 1–4 Vincristine, 0.4 mg/m²/24 hours continuous i.v. on days 1–4 Doxorubicin, 10 mg/m²/24 hours continuous i.v. on days 1–4 Cyclophosphamide, 750 mg/m² i.v. on day 6 Prednisone, 60 mg/m² p.o. on days 1–6 Repeat every 21 days.
MINE	Mesna, 1.33 g/m² mixed with ifosfamide over 1 hour on days 1–3, followed by 500 mg i.v. 4 hours after the ifosfamide Ifosfamide, 1.33 g/m² i.v. over 1 hour on days 1–3 Mitoxantrone, 8 mg/m² i.v. over 15 minutes on day 1 Etoposide, 65 mg/m² i.v. over 1 hour on days 1–3 Repeat every 21 days.

timal preparative regimen (with or without total-body irradiation), and the value of purging have not been resolved. Although allogeneic transplantation eliminates the risk of reinfusing tumor cells, it is associated with significant treatment-related mortality, largely associated with graft-versus-host disease. Clinical results using allogeneic transplantation in this disorder have been highly variable, and its role in the treatment of this disease requires further investigation.

V. Therapy for intermediate-grade lymphomas

    A. Pathologic considerations. The most common intermediate-grade lymphoma is large noncleaved cell lymphoma, a B-cell lymphoma of follicular center cell origin. Also included in the category of intermediate-grade lymphomas are diffuse mixed large cell lymphomas (LCCLs), diffuse small cleaved cell lymphomas (a diverse entity including mantle cell lymphomas and MALTomas), immunoblastic sarcoma of B-cell origin, T-cell rich B-cell lymphomas, and PTCL. It is an oversimplification to consider that all of these disorders behave similarly, and the following discussion of the therapy of intermediate-grade lymphomas is most relevant to large noncleaved cell lymphoma. Other types of intermediate-grade lymphoma for which there is adequate data are discussed in separate sections.

For years, there has been controversy about whether the T-cell lymphomas included in intermediate-grade lymphoma category have a worse prognosis than their B-cell counterparts. The issue has been resolved to some degree by recognizing the heterogeneity of the lymphomas previously regarded as PTCL. With the recognition of T-cell–rich B-cell lymphomas, it has become clear that many lymphomas composed primarily of T cells are actually B-cell lymphomas in which the T cells are a reactive component. In our experience, these lymphomas have a prognosis similar to that of other B-cell lymphomas. Additionally, one of the most common types of PTCL is Ki-1–positive anaplastic large cell lymphoma, a lymphoma that may present as cutaneous disease or as a systemic malignancy. The cutaneous-only form clinically overlaps with lymphomatoid papulosis and often has an indolent course. The systemic forms of Ki-1 anaplastic large cell lymphoma are similar to diffuse large B-cell lymphoma with respect to their ability to be cured by combination chemotherapy. The remaining T-cell intermediate-grade lymphomas have a worse prognosis than their B-cell counterparts and Ki-1 anaplastic large cell lymphoma.

B. **Combination chemotherapy: historical perspective.** In the era of single-agent chemotherapy, the lymphomas classified as "histiocytic lymphoma" (roughly equivalent to large noncleaved cell lymphoma) were associated with a median survival of 6 months, with about 5% to 10% of patients surviving 2 years. The demonstration that COPP combination chemotherapy could produce complete remission in about 40% of cases, with 35% of patients continuing as long-term disease-free survivors, was a major clinical advance. This was quickly confirmed, and slightly improved, with the CHOP regimen, which substituted doxorubicin (hydoxydaunorubicin, Adriamycin) for procarbazine. Numerous regimens have been employed since the introduction of CHOP in the mid-1970s. It is interesting to consider the past 20 years of clinical investigation in terms of the early COPP and CHOP studies.

1. **COPP showed that "histiocytic" lymphoma was curable.** This has been continually been

confirmed with the caveat that LCCL and PTCL may be less curable.

2. **The COPP study showed that 80% of complete remissions are associated with cure.** Patients with LCCL and PTCL probably are at greater risk of relapse, but the 80% estimate is reasonable. In studies in which patients with residual disease by CT scan have been considered complete remissions (the residual is interpreted as scar), the relapse rate is greater than 20%.

3. **The COPP study showed that the 2-year relapse-free survival rate is a good estimate of cure.** Late relapses occur but are uncommon. Determining 2-year relapse-free survival eliminates the problems associated with misinterpreting residual disease as scar. If active disease is present, it will likely lead to clinical progression in this time interval.

4. In the decade following the introduction of COPP and CHOP, **the complete remission rate** reported with newer regimens (Table 23-6), in uncontrolled studies, rose from the 40% observed with CHOP to nearly 80% with MACOP-B. These uncontrolled studies employed younger patients than those included in the CHOP study; older patients were often excluded because of the potential toxicity of newer regimens. Studies of newer regimens also included patients with stage II disease because, after the original CHOP studies, it became well accepted that stage II patients are candidates for chemotherapy rather than radiotherapy. The patient population studied in newer regimens also included higher percentages of patients with mixed-cell lymphoma (LCCL), a lymphoma associated with a high complete remission rate but a low cure rate. Additionally, many of the newer regimens were reported at a time too early to determine whether apparent complete remissions would be durable responses or merely represented favorable misinterpretations of small residual masses found on CT scans. When CHOP was finally compared to m-BACOD, MACOP-B, and ProMACE-CytaBOM in a randomized clinical trial, survival rates were not significantly different among regimens and ranged between 40% and 45% for all regimens. This story provides a critical object lesson to all oncologists who want to rely on comparisons with historical controls.

C. **Combination chemotherapy: current recommendations.** Based on the results of a randomized trial, CHOP has re-emerged as the standard therapy for intermediate-grade lymphoma. Recent studies have looked at dose-intensive therapies, such as

Table 23-6. Combination chemotherapy regimens useful as primary treatment of intermediate-grade lymphomas

Regimen	Drugs and Dosages

CHOP	Cyclophosphamide, 750 mg/m² i.v. on day 1
	Doxorubicin (Adriamycin), 50 mg/m² i.v. on day 1
	Vincristine (Oncovin), 1.4 mg/m² i.v. on day 1
	  (not to exceed 2 mg)
	Prednisone, 100 mg p.o. on days 1–5
	  Repeat every 21 days.

BACOP	Bleomycin, 5 U/m² i.v. on days 15 and 22
	Doxorubicin (Adriamycin), 25 mg/m² i.v. on days 1 and 8
	Cyclophosphamide, 650 mg/m² i.v. on days 1 and 8
	Vincristine (Oncovin), 1.4 mg/m² i.v. on days 1 and 8
	  (not to exceed 2 mg)
	Prednisone, 60 mg/m² p.o. on days 15–28
	  Repeat every 28 days.

m-BACOD	Methotrexate, 200 mg/m² i.v. on days 1 and 8
	Leucovorin, 10 mg/m² p.o. every six hours for
	  eight doses, starting 24 hours after methotrexate
	Bleomycin, 4 U/m² i.v. on day 1
	Doxorubicin (Adriamycin), 45 mg/m² i.v. on day 1
	Cyclophosphamide, 600 mg/m² i.v. on day 1
	Vincristine (Oncovin), 1 mg/m² i.v. on day 1
	Dexamethasone 6 mg/m² p.o. on days 1–5
	  Repeat every 21 days.

ProMACE/
MOPP
	Prednisone, 60 mg/m² p.o. on days 1–14
	Methotrexate, 1,500 mg/m² i.v. on day 14
	Leucovorin, 50 mg/m² i.v. every 6 hours for five doses,
	  starting 24 hours after methotrexate
	Doxorubicin (Adriamycin), 25 mg/m² i.v. on days 1 and 8
	Cyclophosphamide, 650 mg/m² i.v. on days 1 and 8
	Etoposide, 120 mg/m² i.v. on days 1 and 8
	  Repeat every 28 days.
	ProMACE, as above, is given for a variable number of
	  cycles, based on tumor response, then MOPP therapy
	  (see Chapter 22 on Hodgkin's disease) is given for the
	  same number of cycles.

MACOP-B	Methotrexate, 400 mg/m² i.v. weeks 2, 6, and 10;
	  one-fourth dose as i.v. bolus, then three-fourths dose
	  over 4 hours
	Leucovorin, 15 mg p.o. every 6 hours for six doses,
	  starting 24 hours after each methotrexate dose
	Doxorubicin (Adriamycin), 50 mg/m² i.v.
	  weeks 1, 3, 5, 7, 9, and 11
	Cyclophosphamide, 350 mg/m² i.v. weeks 1, 3, 5, 7, 9, 11
	Vincristine (Oncovin), 1.4 mg/m² i.v. weeks 2, 4, 6, 8, 10, 12
	Bleomycin, 10 U/m² i.v. weeks 2, 4, 6, 8, 10, 12
	Prednisone, 75 mg/day p.o. for 12 weeks,
	  taper to zero during weeks 10–12
	Trimethoprim-sulfamethoxazole,
	  1 double-strength tablet b.i.d. daily for 12 weeks

augmented CHOP or the high-intensity, brief duration regimen presented in Table 23-7, as initial treatment of intermediate-grade lymphomas. It has not been proved that routine use of these regimens produces results superior to those achieved with CHOP.

Another approach to the initial therapy of intermediate-grade lymphoma is to consolidate complete remissions with high-dose therapy in conjunction with autologous stem cell transplantation. This approach has improved disease-free survival but has not significantly improved overall survival in patients with intermediate-grade lymphoma. In one randomized study, however, subset analysis found improved survival among patients with high-risk and high-intermediate-risk disease treated with this approach. Further studies are needed to clarify the role of high-dose therapies with or without autologous transplantation in the treatment of this group of lymphomas.

D. **Salvage therapy of intermediate-grade lymphomas: chemotherapy.** Patients who are not cured with initial chemotherapy represent a relatively unfavorable group. Using salvage chemotherapy regimens, such as those shown in Table 23-5, response rates near 50% have been reported. However, complete response rates are generally in the 20% to 30% range, and long-term relapse-free survival has been observed in fewer than 5% of patients treated with salvage chemotherapy.

E. **Salvage therapy of intermediate-grade lymphomas: high-dose chemotherapy in conjunction with autologous transplantation.** Because of the

Table 23-7. High-intensity brief duration regimen for lymphoma

Drug	Dosage
Cyclophosphamide	1500 mg/m^2 i.v. on days 1, 2, and 29
Etoposide	400 mg/m^2 i.v. on days 1, 2, and 3
Etoposide	100 mg/m^2 i.v. on day 29, 30, and 31
Doxorubicin	45 mg/m^2 i.v. on days 29 and 30
Vincristine	1.4 mg/m^2 i.v. on days 8, 22, 36, and 50
Bleomycin	10 units/m^2 i.v. on days 8, 22, 36, and 50
Methotrexate	200 mg/m^2 i.v. on days 15 and 43
Leucovorin	15 mg/m^2 i.v. or p.o. every 6 hours for six doses, starting 24 hours after methotrexate
Prednisone	60 mg/m^2 p.o. on days 1–7 and 29–35

Granulocyte colony-stimulating factor should be administered starting on day 4, and again on day 32, and administered until granulocyte recovery occurs.

limited long-term disease-free survival achieved with salvage combination chemotherapy, the major approach to salvage therapy has become high-dose chemotherapy with or without total-body irradiation in conjunction with peripheral blood stem cell transplantation. Studies comparing bone marrow and peripheral blood as a source of stem cells for autologous transplantation have not been conducted. However, because of the ease of peripheral blood stem cell collection and the long-term viability of peripheral stem cell autografts, peripheral blood stem cell transplantation has become the treatment of choice in intermediate-grade lymphoma. Among patients under the age of 60 years, advances in supportive care, such as the use of granulocyte or granulocyte-macrophage colony-stimulating factor, have decreased the mortality rate associated with this therapy to 5% to 10%. Preparative regimens commonly used in the treatment of intermediate-grade lymphomas are shown in Table 23-8.

Response rates to salvage autologous transplantation have generally depended on the response to prior therapy. Patients who respond to primary therapy and who remain sensitive to standard salvage regimens have response rates approaching 60%. Three-year disease-free survival, and probable cure, is observed in about 30% of such patients. Three-year disease-free survival is observed in about 15% of patients who respond to primary therapy but are resistant to salvage treatment, or among patients who fail

Table 23-8. Preparative regimens used before autologous transplantation in intermediate-grade lymphoma

Regimen	Drug and dosage
Cy-TBI	Cyclophosphamide, 60 mg/kg/day; day −6 and −5
	Total-body irradiation, 12 Gy administered in six fractions of 2 Gy each, 2 fractions daily, days −4, −3, and −2
Cy-VP-TBI	Etoposide, 1,800 mg/m^2 day −7
	Cyclophosphamide, 50 mg/kg/day; days −6, −5, −4
	Total-body irradiation, 10 Gy administered in five fractions of 2 Gy each, two fractions daily, days −3 and −2, one fraction day −1
CBV	Cyclophosphamide, 1,800 mg/m^{2}days −6, −5, −4, −3
	Carmustine (BCNU) 400 mg/m^2 day −2
	Etoposide, 2,400 mg/m^2 day −7
BEAM	Carmustine (BCNU), 300 mg/m^2 day −6
	Etoposide, 200 mg/m^2 days −5, −4, −3, −2
	Ara-C, 200 mg/m^2 days −5, −4, −3, −2
	Melphalan, 140 mg/m^2 day −1

primary therapy but experience at least a partial response to salvage treatment. In patients who are refractory to both primary therapy and salvage therapy, long-term disease-free survival is rare. In view of the expected morbidity and mortality associated with the procedure, our preference is to use allogeneic transplantation in such patients if a donor is available.

F. **Intermediate-grade lymphoma in the elderly.** The incidence of lymphoma increases with age. Thus, the clinician is often faced with an elderly patient with an intermediate-grade lymphoma. Although there are no strict guidelines, elderly people are often defined as those 70 years or older or those between the ages of 60 and 70 years with significant comorbid disease. As with acute leukemia, elderly patients should not be denied potentially curative therapy because of their age. Elderly patients with good performance status and well-controlled comorbid disease are good candidates for potentially curative therapy.

Unfortunately, the optimal regimen or intensity of therapy has not been defined for these patients, who have often been excluded from chemotherapy studies in lymphoma. One option in treating the elderly lymphoma patient is simply to use a standard regimen such as CHOP or CNOP while minimizing toxicity through the use of growth factors, by extending the interval between cycles to 28 days, or both. Intensive therapy of short duration such as DOCE or P-VABEC (Table 23-9) may produce similar results with acceptable toxicity. Regimens based on oral VP-16, such as Vanderbilt VP-16 or PEN (see Table 23-9) are less myelosuppressive. The curative potential of these alternative regimens is not known, and the final selection of a regimen for the elderly patient is usually based on the clinician's estimate of how much toxicity can be tolerated by the individual patient.

VI. **Therapy for high-grade lymphomas**

A. **Small noncleaved cell lymphoma.** This category of lymphoma includes both Burkitt's and Burkitt's-like lymphoma. In the United States, Burkitt's type tends to occur in younger patients and to be associated with more gastrointestinal disease and a lower incidence of bone marrow involvement. Both diseases are high-grade lymphomas and are relatively resistant to standard chemotherapy. Median survivals in the range of 6 to 10 months have been reported. With high-intensity, brief-duration therapy (see Table 23-7), long-term disease-free survival rates approaching 50% can be achieved, but these results are dependent on stage. Patients with central nervous system (CNS) disease, bone marrow involvement, or markedly elevated serum LDH levels have an especially poor prognosis. Because of the poor prognosis, some investigators have advocated the use of high-dose therapy in conjunction with autologous stem cell

Table 23-9.   Combination chemotherapy regimens useful as primary treatment of lymphomas in elderly patients

Regimen	Drugs and dosages
DOCE	Doxorubicin, 40 mg/m² i.v. weeks 1, 2, 7, and 8
	Vincristine, 1.2 mg/m² i.v. weeks 1, 4, and 7
	Cyclophosphamide, 300 mg/m² i.v. weeks 1, 4, and 7
	Etoposide, 50 mg/m² i.v. on day 1 of week 4, then 100 mg/m² p.o. on days 2, 3, 4, and 5 (of week 4)
	Prednisone, 50 mg p.o. daily × 10 days, weeks 1, 4, and 7
	Trimethoprim-sulfamethoxazole, 1 double-strength tablet b.i.d. daily for 8 weeks
	Ketoconazole, 200 mg p.o. daily × 10 days, weeks 1, 4, and 7
	Cimetidine, 600 mg p.o. b.i.d. × 10 days, weeks 1, 4, and 7
	Regimen is given for 8 weeks only.
P-VABEC	Doxorubicin 30 mg/m² IV weeks 1, 3, 5, 7, and 11
	Etoposide 100 mg/m² IV weeks 1, 3, 5, 7, 9, and 11
	Cyclophosphamide 350 mg/m² IV weeks 1, 3, 5, 7, 9, and 11
	Vincristine 1.2 mg/m² IV weeks 2, 4, 6, 8, 10, and 12
	Bleomycin 5 mg/m² IV weeks 2, 4, 6, 8, 10, and 12
	Prednisone 50 mg PO daily × 12 weeks
Vanderbilt Prolonged VP-16	Etoposide, 50 mg/m² p.o. for 21 days
	Methotrexate, 40 mg/m² i.v. weeks 1 and 3
	Leucovorin, 15 mg p.o. every 6 hours for four doses, starting 24 hours after each methotrexate dose
	Prednisone, 60 mg p.o. × 7 days, weeks 1 and 6
	Cyclophosphamide, 500 mg/m² i.v. bolus week 6
	Mitoxantrone, 12 mg/m² i.v. bolus week 6
	Vincristine, 1 mg/m² i.v. week 6
	A second cycle is repeated weeks 9–15.
PEN	Prednisone, 50 mg p.o. on days 1–14
	Etoposide, 50 mg p.o. on days 1–14
	Mitoxantrone, 8 mg/m² i.v. on day 1
	Repeat every 4 weeks.

transplantation as consolidation therapy. However, there is no proof that this approach is associated with significantly improved survival.

B.   Lymphoblastic lymphoma. This entity, which frequently presents with a mediastinal mass and bone marrow involvement, can be regarded as a variant of T-cell acute lymphoblastic leukemia (ALL). Patients may be treated with any of the regimens used in ALL. However, a regimen devised at Stanford University, which employs a CHOP-like induction, CNS prophylaxis, consolidation with methotrexate and L-asparaginase, and later consolidation with methotrexate and 6-mercaptopurine has been associated with excellent results. The 5-year survival rate was 19% in high-risk patients (marrow involvement, CNS involvement, elevated LDH) and 94% in patients without these features. We have employed high-intensity, brief-duration therapy in these patients, but the small number of patients so treated precludes drawing firm conclusions. The role of autologous transplantation as either consolidation or salvage therapy also requires further investigation. At this time, ALL-type therapy remains the standard treatment for these patients.

C. **Peripheral T-cell lymphomas.** When T-cell–rich B-cell lymphomas and the Ki-1–positive anaplastic large cell lymphomas are excluded, the remaining cases of T-cell lymphoma (about 5% of adult lymphomas) are best regarded as high-grade lymphomas. Results with CHOP in high-grade lymphomas are significantly worse than those achieved in intermediate-grade lymphomas. No standard therapy for these disorders exists. We have generally employed high-intensity, brief-duration therapy in these patients and have achieved results equivalent to those achieved in patients with B-cell lymphomas.

VII. **Other pathologic types of NHL**
A. **Mantle cell lymphoma.** These lymphomas are composed of small B lymphocytes, but the cell of origin is the mantle zone cell, which surrounds the lymphoid follicle, and not a follicular center cell. The cells are CD5+ and CD23– and usually have a t(11;14) chromosomal translocation. The prognosis for patients with mantle cell lymphoma is distinctly worse than that for patients with low-grade lymphoma, with median survival times of 3 to 4 years. Even with CHOP therapy, cure is rarely observed. The high incidence of bone marrow involvement limits the use of autologous transplantation. This has led some investigators to advocate the early use of allogeneic transplantation, but even that highly aggressive therapy has not been shown to be associated with high cure rates.

B. **MALTomas.** The term *MALToma* stands for mucosal-associated lymphoid tumors and includes low-grade B-cell tumors of a wide variety of sites, including conjunctiva and the gastrointestinal tract. Maltomas tend to be localized and are associated with a better survival than other low-grade lymphomas. Maltomas of the stomach have been associated with *Helicobacter pylori* infection, with apparent cure following the administration of antibiotics. However, it has not been determined if this truly represents cure of a malignancy by antibacterial therapy or the misdiagnosis of pseudolymphoma as lymphoma.

C. **Anaplastic large cell lymphomas.** These lymphomas are CD30+, are frequently characterized by a t(2;5) chromosomal translocation, and, in most cases, are T-cell lymphomas. However, they are an exception to the general observation that PTCLs are high-grade lymphomas because they have a biology similar to that of intermediate-grade B-cell lymphomas. Additionally, these lymphomas have pathologic features that may lead to their being mistaken for Hodgkin's disease. Those cases that involve only the skin may have an unusually benign clinical course.

D. **Angioimmunoblastic lymphadenopathy.** This lymphoproliferative disorder is characterized by lymphadenopathy, hepatosplenomegaly, and nonspecific hyperglobulinemia. In many patients, the disease evolves to a high-grade T-cell lymphoma. Criteria have not been established to allow hematopathologists to distinguish those patients who will have a relatively benign course from those in whom lymphoma will develop. We treat benign forms of the disease with corticosteroids. In the face of clinical change, progressive adenopathy, organomegaly, or weight loss, we recommend repeat biopsy to assess for evolution to lymphoma. If lymphoma is found, we recommend that the patients be treated for a high-grade process. The median age of these patients is 60 years, however, and patients may be unable to tolerate regimens more aggressive than CHOP.

VIII. **Special considerations in therapy**

A. **CNS prophylaxis.** Involvement of the CNS by NHL has been associated with bone marrow involvement. However, most patients with CNS disease have small noncleaved cell lymphoma or lymphoblastic lymphoma. In patients with these high-grade lymphomas and marrow involvement, we recommend cranial irradiation and intrathecal methotrexate. as would be used in ALL. It is not known if marrow involvement is a risk factor for CNS disease in other histologic types of lymphoma. In patients with intermediate-grade lymphoma and bone marrow involvement, it is reasonable to consider CNS prophylaxis. However, there are no prospective data showing that such therapy decreases the incidence of CNS complications or improves survival.

B. **Lymphomas among patients with human immunodeficiency virus (HIV) infection.** The prevalence of NHL in HIV patients is 3% to 6% with the risk of lymphoma increasing with the duration of infection. The risk of AIDS is also associated with low levels of CD4+ lymphocytes, male homosexuality, a prior diagnosis of Kaposi's sarcoma, cytomegalovirus infection, and oral hairy leukoplakia. Lymphoma is an AIDS-defining illness among patients with HIV infection, and it has been estimated that about one fourth of the cases of lymphoma occurring in the 1990s will be AIDS related. Because of the poor overall prognosis of these patients and their preexistent immunosuppression, chemotherapy regimens characterized by dose reductions (e.g., below the doses given in CHOP, for example) have become the standard approach. Although this may be reasonable for patients with end-stage disease, the prognosis of AIDS is changing, and for many patients with HIV infection, lymphoma is the AIDS-defining illness. It is not known whether standard regimens, such as CHOP, or high-intensity regimens, such as the one shown in Table 23-7, might produce better results in HIV patients who are diagnosed as having lymphoma when their immune systems are relatively intact. CNS evaluation and prophylaxis should be considered in HIV patients with lymphoma.

C. **Extranodal lymphomas.** NHLs arise at extranodal sites in 10% to 20% of cases. In the past, these patients were most often treated with radiation therapy. With the demonstration that chemotherapy is a rational approach to nodal stage I lymphomas, however, many of these patients are being treated with chemotherapy. The optimal approach to extranodal lymphomas is unknown; however, NHL occurs frequently enough at some extranodal sites that specific comments are indicated.

1. **Gastric lymphomas.** The stomach is the most common site of extranodal lymphomas. Gastric MALTomas represent about two thirds of all MALTomas and about one half of gastric lymphomas. Of the remainder of cases of gastric lymphoma, the common histologic type is large noncleaved cell lymphoma. Because of the risk of perforation during treatment, it is often recommended that these patients undergo surgical resection before definitive treatment. This recommendation, however, dates to a period when bulky tumors were encountered at surgery and radiation therapy was the treatment of choice. In the modern chemotherapy era, during which the diagnosis of gastric lymphoma is most commonly made endoscopically, we do not believe that surgical resection is necessary.

2. **Lymphomas of the CNS.** In patients who do not have AIDS, these lymphomas are most often large noncleaved cell or immunoblastic lymphomas. Radiation therapy alone has generally been associated with median survival times of less than 1 year, even when high doses of radiation are employed. Recent trials employing chemotherapy (i.e., high-dose methotrexate or cytarabine) before radiation have produced better results.

In patients who have HIV, large noncleaved cell lymphoma, immunoblastic lymphoma, and small noncleaved cell lymphoma are all common. Because of the limited prognosis of these patients, owing the HIV infection, they generally have been treated with radiation therapy alone. However, as noted previously, in patients whose lymphomas develop early in the course of HIV infection, the role of aggressive chemotherapy is yet to be determined.

3. **Testicular lymphomas.** The most common cause of testicular cancer in elderly men is lymphoma, with large noncleaved B-cell lymphoma being the most common histologic type. Therapy generally consists of orchiectomy, chemotherapy, radiation of the contralateral testis, and CNS prophylaxis.

4. **Nasopharyngeal lymphomas.** More commonly seen in Asia than in the United States, these tumors are often angiocentric tumors of T-cell or natural killer cell origin. Combined-modality therapy (radiation therapy plus combination chemotherapy) plus CNS prophylaxis is generally employed in these poor-prognosis lymphomas.

5. **Cutaneous lymphomas.** The most common type of cutaneous lymphoma is cutaneous or cerebriform T-cell lymphoma (CTCL), also known as *mycosis fungoides,* or, when there is generalized erythema and involvement of the peripheral blood, *Sézary's syndrome.* If disease is apparently limited to the skin, therapy is generally topical (i.e., topical nitrogen mustard, electron-beam radiation therapy, or psoralen in conjunction with ultraviolet irradiation). CTCL is an indolent but lethal disease. It generally exists as plaques, involving only the skin, for many years but eventually progresses to involve skin tumors, adenopathy, or visceral disease, at times in association with a histologic transformation to large cell lymphoma. These latter stages of the disease carry an extremely poor prognosis and are generally treated with combination chemotherapy, such as the regimens used for intermediate-grade lymphoma. B-cell lymphomas may involve the skin, but this is usually a manifestation of disseminated disease. These cases are approached according to histology and stage.

D. **Posttransplantation lymphomas.** Lymphoproliferative disorders, including lymphoma, can complicate organ transplantation and, less commonly, allogeneic bone marrow transplantation. Most patients have extranodal sites of disease, typically the CNS and gastrointestinal tracts. Therapeutic options include withdrawing or decreasing immunosuppression, antiviral therapy (based on the association with Epstein-Barr virus), interferon, monoclonal antibody therapy, donor lymphocyte infusion, or conventional chemotherapy. Surgery is also an option in the case of local disease.

Immunologic manipulations are most likely to be successful when disease is limited in extent and is polyclonal rather than monoclonal. Advanced visceral disease is likely to require chemotherapy, but such therapy has a low success rate (about 20%) and is usually deferred until after immunologic therapies have been employed.

IX. **Conclusion**. The NHLs are a heterogenous group of neoplasms. Therapy is based on patient features (age, performance status, prelymphomatous conditions), pathology, stage, and IPI. Classification of lymphomas continues to evolve, and the new REAL classification system identifies entities based on clinical, morphologic, immunologic, and genetic data, when available. As further progress in the field of molecular genetics is made, it is hoped that classification of NHL will evolve, providing a stronger framework for clinical advances in the management of this disease.

SELECTED READING

Coleman CN, Picozzi VJ, Cox RS, et al. Treatment of lymphoblastic lymphoma in adults. *J Clin Oncol* 1986;4:1628–1637.

DeVita VT, Canellos GP, Chabner B, et al. Advanced diffuse histiocytic lymphoma, a potentially curable disease: results with combination chemotherapy. *Lancet* 1975;1:248–250.

Fisher RI, Gaynor ER, Dahlberg S, et al. Comparison of a standard regimen (CHOP) with three intensive regimens for advanced non-Hodgkin's lymphoma. *N Engl J Med* 1993;328:1002–1006.

Gianni AM, Bregni M, Siena S, et al. High-dose chemotherapy and autologous bone marrow transplantation compared with MACOP-B in aggressive B-cell lymphoma. *N Engl J Med* 1997;336:1290–1297.

Haioun C, Lepage E, Gisselbrecht C, et al. Benefit of autologous bone marrow transplantation over sequential chemotherapy in poor-risk aggressive non-Hodgkin's lymphoma: updated results of the prospective study LNH87-2. *J Clin Oncol* 1997;15:1131–1137.

International Non-Hodgkin's Lymphoma Prognostic Factors Project. A predictive model for aggressive non-Hodgkin's lymphoma. *N Engl J Med* 1993;329:987–994.

Jones SE, Rosenberg SA, Kaplan HS, Kadin ME, Dorfman RF. Non-Hodgkin's lymphomas. II. Single agent chemotherapy. *Cancer* 1972;30:31–38.

Macon WR, Williams ME, Greer JP, et al. T-cell rich B-cell lymphoma. *Am J Surg Pathol* 1992;16:351–363.

Maloney DG, Grillo-Lopez AJ, Badkin DJ, et al. IDEC-C2B8: results of a phase I multiple dose trial in patients with relapsed non-Hodgkin's lymphoma. *J Clin Oncol* 1997;15:3266–3274.

McMaster ML, Greer JP, Greco FA, et al. Effective treatment of small non-cleaved cell lymphoma with high-intensity, brief duration chemotherapy. *J Clin Oncol* 1991;9:941–946.

Miller TP, Dahlberg S, Cassady JR, et al. Chemotherapy alone compared with chemotherapy plus radiotherapy for localized intermediate- and high-grade non-Hodgkin's lymphoma. *N Engl J Med* 1998;339:21–26.

Non-Hodgkin's Lymphoma Classification Project. A clinical evaluation of the international lymphoma study group classification of non-Hodgkin's lymphoma. *Blood* 1997;89:3909–3918.

Non-Hodgkin's Lymphoma Pathologic Classification Project. National Cancer sponsored study of classification of non-Hodgkin's lymphomas: summary and description of a working formulation. *Cancer* 1982;49:2112–2135.

Smalley RV, Andersen JW, Hawkins MJ, et al. Interferon alpha combined with cytotoxic chemotherapy for patients with non-Hodgkin's lymphoma. *N Engl J Med* 1992;327:1336–1341.

Stein RS, Cousar J, Flexner JM, Collins RD. Correlations between immunologic markers and histopathologic classifications: clinical implications. *Semin Oncol* 1980;7:244–254.

Stein RS, Magee MJ, Lenox RK, et al. Malignant lymphomas of follicular center cell origin in man. VI. Large cleaved cell lymphoma. *Cancer* 1987;60:2704–2711.

Weisenburger DD, Armitage JO. Mantle cell lymphoma: an entity comes of age. *Blood* 1996;87:4483–4494.

Young RC, Longo DL, Glatstein E, et al. The treatment of indolent lymphomas: watchful waiting v aggressive combined modality treatment. *Semin Hematol* 1988;25[Suppl 2]:11–16

Zinzani PL, Bendandi M, Martelli M, et al. Anaplastic large cell lymphoma: clinical and prognostic evaluation of 90 adult patients. *J Clin Oncol* 1996;14:955–962.

24

Multiple Myeloma and Other Plasma Cell Dyscrasias

Martin M. Oken

I. **Introduction**
   A. **Types of plasma cell dyscrasias.** Plasma cell dyscrasias, or plasma cell neoplasms, are a group of conditions characterized by unbalanced proliferation of cells that normally synthesize and secrete immunoglobulins. They range from malignant neoplasms, such as multiple myeloma, to monoclonal gammopathy of undetermined significance, a usually benign condition that is sometimes termed *benign monoclonal gammopathy*. Associated with the abnormal cellular proliferation in nearly all instances is the production of homogeneous monoclonal immunoglobulin, referred to either as *myeloma protein* or *M protein,* or of excessive quantities of homogeneous polypeptide subunits of a monoclonal protein. The latter usually appear as monoclonal free light chains excreted into the urine. Frequently, both whole immunoglobulin M protein and free light chains are produced. The plasma cell dyscrasias discussed in this chapter are multiple myeloma, macroglobulinemia (Waldenström's macroglobulinemia), heavy-chain diseases, amyloidosis, and monoclonal gammopathy of undetermined significance.
   B. **M protein.** Unlike most neoplastic diseases, which are followed objectively by serial evaluation of palpable or radiographically measurable tumor masses, most plasma cell dyscrasias are best followed by serial measurements of the monoclonal protein (M protein) elaborated by the tumor. Effective use of this tumor marker is important for the proper evaluation of the disease course of most plasma cell dyscrasias and is usually essential to the determination of response to treatment. The basic immunoglobulin unit comprises two identical heavy chains with a molecular mass of 55,000 daltons linked to two identical light chains with molecular masses of 22,500 daltons. The heavy chains are either γ, α, μ, δ, or ϵ, corresponding to immunoglobulin G (IgG), IgA, IgM, IgD, and IgE, respectively. The light chains exist as either κ or λ subtypes. Serum M protein is a monoclonal whole immunoglobulin and therefore possesses only one heavy-chain type and one light-chain type. Urine M protein consists of free light chains or, in the case of some heavy-chain diseases, free heavy-chain fragments of single specificity. Serum M protein may be quantitatively evaluated by either serum protein electrophoresis or determining the concentration of

the individual immunoglobulins (particularly IgG, IgA, and IgM). Urinary M protein, usually in the form of free light chains, should be characterized by immunoelectrophoresis as monoclonal κ or λ light chain and then followed sequentially, expressed as urinary light-chain excretion in grams per 24 hours. This characterization requires determination of 24-hour urine protein excretion and scanning the urine protein electrophoresis to determine the percentage of urine protein present as free monoclonal immunoglobulin light chain.

II. Multiple myeloma

A. General considerations and aims of therapy

1. **Diagnosis.** Multiple myeloma is a neoplasm of malignant plasma cells invading bone and bone marrow, causing widespread skeletal destruction, bone marrow failure, and problems related to quantitatively abnormal serum or urinary M proteins. The diagnosis of multiple myeloma requires histologic documentation by the demonstration of increased numbers (usually >10%) or abnormal, atypical, or immature plasma cells in the bone marrow in addition to finding serum or urinary M protein or characteristic osteolytic bone lesions. Some patients have multiple plasmacytomas of bone with intervening normal areas of bone marrow. In these patients, a random bone marrow aspirate and biopsy may fail to reveal the tumor, and biopsy of specific bone lesions may be necessary to establish the diagnosis. One variant is the polyneuropathy, organomegaly, endocrinopathy, monoclonal gammopathy (POEMS) syndrome. Patients with POEMS have a better survival than do those with multiple myeloma.

2. **Incidence.** The annual incidence of multiple myeloma is 4 per 100,000 population with a peak occurrence between ages 60 and 70 years. Although as many as 4% of patients with myeloma have indolent or smoldering disease at diagnosis, and an additional 5% have an isolated plasmacytoma of bone, most patients with multiple myeloma require chemotherapy of their disease soon after diagnosis.

3. **Effect of treatment.** The goals of therapy are to improve the duration of survival and to diminish or prevent the serious manifestations of this disease, such as bone pain, pathologic fractures, severe anemia, renal failure, or hypercalcemia. Treatment produces an objective response in at least half of patients as determined by a sustained 50% decline in the levels of serum or urine M protein. Temporary, sometimes long-lasting, alleviation of symptoms occurs in nearly all patients exhibiting an objec-

tive response to treatment and in some additional patients with lesser degrees of objective improvement. Median survival times usually reported for treated patients range from 2 to 3 years and are influenced by response to treatment and by the initial tumor load.

4. **Prognostic factors.** Table 24-1 presents a clinical staging system developed to estimate myeloma tumor cell mass using readily obtained clinical findings. Severe anemia, hypercalcemia, advanced osteolytic lesions, and extremely high M protein production rates are all associated with a high tumor burden and a poor survival prognosis. Renal failure, although not well correlated with tumor burden, is associated with poor prognosis. Advanced age, poor performance status, high serum lactate dehydrogenase level, and plasmablastic subtype have also been established as adverse prognostic signs.

The serum level of β_2-microglobulin correlates with the myeloma tumor burden but is of little value for serially monitoring patients with myeloma. Serum β_2-microglobulin usually falls during response to therapy and may increase during relapse, but it has been inconsistent in detecting fulminant progression in which the serum or urinary M proteins may fail to reflect the increasing tumor mass. The plasma cell–labeling index is a reflection of the proportion of myeloma cells that are synthesizing DNA. Patients with a labeling index higher than 3% who have a high cell mass have a particularly poor survival prognosis. A low labeling index has been associated with more indolent disease and particularly with a stable plateau phase during an objective response to therapy.

When the pretreatment plasma cell–labeling index is combined with serum β_2-microglobulin, one can assign half the patients either to a very favorable prognostic group in which both values are low and the prognosis approaches 6 years, or to a very poor prognostic group in which both values are high and the survival prognosis is less than 2 years. The remaining patients have an intermediate and less well-defined prognosis. Others have used serum levels of C-reactive protein as a reflection of interleukin-6 (IL-6) activity and have combined this with the β_2-microglobulin level to produce an index that divides myeloma patients into low-, intermediate-, and high-risk groups with observed median survival times of 54, 27, and 6 months, respectively. Other adverse prognostic factors include low circulating CD19 B lymphocytes and high serum levels of the IL-6 receptor.

Table 24-1.   Clinical staging system for myeloma

Stage	Criteria	Myeloma cell mass (cells/m²)

I	All of the following:
	1. Hemoglobin >10 g/dL
	2. Serum calcium value normal (≤12 mg/dL)
	3. On radiograph, normal bone structure or solitary bone plasmacytoma only
	4. Low M component production rates
	  a. IgG value <5 g/dL
	  b. IgA value <3 g/dL
	  c. Urine light-chain M component on electrophoresis <4 g/24 h
		$<0.6 \times 10^{12}$ (low)

II	Fitting neither stage I nor III	0.6×10^{12} to 1.2×10^{12} (intermediate)

III	One or more of the following:
	1. Hemoglobin <8.5 g/dL
	2. Serum calcium value >12 mg/dL
	3. Advanced lytic bone lesions
	4. High M-component production rates
	  a. IgG value >7 g/dL
	  b. IgA value >5 g/dL
	  c. Urine light-chain M component on electrophoresis >12 g/24 h
		$>1.2 \times 10^{12}$ (high)

Subclass of any stage		
A	Serum creatinine <2 mg/dL	
B	Serum creatinine ≥2 mg/dL	

Modified from Durie BGM, and Salmon SE. A clinical staging system for multiple myeloma: correlation of measured myeloma cell mass with presenting clinical features, response to treatment and survival. *Cancer* 1975;36:842.

B. **Initial treatment**
1. **General measures.** Complications of myeloma (e.g., hypercalcemia and renal failure) may be present at the time of diagnosis (see Section II.C). These complications should be promptly identified and treated before the start of chemotherapy. Patients who present with smoldering or indolent asymptomatic stage 1A disease may be followed with observation alone until evidence of progression appears. Most patients have more advanced or progressive disease at diagnosis and require chemotherapy. Patients should be maintained on allopurinol, 300 mg/day p.o., through the first 2 months of chemotherapy to prevent urate nephropathy. A general supportive care regimen emphasizing ambulation and hydration should be maintained throughout the initial treatment.
2. **Standard induction chemotherapy recommendations** are based on an Eastern Cooperative Oncology Group (ECOG) prospective, randomized clinical trial comparing moderate (MP) therapy (see Section I.B.2.b) to a more intensive regimen (VBMCP) (see Section I.B.2.a). In that study, VBMCP yielded an objective response rate of 72%, in contrast to a 51% objective response rate with MP. Median survival time was similar for the two treatments at 28 to 30 months, but 26% of VBMCP patients survived 5 years, compared with a 19% 5-year survival rate with MP.
   a. **Most patients should receive VBMCP.** With this regimen, the prednisone schedule is frequently individualized so that slowly responding patients with persistent generalized bone pain or severe anemia may receive low-dose prednisone each day of the first two or three cycles in addition to the higher scheduled prednisone dose on days 1 to 14.
   The VBMCP regimen consists of the following:
   Vincristine, 1.2 mg/m^2 i.v. on day 1 (up to 2.0 mg), *and*
   Carmustine (BCNU), 20 mg/m^2 i.v. on day 1, *and*
   Melphalan, 8 mg/m^2 p.o. on days 1 to 4, *and*
   Cyclophosphamide, 400 mg/m^2 i.v. on day 1, *and*
   Prednisone, 40 mg/m^2 p.o. on days 1 to 7 (all cycles), 20 mg/m^2 p.o. on days 8 to 14 (cycles 1 to 3 only);
   Repeat cycle of VBMCP every 35 days for at least 1 year.

b. **Patients over 70 years old who have poor performance status,** defined as partially or completely bedridden (ECOG grades 2 to 4), do not tolerate VBMCP. These high-risk patients, who compose 10% to 15% of myeloma patients, should instead be treated with MP according to the following schedule:

Melphalan, 8 mg/m^2 p.o. on days 1 to 4, *and*

Prednisone, 60 mg/m^2 p.o. on days 1 to 4.

Repeat cycle every 28 days for at least 1 year.

Because of the similarity in median survival data between VBMCP and MP, the latter regimen can also be considered an alternative to VBMCP for some patients not in the above high-risk group if a less aggressive approach is required. Because of erratic absorption of melphalan in most patients, some investigators recommend cautiously escalating the dose of melphalan on subsequent cycles of chemotherapy until a dose is reached that produces moderate nadir leukocyte counts of 2,000 to 3,000 cells/µL. For reliable absorption, melphalan should be taken on an empty stomach.

3. **Alternative induction chemotherapy.** VBMCP + interferon-α$_2$ (rIFN-α$_2$) represents a promising alternative approach to induction therapy. With this regimen, two initial cycles of VBMCP are given, followed by alternating 3-week cycles of rIFN-α$_2$ with 3-week cycles of VBMCP. The rIFN-α$_2$ is administered in a dosage of 5×10^6 U/m^2 s.c. three times a week for 10 doses each cycle, for a total treatment duration of 2 years. The advantages of this regimen over VBMCP are a higher complete response rate and longer response duration. The disadvantages are the expense and toxicity of IFN. The latter is a minor problem for some, but for others, the fatigue is dose-limiting.

Another induction regimen that provides comparable results to VBMCP is composed of alternating cycles of vincristine, melphalan, cyclophosphamide, and prednisone with vincristine, BCNU, doxorubicin (Adriamycin), and prednisone (VMCP/VBAP). This and a similar regimen lacking VP are described more fully in two selected readings (Durie et al., 1986; MacLennan et al., 1992). A third regimen, VAD, is described later as a salvage treatment option. It may be used as an induction regimen when autologous transplantation is contemplated because it lacks alkylating agents and is therefore less damaging to marrow stem cells.

4. **High-dose therapy with bone marrow or peripheral blood stem cell transplantation.** Allogeneic bone marrow transplantation after high-dose therapy can cure myeloma, but this happens in fewer than 20% of patients according to recent updates. At present, suitable candidates represent only a small portion of patients with myeloma. Early transplantation-related mortality rates of 40% to 45% further limit its usefulness at this time. However, in carefully selected patients under 55 years of age, with a matched related donor and with poor prognostic factors, it is reasonable to consider allotransplantation in first remission.

   High-dose therapy followed by autologous transplantation with bone marrow or peripheral blood stem cells as rescue is unlikely to be curative but, with growth factor support, can be carried out with relative safety and merits consideration as consolidation therapy in first remission or after relapse in patients with responsive disease. Its precise role is yet to be determined and is still the subject of ongoing clinical trials. The one reported trial shows a 52% 5-year survival, with about half of the patients surviving 5 years still in their first remission. Two other major trials are still accruing patients. It has been well demonstrated that patients who would be candidates for transplantation therapy have a better prognosis than the average myeloma patient and that this explains part of the improvement in survival seen in many uncontrolled transplantation reports. The most commonly used preparative regimens include high-dose melphalan, 200 mg/m^2, without total-body radiation. A role for purging the graft of potentially malignant cells seems intuitively likely, but proof of its efficacy in preventing recurrence remains an unmet challenge. Future treatments will target the minimal residual disease that virtually always remains after a successful autologous transplantation.

5. **Duration of therapy and the role of maintenance therapy.** Although no study has conclusively demonstrated benefit by continuing chemotherapy beyond 1 year in responding patients, several investigators have noted earlier reemergence of active myeloma after early cessation of therapy. Therefore, one acceptable approach is to continue the induction regimen for a total duration of 2 years or to maximal response, but to decrease its frequency to one cycle every 6 to 8 weeks during the second year while continuing to follow M protein production

carefully. It is probably safe to stop treatment at 1 year in patients who started therapy with stage I disease and whose disease has remained stable, in plateau phase, for at least 6 months. These patients should be observed carefully, with reevaluation of serum and urine M protein once every 3 months.

Several randomized trials evaluated maintenance therapy with IFN after at least 1 year of induction chemotherapy. Most of these showed significant improvement in response duration but no significant difference in survival. Intriguingly, the nonsignificant survival trends tended to favor the IFN maintenance. A meta-analysis evaluating all controlled trials randomizing for the use of IFN in maintenance or induction in myeloma is to be reported soon and could well resolve this issue. At present, it is reasonable to employ IFN maintenance for those who tolerate its side effects. A preferred regimen is rIFN-α_2, 2 million U/m^2 s.c. three times a week to relapse. This regimen can also be used following transplantation.

6. **Role of radiotherapy.** Solitary plasmacytoma of bone is best treated by local radiation therapy and may not require chemotherapy for months to years. Radiotherapy is also useful as palliative therapy for patients with extraskeletal plasmacytomas, large lytic lesions threatening fracture of long bones, spinal cord or root compression by plasma cell tumor, and certain pathologic fractures. Repeated local irradiation should be avoided when possible in patients with disseminated myeloma because chemotherapy is the only treatment demonstrated to improve survival while controlling systemic manifestations of the disease. Excessive use of radiation therapy can impair marrow reserves and render the patient less able to tolerate subsequent chemotherapy.

C. **Complications of disease or therapy.** Chemotherapy for multiple myeloma typically causes myelosuppression, and packed red blood cell transfusions are often required during the early weeks of treatment and the late refractory period. Toxicity of each chemotherapeutic agent is described in Chapter 5. In addition to these problems, several complications characteristic of multiple myeloma may occur.

1. **Hypercalcemia.** This common complication of multiple myeloma is believed to result from the liberation of bone calcium stimulated by osteoclast-activating factor released by the tumor cells. Presenting symptoms may include anorexia, nausea, vomiting, constipation, and

polyuria, progressing to lethargy, confusion, coma, and death. Dehydration and potentially reversible renal failure frequently occur during hypercalcemic crises. Control of hypercalcemic crises of multiple myeloma is usually accomplished with saline hydration (initially, 200 to 300 mL/hr i.v.), furosemide (20 to 40 mg every 4 to 6 hours) once the hypovolemia has been corrected, and prednisone (40 to 80 mg p.o. daily for 3 to 7 days). When hypercalcemia occurs in previously untreated patients, prompt initiation of chemotherapy of the myeloma, in addition to these measures, usually produces effective, durable control. In some patients, oral inorganic phosphates, calcitonin, pamidronate, or, more exceptionally, plicamycin may be needed and can be used on the following schedules.

   a. **Inorganic phosphate,** such as Neutra-Phos or Fleet Phospho-Soda, at a dose equivalent to 0.5 g of phosphorus p.o. q.i.d. (diluted in water to reduce diarrhea). This may be useful for chronic control of hypercalcemia in some patients.

   b. **Pamidronate,** 90 mg given as a 4-hour i.v. infusion that can be repeated at 7- to 30-day intervals if needed.

   c. **Calcitonin,** 100 to 300 units s.c. every 8 to 12 hours for up to 2 to 3 days. Calcitonin is usually given with prednisone, 10 to 20 mg p.o. two or three times daily to prolong its effectiveness.

   d. **Plicamycin** (mithramycin), 1 mg/m² i.v. every 3 to 7 days. This agent is myelosuppressive and can cause hemostatic disorders and nausea. Its long-term or repeated use in myeloma patients should be avoided except in refractory cases of hypercalcemia.

   e. **Hemodialysis** is effective but seldom needed for hypercalcemia.

2. **Infection.** Myeloma patients are highly susceptible to respiratory and urinary tract infections with common gram-positive and gram-negative bacterial pathogens. Deficiency of normal immunoglobulins, diminished bone marrow reserves, and immobilization due to skeletal disease are important predisposing factors. The weeks immediately following initiation of chemotherapy are a particularly high-risk period for infection. Prompt evaluation of fever or other manifestations of infection is essential. Antibiotic coverage for gram-positive and gram-negative organisms should be instituted while awaiting culture results from pa-

tients whose clinical picture suggests infection. Infection prophylaxis with antibiotics during the first 2 months of chemotherapy may be of help. Use of trimethoprim-sulfamethoxazole (1 double-strength tablet b.i.d.) or ciprofloxacin (500 mg b.i.d.) is under study in this setting. Granulocyte colony-stimulating factor (G-CSF), 5 µg/kg/day s.c., hastens neutrophil recovery by 1 to 3 days in neutropenic febrile patients. More dramatic reduction in the duration of neutropenia may be seen when this agent is used from 24 hours after cytotoxic therapy until full recovery from nadir neutropenia has occurred. Such prophylactic use of G-CSF is justified in patients with prior prolonged neutropenia or infection or who are at exceptionally high risk of infection due to age, intercurrent illness, chemotherapy regimen, or prior history of infection during chemotherapy.

3. **Hyperviscosity** may present as central nervous system impairment, congestive heart failure, ischemia, or bleeding tendency. It is more characteristic of Waldenström's macroglobulinemia than of multiple myeloma, but it may be seen in patients with extremely high IgG or IgA concentrations or in patients whose M protein tends to form aggregates. Treatment of symptomatic hyperviscosity is with plasmapheresis.

4. **Renal dysfunction** may be caused by myeloma kidney, amyloidosis, pyelonephritis, hypercalcemia, hyperuricemia with urate nephropathy, hyperviscosity syndrome, plasma cell infiltration of both kidneys (rare), and renal tubular acidosis. Most of these problems are at least partially reversible if recognized and treated promptly. Renal failure may also result from radiographic contrast material, particularly in a patient whose renal function is already compromised or who is dehydrated. Hypercalcemia and hyperuricemia are especially common potential causes of reversible renal failure and should be ruled out at the onset of the evaluation of a patient with myeloma. In patients with severe renal failure, hemodialysis should be considered as long as chemotherapy offers the potential for a prolonged remission.

5. **Skeletal destruction** is a major cause of disability and immobilization in multiple myeloma. Radiation therapy, surgery, or both may be needed to treat fractures or to prevent impending fractures of weight-bearing bones. In patients who exhibit lytic disease, monthly infusions of pamidronate, 90 mg given over 2 to 4 hours, can decrease or delay destructive skeletal events and improve the patient's comfort.

6. **Anemia.** For patients with refractory disease and chronic symptomatic anemia, treatment with recombinant human erythropoietin frequently diminishes or eliminates the transfusion requirement and returns the hemoglobin to asymptomatic levels. A schedule of 150 to 250 U/kg s.c. two times a week may be used.

7. **Leukemia.** Acute nonlymphocytic leukemia (ANLL) develops in about 4% of myeloma patients who receive chemotherapy. The incidence of ANLL is appreciably greater in patients surviving 4 years or more after the start of chemotherapy. Leukemia in this setting appears to be caused by the interaction of a carcinogenic drug with a predisposed host. ANLL complicating multiple myeloma is usually preceded by sideroblastic anemia as part of a myelodysplastic syndrome.

D. **Recurrence and treatment of refractory disease.** Objective responses to chemotherapy have a median duration of about 2 years. Response duration is influenced by the degree of reduction of tumor burden as reflected by the degree of reduction of myeloma proteins in the serum and urine. Eventually, virtually all patients develop recurrent or refractory disease. These patients pose a difficult clinical problem because of the small number of chemotherapeutic agents with proved activity in myeloma. In patients who relapse months or years after last receiving chemotherapy, remission can frequently be reinduced with the original regimen.

1. **Treatment of disease refractory to melphalan.** Disease that is refractory to melphalan or melphalan plus prednisone regimens may still respond to other alkylating agents. Two regimens that may be considered are as follows:

   a. **VBMCP** (see Section II.B.2.a).

   b. **BCP** may be effective in patients who absorbed oral melphalan poorly.

   Carmustine (BCNU), 75 mg/m^2 i.v. on day 1, *and*

   Cyclophosphamide, 400 mg/m^2 i.v. on day 1, *and*

   Prednisone, 75 mg p.o. on days 1 to 7.

   Repeat every 4 weeks.

   Treatment with these alkylating agent–based regimens can be expected to yield objective responses in about 20% of patients refractory to prior MP therapy. These regimens remain useful as conservative treatment choices for patients in their first relapse or for some patients who have failed initial MP therapy.

2. **Alternative regimens** not based on standard dose alkylating agents include the following:

a. **VAD**

Vincristine, 0.4 mg/day as a continuous i.v. infusion on days 1 to 4, *and*

Doxorubicin (Adriamycin), 9 mg/m^2/day as a continuous i.v. infusion on days 1 to 4, *and*

Dexamethasone, 40 mg p.o. on days 1 to 4, 9 to 12, and 17 to 20.

Repeat cycle every 28 to 35 days until four cycles beyond occurrence of maximum reduction in myeloma protein. Maximum cumulative doxorubicin dose is 540 mg/m^2. To avoid problems related to adrenal steroid excess, the frequency of dexamethasone courses should be decreased after 2 or 3 VAD cycles.

b. **High-dose cyclophosphamide.** Cyclophosphamide, 600 mg/m^2 i.v., is given on days 1 to 4, with this dosage repeated in 1 to 2 months. This aggressive regimen effectively produces pain relief of more than 1 month's duration and yields short-term objective responses in more than 30% of patients with disease that was refractory to prior treatments. Because the regimen is highly myelotoxic (it is employed without dose modification), its use should generally be limited to patients with active, markedly symptomatic refractory disease in institutions equipped to render intensive support, including platelet transfusion and infectious disease consultation. The prophylactic use of G-CSF is reasonable with this regimen. A recommended schedule is filgrastim, 5 µg/kg s.c. daily starting 24 hours after chemotherapy and continuing through the nadir until the granulocyte count exceeds 8,000 to 10,000/µL. Simultaneous use of plicamycin with high-dose cyclophosphamide should be avoided.

c. **Interferon-α_2** (rIFNα_2), 5×10^6 U/m^2 s.c. three times a week. This regimen produces clinical benefit in 35% of patients by objective and symptomatic standards but full objective responses (50% decrease in serum myeloma protein) in only 10%.

d. **High-dose methylprednisolone.** Methylprednisolone, 2 g i.v. three times weekly for 8 weeks, followed by 2 g weekly, produces clinical benefits in about one third of patients. It is particularly useful in patients whose marrow status is severely impaired.

e. **Autologous bone marrow transplantation** has been employed after preparative regimens such as high-dose melphalan plus total-body irradiation to induce good-quality responses in some patients with relapsed myeloma. There are issues related to marrow purge, the intensity of antitumor therapy, age range, expense, and the presence or absence of cure potential for this approach in myeloma.

III.   Waldenström's macroglobulinemia

   A.   General considerations and aims of therapy. This neoplasm is characterized by the proliferation of plasmacytoid lymphocytes that elaborate a monoclonal IgM. In contrast to multiple myeloma, skeletal destruction does not occur, but hepatosplenomegaly and lymphadenopathy are common. The major problems are hyperviscosity syndrome, severe anemia, and occasionally pancytopenia. The median survival time is only about 5 years from diagnosis, partly owing to the advanced age of most affected patients (60 to 75 years old) as well as to the common association with second neoplasms (20% of patients) and chronic or recurrent infections (25% of patients). The primary aims of therapy are to control complications and to decrease their incidence. Although response to chemotherapy has been associated with a more favorable median survival, the actual role of chemotherapy in prolonging survival in this disease has not been fully defined.

   B.   Treatment

      1.   Anemia. Most patients with macroglobulinemia are anemic; however, erythropoietin or transfusions should generally be reserved for those with symptomatic anemia. Overtransfusion is dangerous because of the important contribution of red blood cells to whole blood viscosity.

      2.   Hyperviscosity. Hyperviscosity syndrome requires plasmapheresis for acute management and chemotherapy with alkylating agents for long-term control.

      3.   Chemotherapy. In general, chemotherapy is withheld until symptomatic disease or progressive cytopenia occurs.

         a.   Standard chemotherapy
            Chlorambucil, 2 to 6 mg p.o. daily, *or* Cyclophosphamide, 50 to 100 mg p.o. daily. (Prednisone, 40 to 60 mg p.o. on days 1 to 4 every 4 weeks may be added.)

         b.   Alternatively, a high-dose intermittent chlorambucil plus prednisone regimen may be used every 2 to 3 weeks. Chlorambucil, 30 mg/m^2 p.o. on day 1, *and* Prednisone, 40 mg/m^2 p.o. on days 1 to 4.

         c.   VBMCP (described in Section II.B.2.a).

           d. **Fludarabine**, 25 mg/m^2 i.v. days 1–5 every 3–4 weeks, is effective in up to 40% of patients but may cause prolonged CD4 suppression. This agent is yet to be compared with standard regimens such as intermittent chlorambucil.

       4. **Disease variants.** Some patients with IgM monoclonal proteins have clinical chronic lymphocytic leukemia or lymphoma and should have their treatment directed at that disease. Rare patients with macroglobulinemia have prominent skeletal disease, and their disease should be approached as IgM myeloma and treated similarly to other multiple myelomas.

IV. **Heavy-chain diseases** comprise a group of rare plasma cell dyscrasias in which the abnormal clone of plasma cells or B lymphocytes elaborates an abnormal polypeptide consisting of anomalous γ, α, or μ heavy chains with deleted segments.

    A. **γ Heavy-chain disease** presents as a lymphoma usually with lymphadenopathy, hepatosplenomegaly, and involvement of Waldeyer's ring. The latter may lead to characteristic palatal edema. Bone marrow involvement is the rule. Treatment by local radiotherapy or lymphoma-directed chemotherapy regimens is sometimes effective.

    B. **α Heavy-chain disease** appears to be the most common of the heavy-chain diseases and occurs mainly in people under the age of 50 years. Its most common clinical presentation is in the enteric form, with chronic diarrhea, malabsorption syndrome, and marked lymphoplasmacytic infiltration of the small bowel mucosa. Remissions have been reported using lymphoma chemotherapy regimens and occasionally antibiotics alone.

    C. **μ Heavy-chain disease** is rare, usually presenting as chronic lymphocytic leukemia, and it should be managed as such.

V. **Amyloidosis.** Only primary amyloidosis with or without associated plasma cell or lymphoid neoplasms is considered in this section. With these disorders, the amyloid substance consists of fragments of immunoglobulin light chains and is therefore termed an *amyloid L-chain protein.* This type of amyloid characteristically infiltrates the tongue, heart, skin, ligaments, and muscle, and occasionally the kidney, liver, and spleen. In patients with documented lymphomas or plasma cell neoplasms, treatment is of the underlying neoplasm, but the decline in the amount of amyloid is often minimal. With primary amyloidosis without a demonstrable underlying neoplasm, treatment with MP has been shown to be of moderate benefit when tested in a randomized double-blind study, although the exact role of chemotherapy for this disease is not yet clear. High-dose therapy with stem cell rescue is also under investigation.

VI. Monoclonal gammopathy of undetermined significance **(MGUS)** has been found in up to 3% of people over 70 years of age. It has been termed *benign monoclonal gammopathy;* however, because about 20% of patients with this finding progress to more severe plasma cell dyscrasias, the term *monoclonal gammopathy of undetermined significance* has been introduced as more appropriate. With this condition, patients usually have an M spike of less than 2 g/dL, no bone lesions, no conclusive evidence of myeloma on bone marrow aspirate or biopsy, no anemia or bone marrow failure, and stability of the clinical picture and M protein studies over a period of follow-up. The serum beta-2-microglobulin (B_2M) and the plasma cell–labeling index are both low. Once initial stability has been demonstrated, these patients should be followed at yearly intervals with evaluation of hemoglobin levels and M protein status. No treatment is indicated unless progression to myeloma or symptomatic macroglobulinemia occurs.

SELECTED READINGS

Atral M, Harousseau J-L, Stoppa A-M, et al. A prospective randomized trial of autologous bone marrow transplantation and chemotherapy in multiple myeloma. *N Engl J Med* 1996;335:91–97.

Barlogie B, Smith L, Alexanian R. Effective treatment of advanced multiple myeloma refractory to alkylating agents. *N Engl J Med* 1984;310:1353–1356.

Bataille R, et al. C-reactive protein and beta 2-microglobulin produce a simple and powerful myeloma staging system. *Blood* 1992;80:733–737.

Berenson JR, Lichtenstein A, Porter L, et al. Efficacy of pamidronate in reducing skeletal events in patients with advanced multiple myeloma. *N Engl J Med* 1996;334:488–493.

Blade J, San Miguel JF, Fontanillas M, et al. Survival of multiple myeloma patients who are potential candidates for early high-dose therapy intensification/autotransplantation and who were conventionally treated. *J Clin Oncol* 1996;14:2167–2173.

Case DC, Lee BJ, Clarkson BD. Improved survival times in multiple myeloma treated with melphalan, prednisone, cyclophosphamide, vincristine and BCNU: M-2 protocol. *Am J Med* 1977;68:897–903.

Durie BG, Dixon DO, Carter S, et al. Improved survival duration with combination chemotherapy for multiple myeloma: a Southwest Oncology Group Study. *J Clin Oncol* 1986;4:1227–1237.

Durie BGM, Salmon SE. A clinical staging system for multiple myeloma: correlation of measured myeloma cell mass with presenting clinical features, response to treatment and survival. *Cancer* 1975;36:842–854.

Durie BGM, Salmon SE, Moon TE. Pretreatment tumor mass, cell kinetics and prognosis in multiple myeloma. *Blood* 1980;55:364–372.

Fernand JP, et al. The role of autologous blood stem cells in support of high-dose therapy for multiple myeloma. *Hematol Oncol Clin North Am* 1992;6:451.

Gahrton G, Tura S, Ljungman P, et al. Allogeneic bone marrow transplantation in multiple myeloma. *N Engl J Med* 1991;325:1267–1273.

Greipp PR, Katzmann JA, O'Fallon WM, Kylle RA. Value of beta-2 microglobulin level and plasma cell labeling indices as prognostic factors in patients with newly diagnosed myeloma. *Blood* 1988;72:219–223.

Greipp PR, Lust JA, O'Fallon WM, Katzmann JA, Witzig TE, Kyle RA. Plasma cell labeling index and beta 2-microglobulin predict survival independent of thymidine kinase and C-reactive protein in multiple myeloma. *Blood* 1993;81:3382–3387.

Kyle RA, Lust JA. Monoclonal gammopathies of undetermined significance. *Semin Hematol* 1989;26:176–200.

Lenhard RE, Oken MM, Barnes JM, Humphrey RL, Glick JH, Silverstein MN. High-dose cyclophosphamide: an effective treatment for advanced refractory multiple myeloma. *Cancer* 1984;53:1456–1460.

MacLennan IC, Chapman C, Dann J, Kelly K. Combined chemotherapy with ABCM versus melphalan for treatment of myelomatosis. The Medical Research Council Working Party for Leukemia in Adults. *Lancet* 1992;339:200–205.

Mandelli F, Avvisati G, Amadori S, et al. Maintenance treatment with recombinant interferon alfa-2b in patients with multiple myeloma responding to conventional induction chemotherapy. *N Engl J Med* 1990;322:1430.

Mirallis GD, O'Fallon JR, Talley NJ. Plasma-cell dyscrasia with polyneuropathy. *N Engl J Med* 1992;327:1919–1923.

Oken MM. Standard treatment of multiple myeloma. *Mayo Clin Proc* 1994;69:781–787.

Oken MM. Multiple myeloma. *Med Clin North Am* 1984;68:757.

Oken MM, Pomeroy C, Weisdorf D, et al. Prophylactic antibiotics for the prevention of early infection in multiple myeloma. *Am J Med* 1996;100:624–628.

Oken MM, Harrington DP, Abramson N, et al. Comparison of melphalan and prednisone with vincristine, carmustine, melphalan, cyclophosphamide and prednisone in the treatment of multiple myeloma. Results of Eastern Cooperative Oncology Group Study E2479. *Cancer* 1997;79:1561–1567.

Metastatic Cancer of Unknown Origin

Martin M. Oken

In about 5% of patients with newly diagnosed cancer (excluding nonmelanoma skin cancer), the primary site remains unknown despite a detailed history and physical examination, routine blood chemistries, complete blood count, urinalysis, chest radiograph, and histologic evaluation of the biopsy. The problem of metastatic cancer of unknown origin raises difficult questions for both diagnosis and treatment. Although the median survival time of patients with cancer of unknown origin has been reported to be less than 6 months, subgroups of patients have been defined who have a far better outlook with proper management. With modern therapy, the overall survival of these patients appears to be improving. A major responsibility of the clinician is to identify those patients with a characteristic presentation who might benefit from a specific strategy, and to identify the increasingly large group of patients that might benefit from a trial of chemotherapy.

I. **General considerations and aims of therapy**
   A. **Histology and presenting clinical manifestations.** Adenocarcinoma and undifferentiated carcinoma each comprise up to 40% of all cancers of unknown origin. Fewer than 15% of cancers of unknown origin are squamous cell carcinomas (SCCs), and, at most, 2% to 5% are malignant melanoma. Other histologies that may present as cancer of unknown origin include lymphomas, germ cell tumors, and neuroendocrine carcinomas. These histologies are particularly important to identify because they represent tumors that may be effectively managed with systemic chemotherapy. Nearly half of all patients with unknown primaries and well over half of those with adenocarcinoma present with hepatomegaly, abdominal mass, or other abdominal symptoms. Lymphadenopathy is the presenting clinical manifestation in 15% to 25% of patients. Lower cervical or supraclavicular lymph nodes usually contain adenocarcinoma or undifferentiated carcinoma, and middle to high cervical adenopathy generally represents SCC. Between 10% and 20% of patients present with manifestations of bone, lung, or pleural involvement, whereas fewer than 10% present with evidence of central nervous system disease. Most of the latter group are eventually found to have either lung or gastrointestinal tract primaries.

   Two presentations of advanced carcinoma of unknown primary site have been recognized as more treatable than others: (1) poorly differentiated carcinoma or adenocarcinoma, especially with predominant sites of involvement in the mediastinum, retroperitoneum, lymph nodes, or lungs; and (2) adeno-carcinoma in women predominantly involving the peritoneal surfaces. In these instances, platinum-based chemotherapy regimens designed for germ cell or ovarian cancers have produced many useful objective responses and occasional long-term disease-free survival.

B. Sites of origin. It is sometimes possible to predict the most likely primary sites from the histology and location of the metastatic lesion of unknown origin. Pancreas and lung are the most common ultimately determined sites of origin. Together they represent more than 40% of the adenocarcinomas of unknown origin. Colorectal, gastric, and hepatobiliary carcinoma each represents about 10% of the cancers of unknown origin.

In general, adenocarcinomas or undifferentiated carcinomas presenting with hepatic metastases or left supraclavicular adenopathy are eventually demonstrated to be of gastrointestinal origin. SCCs that present in the supraclavicular or low cervical lymph nodes are usually from lung primaries, whereas similar lesions of higher cervical nodes are more likely to have originated from occult primary lesions in the head and neck region.

The pattern of metastatic involvement associated with occult primary tumors differs from that associated with overt primaries. For example, occult lung cancer rarely involves bone, a common site of metastasis from overt lung cancer; however, bone metastases appear to be more common in patients with gastrointestinal cancer who have occult primaries than in those who have overt primaries.

C. Aims of diagnostic evaluation. The first objective in the management of a patient newly diagnosed with cancer of unknown origin is to plan the appropriate diagnostic evaluation. There are three chief aims of this evaluation.

1. Identify a tumor in which cure or effective disease control is possible.
2. Determine if the tumor is regionally confined or widely metastatic.
3. Identify any complication for which immediate local therapy is indicated.

D. Goal of treatment. In patients with tumors for which effective systemic therapy is available and in patients with disease regionally confined to peripheral lymph nodes alone, active management with the goal of prolongation of life through extended disease control or cure should be considered. These patients represent about 25% of patients with occult primaries. For the remaining patients, the chance of prolonging life has been less likely, but with newer therapy, it might be improving. Treatment should also address palliation of symptoms and preservation of the best possible quality of life.

II. Diagnostic evaluation

A. **Analysis of the biopsy specimen**. If possible, the pathologist should receive fresh, unfixed material to allow electron microscopy, histochemistry, immuno-histology, and hormone receptor studies to be done, if needed, after routine examination. Careful review of the biopsy material should be undertaken to classify the tumor conclusively as SCC, adenocarcinoma, or other identifiable histology. Up to 40% of cancers of unknown origin are undifferentiated or poorly differentiated tumors based on evaluation of hematoxylin and eosin–stained material. Electron microscopy, when available, may be useful for the further classification of these tumors through the identification of desmosomes and intercellular bridges (SCC); tight junctions, microvilli, and acinar spaces (adenocarcinoma); premelanosomes (amelanotic melanoma); neurosecretory granules (small cell or neuroendocrine carcinoma); and absence of junctions (lymphoma). Immunohistology is an indispensable part of the evaluation of carcinoma of unknown primary site. Immunohistochemical studies on the tumor may be used to demonstrate the presence of prostatic acid phosphatase or prostate-specific antigen (prostate carcinoma), human chronic gonadotropin (β-hCG: germ cell tumors), α-fetoprotein (germ cell tumors or hepatocellular carcinoma), or monoclonal immunoglobulin (lymphoma, plasmacytoma). Immunoglobulin or T-cell–receptor gene rearrangements may be helpful in identifying tumors of lymphoid origin. Undifferentiated carcinomas or adenocarcinomas in women should be evaluated for estrogen and progesterone receptors. Mucin positivity is helpful in eliminating the possibility of renal cell carcinoma.

Clearly, the use of many of these specialized studies must be balanced against their expense. If judiciously applied, they can aid in the identification of some of the undifferentiated or poorly differentiated tumors of unknown origin and help to focus their subsequent diagnostic evaluation and management.

One exception to the policy of seeking a definitive histologic diagnosis as the first step in evaluating a tumor of unknown origin is when the patient presents with a potentially resectable neck mass (other than supraclavicular adenopathy) and no other apparent lesion. In these patients, a head and neck primary should be sought by detailed head and neck examination, radiographs of the sinuses, and, if necessary, panendoscopy under general anesthesia to include laryngoscopy, bronchoscopy, esophagoscopy, and nasopharyngoscopy with blind biopsy of the base of the tongue, piriform sinuses, nasopharynx, and tonsillar fossae if no gross primary is found. A computed tomography (CT) scan of the head and neck may also be of value. If this work-up is not diagnostic, biopsy of the neck mass is undertaken. This order of evaluation is chosen so that if a resectable SCC of the head and neck is found, the neck mass can be removed as part of the curative procedure.

B. **Squamous cell carcinoma.** For SCCs with apparent involvement of only one lymph node group, the possibility of long-term survival exists if proper treatment is carried out. The diagnostic evaluation depends on the lymph node region involved. The most common lymph node presentation for SCCs of unknown origin is in the cervical or supraclavicular region. Cervical lymph node metastases above the supraclavicular region usually originate from head and neck primary lesions. The diagnostic approach to these lesions is discussed in the preceding section. Because surgery, irradiation, or both, with curative intent, are employed if disease is localized to this region, distant metastases should be excluded with a bone scan, a chest radiograph, and in some instances, a chest CT scan. SCC of supraclavicular lymph nodes is usually of lung or esophageal origin and seldom represents regionally confined disease. Evaluation is the same as that for disease that extends beyond regional lymph nodes.

SCC in axillary or inguinal lymph nodes is rarely associated with an occult primary. Regional skin and lung should be examined as possible primary sites with axillary disease, whereas the skin, anus, and genitalia should be carefully examined when the presentation is SCC in the inguinal nodes.

SCC with generalized lymphadenopathy or, more commonly, with disease that extends beyond the lymph nodes represents disease that cannot be satisfactorily controlled by present-day techniques. The search for the primary lesions should be done mainly by a chest radiograph and careful physical examination of the appropriate organs. Serum chemistries, including the calcium level, should be determined. Further diagnostic studies are needed only if indicated by signs, symptoms, or abnormalities on the initial studies.

C. **Adenocarcinoma and poorly differentiated carcinoma.** Women with adenocarcinoma or poorly differentiated carcinoma of unknown origin should undergo mammography, careful pelvic examination, and hormone receptor evaluation of the tumor. In men, serum acid phosphatase, prostate-specific antigen, β-hCG, and α-fetoprotein should be determined to help exclude prostate and germ cell tumors, respectively. All patients should have stools and urine examined for occult blood, and the serum should be tested for abnormalities in the liver chemistries, creatinine, and electrolytes. With disease apparently confined to axillary lymph nodes, mammography is particularly important in women and should be considered in some men as well. Undifferentiated carcinoma found only in middle to high cervical lymph nodes should be evaluated in the same manner as described in Section II.B for cervical SCC.

Traditional contrast studies, such as intravenous pyelogram, barium enema, and upper gastrointestinal series, are not indicated unless specifically suggested by signs or symptoms (e.g., occult blood in the stool). Abdominal CT scan with intravenous contrast is a reasonable option in view of the frequency with which it detects carcinoma of the pancreas or hepatobiliary cancer in this setting.

D. **Malignant melanoma.** The finding of malignant melanoma confined to a single lymph node group and without a detectable primary lesion represents stage II disease and is associated with a 30% 5-year survival rate after lymphadenectomy. Evaluation to exclude more extensive disease should include a history, physical examination (emphasizing skin and ophthalmoscopic examination), chest radiograph, liver chemistries, liver scan, and brain CT scan.

III. Treatment

A. **General strategy.** The importance of identifying tumors that may be treated effectively, such as lymphomas, germ cell tumors, trophoblastic tumors, and breast, prostate, ovarian, and neuroendocrine carcinomas, is readily apparent. Once identified, these lesions should be treated as described in their respective chapters. In patients whose primary lesion remains obscure, a therapeutic distinction must be made between those with disease confined to one lymph node region and those with more widespread disease or involvement of visceral organs. In the former, some may be treated with curative intent, whereas in the latter, the aims of treatment are palliative.

B. **Squamous cell carcinoma.** Patients with SCC confined to the cervical lymph nodes above the supraclavicular region should receive full-course radiotherapy to a field extending from the base of the skull to the clavicles. Alternatively, they may be treated with radical lymph node dissection followed by radiation therapy. In either case, the irradiation is designed to include any possible head and neck primary carcinoma. Survival of patients so treated is at least as good as that for patients with known head and neck primaries. More limited lymph node dissection or regional irradiation may also be indicated for SCC confined to unilateral involvement of the axillary or inguinal nodes.

More widespread SCCs of unknown origin are treated with a palliative intent. No treatment except for local radiotherapy to symptomatic lesions is the standard approach. In patients with symptomatic or progressive disease who desire chemotherapy, regimens designed mainly for head and neck or non–small cell lung cancer should could be considered.

1. **DF**

   Cisplatin, 100 mg/m² i.v. on day 1, *and*

   Fluorouracil, 1,000 mg/m² as a continuous 24-hour i.v. infusion for 4 days (days 1 to 4)

   Repeat every 3 weeks.

2. **MBP**

   Methotrexate, 40 mg/m² i.m. on days 1 and 15, *and*

   Bleomycin, 10 units i.m. on days 1, 8, and 15, *and*

   Cisplatin, 50 mg/m² i.v. on day 4

   Repeat every 3 weeks.

3. **Various combinations of cisplatin or carboplatin with paclitaxel** as outlined in Chapter 8 on lung cancer.

   Do not use regimens 1 or 2 if the serum creatinine level is more than 1.5 mg/dL. The cumulative dose of bleomycin should not exceed 300 units. Use proper hydration with cisplatin as described elsewhere in this text.

C. **Adenocarcinoma and poorly differentiated carcinoma.** In women, if these carcinomas are confined to the unilateral axillary lymph nodes, they should be considered possible breast cancer and treated accordingly as stage II disease (see Chap. 11). A woman with adenocarcinoma or poorly differentiated carcinoma predominantly confined to the peritoneal surface should be considered for a cisplatin-based ovarian cancer regimen. Undifferentiated carcinoma confined to the middle or high cervical lymph nodes should be treated actively as SCC (see Section II.B). Men with adenocarcinoma of unknown primary and a positive tumor or serum Prostate specific antigens (PSA) should have a trial of hormonal therapy.

   Patients with more advanced adenocarcinoma or poorly differentiated carcinoma in whom the evaluation previously described in Section II.C does not suggest breast, prostate, or other highly treatable primary should be managed according to the histology. Cisplatin-based combination chemotherapy is valuable in the treatment of poorly differentiated carcinoma and poorly differentiated adenocarcinoma. In these patients, the germ-cell regimen of bleomycin, etoposide, and cisplatin (BEP), or EP (with or without the bleomycin), has been studied in a series of 220 patients. This combination may produce more than a 60% objective response rate and more than a 20% complete response rate with up to a 13% long-term survival rate. This regimen is fully described in Chap. 13.

   Patients with widespread adenocarcinoma that is well or moderately well differentiated may be more responsive to systemic therapy than previously thought. The combination of paclitaxel, carboplatin, and oral etoposide yields objective responses in 45% of patients, and the DM regimen may produce partial responses in about one third of patients.

1. **PCE**

   Paclitaxel, 200 mg/m² as a 1-hour i.v. infusion on day 1, *and*

   Carboplatin, at an area under the curve (AUC) of 6 i.v. over 30 to 60 minutes on day 1, *and*

   Etoposide, 50 and 100 mg p.o. on alternate days for days 1 to 10

   Repeat every 3 weeks

   Follow the usual paclitaxel desensitization regimen with dexamethasone, H_1- and H_2-histamine receptor antagonists.

2. **DM**

   Doxorubicin (Adriamycin), 50 mg/m² i.v. on days 1 and 22, *and*

   Mitomycin, 20 mg/m² i.v. on day 1

   Repeat every 42 days.

   Do not exceed a 540-mg/m² cumulative dose of doxorubicin.

   Both regimens are worthy of consideration in patients with good performance status because occasional durable responses have occurred. Both reports are based on limited accrual phase II studies. Responding patients show improvement within two cycles, and chemotherapy should be stopped after two cycles if no improvement is seen. PCE is also effective in patients with poorly differentiated adenocarcinoma and poorly differentiated carcinoma and may be considered as an alternative to BEP.

D. **Malignant melanoma.** For disease confined to a single lymph node group, radical lymph node dissection yields long-term survival in 30% of treated patients. Treatment of disseminated melanoma is discussed in Chap. 15.

E. **Neuroendocrine carcinoma.** Poorly differentiated neuroendocrine carcinoma may represent up to 13% of cases of poorly differentiated carcinoma or adenocarcinoma. The diagnosis is secured by recognition of neurosecretory granules on electron microscopy. Localized lesions are uncommon and should be treated with surgery or radiation therapy. Metastatic disease frequently responds to platinum-based chemotherapy, such as etoposide plus cisplatin.

SELECTED READINGS

Abbruzzese JL, Abbruzzese MC, Hess KR, et al. Unknown primary carcinoma: natural history and prognostic factors in 657 consecutive patients. *J Clin Oncol* 1994;12:1272–1284.

Altman E, Cadman E. An analysis of 1539 patients with cancer of unknown primary site. *Cancer* 1986;57:120–124.

Greco FA, Vaughn WK, Hainsworth JD. Advanced poorly differentiated carcinoma of unknown primary site: recognition of a treatable syndrome. *Ann Intern Med* 1986;104:547–556.

Hainsworth JD, Greco FA. Treatment of patients with cancer of an unknown primary site. *N Engl J Med* 1993;329:257–263.

Hainsworth JD, Erland JB, Kalman LA, Schroeder MT, Greco FA. Carcinoma of unknown primary site: treatment with one-hour paclitaxel, carboplatin, and extended schedule etoposide. *J Clin Oncol* 1997;15:2385–2393.

Hainsworth JD, Johnson DH, Greco FA. Poorly differentiated neuroendocrine carcinoma of unknown primary site: a newly recognized clinicopathologic entity. *Ann Intern Med* 1988;109:364–371.

Hainsworth JD, Johnson DH, Greco FA. Cisplatin-based combination chemotherapy in the treatment of poorly differentiated carcinoma and poorly differentiated adenocarcinoma of unknown primary site: results of a 12-year experience. *J Clin Oncol* 1992;10:912–922.

Lenzi R, Hess KR, Abbruzzese MC. Poorly differentiated carcinoma and poorly differentiated adenocarcinoma of unknown origin: favorable subsets of patients with unknown-primary carcinoma. *J Clin Oncol* 1997;15:2056–2066.

Moertel CG. Adenocarcinoma of unknown origin. *Ann Intern Med* 1979;91:646–647.

Neumann KH, Nystrom JS. Metastatic cancer of unknown origin: nonsquamous cell type. *Semin Oncol* 1982;9:427.

Strnad CM, Grosh WW, Baxter J, et al. Peritoneal carcinomatosis of unknown primary site in women: a distinctive subset of adenocarcinoma. *Ann Intern Med* 1989;11:213–217.

Woods RL, Fox RM, Tuttersall MH, Levi JA, Brodie GN. Metastatic adenocarcinomas of unknown primary site: a randomized study of two combination chemotherapy regimens. *N Engl J Med* 1980;303:87–89.

26

Human Immunodeficiency Virus–Associated Malignancies

Lynne Jahnke and Jamie H. Von Roenn

I. **Introduction**

Four malignancies are considered acquired immunodeficiency syndrome (AIDS)-defining illnesses: Kaposi's sarcoma (KS), primary central nervous system lymphoma (PCNSL), non-Hodgkin's lymphoma (NHL), and cervical cancer. Although other malignancies appear to have an increased incidence in human immunodeficiency virus (HIV)-infected patients (e.g., squamous cell anal cancer and Hodgkin's disease), their precise relationship to HIV infection has not yet been established. The management of any cancer in an HIV-infected patient requires an integrated team approach. Treatment of the underlying HIV infection must be incorporated into the overall treatment plan, in addition to aggressive prophylaxis and treatment of opportunistic infections, maintenance of general health and nutrition, and psychosocial support.

II. **Kaposi's sarcoma**

A. **Epidemiology.** KS is the most common HIV-associated malignancy. The prevalence of KS in HIV-infected patients remained stable at 25% to 35%, although the incidence of KS as an AIDS-defining illness has decreased from about 33% of patients in the early 1980s to only 14% in the 1990s. In recent years, KS more often presents as a late, non-AIDS–defining manifestation of HIV infection. Although immunosuppression is an important risk factor for KS, it is 300 times more common in HIV-infected patients than in other immunocompromised patients. Greater than 90% of cases of epidemic KS occur in bisexual or homosexual men. The association of KS with a history of sexually transmitted diseases and high level of sexual activity, and the development of KS in a handful of well-studied homosexual men without HIV infection, has led many investigators to suspect that a sexually transmitted cofactor contributes to the development of KS. Current evidence suggests that the recently discovered human herpes virus type 8 (HHV-8) is important in the pathogenesis of KS. HHV-8 DNA is identified in more than 90% of KS biopsies. Serologic studies demonstrate detectable antibodies to HHV-8 in 55% to 85% of KS patients. Furthermore, antibodies to HHV-8 have been associated with the subsequent development of KS.

B. **Presentation and detection.** The natural history of KS is extremely variable. KS most often presents as a pink or brownish-purple papule or plaque on the skin or mucous membranes. Lesions are frequently symmetric and follow Langer's lines. KS can present anywhere but has a predilection for the retroauricular areas, soles of the feet, extremities, genitalia, and face. In addition to their cosmetic unacceptability, KS lesions can cause significant morbidity and organ dysfunction. Dermal lymphatic involvement, most commonly involving the lower extremities, genitalia, and periorbital area, can cause painful and disfiguring lymphedema. The edema is often out of proportion to the visible skin involvement. Oral cavity lesions occur in about 45% of patients with cutaneous KS and as the first site of disease in 15% of patients. Oral lesions can interfere with speech and eating. Gastrointestinal involvement, present in up to half of patients, is often asymptomatic but can cause pain, diarrhea, and bleeding. Pulmonary involvement is the most common life-threatening manifestation of KS. It may be difficult to differentiate from opportunistic infection because the chest radiograph may show a reticulonodular or nodular infiltrate, with or without pleural effusions. Bronchoscopy is useful to visualize the characteristic erythematous plaque-like bronchial lesions of KS. However, biopsy is rarely done because of the risk of bleeding from these highly vascular tumors. Thallium and gallium scans may be useful to differentiate KS from an opportunistic pulmonary infection.

C. **Staging.** KS is a multicentric tumor and hence does not easily fit the usual TNM categorization. Because the overall prognosis is more closely related to the degree of underlying immune dysfunction than to sites of disease involvement, the AIDS Clinical Trials Group (ACTG) developed a staging system that reflects various prognostic factors (Table 26-1). Patients are defined as good or poor risk on the basis of tumor burden, sites of involvement, CD4 lymphocyte count, history of opportunistic infections, systemic symptoms, and performance status. A recent study validating the ACTG staging system identified tumor burden as a significant predictive factor only in patients with a CD4 count of at least 200 cells/μL. The presence of systemic symptoms was not a predictor of outcome, and a CD4 count of 150 cells/μL, rather than 200 cells/μL, was a better descriminant of outcome.

The initial evaluation of a patient with KS should include a careful physical examination, including a rectal examination with Hemoccult testing. The history should focus on the rate of progression of KS, lesion-associated symptoms (pain, edema, disfigurement), as well as the history of HIV treatment, HIV-related opportunistic infections, the rate of decline in CD4 lymphocyte counts, and viral load. Even though the lesions are characteristic, a biopsy should be done to exclude other cutaneous processes. A baseline chest radiograph is important to look for asymptomatic visceral disease. Computed tomography (CT)

Table 26-1. AIDS clinical trials group staging for epidemic Kaposi's sarcoma*

| Disease status | Relative risk | |
	Good risk (0) (All of the following)	Poor risk (1) (Any of the following)
Tumor (T)	Confined to skin, minimal oral disease, or both	Edema; extensive oral ulcers; visceral and gastrointestinal disease
Immune Status (I)*	CD4 count $\geq 150/\mu$L	CD4 count $< 150/\mu$L
Systemic Illness (S)	No prior opportunistic infection or thrush; no B symptoms	Prior opportunistic infection or thrush; B symptoms; performance status $< 70\%$; other HIV-related illnesses

* Modified by recent validation study.

scans are not indicated unless the patient's symptoms suggest abdominal disease. Upper endoscopy and colonoscopy are not indicated in the absence of unexplained gastrointestinal bleeding or symptoms. Medications should be reviewed to ensure that patients are receiving appropriate highly active antiretroviral therapy and prophylaxis for opportunistic infections as well as to identify potentially myelosuppressive drugs that may complicate the use of chemotherapeutic agents (e.g., trimethoprim-sulfamethoxazole, sulfadiazine, zidovudine).

D. Treatment. Effective treatment of KS is dependent on clear communication between the doctor and patient with regard to the risks and benefits of the proposed therapy, its interaction with HIV treatment, and the patient's overall expectations. KS is not a curable tumor. Treatment has not clearly been shown to prolong survival. The first decision to be made is whether to initiate therapy. Indications to initiate treatment for KS include prevention of disease progression, cosmesis, palliation of symptoms, and visceral disease. In general, local therapies are used for minimal, primarily cosmetically disturbing KS or for patients with severe multisystem compromise who may not tolerate systemic treatment. Systemic therapy is indicated for bulky, rapidly progressing, symptomatic or life-threatening disease (Table 26-2). The determination of appropriate therapy is based on an evaluation of both tumor and immune status.

1. Local therapy. Limited numbers of small lesions can be treated by radiotherapy, cryother-

Table 26-2.   Treatment guidelines for Kaposi's sarcoma

Disease status of KS	HIV disease status	Treatment options
Minimal cutaneous disease	CD4 count < 200/µL; prior OI; B symptoms	Local therapy
	CD4 count ≥ 200/µL; no prior OI; no B symptoms	Interferon and antivirals or local therapy
Cosmetically disturbing disease	Any	Local therapy
Extensive cutaneous disease	CD4 count < 200/µL; prior OI; B symptoms	Chemotherapy
	CD4 count ≥ 200/µL; no prior OI; no B symptoms	Interferon and antivirals or chemotherapy
Localized bulky or painful disease	Any	Radiation therapy or chemotherapy
Tumor-associated edema	Any	Chemotherapy
Symptomatic visceral disease	Any	Chemotherapy

KS, Kaposi's sarcoma; OI, opportunistic infection.
Adopted with permission from Susan Krown, M.D.

apy, or intralesional injection. Surgery is occasionally useful for an isolated pedunculated lesion. Cryotherapy with liquid nitrogen can lead to hypopigmentation, which may be cosmetically unacceptable to dark-skinned patients. Intralesional therapy with vinblastine or interferon (IFN) can be effective but is limited by the need for multiple injections (Table 26-3). After the injection of oral lesions, patients typically slough the oral mucosa in 24 to 48 hours,

Table 26-3.   Intralesional chemotherapy for Kaposi's sarcoma

Chemotherapy Regimen*	
Vinblastine (0.2 mg/mL)	0.1 mL per 0.5 cm of surface area of lesion (maximum, 4 mL)
Interferon-α	$3–5 \times 10^6$ units three times per week for 4 weeks

* Appropriate local anesthesia should be given before injection.

for which narcotic analgesics should be empirically provided. Intralesional IFN-α is occasionally effective even in patients who have failed systemic IFN. Radiation therapy is effective for local control of KS. Depending on the dose and schedule, radiation therapy results in the most satisfying cosmetic result and longest duration of benefit of all the available local interventions.

2. **Systemic therapy**
   a. **Biologic response modifiers.** IFN-α is the best studied biologic response modifier. A clear-cut dose-response relationship has not been established. Responses have been reported with doses ranging from 1 million units per day to 36 million units three times per week (see Table 26-4 for recommended dosing). Immune function, as measured by CD4 lymphocyte counts, is the best predictor of response to IFN as a single agent. Patients with CD4 lymphocyte counts of more than 400 cells/μL have an overall response rate of 45%, whereas patients with CD4 lymphocyte counts of less than 100 cells/μL respond less than 10% of the time. Although it may take greater than 8 weeks to respond, the responses are often durable, with a median response duration of 1 to 2 years. IFN is best prescribed in combination with antiretroviral agents. IFN plus azidothymidine (AZT) results in a response rate of greater than 40%, with responses seen even in patients with CD4 counts below 100 cells/μL. Ongoing trials are evaluating IFN in combination with other less myelosuppressive antiretroviral agents. Most practitioners begin with anti-

Table 26-4. Selected systemic treatment regimens for Kaposi's sarcoma

Biologic response modifiers	
Interferon-α	$1–10 \times 10^6$ million u/day s.c.
Chemotherapy	
Liposomal doxorubicin (Doxil)	20 mg/m^2 i.v. every 3 wk
Liposomal daunorubicin (DaunoXome)	40 mg/m^2 i.v. every 2 wk
Paclitaxel	100 mg/m^2 i.v. over 3 h every 2 wk, *or* 135 mg/m^2 i.v. over 3 h every 3 wk

retroviral therapy and relatively low-dose IFN-α, 1 to 5 million units s.c. daily, and increase to 10 million units s.c. daily, if well tolerated.

b. **Chemotherapy.** Chemotherapy provides rapid palliation of KS-related symptoms for most patients. Liposomal anthracyclines (e.g., daunorubicin [DaunoXome], liposomal doxorubicin [Doxil]) are currently considered the chemotherapeutic agents of choice for advanced KS. Multiple randomized trials of bleomycin and vincristine, with or without doxorubicin (Adriamycin), compared with one of the liposomal anthracyclines have consistently demonstrated less toxicity and equal or better response rates and response durations with the liposomal anthracyclines. For second-line therapy, paclitaxel, 100 mg/m² every 2 weeks or 135 mg/m² every 3 weeks, has produced response rates of 50% to 70% associated with significant palliation of tumor-related symptoms.

Patients often require growth factor support between cycles. Granulocyte colony-stimulating factor, 5 μg/kg s.c. given days 7 to 12 of a 14-day treatment cycle, is often sufficient to preserve adequate neutrophil counts to prevent infection and allow timely administration of therapy. An absolute neutrophil count of 750/μL is adequate to deliver therapy with liposomal anthracyclines.

The duration of treatment is variable. Treatment should be continued until the maximal response is obtained; however, intercurrent illness often interrupts therapy. Although lesions frequently progress after therapy is discontinued, an effective maintenance therapy has not yet been defined. Early data suggest, however, that maximal viral suppression with highly active antiretroviral therapy may suppress KS tumor regrowth after discontinuation of chemotherapy.

III. **Non-Hodgkin's lymphoma**

A. **Background.** HIV-seropositive patients have a 5-10% lifetime risk of developing NHL. In a small proportion of patients (2% to 3%), NHL is the AIDS-defining event; but for most, NHL is a late manifestation of HIV infection, arising in the milieu of prolonged immunosuppression. HIV-associated NHLs are high-grade B-cell lymphomas similar to those seen in other immunocompromised patients.

B. **Presentation and detection.** The most common presentations for HIV-associated NHL are constitutional symptoms (fevers, night sweats, and weight loss) or a rapidly enlarging mass. Extranodal presentations are common and occur in 75% to 95% of patients. The most common extranodal sites of involvement are the gastrointestinal tract, bone marrow, central nervous system (CNS), and liver. Very unusual sites have been seen as well, including the ear lobe, heart, and bile ducts. Seventy-five percent of patients present with advanced disease (stage III or IV).

C. **Staging.** The Ann Arbor staging classification is commonly used to stage HIV-related NHL (see Chap. 23); however, no direct correlation between stage and prognosis exists. Prognosis is more closely related to immune function. In one study, patients with CD4 lymphocyte counts of less than 100 cells/μL had a median survival of 4.1 months, whereas patients with CD4 lymphocyte counts greater than 100 cells/μL had a median survival of 24 months. Similarly, in a retrospective review of 60 patients, two prognostic subgroups were identified based on immune function, performance status, and bone marrow involvement (Table 26-5).

   Complete staging evaluation should include CT scans of the head, chest, abdomen, and pelvis; bilateral bone marrow biopsies; and lumbar puncture with cerebrospinal fluid (CSF) sent for protein and cytologic evaluation. Even in the absence of bone marrow involvement, 40% of patients have CNS involvement; therefore, all patients should undergo CSF evaluation regardless of clinical stage.

D. **Treatment**
   1. **General approach.** The best therapy for HIV-associated NHL remains to be defined. Fortunately, many clinical trials are ongoing to improve our understanding and treatment of this

Table 26-5. Prognostic stratification for HIV-associated non-Hodgkin's lymphoma (NHL)

Good Prognosis: Median survival = 11.3 mo

No prior AIDS diagnosis, *and*
Karnofsky performance status >70%, *and*
No bone marrow involvement

Poor Prognosis: Median survival = 4.0 mo

Prior AIDS diagnosis, *or*
Karnofsky performance status <70%, *or*
Bone marrow involvement

From Levine

disease. Therapy must be tailored to the overall
condition of each individual patient. In contrast
to non–HIV-related lymphoma, in which dose
intensity is important, increased dose intensity
is associated with decreased survival in HIV-
associated NHL. Patients treated with dose-
intensive therapy have an increased incidence
of opportunistic infections and an increased
rate of CNS relapse. Using a variety of "standard" lymphoma regimens, complete responses
are seen in about 50% of patients, of whom 25%
to 50% relapse within 6 months after completing therapy. Overall median survival time is
5 to 6 months. Half of the deaths are due to intercurrent opportunistic infections, and half are
due to progressive lymphoma.

2. **Systemic therapy.** Because of the high incidence of opportunistic infections, the limited
bone marrow reserve of these patients, and the
poor outcome with dose-intensive treatment, the
ACTG compared standard m-BACOD (Table
26-6) to low-dose (50% doses of cyclophosphamide and doxorubicin) m-BACOD in patients
with HIV-associated NHL. There was no difference in the complete response rate or median

**Table 26-6. Selected chemotherapy
regimens for HIV-associated non-Hodgkin's lymphoma**

Low dose m-BACOD	
Bleomycin	4 mg/m^2 i.v. day 1
Doxorubicin	25 mg/m^2 i.v. day 1
Cyclophosphamide	300 mg/m^2 i.v. day 1
Vincristine	1.4 mg/m^2 i.v. day 1 (not to exceed 2 mg total)
Dexamethasone	3 mg/m^2 p.o. days 1–5
Methotrexate	500 mg/m^2 i.v. day 15
Leucovorin	25 mg p.o. every 6 h for four doses, day 16 beginning exactly 24 h after methotrexate
CHOP	
Cyclophosphamide	750 mg/m^2 i.v. day 1
Doxorubicin	50 mg/m^2 i.v. day 1
Vincristine	1.4 mg/m^2 i.v. day 1, not to exceed 2 mg total
Prednisone	100 mg/m^2 p.o. days 1–5
CDE Chemotherapy	
Cyclophosphamide	200 mg/m^2/24 h CIV days 1–4
Doxorubicin	12.5 mg/m^2/24 h CIV days 1–4
Etoposide	60 mg/m^2/24 h CIV days 1–4

CIV, continuous intravenous infusion.

survival between the two groups, but the low-dose group had significantly less hematologic toxicity. This led to the recommendation of low-dose treatment, particularly for patients with CD4 counts of less than 200 cells/µL.

Based on data suggesting that longer exposure of tumor cells to drugs may enhance drug efficacy, a 4-day infusional regimen of cyclophosphamide, etoposide, and doxorubicin (CDE) has been evaluated in HIV-associated NHL. Early results are encouraging, and a confirmatory multi-institutional trial of this regimen is underway.

In patients who are not eligible for a randomized clinical trial, standard-dose CHOP, low-dose m-BACOD, and infusional CDE are reasonable therapeutic options (see Table 29-6). In the era of highly active antiretroviral therapy, it is not clear what dose of therapy should be recommended. For patients with good performance status and relatively preserved immune function, standard-dose treatment is most commonly recommended. Although treatment with highly active antiretroviral agents is important, the protease inhibitors may significantly alter the metabolism of chemotherapeutic agents and increase their toxicity. Recommendations for dose modifications based on these pharmacologic interactions are not yet available. Careful observation for increased or unusual toxicities is essential. Growth factor support is usually needed because this patient population often has decreased bone marrow reserve secondary to the HIV infection, to bone marrow infiltration by lymphoma, or to concurrent drug therapies. Aggressive prophylaxis against opportunistic infections is important. Regardless of CD4 lymphocyte count, all patients should receive prophylaxis for *Pneumocystis carinii* pneumonia during treatment of a high-grade lymphoma (Table 26-7).

3. **CNS prophylaxis.** CNS prophylaxis is recommended for patients with small noncleaved cell tumors or epidural, bone marrow, or paranasal sinus involvement. CNS prophylaxis should include four weekly treatments of either preservative-free methotrexate (12 mg) or cytosine-arabinoside (50 mg). In patients with documented meningeal disease, intrathecal therapy should be given three times per week until the CSF clears, then weekly for 8 weeks and monthly for 10 months. An Ommaya reservoir should be placed to facilitate therapy.

4. **Follow-up.** In this era of cost-containment, repeat staging studies are often controversial. De-

**Table 26-7. Prophylaxis regimens
for *Pneumocystis carinii* pneumonia**

Trimethoprim-sulfamethoxazole (Bactrim DS), 1 tablet p.o., M, W, F, *or*

Pentamidine, 300 mg in 6 mL sterile water by aerosol, every 4 wk, *or*
Dapsone, 100 mg po daily*

* Exclude glucose-6-phosphatase deficiency by quantitative spectrophotometry in high-risk patients before initiating therapy.

spite this zeal to minimize testing, documentation of a complete response as early as clinically warranted is important to minimize the duration of therapy in this already immunocompromised group of patients. Treatment should be continued for a minimum of four cycles, or for two cycles after attainment of complete response.

5. **Salvage therapy.** Some patients who relapse after initial treatment have been successfully treated with an alternate NHL regimen. There are currently no specific recommendations for salvage therapy.

IV. **Primary CNS lymphoma**

A. **Background.** PCNSL represents 10% to 20% of all cases of HIV-associated NHL. Unlike systemic HIV-associated NHL, which can occur at earlier stages of HIV infection, PCNSL typically occurs in profoundly immunocompromised patients with CD4 lymphocyte counts of less than 50 cells/µL. The Epstein-Barr virus (EBV) genome is identified in virtually all investigated cases of HIV-associated PCNSL. This supports the belief that EBV may have a direct etiologic role in the development of this disease.

B. **Presentation and detection.** The diagnosis of PCNSL is often difficult to make. Most patients present with a focal neurologic deficit. CT scan or magnetic resonance imaging (MRI) of the head typically shows single or multiple contrast-enhancing masses with surrounding edema. These lesions are often in a periventricular location and may be difficult to distinguish from those of toxoplasmosis. CSF cytology is rarely diagnostic, and stereotactic biopsy is often recommended to establish a tissue diagnosis. Because 95% of HIV-positive patients with toxoplasmosis have serologic evidence of *Toxoplasma* species infection, the *Toxoplasma* titer can be useful to determine a course of action.

- If the *Toxoplasma* titer is negative, stereotactic biopsy should be considered.
- If the *Toxoplasma* titer is positive and the patient is either clinically unstable or the clinician feels

uncomfortable without a tissue diagnosis based on the clinical scenario, stereotactic biopsy should be considered.

- If, however, the *Toxoplasma* titer is positive and the patient is clinically stable, a 1- to 2-week trial of empiric therapy for a presumptive diagnosis of toxoplasmosis may be appropriate. If there is no evidence of clinical or radiologic improvement, or if there is evidence of clinical decompensation, stereotactic biopsy should be considered.

This approach requires close and frequent monitoring for signs of neurologic deterioration or progression. A newer potential alternative to the above is the use of EBV polymerase chain reaction (PCR) in the spinal fluid as a diagnostic clue. The presence of EBV by PCR in the CSF is highly specific for primary PCNSL. This, in the context of both a suggestive MRI or CT of the brain and a positive thallium scan, may be considered highly suggestive of PCNSL in the absence of a tissue diagnosis.

C. **Treatment.** Whole-brain radiation therapy is the standard therapy. Temporary control and improvement of neurologic deficits occurs in 70% of patients. A range of radiation doses (2000 to 6000 cGy) has been used. In one retrospective review, survival was found to be a function of performance status, not the total radiation dose administered. Median survival is only 2 to 5 months. In responding patients, the usual cause of death is opportunistic infection, not progressive lymphoma. Therefore, patients need prophylaxis for multiple infectious pathogens. Treatment with combined modality therapy (CHOP plus radiation therapy) based on the experience in non–HIV-related PCNSLs, was evaluated and did not demonstrate superior results to radiation therapy alone.

V. **Cervical cancer**
A. **Background.** It was not until 1993 that cervical cancer became an AIDS-defining illness. As in non–HIV-infected women, the development of cervical squamous carcinoma has been directly linked to prior infection with human papilloma virus (HPV). Although both HIV and HPV are sexually transmitted diseases, other immunosuppressed populations also have an increased incidence of HPV infection, suggesting that immune competence is a deterrent to the development of HPV coinfection. The presence of HPV, especially types 16, 18, and 31, is correlated with a higher incidence of cervical intraepithelial neoplasia (CIN).
B. **Presentation and detection.** Presentation is similar to that of non–HIV-related cervical cancer, except the disease is often more aggressive in HIV-infected patients, and advanced disease is more common. Routine Papanicolaou's (Pap) smears may not be sensitive enough to detect this aggressive neoplasm. It has

been recommended that colposcopy, not Pap smears, be the standard for following HIV-infected women at high risk of CIN. Because CIN may progress at a faster rate in HIV-infected women, annual screening may not detect "curable" disease. Women with rapidly progressing CIN should probably be tested for HIV.

C. **Staging.** The FIGO staging system, used for non–HIV-infected patients, is used in this population as well (see Chap. 16). Stage for stage, however, the prognosis appears worse in HIV-infected women owing to their compromised immune function.

D. **Treatment.** In a small study, women with CD4 lymphocyte counts of less than 500 cells/μL did significantly worse than women with intact immune function. Until these results are confirmed in larger trials, HIV-positive women with invasive cervical cancer should be treated in the same manner as women without HIV infection.

VI. **Other malignancies**. Hodgkin's lymphoma, testicular carcinoma, and anal cancers are also seen frequently in HIV-infected patients. Anecdotally, these malignancies appear more aggressive than their usual counterpart in immunocompetent patients, but no large trial has yet confirmed either increased virulence or increased incidence. It is interesting to speculate that EBV may play a role in the development of Hodgkin's disease. The role of HPV in the development of anal cancers has been well described. We recommend treatment of these malignancies with standard therapy. However, close attention should be paid to the prophylaxis and treatment of opportunistic pathogens as well as to the appropriate use of antiretroviral agents.

SELECTED READINGS

Formenti SC, Gill PS, Lean E, et al. Primary central nervous system lymphoma in AIDS: results of radiation therapy. *Cancer* 1989;63:1101–1107.

Forsyth PA, DeAngelis LM. Biology and management of AIDS-associated primary CNS lymphomas. *Hematol Oncol Clin North Am* 1996;10:1125–1134.

Gill PS, Wernz J, Scadden DT, et al. Randomized phase II trial of liposomal daunorubicin (DaunoXome) versus doxorubicin, bleomycin, vincristine (ABV) in AIDS-related Kaposi's sarcoma. *J Clin Oncol* 1996;14:2353–2364.

Goldstein JD, Dickson DW, Moser FG, et al. Primary central nervous system lymphoma in acquired immune deficiency syndrome: a clinical and pathologic study with results of treatment with radiation. *Cancer* 1991;67:2756.

Kaplan L, Strauss D, Testa M, et al. Low-dose compared with standard dose m-BACOD chemotherapy for non-Hodgkin's lymphoma associated with human immunodeficiency virus infection. *N Engl J Med* 1997;336:1164–1648.

Knowles DM. Etiology and pathogenesis of AIDS-related non-Hodgkin's lymphoma. *Hematol Oncol Clin North Am* 1996;10:1081–1109.

Krown SE, Testa MA, Huang J. AIDS-related Kaposi's sarcoma: prospective validation of the AIDS Clinical Trials Group staging classification. *J Clin Oncol* 1997;15:3085–3092.

Levine AM, Sullivan-Halley J, Pike MC, et al. Human immunodeficiency virus-related lymphoma: prognostic factors predictive of survival. *Cancer* 1991;68:2466–2472.

Levine AM, Wernz JC, Kaplan L, et al. Low-dose chemotherapy with central nervous system prophylaxis and zidovudine maintenance in AIDS-related lymphoma. *JAMA* 1991;266:84–88.

Maiman M, Fruchter RG, Guy L, et al. Human immunodeficiency virus infection and invasive cervical carcinoma. *Cancer* 1993;71: 402–406.

Maiman M, Tarricone N, Vieira J, et al. Colposcopic evaluation of human immunodeficiency virus-seropositive women. *Obstet Gynecol* 1991;78:84–88.

Miles SA. Pathogenesis of AIDS-related Kaposi's sarcoma: evidence of a viral etiology. *Hematol Oncol Clin North Am* 1996;10:1011–1021.

Mitsuyasu RT. Interferon alpha in the treatment of AIDS-related Kaposi's sarcoma. *Br J Haematol* 1991;79[Suppl 1]:69–73.

Northfelt DW. Treatment of Kaposi's sarcoma. *Drugs* 1994;48:569–582.

Robinson WR, Morris CB. Cervical neoplasia: pathogenesis, diagnosis and management. *Hematol Oncol Clin North Am* 1996;10: 1163–1176.

Schafer A, Friedmann W, Mielke M, Schwartlander B, Koch MA. The increased frequency of cervical dysplasia-neoplasia in women infected with the human immunodeficiency virus is related to the degree of immunosuppression. *Am J Obstet Gynecol* 1991;164: 593–599.

Saville MW, Lietzau J, Pluda JM, et al. Treatment of HIV-associated Kaposi's sarcoma with paclitaxel. *Lancet* 1995;346:26–28.

Sparano JA, Wiernik PH, Strack M, Leaf A, Becker N, Valentine ES. Infusional cyclophosphamide, doxorubicin and etoposide in HIV-1 and HTLV-1-related non-Hodgkin's lymphoma: a highly active regimen. *Blood* 1993;81: 2810–2815.

Stelzer KJ, Griffin TW. A randomized prospective trial of radiation therapy for AIDS-associated Kaposi's sarcoma. *Int J Radiat Oncol Biol Phys* 1993;27:1057–1061.

Selected Aspects of Supportive Care of Patients with Cancer

27

Acute Reactions and Short-Term Side Effects of Cancer Chemotherapy

Janelle M. Tipton and Roland T. Skeel

Systemic cancer chemotherapy agents control tumor growth by interfering with the proliferation of cancer cells. Because cell replication is characteristic of normal cells as well as cancer cells, chemotherapeutic agents often have undesirable effects on normal tissue. Rapidly dividing normal cells that are vulnerable to damage include cells of the bone marrow, hair follicles, and mucous membranes. Other toxicities that are particular to the individual agents and not dependent on cell growth can occur. The side effects may be acute or chronic, self-limited or permanent, and mild or potentially life-threatening. Management of these side effects is of utmost importance because they can affect the tolerability and continuation of therapy in addition to overall quality of life.

I. **Acute Reactions**
   A. **Extravasation.** Extravasation is defined as the leakage or infiltration of drug into the subcutaneous tissues. *Vesicant* drugs that extravasate are capable of causing tissue necrosis or sloughing. *Irritant* drugs cause inflammation or pain at the site of extravasation.
      1. **Vesicant agents** that are commonly used include dactinomycin (actinomycin D), daunorubicin (daunomycin, Cerubidine), doxorubicin (Adriamycin), idarubicin (Idamycin), mitomycin (Mutamycin), mechlorethamine hydrochloride (nitrogen mustard, Mustargen), vinblastine (Velban), vincristine (Oncovin), vindesine (Eldisine), and vinorelbine (Navelbine).
      2. **Irritant agents** that are commonly used include carmustine (BCNU, BiCNU), dacarbazine (DTIC), etoposide (VP-16, VePesid), liposomal doxorubicin (Doxil), mitoxantrone (Novantrone), paclitaxel (Taxol), and teniposide (VM-26). Case reports have also indicated that in large extravasations of concentrated solutions, cisplatin (Platinol) and fluorouracil (5-FU) may be considered irritants.
      3. **Management of extravasation** is controversial, with some disagreement in the literature regarding antidotes. In addition, many of the studies concerning extravasation management have been in animals. Less than 6% of patients receiving peripheral intravenous chemotherapy experience vesicant extravasations. The most

effective management of extravasation is prevention. Nurses who administer chemotherapy need to stay abreast of extravasation guidelines in an effort to prevent or minimize the serious complications of extravasation. A complaint such as burning or pain at the site of vein cannulation should be considered a symptom of extravasation until proved otherwise. It is advantageous to have orders for extravasation management for common vesicant and irritant chemotherapy agents before administration. Extravasation kits with the necessary drug antidotes and supplies are also helpful to have available.

   a. **General procedures.** If an extravasation is suspected, the following actions should be taken:

      1. Stop administration of the chemotherapy agent.

      2. Leave the needle in place and immobilize the extremity.

      3. Aspirate any residual drug in the tubing, the needle, or the suspected extravasation site.

      4. Remove the needle.

      5. Avoid applying pressure to the extravasation site.

      6. Inject appropriate antidote drug for the specific chemotherapy drug that extravasated, as indicated.

      7. Apply warm or cold compresses as appropriate for the specific drug used.

      8. Elevate the arm.

      9. Notify the responsible physician of the occurrence and discuss the need for further intervention and photographing of the suspected area of extravasation.

   b. **Recommended procedures for specific agents.** Antidotes and dosages for specific chemotherapeutic agents listed in Table 27-1 are based on current data in the literature. Little information is available on antidotes for other chemotherapy agents. As new investigational agents emerge, it is important to examine the literature for possible extravasation guidelines.

B. **Hypersensitivity and anaphylaxis.** Specific drugs with the potential for hypersensitivity with or without an anaphylactic response should be administered under constant supervision of a nurse knowledgeable about chemotherapy and with a physician readily available, preferably during the daytime hours. An allergy history should be documented but may not predict an allergic reaction to chemotherapy. The

Table 27-1.   Antidotes for vesicant and irritant drugs

Chemotherapy agent	Pharmacologic antidote	Nonpharmacologic antidote	Method of administration
Mechlorethamine (nitrogen mustard)	Sodium thiosulfate	None	Prepare 1/6 molar solution: If 10% Na thiosulfate solution, mix 4 mL with 6 mL sterile water for injection. Through existing i.v. line, inject 2 mL for every 1 mg extravasated. Inject s.c. if needle is removed.
Vincristine (Oncovin) Vinblastine (Velban) Vindesine (VP-16) Etoposide (VP-16) Teniposide (VM-26) Vinorelbine (Navelbine)	Hyaluronidase (Wydase)	Warm compresses, 15–20 min at least four times/day for the first 24–48 h and elevate	Prepare hyaluronidase, 150 units/mL with 1–3 mL saline. Inject through existing i.v. line, 1 mL for each 1 mL infiltrated. Inject s.c. if needle is removed.
Doxorubicin (Adriamycin) Daunorubicin (Daunomycin) Idarubicin (Idamycin)	None	Topical cooling	Apply cold pad with circulating ice water, ice pack, or cryogel pack for 15–20 min at least four times/day for first 24–48 h. Some research studies suggest benefit of 99% dimethyl sulfoxide (DMSO) 1–2 mL applied to site every 6 h.

drug most commonly associated with anaphylaxis is L-asparaginase. Other drugs for which hypersensitivity reactions may occur include bleomycin (with lymphoma), paclitaxel, cisplatin, melphalan (given intravenously), doxorubicin, and docetaxel. If a drug is known to have an increased incidence of hypersensitivity response, a test dose or skin test may be performed. This is generally done only with bleomycin and asparaginase. The hypersensitivity reactions experienced by patients receiving cancer chemotherapy agents are typically type I reactions. The reactions characteristically occur within 1 hour of receiving the drug but can occur up to 24 hours after exposure. The manifestations of a type I reaction include urticaria, bronchospasm, and anxiety, but can progress to cardiovascular collapse and shock. Patients may also be premedicated prophylactically with corticosteroids, histamine antagonists (both classic H_1-receptor antagonists such as diphenhydramine and H_2-receptor antagonists such as ranitidine), or both to prevent possible reactions. Emergency equipment that should be immediately accessible includes oxygen, an AMBU respiratory assist bag, and intubation equipment. The following parenteral drugs must also be stocked in the treatment area: epinephrine, 1:1,000 or 1:10,000 solution; diphenhydramine, 25 to 50 mg; methylprednisolone, 250 mg (or hydrocortisone, 250 mg); and dexamethasone, 10 to 20 mg.

The development of an anaphylaxis clinical guideline may be helpful in preparing for the potential anaphylactic reaction, reducing delays in response time to an anaphylactic event, and standardizing the management of an anaphylactic reaction with preprinted orders. An example of a grading scale that may be used with anaphylactic symptoms is given in Table 27-2. This grading scale could be used in conjunction with anaphylaxis preprinted orders. A sample anaphylaxis preprinted order sheet or guideline is presented in Table 27-3.

II. **Nausea and vomiting.** Patients who are about to begin chemotherapy are often concerned and apprehensive about nausea and vomiting. Nausea and vomiting can be distressing enough to the patient to cause extreme physiologic and psychological discomfort, culminating in withdrawal from therapy. With the advent of more effective antiemetic regimens in the past 10 years, many improvements in the prevention and control of nausea and vomiting have led to a better quality of life for patients receiving chemotherapy. The goal of therapy is to prevent the three phases of nausea and vomiting: that which occurs before the treatment is administered (anticipatory), that which follows within the first 24 hours after the treatment (acute), and that which occurs more than 24 hours after the treatment (delayed). It is also important to assess nausea and vomiting separately because they are different

Table 27-2.   Grading scale for anaphylactic symptoms

Grade	Definition
1	Localized reaction with hives <6 cm
2	Generalized reaction with multiple, widely spread hives each <6 cm, *or* a severe localized reaction with hives measuring >6 cm
3	Severe bronchospasm, difficulty breathing, chest tightness, cough, chills, vomiting, tachycardia, agitation, serum sickness
4	Anaphylaxis, severe hypotension, shock, *or* any of the above symptoms plus hypotension and shock (cardiovascular collapse)

events and may have different causes. Factors related to the chemotherapy that can affect the likelihood and severity of symptoms include the specific agents used, the doses of the drugs, and the schedule and route of administration.

A. **Emetic potential of the drug.** To plan an effective approach to control nausea and vomiting, the chemotherapeutic agents are grouped according to their emetic potential (Table 27-4). This type of categorization is helpful in making decisions regarding possible antiemetics to be used and how aggressive the antiemetic regimen should be for patients receiving chemotherapy for the first time or in subsequent treatments.

B. **Antiemetic drugs.** Agents that have been effective in preventing and treating nausea and vomiting (Table 27-5) come from various pharmacologic classes. They work by different mechanisms that may relate to the pathophysiologic processes causing nausea and vomiting. For many years, the mainstays of antiemetic therapy have been agents that block dopamine receptors. These agents have been somewhat effective but have limited value for highly emetogenic agents and, in escalating doses, have caused problematic side effects. Within in the past 10 years, it was discovered that agents that block predominately the serotonin (5-hydroxytryptamine) subtype 3 (5-HT3) receptors, rather than the dopamine receptors, have greater efficacy in the prevention of nausea and vomiting. It is important to use an antiemetic regimen sufficient to prevent nausea and vomiting to the greatest degree possible to avoid the development of conditioned responses and failure of antiemetic therapy.

C. **Combination antiemetic therapy.** Several antiemetic regimens are effective, but their design should be based on several general principles:

   1. Combinations of antiemetics have been shown to be more effective than single agents. It is common to use two or more antiemetics to prevent or manage nausea and vomiting.

Table 27-3.   Anaphylaxis precaution guideline preprinted orders

1. Patient height_____(cm) weight_____(kg)   BSA_____
   _____(in)   _____(lbs)

2. The following medications will be at the patient's bedside:
   a. Diphenhydramine (Benadryl), 50 mg i.v.
   b. Epinephrine (1:10,000), 10 mL/single dose vial (or 1 mL of 1:1000) = 1 mg/vial
   c. Methylprednisilone (Solu-Medrol), 250 mg i.v. (or equivalent hydrocortisone)

3. **Observe for signs and symptoms of a grade 1 or 2 reaction:**

Grade 1: Localized reaction with hives <6 cm
Grade 2: Generalized reaction with multiple, widely spread hives each <6 cm, *or* a severe localized reaction with hives measuring >6 cm

   a. **If the patient develops any of the above symptoms,** maintain i.v. access with i.v. fluids or NS at 100 mL/m^2/h _____mL/h.
   b. Notify the attending physician or house officer immediately of any signs or symptoms of a reaction of any severity.
   c. Administer the following medications for a **grade 1 or 2 reactions**
      Diphenhydramine (Benadryl), _____mg (1 mg/kg) i.v. push (maximum dose, 50 mg)
      Hydrocortisone, _____mg (2 mg/kg) i.v. push (maximum dose, 250 mg)

4. **Observe for signs and symptoms of a grade 3 or 4 reaction:**

Grade 3 Severe bronchospasm, difficulty breathing, chest tightness, cough, chills, vomiting, tachycardia, agitation, serum sickness
Grade 4 Anaphylaxis, severe hypotension, shock, *or* any of the above symptoms plus hypotension and shock (cardiovascular collapse)

   a. **If the patient develops any of the above symptoms,** maintain i.v. access with i.v. fluids or NS at 100 mL/m^2/h _____mL/h.
   b. Notify the attending physician or house officer immediately of any signs or symptoms of a reaction of any severity.
   c. Administer the following medications for a **grade 3 or 4 reaction:**
      Epinephrine (1:10,000 = 0.1 mg/mL), _____mL (0.01 mg/kg = 5–10 mL) slow i.v. push (maximum, 10 mL/single dose vial) May repeat two times per physician's order.
      Follow epinephrine with:
         Diphenhydramine (Benadryl), _____mg(1 mg/kg) i.v. push (maximum dose, 50 mg)
         Methylprednisilone, _____mg (2 mg/kg) i.v. push (maximum dose, 250 mg)

5. Administer oxygen and pulse oximetry as needed for respiratory difficulty.

6. Obtain vital signs every 2–5 min until patient is stable.

**Table 27-4.   Emetogenic potential for
commonly used chemotherapeutic agents***

Highly emetogenic agents (75% or greater potential for nausea, vomiting, or both)	Moderately emetogenic agents (50%–75% potential for nausea, vomiting, or both)	Mildly emetogenic agents (25%–50% potential for nausea, vomiting, or both)
Carmustine	Carboplatin	Asparaginase
Cisplatin (>40 mg/m^2)	Cisplatin (<40 mg/m^2)	Bleomycin
Cyclophosphamide (>1 g/m^2)	Cyclophosphamide (200 mg/m^2 to 1 g/m^2)	Busulfan
Cytarabine (>1 g/m^2)	Cytarabine (200mg/m^2 to 1 g/m^2)	Chlorambucil
Dacarbazine (days 1 and 2)	Daunorubicin	Cladribine
Dactinomycin	Doxorubicin (<60 mg/m^2)	Cyclophosphamide (<200 mg/m^2)
Doxorubicin (>60 mg/m^2)	Etoposide	Cytarabine (<200 mg/m^2)
Ifosfamide (>1.2 g/m^2)	Gemcitabine	Docetaxel
Mechlorethamine	Idarubicin	Fludarabine
Methotrexate (>1.2 g/m^2)	Ifosfamide (<1.2 g/m^2)	Fluorouracil
Mitomycin (>15 mg/m^2)	Irinotecan	Hydroxyurea
Streptozocin	Methotrexate (100 mg/m^2 to 1.2 g/m^2)	Liposomal doxorubicin
	Mitomycin (<15 mg/m^2)	Melphalan
	Mitoxantrone	Methotrexate (<100 mg/m^2)
	Topotecan	Paclitaxel
	Vinorelbine	Thioguanine or mercaptopurine (6-MP)
		Thiotepa
		Vinblastine
		Vincristine

* High-dose therapy requiring progenitor cell support is not included in this table.

2. Preemptive treatment and scheduled administration are also necessary to prevent nausea and vomiting early in therapy and to manage potential delayed nausea and vomiting for several hours or days. Table 27-6 shows examples of antiemetic regimens that may be used when the chemotherapy has a high, moderate, and low emetic potential.

D. Nonpharmacologic interventions. Patients who are likely to experience or have experienced anticipatory nausea and vomiting related to chemotherapy may benefit from the use of nonpharmacologic interventions in addition to the pharmacologic agents taken. The use of guided imagery, massage therapy, music therapy, and self-hypnosis show some effec-

Table 27-5.   Management of acute chemotherapy-induced nausea and vomiting

Agent	Route of administration	Dose	Comments
Phenothiazines			
Prochlorperazine (Compazine)	p.o.	10 mg q 4–6 h	Some extrapyramidal symptoms (EPS)
	p.o. (sustained release)	15–30 mg q 12 h	Potential for postural hypotension when given i.v.
	i.m. or i.v.	2–10 mg q 4–6 h	
	p.r.	25 mg q 8–12 h	
Thiethylperazine (Torecan)	p.o	10 mg q 6–8 h	Some EPS
	i.m. or p.r.		
Trimethobenzamide (Tigan)	p.o.	250 mg q 4–6 h	Some EPS
	i.m. or p.r.	200 mg q 4–6 h	
Butyrophenones			
Haloperidol (Haldol)	i.m. or p.o.	2–5 mg q 2–4 h	Some EPS
	i.v.		
Droperidol (Inapsine)	i.v. or i.m.	0.5–2.5 mg q 4 h	Causes sedation, EPS, hypotension
Substituted Benzamide			
Metoclopramide (Reglan)	p.o.	10–40 mg q.i.d. to 1–2 mg/kg dose at 2-h intervals	EPS common in higher doses; should be given with diphenhydramine; EPS worse with younger patients; may have diarrhea in higher doses
	i.v.		

Benzodiazapines

Lorazepam (Ativan)	p.o. or s.l.	1–2 mg q 4–6 h	Causes sedation, amnesia, and confusion
	i.v.	0.5 to 2 mg q 4–6 h	
Corticosteroids			
Dexamethasone (Decadron)	i.v.	4–20 mg (10–20 mg × 1, otherwise q 4–6 h	Potential for agitation, delirium
	p.o.	4–8 mg q 4 h	
Serotonin (5-HT₃) Antagonists			
Ondansetron (Zofran)	i.v.	8–32 mg × 1	For highly emetogenic chemotherapy
		0.15 mg/kg, q 4 h × 3	Lower doses effective for less emetogenic regimens
	p.o.	8 mg q 8 h	
Granisetron (Kytril)	i.v.	10 μg/kg × 1	Similar to ondansetron
	p.o.	2 mg before or 1 mg q 12 h	
Dolasetron (Anzemet)	i.v. or p.o.	100 mg before (once daily)	Similar to the above
Cannabinoids			
Dronabinol (Marinol)	p.o.	2.5–10 mg q 4–6 h	Causes sedation, may be habit-forming, a controlled substance

**Table 27-6.   Examples of regimens for
antiemetic prevention and management of
chemotherapy-induced nausea and vomiting**

Level I: Patients receiving a mildly emetogenic agent

Prochlorperazine, 10 mg p.o. before chemotherapy, then 10 mg p.o.
 q 4–6 h p.r.n.
With or without
Dexamethasone, 4 mg p.o. before chemotherapy, *and*
Lorazepam, 1 mg p.o. q 4–6 h p.r.n.

**Level II: Patients Receiving a Moderately Emetogenic Agent or
Patients Receiving a Mildly Emetogenic Agent Who Have Failed to
Respond to or Are Intolerant of at Least Two Level 1 Regimens**

Dolasetron,* 100 mg p.o. or i.v. before chemotherapy, *and*
Dexamethasone, 8 mg p.o. or 10 mg i.v. before chemotherapy
With or without
Lorazepam, 1 mg p.o. or i.v. before q 4–6 h p.r.n., *and*
Prochlorperazine, 10 mg p.o. q 4–6 h p.r.n.
*Alternatives (5-HT₃)
  Ondansetron, 10 mg i.v. × 1 before chemotherapy, *or*
  Granisetron, 10 µg/kg i.v. or 1 mg p.o. before chemotherapy

**Level III: Patients receiving a highly emetogenic agent patients
receiving 2 or more moderately emetogenic agents, patients who
have failed a level 2 regimen**

Dolasetron,* 100 mg p.o. or i.v. before chemotherapy, *and*
Dexamethasone, 8 mg p.o. or 10–20 mg i.v. before chemotherapy, *and*
Lorazepam, 1 mg p.o. or i.v. before chemotherapy, then q 4–6 h p.r.n.
In Addition, for Delayed Nausea and Vomiting:
Metoclopramide, 40 mg p.o. q 6 h × 4 days, *or*
Compazine spansules, 15–30 mg p.o. q 12 h × 4 days, *with*
Dexamethasone, 4 mg p.o. q 6 h × days, then 4 mg p.o. q 12 h × 1 day
*Alternatives (5-HT₃ antagonists)
  Ondansetron 32 mg i.v. before chemotherapy
  Granisetron, 10 µg/kg i.v. or 2 mg p.o. before chemotherapy

tiveness in preventing nausea and vomiting. These forms of distraction assist patients in maintaining a feeling of control over their treatment effects. Patients who are able to have little or no nausea and vomiting with their first chemotherapy treatment often assert that positive thinking is helpful as well. Patients may also prepare for their chemotherapy treatments by eating foods that do not have offensive odors or spicy taste. Clear liquids, foods served at room temperature, soda crackers, and carbonated beverages are sometimes good suggestions. Some patients prefer to receive their therapy at night, so as to sleep during the periods when nausea and vomiting may occur.

III. Other short-term complications related to cancer chemotherapy

A. Stomatitis and other oral complications. The oral mucosa is vulnerable to the effects of chemotherapy and radiotherapy because of its rapid growth and cell turnover rate. Radiotherapy also interferes with the production of saliva and may increase oral complications because of a consequent reduction in the protective effect of the saliva. It is crucial to manage oral complications effectively because patients may experience considerable discomfort or develop secondary infections from the disruption of the oral mucosa. The likelihood of the development of stomatitis from a drug is dependent on the agent, the dose, and the schedule of administration. Continuous rather than intermittent administration is more likely to cause stomatitis with the antimetabolites.

1. Specific chemotherapy agents that may cause stomatitis include the following:

Antimetabolites: methotrexate, fluorouracil, cytarabine, irinotecan

Antitumor antibiotics: doxorubicin, dactinomycin, mitomycin, bleomycin

Plant alkaloids: vincristine, vinblastine, etoposide

Others: alkylating agents in high doses

Biologic agents: interleukins, lymphokine-activated killer cell therapy

2. Prevention and early detection. If oral complications are anticipated, it is important to implement a good oral hygiene program before the initiation of therapy. Maintaining good nutrition and dental hygiene is also a primary preventive measure. Systemic oral assessments should be integrated into the physical examination at regular intervals (e.g., one or two times a day). Special attention should be given to the tongue, the gingiva, the buccal mucosa, the soft palate, and the lips. It is also important to assess the patient for soreness, functional ability to swallow, and any effects on eating.

3. Management of oral complications. Although the primary goal is prevention, once oral complications develop, the focus of care should shift to the continuation of good oral hygiene and treatment of symptoms. Agents used for oral care are categorized according to function: cleansing agents, lubricating agents, and analgesic agents. Table 27-7 lists several commonly used agents. Commercial mouthwashes and lemon glycerin swabs are not recommended for use because of their irritating and drying effects. A common oral care agent used is chlorhexidine, 15 mL, which is swished and expectorated twice a day. If painful ulcerations do

Table 27-7.   Agents for oral care

Agent	Indications and comments
Cleansing Agents	
Normal saline solution (½ tsp salt in 8 oz water)	Economical, nondamaging
Hydrogen peroxide (mix with normal saline or tap water)	Germicidal, débriding
Sodium bicarbonate	Nonirritating, débriding
Chlorhexidine (15 mL swish and spit b.i.d.)	May decrease infection
Lubricating agents	
Saliva substitutes	Decreases dryness
Water or oil-based lubricants	Useful emollient; oil-based lubricants should not be used in the mouth because of danger of aspiration
Analgesic Agents	
a. Healing and coating agents	
Sulcralfate	Binds to mucosa, forms protective coating
Vitamin E	Protection to mucosa, healing properties
Antacids	Enhance comfort, coat mucosa
Allopurinol	May decrease intensity of mucositis
b. Topical anesthetics	
Lidocaine viscous	Transient pain relief, absorbed systemically
Diclonime hydrochloride	Transient pain relief
Benzocaine	Transient pain relief
Zilactin	Burns on application
c. Systemic analgesics	
Nonsteroidal antiinflammatory drugs	Take before meals and as needed
Narcotic analgesics	

develop, topical relief may be obtained by using a stomatitis mixture containing diphenhydramine (Benadryl) elixir, 5 mL, antacid (Maalox), 30 mL, and viscous lidocaine (Xylocaine), 5 mL. Systemic pain control measures, such as oral or parenteral narcotics, should be implemented if topical analgesics are ineffective.

4. **Xerostomia** that follows radiation therapy to the mouth area may require treatment with artificial saliva. It may also be benefited by the

administration of pilocarpine, 5 to 10 mg p.o. t.i.d., before meals. Before the initiation of radiation therapy to the head and neck area, dental consultation is necessary to evaluate oral hygiene, the state of repair of the teeth, and the health of the gums.

5. **Secondary oral infections** should be treated promptly and as accurately as possible. Fungal infections may be treated with nystatin (Mycostatin) suspension, clotrimazole troches, or oral fluconazole. Viral infections may be reactivated after chemotherapy and are commonly treated with oral or intravenous acyclovir. The benefit of prophylactic use of antiviral agents or antifungal agents is not well established. However, in patients with a known history of cold sores or positive herpes simplex virus titers, it may be advantageous to administer prophylactic acyclovir.

Patients with dentures may be encouraged to remove them during the period after chemotherapy when they are at risk for infection, except at mealtime. In addition, the dentures should be cleansed before use. Although removal of the dentures may be detrimental to the patient's self-esteem, irritation of the dentures may lead to inflammation, ulceration, and secondary infection.

B. **Alopecia.** Chemotherapy-induced hair loss is not necessarily a serious physiologic complication, but psychologically, it can be one of the most devastating side effects. Partial or total hair loss can contribute to a perceived negative body image owing to the emphasis placed on the hair and overall appearance in society. The hair loss from chemotherapy, which often occurs 2 to 3 weeks after chemotherapy, is usually temporary, and hair growth returns in about 1 to 2 months after the treatment is completed. The new hair may have a different texture or color than its pretreatment characteristics.

1. **Specific chemotherapy agents** with a high potential of causing alopecia include doxorubicin, cyclophosphamide, ifosfamide, vincristine, and paclitaxel. Other drugs capable of causing alopecia include bleomycin, dactinomycin, daunorubicin, etoposide, vinblastine, methotrexate, and mitoxantrone.

2. **Nursing interventions** start with informing and preparing the patient for the possibility of alopecia. It is helpful to encourage purchasing wigs and other headwear before the alopecia occurs so that the hair color and style may used in selecting a wig as well as allowing time for adjustment. It is important to encourage discussion of feelings regarding the hair loss for both

men and women and to recognize their concerns and fears. Scalp hypothermia has been used in the past as an attempt to restrict the circulation to the scalp, with the goal of minimizing alopecia. Because of the concern for scalp metastases and sanctuary sites, scalp hypothermia is no longer recommended.

C. **Diarrhea.** Among the many causes of diarrhea in patients with cancer are chemotherapy, radiotherapy, the cancer itself, medications, supplemental feedings, and anxiety. Infectious causes (e.g., *Clostridium difficile* or other enterocolitis-causing bacteria) always need to be considered in the hospitalized neutropenic patient receiving antibiotics. Prolonged diarrhea can lead to discomfort, severe electrolyte imbalances and dehydration, altered social life, and poor quality of life.

1. **Chemotherapy and biologic agents** may contribute to the development of diarrhea and most commonly include the antimetabolites, such as fluorouracil, methotrexate, cytarabine, and azacitidine. In addition, agents such as dactinomycin, floxuridine, hydroxyurea, idarubicin, irinotecan, the nitrosoureas, and paclitaxel relatively frequently cause diarrhea. When diarrhea from fluorouracil, floxuridine, or irinotecan is present while on therapy, it is a sign of toxicity that must be monitored closely and could escalate to severe levels at which the drug may need to be held or discontinued. With the increased use of biologic agents, diarrhea has been noted with interferon-α and interleukin-2. High-dose chemotherapy regimens used in stem cell transplantation may also be associated with severe diarrhea.

2. **Assessment** of a patient experiencing diarrhea should begin with a baseline history of usual elimination patterns, pattern of symptoms, and concurrent medications. In particular, the duration of the diarrhea and frequency of stool passage should be noted with reference to a stool diary if indicated. The physical examination may disclose abdominal tenderness, signs of dehydration, and disruption in perianal or peristomal skin integrity. Laboratory data may be obtained to assess serum chemistries, complete blood count, and stool samples for *C. difficile* toxin and other enteropathic bacteria.

3. **Management** of treatment-related diarrhea is often symptomatic and requires little or no alteration in cancer therapy. Agents that decrease bowel motility should not be used for longer than 24 hours unless significant infections have been excluded. In the absence of obvious inflammation and infection, it is appropriate to treat most patients with nonspecific treatment for

diarrhea, including opioids (loperamide, diphenoxylate, and codeine), anticholinergics (atropine, scopolamine), or both. More recently, it has been recognized that octreotide is often effective in controlling chemotherapy-related diarrhea and diarrhea associated with the carcinoid syndrome. Table 27-8 lists common agents used to treat diarrhea. Nonpharmacologic measures that may also assist in the prevention and management of diarrhea are a low-residue diet and increased fluids. If the diarrhea is severe, intravenous hydration is necessary to prevent serious hypovolemia, electrolyte disturbances, and shock.

D. **Constipation.** In patients whose cancer has resulted in debility or immobility, or in those who require narcotic analgesics, constipation can be a particular problem. Constipation may also develop in patients who have received neurotoxic chemotherapy agents, including the vinca alkaloids, etoposide, and cisplatin, each of which may cause autonomic dysfunction. Decreased bowel motility due to intraabdominal disease, hypercalcemia, or dehydration can also contribute to constipation. Chronic constipation in patients with cancer is a problem that is more easily prevented than treated. A diet high in bulk fiber, fresh fruits and vegetables, and adequate fluid intake may help to minimize constipation. Pa-

Table 27-8. **Pharmacologic management strategies for diarrhea**

Agent	Comments
Kaolin pectin (Kaopectate)	30–60 mL p.o. after each loose stool
Loperamide (Imodium)	2 capsules (4 mg) p.o. 4 h initially, then add 1 capsule (2 mg) after each loose stool; should not exceed 16 capsules daily
Diphenoxylate hydrochloride, antropine sulfate (Lomotil)	1–2 tablets p.o. 4 h; should not exceed 8 tablets daily; there may be anticholinergic effects due to atropine
Paregoric	1 tsp p.o. 4 times a day; may alternate with Lomotil
Octreotide	May be useful for fluorouracil-induced diarrhea; starting dose: 0.05–0.1 mg s.c. t.i.d; may be increased to 1.8 mg/day in refractory diarrhea

tients started on narcotic analgesics should also begin a bowel regimen, first with mild stool softeners and bulk laxatives, and then proceeding to stimulants or osmotic laxatives if the milder regimen is not effective. A bowel regimen example for a patient at risk for constipation is as follows:

1. Docusate sodium, 100 mg b.i.d. alone, or with casanthranol (Peri-Colace), 1 capsule b.i.d.
2. If no bowel movement, add:
   a. Senna at bedtime (dose varies with the preparation), *or*
   b. Milk of magnesia, 30 mL at bedtime
3. If no bowel movement with the above, may add:
   a. Biscodyl, 1 to 3 tablets or one 1 10-mg suppository, at bedtime, *or*
   b. Lactulose, 1 to 4 tablespoons daily
4. Other, more aggressive alternatives include:
   a. Cisapride, 10 to 20 mg p.o. q.i.d.
   b. Fleet enema
   c. Magnesium citrate, 1 bottle
   d. Tap-water enema

E. **Altered nutritional status.** Patients with cancer often experience progressive loss of appetite and sometimes severe malnutrition during the course of the disease and treatment. Malnutrition may result from a side effect of the therapy or a direct effect of the cancer (e.g., gut obstruction or hepatic or brain metastases). The resulting effects of malnutrition are a poorer response to therapy, increased incidence of infections, and an overall worsening of patient well-being. Many times, one of the presenting signs that leads to the diagnosis of cancer is weight loss; therefore, the patient is most likely already experiencing some alteration in nutritional status. Malnutrition is reported to occur in 50% to 80% of patients with advanced disease. Nutritional management of the patient with cancer involves early intervention using a supportive health care team.

1. **Effects of chemotherapy and radiation therapy on nutrition.** Chemotherapy has a major effect on nutritional status because of the direct insult on the gastrointestinal tract. Among the gastrointestinal effects are anorexia, nausea, vomiting, taste alterations, stomatitis, esophagitis, colitis, constipation, and diarrhea. Not only are the effects physiologic in nature, but also the added psychologic impact of the disease and therapy can result in anxiety and depression, which can contribute to the lack of interest in food.

2. **Nutritional assessment.** Early in the patient's treatment, a thorough nutritional assessment should be completed by the health care team. The assessment should include diet history,

nutrient intake, anthopometric measurements (height, weight, and skinfold thickness and mid-arm circumference if possible), laboratory tests for anemia and serum albumin, and an evaluation of activity and functional status. A good nutritional assessment may help to identify patients who are already at risk of malnutrition or those who may be prone to develop problems during the course of the illness and treatment.

3. **Nutritional intervention.** Nutritional intervention should be considered during the initial and ongoing assessments. Situations that warrant nutritional intervention include involuntary weight loss (more than 10% within the past 6 months, especially when combined with weakness and fatigue), history of recent physiologic stress, serum albumin below 3.2 g/dL, or severe immunocompromise. Nurses, dietitians, and even family members can identify problems and may be the first to act to promote weight gain. Various approaches to help increase weight are changes in diet; symptomatic treatment of nausea and vomiting, stomatitis, and other gastrointestinal effects of chemotherapy; and supplemental nutrition.

   a. **Nutritional supplements.** Several nutritional supplements are commercially available for oral use. One benefit of nutritional supplements is that they are a concentrated form of nutrition for protein and calories. Some of the disadvantages are the unappealing taste and the high cost to the consumer. Some patients and their families are able to develop some creative high protein and calorie supplements using household items with some suggestions from the health care team.

   b. **Tube feedings.** Enteral nutrition through a nasogastric or gastrostomy tube may be an alternative if oral intake is not possible. Enteral feedings are the recommended route if the gastrointestinal tract is functional. Advantages of enteral feeding include lower cost and fewer complications than with parenteral feedings, and maintenance of normal gastrointestinal function. Some care and maintenance are involved with feeding tubes, and patients and their families need to be given information regarding available options for feeding.

   c. **Total parenteral nutrition (TPN).** Parenteral nutrition should be considered in patients who do not have a functioning gastrointestinal tract or in those for whom supplemental nutrition is anticipated for a short period of time. Patients who receive TPN usually require the insertion of a central venous catheter, which may result in other iatrogenic complications, such as pneumothorax, vein thrombosis, and catheter-related infections. In many situations, TPN used in the patient with cancer increases morbidity, especially from infection, without improving survival. Thus, TPN has considerable economic, ethical, and medical consequences that must be evaluated in conjunction with the patient's overall prognosis.

4. **Pharmacologic interventions.** A recent area of interest is pharmacologic appetite stimulation. One of the agents currently used is megestrol acetate oral suspension, 800 mg/day (20 mL/day). Agents such as megestrol acetate have documented evidence in promoting increased weight gain in some patients, and at least a decreased weight loss in others.

F. **Neurotoxicity.** The incidence of neurotoxicity associated with chemotherapy is increasing, potentially because of the greater use of high-dose chemotherapy and newer drugs causing neurotoxicity used in combination. In many cases, early detection and treatment of neurotoxicity (i.e., reduction of drug dose or discontinuation) allows for the reversal of symptoms. The neurotoxic symptoms may manifest as altered level of consciousness or coma, cerebellar dysfunction, ototoxicity, or peripheral neuropathy, which may be temporary but can cause significant changes in functional ability that persist as a long-term effect. It is also important to assess renal function because poor renal function may reduce clearance of the chemotherapy agent, leading to increased neurotoxicity.

1. **Chemotherapy and biologic agents** with known potential for neurotoxicity include high-dose cytarabine, high-dose methotrexate, vincristine, vinblastine, vinorelbine, ifosfamide, cisplatin, carboplatin, paclitaxel, procarbazine, interleukin-2, and the interferons.

2. **Prevention and early detection** of neurotoxicity is key to prevention of permanent neurologic damage. Assessment of symptoms of neurotoxicity should be documented on a routine basis. In certain treatment regimens, altering the drug order can markedly decrease the symptoms.

3. **Management** of peripheral neurotoxicity is being studied, with the goal of slowing, halting, and reversing the neuropathy. One agent that has shown promise in early trials is the cytoprotectant amifostine.

SELECTED READINGS

Cascinu S, Fedeli A, Fedeli SL, Catalano G. Octreotide versus loperamide in the treatment of fluorouracil-induced diarrhea: a randomized trial. *J Clin Oncol* 1993;11:148–151.

Hesketh P, Kris M, Grunberg S, et al. Proposal for classifying the acute emetogenicity of cancer chemotherapy. *J Clin Oncol* 1997;15:103–109.

Hesketh P, Navari R, Grote T, et al. Double-blind, randomized comparison of antiemetic efficacy of intravenous dolasetron and ondansetron in the prevention of acute cisplatin-induced emesis. *J Clin Oncol* 1996;14:2242–2249.

Kemp G, Rose P, Lurain J, et al. Amifostine pretreatment for protection against cyclophosphamide-induced and cisplatin-induced toxicities: results of a randomized control trial in patients with advanced ovarian cancer. *J Clin Oncol* 1996;14:2101–2112.

Oncology Nursing Society. *Cancer Chemotherapy Guidelines and Recommendations for Practice.* Pittsburgh: Oncology Nursing Press, 1996.

Weiss RB. Hypersensitivity reactions. *Semin Oncol* 1992;19(5):458–77.

Infections: Etiology, Treatment, and Prevention

Rodger D. MacArthur

Infection is a major source of morbidity and mortality among patients with cancer, despite recent advances in prevention and treatment. In many series, infection is the most frequent cause of death, exceeding all other causes combined. Granulocytopenia, cellular immune dysfunction, humoral immune dysfunction, and splenectomy can each predispose patients to certain types of infections. In addition, mucosal or integumentary damage, prolonged hospitalization, lack of ambulation, malnutrition, neurologic dysfunction, and local tumor effect all contribute to the risk of infection.

Most bacterial and fungal infections in cancer patients arise from the patients' own flora. Environmental reservoirs may also contribute to infection in certain circumstances. Prolonged hospitalization and antibiotic use tend to favor the acquisition of resistant strains of organisms. Careful hand washing by health care workers is the most important means of reducing the occurrence of infection. Reverse isolation of patients can be justified only rarely. The prompt initiation of therapy with broad-spectrum antibiotics in documented and suspected bacterial infections is essential. The addition of antifungal therapy should be considered in patients who do not respond within a reasonable period of time to antibiotics. Daily reevaluation of all patients is critical. Appropriate diagnostic studies (e.g., computed tomography [CT] scans, bronchoscopy, cultures) should be obtained earlier, rather than later, in the evaluation of any febrile patient with cancer.

I. **Reasons for infection**
   A. **Granulocytopenia**
      1. **General comments.** Acute leukemias or lymphomas after chemotherapy are prototypical malignancies in which infection resulting from granulocytopenia is seen. An increase in the incidence of infection can be expected when the granulocyte count is less than 500/µL. A substantial increase in both the incidence and severity of infection occurs when there are fewer than 100 granulocytes/µL. Infection early in the course of granulocytopenia typically is caused by relatively nonresistant endogenous bacteria. Fungal infections and infection with resistant bacteria most often occur during prolonged periods of granulocytopenia.
      2. **Sites of infection.** Damage to skin and mucosal membranes (e.g., from venipuncture or chemotherapy) greatly increases the risk of infection in granulocytopenic patients. Thus, the integument, periodontium, oropharynx, colon, and

perianal area are common foci from which organisms can seed the bloodstream and disseminate. Pneumonia typically is caused by bacteria that have colonized the oropharynx.

3. **Microbiology**

   a. **General comments.** The epidemiology of organisms causing infections in cancer patients has changed in the past 10 to 15 years. The number of infections caused by gram-positive bacteria and fungi has increased markedly; the number of infections caused by gram-negative bacteria has remained constant but has decreased as a percentage of all infections. The most likely explanation for the increase in gram-positive infections is the increased use of indwelling venous catheters. The specific bacteria most commonly associated with infections tend to vary from institution to institution and often vary within institutions over time. The sensitivity patterns of bacteria to antibiotics also vary widely among institutions. Hospital-specific organism sensitivity and resistance data are typically updated at least yearly and can be invaluable in selecting an appropriate initial antibiotic regimen.

   b. **Gram-negative bacteria.** *Escherichia coli, Klebsiella pneumoniae,* and *Pseudomonas aeruginosa* predominate, although the incidence of infection with *P. aeruginosa* has decreased in recent years for unknown reasons. *Enterobacter* species, *Acinetobacter* species, *Serratia marcescens, Burkholderia (Pseudomonas) cepacia,* and *Stenotrophomonas (Xanthomonas) maltophilia* are less common, but still important, pathogens.

   c. **Gram-positive bacteria.** Infection with either *Staphylococcus epidermidis* or *Staphylococcus aureus* is now almost as common as infection with gram-negative bacteria. *Corynebacterium jeikeium* occasionally is found in association with catheter infections.

   d. **Fungi.** *Candida* species (primarily *albicans* and *tropicalis*), *Aspergillus* species and the agents of mucormycosis are the important pathogens. Recently, the incidence of infection with *Candida krusei* has increased at many centers. *Pseudallescheria boydii, Fusarium* and *Alternaria* species, *Trichosporon* species, and other "unusual" fungi are seen less frequently but should not be assumed to be contaminants when isolated.

B. **Cellular immune dysfunction**
   1. **General comments.** Cellular immune dysfunction and its associated infections can result either from the underlying disease or from antineoplastic agents and corticosteroids. Hodgkin's disease and acute lymphocytic leukemia (ALL) in long-term remission are characteristic malignancies in which cellular immune dysfunction–related infection is encountered.
   2. **Microbiology**
      a. **Bacteria.** *Legionella pneumophila* is of special concern, as are the *Nocardia* species. Nocardiosis typically presents with one or more lesions in the lung, skin, and brain. Infections caused by *Salmonella* species and *Listeria monocytogenes* are considerably less common.
      b. **Mycobacteria.** *Mycobacterium avium–intracellulare* is being seen with increasing frequency in patients with non-Hodgkin's lymphomas receiving intensive cytotoxic therapy. The incidence of infection with *Mycobacterium kansasii* is increased in patients with hairy-cell leukemia. *Mycobacterium tuberculosis* is surprisingly unusual in patients with cancer with altered cell-mediated immunity.
      c. **Fungi.** *Cryptococcus neoformans* is seen frequently. Meningitis is the most common presentation, but pulmonary and cutaneous infections also occur. The incidence of *Histoplasma capsulatum* and *Coccidioides immitis* is geographically dependent. Infections caused by the former are seen in the central river valley regions of the United States, whereas infections caused by the latter are seen in the southwestern United States. Pneumonia is the most common presentation with each of these fungi. *Pneumocystis carinii,* which is genotypically more similar to fungi than to protozoa, is a common cause of pneumonia, especially in children with ALL.
      d. **Viruses.** Varicella zoster virus (VZV), causing either varicella or zoster, is particularly common in this group of patients. Varicella can be life-threatening in children with ALL, causing pneumonitis, purpura fulminans, and encephalitis. Oropharyngeal or esophageal lesions due to herpes simplex virus (HSV) can predispose to infection with bacterial or fungal pathogens. Cytomegalovirus (CMV) is seen most often in patients undergoing bone marrow transplantation and typically results from re-

activation of virus previously acquired by either donor or recipient. Interstitial pneumonia is the most common disease manifestation of CMV infection. The current incidence of CMV disease in CMV-seropositive bone marrow transplant recipients is between 2% and 10%. In CMV-seronegative recipients, the incidence of disease approximates 0% if the donor is also CMV-seronegative and CMV-seronegative blood product support is used. Respiratory syncytial virus (RSV), adenovirus, parainfluenza virus, and influenza virus occasionally cause pneumonia in bone marrow transplant recipients.

e. **Protozoa and helminths.** Infection with *Toxoplasmosis gondii* presents as either chorioretinitis or cerebral abscesses. *Strongyloides stercoralis* can cause diarrhea or life-threatening disseminated infections. Diffuse pulmonary infiltrates, shock, and sepsis from enteric gram-negative bacilli are the typical features of disseminated strongyloidiasis.

C. **Humoral immune dysfunction**

1. **General comments.** Agammaglobulinemic or hypogammaglobulinemic patients are susceptible to infections because they often lack opsonizing antibodies to the common encapsulated pyogenic bacteria. Many of these patients are also deficient in functional complement activity. Multiple myeloma and chronic lymphocytic leukemia are prototypical neoplasms with humoral immune dysfunction.

2. **Microbiology.** *Streptococcus pneumoniae* predominates. In addition, decreased complement activity increases the risk of infection by *Haemophilus influenzae, Neisseria meningitidis,* and *Escherichia coli.*

D. **Splenectomy**

1. **General comments.** The spleen is the organ most efficient at removing nonopsonized bacteria. Specific opsonizing antibodies are required for effective killing of the encapsulated bacteria. Thus, splenectomized patients are at risk of overwhelming sepsis when infected with a strain of encapsulated bacteria against which they have never had an opportunity to make antibodies.

2. **Microbiology.** Infections are usually caused by *S. pneumoniae* and, to a lesser extent, by *H. influenzae* and *N. meningitidis.*

E. **Other factors**

1. **Indwelling vascular catheters** increase the risk of bacterial and fungal infections. The risk

increases with the length of time they have been in place. Concurrent granulocytopenia magnifies the infection risk.

2. **Nonambulation and length of stay** have been identified as independent risk factors for infection in most studies. Other factors, such as previous antibiotic use and the presence of a Foley catheter, are correlated with nonambulation and length of stay but are not independent risk factors for infection.

3. **Malnutrition and neurologic dysfunction.** It is controversial whether malnutrition is an independent risk factor for immunosuppression. On the other hand, malnourished patients who require enteral feedings are certainly at increased risk for aspiration. Loss of the gag reflex also increases the risk of aspiration. Loss of sensation facilitates the development of cutaneous ulcers.

4. **Local tumor effect.** Complete or partial obstruction by tumor may lead to infection behind the obstruction. Two examples of this phenomenon are postobstructive pneumonia in a patient with bronchogenic cancer and ascending cholangitis in a patient with an intraabdominal lymphoma.

II. **Treatment of infection**

A. **Clinical findings that suggest the diagnosis of infection**

1. **Symptoms**

   a. **General.** Malaise, fatigue, confusion, or other nonspecific or subtle symptoms may be the first indication of infection. Any unexplained change in the patient's condition should be evaluated clinically and microbiologically.

   b. **Localizing.** Symptoms referable to a particular organ system are particularly worrisome and demand an immediate and thorough evaluation.

2. **Signs**

   a. **Fever** is the single most important indicator of infection in cancer patients. Often, it is the only abnormal finding. It is dangerous to assume that an unexplained fever is due to the underlying malignancy. Similarly, it is unwise to rely exclusively on fever to diagnose infection: debilitated or elderly patients occasionally are afebrile in the presence of infection. In general, a single oral temperature reading of more than 38.5°C, or two or three oral temperature readings higher than 38.0°C within 24 hours, strongly suggests the presence of infection.

b. **Hypotension and shock** occur with a variety of infections; they are not specific for infections caused by gram-negative bacteria.

c. **Tachycardia,** especially if new or unexplained, can also suggest infection.

d. **Inflammation,** if present, suggests underlying infection. Note, however, that granulocytopenic patients often fail to show a normal inflammatory response to infection. Consequently, bacterial pneumonia can present without an identifiable infiltrate on chest radiograph, or even without significant sputum production. Similarly, abscess formation is often minimal or absent despite significant local or systemic infection.

e. **Leukocytosis,** especially when accompanied by an increase in neutrophils or band-form neutrophils, suggests infection. Of course, patients who are leukopenic from chemotherapy do not show this response. Toxic granulation of neutrophils also suggests infection.

B. **Evaluation of patients with suspected infection**

1. **General.** A thorough, daily evaluation of all patients with cancer is necessary to diagnose and treat infections properly. Areas that should not be overlooked include the retinae, ears and sinuses, mouth, skin, catheter sites, axillae, perineum, perianal region, and extremities.

2. **Cultures**

   a. **General approach.** Multiple cultures from multiple sites need to be obtained whenever infection is suspected. All culture material needs to be delivered promptly to the microbiology laboratory. Any change in a patient's condition suggestive of new infection should warrant repeat culturing, even if a pathogen had been isolated previously. Blood, urine, and respiratory cultures typically are obtained with each evaluation. Specimens from other sources are obtained depending on specific circumstances.

   b. **Blood**

      (1) **Technique.** Two sets (aerobic and anaerobic bottles) should be drawn in every 24-hour period in which infection is suspected to be present, until a diagnosis is made. At least 5 mL of blood should be injected into each culture bottle.

      (2) **Central venous catheters.** If these indwelling devices are present, it is important to obtain additional cultures through each port of the device

in addition to obtaining peripheral specimens in the usual manner.

(3) Resin bottles. Culture bottles containing an antibiotic-binding resin or other antibiotic-binding substance should be included with each culture set for patients who are receiving antibiotics at the time of evaluation.

c. **Urine.** Clean-catch or straight-catheterization specimens are preferred. Urine that has been present in a closed collection system for more than 1 hour should not be sent for culture. If necessary, urine can be obtained from the catheter tubing using a syringe and a small-gauge needle.

d. **Respiratory specimens**

(1) Spontaneously expectorated sputum and endotracheal aspirates. A good specimen should have fewer than 10 squamous epithelial cells per low-power (100×) field.

(2) Induced sputum. The yield on bacterial culture of respiratory specimens can be increased by using 3% saline delivered to the patient's respiratory tract through an ultrasonic nebulizer. *P. carinii* infection is often diagnosed by this technique in centers experienced with its use, thereby sparing patients the need for bronchoscopy. Three percent saline can cause significant bronchospasm and should be administered cautiously only by trained personnel.

(3) Transtracheal aspiration. This procedure is used rarely. More commonly, patients undergo bronchoscopy or open-lung biopsy if pulmonary pathology is suspected and the first two techniques fail to provide an answer.

(4) Nasal washings. Nonbacteriostatic fluid (e.g., saline) delivered to the nares through a bulb syringe and then quickly aspirated back into the syringe is an effective way to obtain virus for culture. The fluid can be transported to the laboratory in any closed container, but needs to be done so promptly. It is important to let the laboratory know which viruses are suspected. Unfortunately, the yield of nasal washings is often much lower than that of bronchoscopy-obtained fluid, primarily because of physician inexperience with the nasal washing technique.

e. **Cerebrospinal fluid (CSF)**
    (1) **Criteria.** A lumbar puncture should be performed in any patient who has an abnormal or a changed neurologic examination. A lumbar puncture should be strongly considered in any patient in whom no other source can be found to explain the suspected infection.
    (2) **Studies.** CSF should always be sent for Gram stain, bacterial cultures, cell count with differential, glucose, and protein. A cryptococcal antigen titer should be performed if the patient has reasons for cellular immune dysfunction. Acid-fast bacillus (AFB) stains and cultures are probably not indicated routinely.

f. **Stool**
    (1) ***Clostridium difficile.*** This toxin-producing anaerobic bacterium is a common cause of diarrhea in patients who have been on antibiotics. A mild-to-moderate leukocytosis, as well as a temperature reading above 38.0°C, typically is part of the syndrome. All patients with diarrhea should have stool sent for a cytotoxic assay for *C. difficile* toxin. Rapid antigen detection tests are not as reliable.
    (2) **Bacterial cultures.** A stool culture should be sent to the microbiology laboratory from patients in whom the diagnosis of infectious diarrhea is suspected. Occasionally, *Salmonella species* and *L. monocytogenes* are causes of nosocomial diarrhea or sepsis.
    (3) **Fecal leukocytes.** The presence of white blood cells in the stool suggests an invasive inflammatory process of the colon. Fecal leukocytes are seen with *Shigella* species, *Campylobacter* species, invasive *E. coli,* and, variably, *Salmonella* species and *C. difficile.* A methylene blue stain of the stool should be ordered routinely along with the culture.
    (4) **Ova and parasites.** Diarrhea that develops more than 3 days after the patient's hospitalization almost never has a parasitic cause. The routine ordering of this test should be discouraged. The important exception is in geographic regions in which *S. sterco-*

ralis is endemic (e.g., southeastern United States).

g. **Viral cultures**

(1) **HSV and VZV.** Suspicious vesicular lesions need to be cultured for HSV or VZV. Fluid-filled lesions should be carefully unroofed. A swab should then be rubbed on the base of the lesion and sent in viral transport media to the laboratory within 30 minutes. These specimens need to be promptly inoculated into tissue culture or stored at 4 to 9°C for no more than 18 hours.

(2) **CMV.** Blood and urine cultures frequently are positive in bone marrow transplant patients who have CMV interstitial pneumonia but are not synonymous with disease. Isolation (culture) of CMV from pulmonary specimens is suggestive of disease if a concurrent chest radiograph or CT scan reveals an interstitial pattern. Evidence of tissue invasion by histologic and histochemical techniques confirms the diagnosis of CMV disease.

h. **Other.** Biopsy or aspirate cultures from any accessible suspected site of infection should be obtained as soon as possible. The risk of complications from such procedures (e.g., infection, bleeding) must be weighed against the possible gains.

3. **Imaging studies**

a. **Radiographs.** A chest radiograph should be obtained routinely in any patient suspected of having an infection. Sinus films are also frequently important.

b. **Computed tomography.** CT scans of the chest, abdomen, brain, head and neck, spine, and other areas can add considerable information to the diagnostic work-up. The ordering of these tests needs to be individualized to the specific clinical situation.

c. **Ultrasonography.** An echocardiogram should be obtained when endocarditis is suspected. Ultrasonography is also good at detecting ascites and biliary, hepatic, and pancreatic pathology. A portable (bedside) ultrasound can be useful in critically ill patients who are too sick to be transported to the radiology department.

d. **Nuclear medicine.** Unfortunately, radionuclide scanning using indium-labeled granulocytes or gallium is often nondiagnostic. False-positive and false-negative results occur too frequently to recommend these tests on a routine basis.

4. **Invasive studies**

   a. **Bronchoscopy.** Bronchoalveolar lavage (BAL) for *P. carinii* and other fungi and for CMV, RSV and other viruses should be considered for patients at risk for one of these organisms. The adequacy of the specimen can be ascertained by noting the presence of alveolar macrophages on subsequent stains. Specimens also should be sent for Gram stain, AFB stain and culture, and bacterial culture.

   b. **Skin biopsy.** Suspicious dermatologic lesions should be sampled and sent for bacterial, fungal, and AFB cultures and for methenamine silver staining for fungi.

   c. **Open-lung biopsy.** A persistent unexplained infiltrate on chest radiograph is often evaluated best with this approach. Morbidity is low in patients with adequate platelets and normal coagulation indices.

   d. **Bone marrow biopsy.** Specimens should be sent for AFB stains and culture.

   e. **Percutaneous liver biopsy.** Occasionally, this procedure is helpful in diagnosing bacterial or fungal pathogens (e.g., *Candida* species) if abnormalities referable to this organ are suspected based on imaging studies or serum chemistries.

   f. **Exploratory laparotomy.** Even multiple imaging studies sometimes fail to reveal intraabdominal abscesses. A positive blood culture and abdominal tenderness should be clues to this diagnosis. An exploratory laparotomy might be required if symptoms persist. Alternatively, surgery may need to be considered if intraabdominal abnormalities detected by other studies fail to resolve with therapy.

5. **Miscellaneous studies**

   a. **A complete blood count** with differential should be performed on every patient suspected of having an infection.

   b. **Liver function tests** are often abnormal in generalized sepsis or during infections involving the organ itself.

   c. **Urinalysis** can help differentiate infection from contamination: the absence of white blood cells suggests the latter diagnosis. Note, however, that white blood cells may be absent in neutropenic patients.

   d. **Sedimentation rate.** This nonspecific test is rarely useful and is seldom indicated.

e. **Serology.** In general, serologic tests are of little value in diagnosing acute infections.

f. **Antigen and antibody rapid-detection tests.** Direct fluorescent antibody testing of sputum for *L. pneumophila* and other *Legionella* species can provide a diagnosis more rapidly than culture, although the sensitivity of this test is somewhat lower than that of culture at most large centers. A urine antigen detection test for *L. pneumophila,* serogroup 1, has sensitivity that rivals culture, but detects only the most common serogroup of *L. pneumophila* and not other *Legionella* species. Urine and serum antigen tests also are available in some centers for *H. capsulatum* and may be useful both for diagnosis and for following response to therapy. Antigen tests for other fungi lack sufficient sensitivity to be clinically useful at this time.

g. **DNA probes.** DNA hybridization tests for ribosomal RNA that is genus specific exist for *Legionella* species, *H. capsulatum,* various mycobacteria, and other organisms. The sensitivity of these tests equals but does not exceed that of other diagnostic techniques. The major advantage of the DNA probes is their ability to determine the identity of organisms growing in culture sooner than is possible by traditional methods.

h. **Polymerase chain reaction (PCR).** Quantitative PCR for CMV is being investigated as a means of determining which patients are at greatest risk of developing disease. PCR techniques have also been used to diagnose HSV encephalitis because the yield of CSF culture for this virus is extremely poor.

C. **Therapy**

1. **Empiric therapy**

a. **Timing.** Two or three oral temperature elevations above 38°C, or one elevation above 38.5°C, suggest infection. Patients with fewer than 500 neutrophils/µL should be started on antibiotics at this time. Nonneutropenic patients may also require antibiotics, but that decision should be individualized based on other findings.

b. **Neutropenic coverage.** Prompt initiation of empiric antibiotic therapy has been shown to reduce mortality. Despite some success with monotherapy, the use of combination therapy remains the standard of care for neutropenic patients.

(1) **Recommended regimens.** Two antipseudomonal antibiotics should be included (Table 28-1 and Fig. 28-1). The usual approach is to combine an antipseudomonal β-lactam with an aminoglycoside. Current popular combinations are piperacillin (or piperacillin-tazobactam) or ceftazidime plus either tobramycin or amikacin. Other regimens are possible; the one that is chosen should reflect local sensitivity patterns.

(2) **Double β-lactam combinations.** These regimens have the potential advantage of avoiding aminoglycoside nephrotoxicity and ototoxicity. Unfortunately, cross-resistance to all β-lactams occurs commonly with many gram-negative organisms. Resistance to the aminoglycosides has been much slower to develop, especially resistance to tobramycin and amikacin.

(3) **Duration.** Antibiotics should be continued for a full 14-day course in patients who remain neutropenic, even

---

Table 28-1. Recommended initial antibiotic regimens for neutropenic patients with normal renal function

Combination therapy

1. Piperacillin, 3 g q 6 h + tobramycin 2 mg/kg q 8 h, *or*
2. Piperacillin-tazobactam, 3.375 g q 6 h + tobramycin as above, *or*
3. Ceftazidime, 2 g q 8 h + tobramycin as above

Monotherapy (generally not recommended)

1. Ceftazidime, 2 g q 8 h, *or*
2. Imipenem, 750 mg q 6 h

Note: 1. Vancomycin, 1 g q 12 h can be *added* to any of the above regimens for better gram-positive coverage
2. Amikacin at 8–10 mg/kg q 12 h can be *substituted* for tobramycin at institutions with significant bacterial resistance rates to tobramycin
3. Tobramycin can be dosed at 5 mg/kg q 24 h and amikacin dosed at 15–20 mg/kg q 24 h, without apparent increased toxicity in recent studies

Antifungal therapy with amphotericin

1. For candidiasis and initial empiric therapy: 0.5–0.7 mg/kg/day
2. For cryptococcosis or histoplasmosis: 0.6–0.8 mg/kg/day
3. For resistant candidiasis or persistent fever: 0.8–1.2 mg/kg/day
4. For aspergillosis: 1.0–1.5 mg/kg/day

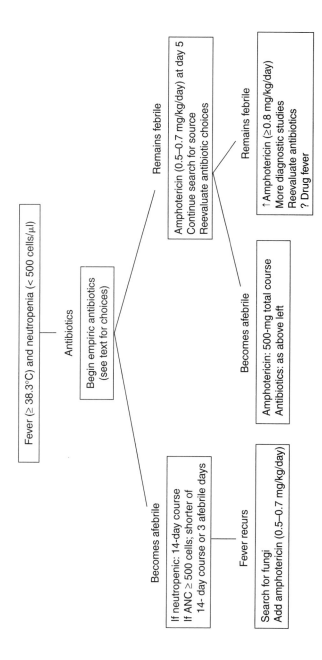

Fig. 28-1.   Therapeutic approach to the febrile neutropenic patient. ANC 5 absolute neutrophil count.

if they become afebrile during therapy. This approach is a compromise: stopping antibiotics too quickly in neutropenic patients results in an unacceptably high percentage of the patients requiring subsequent courses of antibiotics, whereas continuing the antibiotics until granulocyte counts are more than 500/μL may increase the risk of antibiotic-associated toxicities and the development of resistance. Patients who show recovery of their granulocyte counts to more than 500/μL before completion of a 14-day course of antibiotics can have their antibiotics discontinued after they have been afebrile for at least 72 hours.

    (4) **Antifungal therapy.** Amphotericin B, at a dose of 0.5 to 0.7 mg/kg/day, should be started if neutropenic patients remain febrile despite broad-spectrum antibiotic coverage for more than 5 to 7 days. Although the optimal total dose and duration of antifungal therapy are unknown, it seems prudent to continue antifungal therapy to a total dose of 500 mg, assuming that the patient responds to therapy by becoming afebrile. If the patient does not become afebrile within several days of initiating antifungal therapy, the dose of amphotericin should be increased to at least 0.8 mg/kg/day to cover fungi such as *Aspergillus* species. The imidazole derivatives ketoconazole and itraconazole have not been found to be suitable replacements for amphotericin B. On the other hand, fluconazole at doses of 400 to 800 mg/day has shown promise in at least one randomized clinical trial compared with amphotericin B. However, *Candida krusei* and some other non-*albicans* species of *Candida* are resistant to fluconazole. The lipid complex (liposome) formulations of amphotericin B have been shown to have less nephrotoxicity than amphotericin B, with similar efficacy in nonrandomized clinical trials. Randomized comparisons of the lipid formulations with standard amphotericin B are ongoing.

  c. **Aminoglycoside dosing.** A loading dose of 2 mg/kg of tobramycin, or 7.5 mg/kg of amikacin, should be given initially. High peak serum levels (e.g., 7 to 8 µg/mL of tobramycin) have been shown to be beneficial in treating infections in neutropenic patients. To avoid unacceptably high trough levels, it is often necessary to decrease the dosing frequency and increase the amount given with each dose. A reasonable approach is to give slightly less than a loading dose (e.g., 1.7 to 2 mg/kg of tobramycin) with each dose and to adjust only the dosing interval by monitoring peak and trough levels. Alternatively, once-daily dosing of tobramycin (5 mg/kg/day) and amikacin (15 mg/kg/day) has been shown to be as effective as traditional dosing schedules, with no increase in nephrotoxicity or ototoxicity in patients with normal renal function.

d. **Gram-positive coverage.** The addition of an antistaphylococcal antibiotic to the initial empiric regimen should be considered in patients with indwelling vascular catheters. Vancomycin is preferred because of its efficacy against methicillin-resistant *S. aureus, S. epidermidis,* and *C. jeikeium.* Patients with integumentary damage from any cause also should receive an antistaphylococcal antibiotic.

e. **Additional coverage.** Patients at risk for pneumonia caused by *P. carinii* or *Legionella* species should have trimethoprim-sulfamethoxazole and erythromycin, respectively, included in their antibiotic regimens, if evidence for pulmonary infection exists. Anaerobic coverage (e.g., metronidazole or clindamycin) should be considered in patients with necrotizing gingivitis or perianal tenderness.

2. **Definitive therapy**
   a. **Antibiotics**
      (1) **General.** Reevaluation of the empiric antibiotic regimen is mandatory when the identity and sensitivity pattern of an isolated pathogen become available.
      (2) **Gram-negative infections.** Neutropenic patients should be treated with two antibiotics, each effective against the isolated organism. Nonneutropenic patients with *P. aeruginosa* pneumonia also should receive therapy with two antibiotics, at least initially.
      (3) **Gram-positive infections.** One antibiotic is sufficient, but coverage against gram-negative organisms

should be continued in neutropenic patients, as discussed previously.

b.   Specific infections

(1)   Catheter-related sepsis. Staphylococcal infections predominate. Removal of infected indwelling intravascular devices is optimal, but not always possible. Eradication of infection can often be accomplished with long-term antibiotics alone. There is about a 70% to 80% chance of curing a *S. epidermidis* infection with 3 to 4 weeks of antibiotics administered through each port of the device. The chance of success drops to 30% to 50% for gram-negative and *S. aureus* infections. Fungal infections require immediate removal of the catheter. Tunnel infections also generally require catheter removal.

(2)   *Candida* species infections

(a)   Significance. Isolation of *Candida* species from sputum, urine, stool, or drainage fluid is not necessarily synonymous with infection. On the other hand, isolation of *Candida* species from three or more nonblood sites has been shown to correlate with disseminated candidiasis in neutropenic patients. Isolation of this organism from the blood is always significant. The presence of macronodular skin lesions shown on biopsy to be consistent with candidal infection is synonymous with dissemination.

(b)   Therapy. Amphotericin B remains the treatment of choice. The optimum dose and duration are unknown, especially in patients who remain neutropenic. Most centers use doses of 0.5 to 0.7 mg/kg/day, to a total dose of at least 500 mg for documented infections. The addition of 5-fluorocytosine (flucytosine) at doses of 25 mg/kg every 6 hours is often synergistic and may increase response rates. This agent is potentially bone marrow suppressive, and serum levels should be monitored. Fluconazole, at doses of 400 to 800 mg/day, shows promise against *Candida albicans* infection but is ineffective against *Candida krusei* and certain other non-*albicans* species of *Candida.*

(c) **Dissemination.** Candidemia or other evidence of dissemination should prompt a search for deep organ involvement. Weekly funduscopic examinations are essential in such circumstances. When deep organ involvement is present, therapy with amphotericin B should be continued to a total of at least 1 to 2 g. Surgery, when feasible, may improve survival in selected cases of deep organ involvement.

(3) *Aspergillus* **species infections.** Even a single positive culture for one of the *Aspergillus* species warrants the initiation of therapy. Pulmonary involvement is the most common disease manifestation, but thrombosis of major blood vessels and widespread dissemination occur in neutropenic patients. Aggressive therapy is necessary to reduce mortality: early initiation of amphotericin B at doses of 1 to 1.5 mg/kg/day is recommended. A total course of 2 g is typical.

(4) **HSV and VZV infections.** Early initiation of therapy helps to prevent dissemination. The dose of acyclovir for HSV infections in immunocompromised patients with normal renal function is 6.25 mg/kg every 8 hours, administered intravenously. VZV infections require 12.5 mg/kg of acyclovir every 8 hours. Serum levels following an oral dose average about 25% of levels obtained after an intravenous dose; for this reason, oral acyclovir typically is not used for acute HSV or VZV infections in cancer patients. High-dose oral regimens (800 mg five times daily) have been tried with some success, but gastrointestinal distress is a common side effect. Neither valacyclovir nor famciclovir has been studied adequately in cancer patients.

(5) **CMV interstitial pneumonia.** CMV interstitial pneumonia occurs at a

median of 50 to 60 days after bone marrow transplantation. The 6-month mortality rate still exceeds 30%, despite recent improvements in therapy. The current treatment of choice is the combination of ganciclovir at a dose of 5 mg/kg i.v. every 12 hours plus immune globulin, 500 mg/kg i.v. every other day for 21 days, followed by the combination of ganciclovir, 5 mg/kg i.v. every day (5 days/week) plus immune globulin, 500 mg/kg i.v. once weekly for the duration of major immunosuppressive therapy. Significant bone marrow toxicity can occur with ganciclovir use, and CMV resistance to ganciclovir has been reported. Unfortunately, the use of foscarnet, with its associated nephrotoxicity, causes problems in these patients, who typically are on concomitant cyclosporin A.

(6) **RSV pneumonia.** The mortality rate for this difficult-to-treat infection in bone marrow transplant recipients exceeds 50% in many centers. The combination of aerosolized ribavirin, administered as a small-particle aerosol into a tent or mask continuously for 18 h/day for 2 to 5 days, plus immune globulin, 500 mg/kg i.v. every other day for the duration of ribavirin therapy, may be more effective than ribavirin alone.

(7) *Nocardia* **species infections.** Altered cell-mediated immunity, whether intrinsic or corticosteroid induced, is the main risk factor for infection with these organisms. The treatment of choice remains oral sulfadiazine, 6 to 8 g/day. Therapy should be continued for at least 3 months, and regimens of 6 to 12 months are not uncommon. Trimethoprimsulfamethoxazole (intravenous or oral), sulfisoxazole, and triple-sulfonamide combinations are likely to be as efficacious as sulfadiazine. Minocycline is an alternative for patients with sulfa allergies, and imipenem has shown impressive in vitro activity.

c. **Biologic response modifiers**

(1) **Granulocyte transfusions.** Beneficial results have not been seen consistently in controlled trials. Transfusion reactions, allosensitization to HLA

antigens, and transfusion-associated CMV infection occur frequently and further limit the usefulness of this approach. An increased incidence of severe pulmonary reactions, especially when transfusions are given to patients receiving amphotericin B, has also been noted.

(2) **Colony-stimulating factors.** Controlled trials with granulocyte macrophage and granulocyte colony-stimulating factor have shown that these products can shorten the duration of neutropenia, decrease neutropenia-associated infections, and reduce hospital length of stay and total cost for many malignancies requiring intensive (bone marrow–suppressive) chemotherapy. The use of these products has become standard in many malignancies when neutropenia is expected to last 7 to 10 days or more.

(3) **Passive immunization**

(a) **Monoclonal antibodies.** Immunization with high-titer antibody directed against the core glycolipid of gram-negative organisms (J-5 antisera) appears to reduce mortality from infection, presumably by neutralizing endotoxin. Preparation of the antisera is difficult and expensive, and the technique remains primarily a research tool at this time. Successful immunization with a "cocktail" of antibodies directed against different antigenic determinants of gram-negative bacilli has not been achieved.

(b) **Pooled immunoglobulin preparations.** These preparations contain antibodies to many potential pathogens. Results of early controlled trials have been disappointing.

(c) **Tumor necrosis factor-α (TNF-α) antiserum.** TNF-α has been shown to be a central mediator of endotoxic shock. However, antibody to TNF-α has failed to reduce mortality in multiple, large, randomized clinical trials. Newer data suggest that TNF-α might even have a beneficial effect on host defenses as an activator of macrophages. Better targeting of patients likely to benefit from blocking TNF-α (e.g., those with elevated serum levels of interleukin-6) has been suggested as a way of reducing mortality from the sepsis syndrome. Such clinical trials are ongoing.

(d) **Interleukins and interferon.** Activation of monocytes and neutrophils by these substances might be expected to reduce mortality from certain kinds of infections. Unfortunately, systemic side effects limit the usefulness of this approach.

III. Prevention of infection
A. Environmental manipulations
1. **Hand washing.** Numerous studies have confirmed that scrupulous adherence to good hand-washing technique reduces infections. Patients should be told to remind their physicians to wash their hands before allowing them to proceed with the examination. In addition, neutropenic patients should have hand-washing signs placed outside of their rooms as a reminder to all personnel.

2. **Protective isolation**
   a. **Definition.** The concept of a "total protected environment" includes the use of laminar airflow rooms; sterilization of all objects placed in those rooms; gowning, masking, and gloving of personnel before entering the rooms; decontamination of the skin and gut with antimicrobials; and special food preparation to reduce the number of microorganisms present on the food.
   b. **Disadvantages.** This approach is expensive; is cumbersome for patients, their families, and hospital personnel; and decreases perceived quality of life. It is also difficult to justify: recent studies have not shown a significant advantage of protective isolation when compared with other preventive techniques.

3. **Reservoir recognition and removal**
   a. **Foods.** Fresh fruits, vegetables, and non-processed dairy products are frequently contaminated with gram-negative bacteria, especially *P. aeruginosa, E. coli,* and *K. pneumoniae.* Adherence to a cooked diet during periods of neutropenia helps to reduce the risk of infection with these organisms.

        b. Objects. Faucet aerators, sinks, shower heads, and flowers are known to harbor bacteria. However, most epidemiologic studies have not found these objects to be significant causes of infection. No special precautions, except for good hand-washing technique, are necessary.

        c. Construction. The incidence of infections caused by *Aspergillus* species is increased in areas of construction. Patients at risk should be moved to other areas of the hospital during periods of renovation.

B. Surveillance cultures. Routine bacterial surveillance cultures are rarely of benefit. In centers where *Aspergillus* species infection is a significant problem, periodic fungal cultures of the nares for this fungus might be useful for early detection.

C. Prophylaxis

  1. Antibiotics

    a. Nonabsorbable agents

      (1) Rationale. Oral vancomycin, gentamicin, and nystatin have been used in attempts to suppress gut flora and lessen the importance of this reservoir of infection.

      (2) Disadvantages. The combination of antibiotics is poorly tolerated by patients; increased bacterial resistance develops, especially to gentamicin; the regimens do not provide protection against bacteria originating from other body sites; and some controlled studies have failed to demonstrate decreased infection rates.

      (3) Recommendations. These oral nonabsorbable antibiotics should not be used at this time.

    b. Quinolones

      (1) Efficacy. Both norfloxacin and ciprofloxacin have been shown to reduce the incidence of infection (but not mortality) in neutropenic cancer patients.

      (2) Mechanism of action. The quinolones suppress gram-negative and gram-positive aerobic gut flora and also achieve therapeutic serum and tissue levels against many bacteria.

      (3) Recommendations. Side effects have been minimal, and resistance has been slow to develop. Some cancer centers now routinely place patients on a regimen of 400 mg of norfloxacin twice daily before beginning chemotherapy when prolonged neutropenia is anticipated. The quinolones are not approved for use in children.

   c. **Trimethoprim-sulfamethoxazole.** The use of this agent has fallen out of favor for bacterial prophylaxis because of its potential for bone marrow suppression and other side effects. Increased bacterial resistance and break-through infections have also been observed.

2. **Antifungals.** Prophylaxis, usually against *Candida* species, has been attempted with a number of antifungal agents. Disadvantages include the potential for emergence of resistant strains and the lack of correlation between decreased colonization rates and the rate of invasive fungal disease. It has become standard in many centers to use fluconazole, 100 mg once daily, in bone marrow transplant recipients and anyone else with actual or expected profound neutropenia. The duration of therapy is typically for the entire duration of neutropenia.

3. **Antivirals.** Both intravenous (6.25 mg/kg twice daily) and oral acyclovir (400 to 800 mg two or three times daily) can prevent recurrences of HSV infections. Acyclovir is ineffective for treatment of CMV infection but may have some limited prophylactic efficacy against CMV. Ganciclovir, 5 mg/kg i.v. twice daily for 5 days before bone marrow transplantation, then once daily until 100 days after transplantation, reduces the incidence of CMV interstitial pneumonia but not overall mortality at 6 months. CMV disease can be expected to occur in 10% to 15% of bone marrow transplant recipients within 60 days after discontinuation of prophylactic ganciclovir therapy. A strategy of preemptive ganciclovir use in those bone marrow transplant recipients with positive BAL cultures for CMV 35 days after transplantation who were not receiving ganciclovir prophylaxis reduced both the incidence of CMV interstitial pneumonia and the mortality rate at 180 days. The optimal approach to prevent CMV disease in bone marrow transplant recipients is not known at this time.

4. **Antiparasitics**

   a. *Pneumocystis carinii*. Trimethoprim-sulfamethoxazole, 1 double-strength tablet given twice daily on 2 or 3 consecutive days, is effective prophylaxis against this organism. Monthly aerosolized pentamidine may also be of value.

   b. *Strongyloides stercoralis.* Patients living in endemic areas should have stool cultures evaluated and treatment initiated (if

necessary) before beginning immunosuppressive therapy.
  D. **Immunization**
    1. **Vaccines.** Live attenuated viral vaccines should not be used in immunocompromised patients. The efficacy of vaccines against *S. pneumoniae* and *H. influenzae* in immunocompromised patients is suspect. Nevertheless, many authorities recommend their use before immunosuppressive therapy.
    2. **Biologic response modifiers**
        a. **Pooled immunoglobulin.** These preparations, given intravenously at doses of 0.1 to 0.2 g/kg at monthly intervals, have been used in patients with chronic lymphocytic leukemia, multiple myeloma, and other malignancies. Controlled trials appear to indicate some reduction in bacterial infections, but the preparations are expensive, and lifelong therapy is required.
        b. **Monoclonal antibodies.** Prophylactic administration of antibodies directed against virulence determinants of gram-negative bacteria (e.g., J-5 antisera) may be of value in reducing the incidence of infection. However, mortality has been unaltered in early clinical trials.
    3. **VZV immune globulin** (1 vial/10 kg body weight, to a maximum of 5 vials) is effective in reducing morbidity and mortality in seronegative immunocompromised patients exposed to VZV. The product should be given intramuscularly within 96 hours of exposure.
  E. **Miscellaneous.** Intravenous catheters (nonsurgically placed) should be changed at least every 72 hours. Rectal temperatures, rectal suppositories, and unnecessary rectal examinations should be avoided in neutropenic patients.

SELECTED READINGS
Berkman SA, Lee ML, Gale RP. Clinical uses of intravenous immunoglobulins. *Ann Intern Med* 1990;112:278–292.
Crawford J, Ozer H, Stoller R, et al. Reduction by granulocyte colony-stimulating factor of fever and neutropenia induced by chemotherapy in patients with small-cell lung cancer. *N Engl J Med* 1991;325:164–170.
EORTC International Antimicrobial Therapy Cooperative Group. Ceftazidime combined with a short or long course of amikacin for empirical therapy of gram-negative bacteremia in cancer patients with gram-negative bacteremia in cancer patients with granulocytopenia. *N Engl J Med* 1987;317:1692–1698.
Goodrich JM, Mori M, Gleaves CA, et al. Early treatment with ganciclovir to prevent cytomegalovirus disease after allogeneic bone marrow transplantation. *N Engl J Med* 1991;325:1601–1607.

Goodrich JM, Bowden RA, Fisher L, et al. Prevention of cytome-galovirus disease after allogeneic marrow transplant by ganciclovir prophylaxis. *Ann Intern Med* 1993;118:173–178.

Hughes WT, Armstrong D, Bodey GP, et al. From the Infectious Dis-eases Society of America: guidelines for the use of antimicrobial agents in neutropenic patients with unexplained fever. *J Infect Dis* 1990;161:381–396.

Klastersky J, Zinner SH, Calandra T, et al. Empiric antimicrobial ther-apy for febrile granulocytopenic cancer patients: lessons from four EORTC trials. *Eur J Cancer Clin Oncol* 1988;24[Suppl 1]:S35–S45.

MacArthur RD, Bone RC. Sepsis, SIRS, and septic shock. In: Bone RC, eds. *Pulmonary and critical care medicine,* vol 3, 4th ed. St. Louis: Mosby-Year Book, 1997:1–12.

Nichols CR, Fox EP, Roth BJ, et al. Incidence of neutropenic fever in patients treated with standard-dose combination chemotherapy for small-cell lung cancer and the cost impact of treatment with gran-ulocyte colony-stimulating factor. *J Clin Oncol* 1994;12:1245–1250.

Pizzo P. Considerations for the prevention of infectious complications in patients with cancer. *Rev Infect Dis* 1989;11[Suppl 7]:S1551–S1563.

Pizzo P. Management of fever in patients with cancer and treatment-induced neutropenia. *N Engl J Med* 1993;328:1323–1332.

Steward WP. Granulocyte and granulocyte-macrophage colony-stimulating factors. *Lancet* 1993;342:153–157.

Disorders of Hemostasis and Transfusion Therapy

Mary R. Smith and Nurjehan Khan

Disorders of the hemostatic mechanisms are common in patients with malignancy. Abnormalities associated with thromboembolic events cause significantly more morbidity and mortality than disorders leading to hemorrhage.

I. **Thromboembolism in cancer**
   A. **Pathophysiology.** The thromboembolic risk associated with neoplasia reflects an imbalance between platelet number, platelet function, levels of coagulation factors, and generation of thromboplastins, compared with the levels of inhibitors of hemostasis and fibrinolytic activity. Thrombosis may be minor and localized, or widespread and associated with multiple-organ damage. There may also be hemorrhage of varying degrees of severity in association with the thromboembolic events.
   1. **Factors that may affect the risk of thromboembolism** vary widely from patient to patient and include the following:
   Specific type of tumor
   Nutritional status of the patient
   Type of chemotherapy
   Response to chemotherapy (e.g., tumor lysis syndrome)
   Liver and renal function
   Patient immobility and venous stasis
   2. **Factors that can initiate thrombus formation** are common to many cancers:
   Circulating tumor cells adhere to the vascular endothelium and form a nidus for clot formation.
   Tumors may penetrate the vessel, destroying the endothelium and promoting clot formation.
   Neovascularization associated with many tumors may stimulate clotting.
   Arterial thrombosis associated with tumors may result from vasospasm.
   A systemic hypercoagulable state develops (e.g., decreased protein C).
   External compression of vessels by tumor masses impedes blood flow and leads to stasis and clot development.
   3. **Platelet abnormalities associated with an increased risk of thromboembolism** include thrombocytosis and increased platelet adhesion and aggregation. Tumors may produce

substances that cause increased platelet aggregation with subsequent release of platelet factor 3 and ensuing acceleration of coagulation.

B. **Clinical syndromes.** A variety of noteworthy clinical syndromes are associated with the "hypercoagulable state" of malignancy and of its treatment.

   1. **Disseminated intravascular coagulation (DIC).** DIC is a syndrome with many signs, symptoms, and laboratory abnormalities (Table 29-1). As many as 90% of patients with metastatic neoplasms have some laboratory manifestation of DIC, but only a small fraction of these patients suffer morbidity from the coagulation process or subsequent depletion of coagulation factors and consequent bleeding due to DIC. The initiating factor for DIC is apparent in some situations, but unknown in others.

   Among the common initiators of DIC are the following:

   Thromboplastic substances in granules from promyelocytes of acute promyelocytic leukemia (DIC may worsen with therapy). There is a

Table 29-1.   Laboratory diagnosis of disseminated intravascular coagulation (DIC)

Laboratory tests	Acute DIC	Chronic DIC
Screening		
PT, aPTT	Usually prolonged	Normal
Platelets	Usually decreased	Normal or slightly decreased
Fibrinogen	Usually decreased but may be normal*	Usually normal*
Confirmatory[†]		
Fibrin monomer	Positive	Positive
FDP	Strongly positive	Positive
D-Dimer	Positive	Positive
Thrombin time	Normal or abnormal	Usually normal
Factor assays	Decreased factors V and VIII	Normal factors V and VIII
Antithrombin III	May be reduced	Usually normal

PT, prothrombin time; aPTT, activated partial thromboplastin time; FDP, fibrinogen degradation products.
* Fibrinogen is usually elevated in advanced malignancy or acute leukemia that is not complicated by DIC. Thus, a normal fibrinogen level may actually be decreased for the physiologic state of the patient.
[†] Changes indicated are confirmatory if present; the absence of the indicated findings in some of the confirmatory tests does not exclude the diagnosis.

significant concomitant fibrinolysis in many patients.

Sialic acid from mucin produced by adenocarcinomas of the lung or gastrointestinal tract

Trypsin released from pancreatic cancer

Impaired fibrinolysis associated with hepatocellular carcinoma

DIC in any patient may be fostered by sepsis or other causes of the systemic inflammatory response syndrome (SIRS).

2. **Lupus anticoagulant in neoplastic disease.** The lupus anticoagulant is an antiphospholipid antibody (immunoglobulin G or M). Antiphospholipid antibodies are reported to be associated with a number of malignant disorders, including hairy-cell leukemia, lymphoma, Waldenström's macroglobulinemia, and epithelial neoplasms. The lupus anticoagulant leads to a prolonged activated partial thromboplastin time (aPTT) but is paradoxically associated with an increased risk of thrombosis.

3. **Trousseau's syndrome (tumor-associated thrombophlebitis).** Suspect the possibility of neoplasia in the following circumstances:

An unexplained thromboembolic event occurs after the age of 40

Thromboses occur in unusual sites

The thromboses affect superficial as well as deep veins

The thromboses are migratory

The thromboses tend not to respond to the "usual" anticoagulant therapies

An unexplained thrombosis occurs more than once

4. **Thrombotic events that occur after surgery** for tumors of the lung, ovary, pancreas, or stomach.

5. **Nonbacterial thrombotic endocarditis** may be found in association with carcinoma of the lung. These thrombi are formed from accumulations of platelets and fibrin. The mitral valve is the most frequent site of origin of these thrombi, which frequently embolize.

6. **Thrombotic thrombocytopenic purpura (TTP).** TTP is a poorly understood syndrome characterized by thrombocytopenia, acute hemolysis, fever, fluctuating neurologic signs and symptoms, and acute renal failure. TTP and the hemolytic-uremic syndrome (thrombocytopenia, hemolysis, and acute renal failure) have been associated with untreated malignancies as well as with a number of drugs used for treating malignant disease. The agent most often reported is mitomycin, but other drugs, including

bleomycin, cisplatin, cyclophosphamide, and vinca alkaloids, may also be associated with these syndromes. TTP may be difficult to diagnose in this setting because the chemotherapy suppresses platelet production, some agents may impair renal function, and many of the features of DIC are similar to those of TTP. Careful review of the peripheral blood smear is required to identify the changes in red blood cells (RBCs) that are associated with a microangiopathic hemolytic process. The prognosis of patients with TTP is poor, and its therapy has been varied. Plasmapheresis and transfusion with fresh-frozen plasma appear to be the best modalities of therapy.

7. **Thromboembolism associated with chemotherapy**

   a. The use of **central arterial or venous catheters** has markedly facilitated the delivery of chemotherapy, but all such catheters are associated with a significant risk of vascular thrombosis. The empiric use of low doses of warfarin (1 mg/day) decreases the risk of thrombosis without inducing a hemorrhagic state. It is not necessary to follow the prothrombin time (PT) with low-dose warfarin.

   b. Many **chemotherapy agents** cause significant chemical phlebitis. The most common offending agents are mechlorethamine (nitrogen mustard), anthracyclines, nitrosoureas, mitomycin, fluorouracil, dacarbazine, and epipodophyllotoxins.

   c. L-Asparaginase inhibits the synthesis of proteins, including coagulation factors. This inhibition may cause either hemorrhage or thrombosis. Patients with preexisting hemostatic disorders are at particular risk for complications when using L-asparaginase. L-Asparaginase also decreases antithrombin III (AT-III) activity.

   d. **Tamoxifen** has been associated with thromboembolic events. This effect may be magnified when tamoxifen is combined with chemotherapeutic agents.

   e. **Estrogens** may increase the risk of thromboembolism. This is likely due, at least in part, to a decrease in protein S and an increase in coagulation factors.

   f. **Superior vena cava syndrome** is nearly always associated with thrombosis in the thoracic venous system cephalad to the site of obstruction and may lead to upper extremity thrombosis.

C. **Principles of therapy for thrombosis associated with neoplasia**
   1. **Discrete vascular thrombosis**
      a. **General guidelines.** Therapy should be directed at controlling the neoplasm. As an anticoagulant, heparin is superior to warfarin in these patients. Warfarin and antiplatelet drugs have been used with varying degrees of success in some patients with thromboembolism associated with tumors. The use of heparin, warfarin, and antiplatelet agents alone or in combination may be associated with normalization of hemostatic parameters. Despite this, patients with malignant disease are often resistant to anticoagulant therapy and may continue to have thrombotic events even while receiving what appears to be adequate anticoagulant therapy. Great care must be exercised in the use of both heparin and warfarin in patients with malignant disease because hemorrhage into areas of necrotic tumor can be hazardous. The use of anticoagulant therapy is generally contraindicated in patients with central nervous system metastases. Bulky disease is a relative contraindication, especially if central necrosis of the tumor is suspected, and particularly if the lesion is in the mediastinum or pleural spaces.

      The decision to treat thromboembolism occurring in a patient with malignancy may be difficult. One must carefully weigh the risks of therapy against expected benefits. The decision is also influenced by the patient's life expectancy, concurrent therapy, and the type of malignancy.

      b. **Heparin.** Low doses of heparin (5,000 units given subcutaneously every 12 hours) can be used to protect patients with malignant disease from thromboembolism during perioperative periods. Heparin may be used as the initial or long-term therapy for thromboembolic events in patients with malignant disease. Heparin may be administered either intravenously or by the subcutaneous route. Generally, the intravenous route is preferred for initial therapy so that the anticoagulant effect begins at once and adjustment of doses can be easily achieved. An initial dose of 5,000 units (70 U/kg) of heparin is given as an intravenous bolus followed by 1,000 to 1,200 units (15 U/kg) per hour as a continuous infusion. One should check the aPTT 1 hour after the heparin bolus to ensure that the patient is heparinizable (i.e., not AT-III deficient), 6 hours after beginning therapy, and 6 hours after any change in the dose of heparin. Some patients with malignant disease may appear to be refractory to heparin; in all likelihood, this reflects low levels of AT-III, owing to poor production or increased consumption, both of which may occur in patients with malignant disease. (*Note:* Infusion therapy with L-asparaginase has been associated with reduced levels of AT-III.) As long as the AT-III activity is above 50% of normal, it is usually possible to achieve the desired anticoagulant effect if adequate doses of heparin are given. If AT-III activity is less than 50% of normal, AT-III may be replaced using AT-III concentrates or fresh-frozen plasma.

Heparin may be administered by the subcutaneous route for both the acute and the chronic management of thromboembolism associated with malignancy. Using the subcutaneous route may be less desirable when treating acute events because the onset of anticoagulant effect is somewhat slower (2 to 3 hours), and adjusting the therapeutic effect may be more difficult. Subcutaneous heparin can be considered for chronic therapy provided that the patient can manage the twice-daily injection and weekly monitoring of the aPTT. In a patient who has been receiving intravenous heparin, half the total dose of intravenous heparin received in the previous 24 hours should be given subcutaneously twice a day (e.g., 1,000 U/h by intravenous infusion equals 12,000 units s.c. b.i.d.). For the patient being started on subcutaneous heparin, the initial dose is 7,500 to 10,000 units s.c. b.i.d. The partial thromboplastin time (aPTT) should be checked 6 hours after the third dose of heparin. Otherwise, the aPTT should be checked 6 hours after a subcutaneous dose of heparin. The goal for the aPTT should be similar to that of intravenous heparin, namely, 1.5 to 2 times the patient's baseline aPTT.

c. **Warfarin** is often selected as the therapy of choice for the chronic management of thromboembolic events associated with malignant disease. The use of warfarin in this setting is of concern because patients with malignant disease are frequently taking multiple medications that can alter the patient's response to warfarin. An additional concern about the use of warfarin in patients with malignancy is the development of purpura fulminans. This complication may be due to lower than normal protein C levels in patients who had DIC before initiation of warfarin therapy. Warfarin should not be used if there is laboratory evidence of DIC.

Despite these caveats, warfarin is often used for the prevention and treatment of clotting problems in patients with cancer. For most patients, an international normalized ratio (INR) of 2 to 3 is required; for patients with mechanical prosthetic valves, recurrent systemic embolism, or lupus anticoagulant with thrombosis, an INR of 2.5 to 3.5 is necessary (Table 29-2). Table 29-2 also gives the recommended vitamin K dose necessary to reduce the INR to therapeutic levels in patients who are taking warfarin and have INR values higher than 4.5. Care must be taken to balance the risks of bleeding in patients

Table 29-2.   Clinical indications, international normalized ratio (INR) goals

Using the INR for anticoagulation monitoring

A. Clinical indications requiring an INR of 2.0–3.0
   Prophylaxis
      Postoperative deep vein thrombosis (general surgery)
      Postoperative deep vein thrombosis during hip surgical procedures and fractures
      Myocardial infarction to prevent venous thromboembolism
      Transient ischemic attacks
      Tissue heart valves
      Atrial fibrillation
      Valvular heart disease
      Recurrent deep vein thrombosis and pulmonary embolism
      Arterial disease including myocardial infarction
   Treatment
      Venous thrombosis
      Pulmonary embolism
B. Clinical indications requiring an INR of 2.5–3.5
   Prophylaxis
      Mechanical prosthetic valves
      Recurrent systemic embolism
      Lupus anticoagulant with thrombosis

Table 29-3.   Vitamin K₁ administration for patients on warfarin

Doses of vitamin K₁ to reduce INR in patients on warfarin

INR	Vitamin K₁ dosage (slow IVP)*	Time expected for response to vitamin K or to repeat INR
>4.5 but <6	None, hold warfarin	24 h
>6 but <10	0.5–1.0 mg; may repeat dosage if INR still high at 24 h	Reduction of INR expected at 8h: therapeutic INR expected at 24–48 h
>10 but <20	3–5 mg; may repeat dosage if INR is still high at 6–12 h	Reductions of INR expected at 6 h: repeat INR every 6–12 h
>20	10 mg; may repeat dosage if INR is still high at 6–12 h; (consider fresh-frozen plasma)	Reduction of INR expected at 6 h; repeat INR every 6–12 h

* If patient is bleeding, a procedure is planned, or patient has just had a procedure, consider the use of fresh-frozen plasma.
Modified from J. Hirsh et al. Oral anticoagulants.
Mechanism of action, clinical effectiveness, and optimal therapeutic range. *Chest* 102 [Suppl.]:312, 1992.

with elevated INRs—with or without thrombocytopenia—against the risks of clotting and thrombosis if the reversal of the anticoagulation is too vigorous.

d.   **The use of platelet-inhibiting drugs**, such as aspirin, other nonsteroidal anti-inflammatory agents, or dipyridamole, has met with varying degrees of success in the prevention of repeated thromboembolic events in patients with malignant disease. Care must be taken with the use of such drugs, especially in thrombocytopenic patients, because the risk of bleeding associated with thrombocytopenia is increased.

e.   **Fibrinolytic therapy**. Systemic malignancy is a relative contraindication to fibrinolytic therapy.

f.   **Vascular interruption devices**, such as Greenfield filters, may be used in patients who cannot tolerate anticoagulant therapy or who develop emboli while on adequate anticoagulant therapy.

2. **DIC.** Therapy for DIC includes the following:
   Urgently **correct shock** (if present).

   Treat the underlying disease process.

   Replace depleted blood components (e.g., platelets, cryoprecipitate for fibrinogen and factor VIII, fresh-frozen plasma for other factors) if clinically significant bleeding is present.

   Consider the use of **heparin only in the following situations:**
   - In patients with acute promyelocytic leukemia (see Chap. 19).
   - When there is evidence of ongoing end-organ damage due to microvascular thrombosis
   - If venous thrombosis occurs
   - These latter two complications of DIC are most likely to occur as a component of the SIRS, and the treatment of the underlying cause of the SIRS is necessary in addition to treatment with heparin. There is no evidence that chronic warfarin therapy is of value for treating the chronic DIC seen in some patients with neoplasia if thromboses are absent. Warfarin may predispose to the development of purpura fulminans in the presence of chronic DIC.

II. **Bleeding in patients with cancer**
   A. **Tumor invasion**. It is well recognized that bleeding may be a warning sign of cancer. Bloody sputum may indicate carcinoma of the lung, blood in the urine may be a sign of carcinoma of the bladder or kidney, blood in the stool may be due to carcinoma of the alimentary tract, and postmenopausal vaginal bleeding may be caused by endometrial carcinoma. In each of these instances, bleeding can be directly related to the invasive properties of cancer and disruption of normal tissue integrity.
   B. **Hemostatic abnormalities.** Often bleeding in patients with cancer is not due to the direct effects of the neoplasm but rather to indirect effects of the cancer or its therapy on one of the components of the hemostatic system. Because of the frequency and the special management problems caused by abnormalities in the hemostatic system in patients with cancer and the frequency with which these problems occur, it is important to consider the possible causes and corrective measures in detail.
      1. **Increased vascular fragility** may be due to chronic corticosteroid therapy, chronic malnutrition, or "senile purpura." Bleeding is usually not severe, but bruising, particularly around in-

travenous sites, is common. Hemostatic therapy is not necessary.

2. **Thrombocytopenia** may occur for a variety of reasons. Some of the more common causes are as follows:

   a. **Chemotherapy and radiotherapy** regularly cause depression of platelet production. Serial blood cell counts must be monitored while patients are being treated.

   b. **Bone marrow invasion or replacement** causing thrombocytopenia is commonly seen only with leukemias or lymphomas but may occur in other cancers that invade the bone marrow.

   c. **Splenomegaly with splenic sequestration** is most common with leukemia or lymphoma.

   d. **Folate deficiency** with decreased platelet production is common in patients with cancer because of poor nutrition. Dietary history should provide the clues to the diagnosis.

   e. **Immune thrombocytopenic purpura (ITP)**. Patients with lymphoproliferative malignancies (e.g., chronic lymphocytic leukemia, Hodgkin's disease) often develop ITP. ITP may also be the presenting symptom of a nonhematologic malignancy. Usually, the ITP improves with prednisone, 1 mg/kg/day, followed by treatment of the malignancy.

   f. **Drug-induced immune thrombocytopenia**. Many nonchemotherapy medications used to treat patients with malignancy can cause immune thrombocytopenia. Offending agents to consider are heparin, vancomycin, H_2-receptor antagonists, penicillins, cephalosporins, interferon, and sulfa-containing antibiotics, diuretics, or hypoglycemic agents.

   g. **Graft-versus-host disease** developed after bone marrow transplantation may produce a chronic (often isolated) immune-mediated thrombocytopenia. The platelet count may respond to increased immunosuppression.

3. **Abnormalities of platelet function** must be suspected in patients who have a normal or near normal platelet count but signs or symptoms of bleeding and a documented prolonged bleeding time. Most cases are secondary to drug effects, including aspirin and other nonsteroidal antiinflammatory agents, antibiotics (e.g., ticarcillin), antidepressants (e.g., tricyclic drugs), tranquilizers, and alcohol. Consider any drug that the

patient is taking as a possible offender until proved otherwise. The presence of fibrin degradation products is a common cause of platelet dysfunction in patients with malignancy who also have DIC. Platelet dysfunction may occur in patients with malignant paraproteinemias as a result of the coating of the platelet surfaces by the immunoglobulin. When renal failure develops or is present in such patients, the platelet dysfunction is magnified.

4. **Coagulation factor deficiencies** may develop in patients with malignancy for several reasons:

   Acute (decompensated) DIC depletes most clotting factors but to variable degrees.

   Liver failure causes deficiency of all clotting factors except factor VIII.

   Malnutrition leads to deficiency of factors II, VII, IX, and X (the vitamin K–dependent factors).

   Fibrinolysis may be due to the release of urokinase in prostate cancer or secondary to DIC. This may produce hypofibrinogenemia as well as fibrin split products, which act as circulating anticoagulants.

   Functionally abnormal clotting factors are occasionally seen. The most commonly diagnosed abnormality is dysfibrinogenemia.

5. **Acquired circulating anticoagulants** may develop in patients with a number of different tumors. Many of these anticoagulants are heparinoid in nature. The most common associations are with carcinoma of the lung and myeloma. Other anticoagulants act as antithrombins; in this case, the most common association is with carcinoma of the breast.

6. **Chemotherapy-induced bleeding:**

   Mithiamycin, although rarely used now, may lead to platelet dysfunction and a reduction in multiple coagulation factors. Hemorrhage due to these effects may occur in up to half of patients treated with mithramycin.

   Anthracyclines may be associated with primary fibrinolysis or fibrinogenolysis and hemorrhage.

   Dactinomycin is a powerful vitamin K antagonist that causes defective synthesis of all vitamin K–dependent proteins (factors II, VII, IX, and X, protein C, and protein S).

   Melphalan, cytarabine, doxorubicin, vincristine, and vinblastine are all associated with platelet dysfunction.

III. **Laboratory evaluation of hemostasis in patients with malignancy.** About half of all patients with cancer and about 90% of those with metastases manifest abnormalities of one or more routine coagulation parameters. These abnormalities may be minor early in the patient's disease, but as the disease progresses, the hemostatic abnormalities become more pronounced. Serial coagulation tests may offer the clinician a clue to response to therapy or recurrence of malignant disease. Serial evaluations of coagulation tests are of more value in patients with no symptoms of hemostatic disruption than is a single determination.

A. Screening tests for bleeding. The following tests provide an adequate screening battery:

Platelet count	aPTT
Bleeding time	Thrombin time
PT	Fibrinogen level

B. Interpretation of screening laboratory studies. Abnormal results of the screening tests reflect hematologic problems caused by blood vessels, platelets, or coagulation factors. The following list provides clues to the interpretation of the screening test results that help determine the most likely cause or causes of the patient's bleeding.

    1. Platelet count

        Normal is 150,000 to 450,000/μL.

        If **thrombocytopenia** is less than 100,000/μL, consider the following:

            Bone marrow failure
            Increased consumption of platelets
            Splenic pooling of platelets

        Thrombocytosis with a platelet count of more than 500,000/μL has the following characteristics:

            It is common in patients with neoplasms.
            It may be seen in association with iron deficiency (e.g., secondary to gut neoplasm).
            It usually poses no risk of arterial thrombosis unless the patient has a myeloproliferative disorder.

    2. Bleeding time. This is a useful screening test if the platelet count is normal and platelet dysfunction is suspected.

        A normal bleeding time requires normal platelet number, normal platelet function, and normal function of the blood vessels and connective tissues.

        A prolonged bleeding time may be due to thrombocytopenia, abnormal platelet function, and rarely, inadequate vessel function. The bleeding time may be spuriously prolonged in elderly people with "tissue-paper" skin. The following formula is a rough rule of thumb to be used to estimate what the bleeding time should be in patients who have platelet counts between 10,000 and 100,000/μL. Although it was derived using the Mielke template, the principle should still hold for contemporary bleeding time devices.

Bleeding time = 30 − (platelet count/μl ÷ 4,000)

3. **Prolonged PT.** This is seen in the presence of the following:

    Deficiency of one or more of the following clotting factors: VII, X, V, II (prothrombin), or I (fibrinogen); oral anticoagulant therapy leads to a deficiency of factors II, VII, IX, and X

    Circulating anticoagulants against factor VII, X, V, or II

    Dysfibrinogenemia

4. **Prolonged aPTT**

    Deficiency of any of the following clotting factors: XII, XI IX, VIII, X, V, II, or I. Factor XII deficiency is not associated with bleeding. Fletcher and Fitzgerald factor deficiencies (both rare) may also prolong the aPTT.

    Circulating anticoagulants directed against the above-mentioned factors or the lupus inhibitor.

    Anticoagulant therapy with the following:

    Heparin

    Oral anticoagulants

5. **Prolonged thrombin time.** Prolongation of the thrombin time may be due to the following:

    Hypofibrinogenemia (fibrinogen < 100 mg/dL)

    Some forms of dysfibrinogenemia

    Fibrin–fibrinogen split products

    Heparin therapy

    Paraproteins

    If the thrombin time is prolonged, further studies to clarify the cause may be required.

6. **Low fibrinogen level.** When evaluating the results of a fibrinogen assay, one must be familiar with the assay method used. Many laboratories use immunologic assays, which measure both functionally normal and abnormal fibrinogens. If such an assay is in use, the thrombin time can be used to evaluate the functional integrity of the fibrinogen. A low functional fibrinogen level means that production is decreased, consumption is increased, or a dysfibrinogen is present. Fibrinogen is an acute-phase reactant and is often elevated with advanced malignancy. A fibrinogen level in the normal range may actually be relatively low for the patient's physiologic state and thus may be a sign of DIC (see Table 29-1).

C. **Laboratory findings in patients with DIC.** Acute DIC is often associated with significant hemorrhage, whereas chronic DIC may be asymptomatic or associated with thromboses. Screening and confirmatory laboratory tests are shown in Table 29-3.

Table 29-3. Coagulation tests that may show an abnormality in patients with cancer without clinical bleeding or thrombosis

Test	Common result in patients with malignancy
Antithrombin III	Decreased
β-Thromboglobulin	Increased
Cryofibrinogen	Present
D-Dimer	Increased
Factor VIII	Increased
Fibronectin	Decreased
Fibrin monomer (soluble)	Present
Fibrinogen	Increased
Fibrin(ogen) degradation products	Present
Fibrinopeptide A	Increased
Fibrinopeptide B	Increased
Plasmin	Increased
Plasminogen	Decreased
Platelet count	Increased or decreased
Platelet factor 4	Increased
Protein C	Decreased

IV. Treatment of hemorrhagic syndromes in patients with malignant disease
   A. Transfusion therapy
      1. General guidelines
         a. Regard elective transfusion with allogeneic blood as an outcome to be avoided. Consider the factors that will influence the use of blood products, including the following:

Alternative forms of therapy that could control bleeding (e.g., topical measures or desmopressin.

How symptomatic is the patient? Do not treat an abnormal laboratory test in a symptom-free patient. For example, patients with chronic DIC may demonstrate prolongation of both the PT and aPTT and mild to moderate thrombocytopenia. If there is no demonstrable bleeding, transfusion therapy is not necessary.

         b. Use the specific blood component needed by the patient
         c. Minimize complications of transfusion by using the following:

Only the amount and type of blood product indicated for the patient in the specific clinical setting.

Special filters, irradiated blood, or both when indicated.

2. **Blood component therapy**
   a. **Platelet transfusions**
      (1) **Available forms of platelets for transfusion.** Platelets may be ordered and transfused in various ways. Because most patients with an underlying malignancy have the potential for needing long-term platelet support, platelet products should be leukocyte reduced from the initiation of transfusion (see Section IV.A.3). In general, patients who need platelet support can be started with random donor platelets. Given the added expense and the limited pools of platelet pheresis donors in many centers, single donor and HLA-matched platelets should be reserved for patients who have become refractory to random-donor platelets [see Section IV.A.2.a.(4)]. There are no solid data to suggest that starting with platelet pheresis products decreases the incidence of alloimmunization. In fact, the Trial to Reduce Alloimmunization to Platelets Study Group study did not show any benefit in the use of platelet pheresis over platelet concentrates. Conversely, patients who are candidates for bone marrow transplantation should receive single-donor platelets (if available) from the initiation of platelet therapy. Patients who are candidates for transplantation with bone marrow from an HLA-matched sibling should not receive apheresis products from the potential donor before the transplantation.

         (a) **Random-donor platelets or platelet concentrates.** Five to six units (usually pooled in one bag) are considered an adequate dose for a 70-kg adult.

         (b) **Platelets obtained by pheresis (single-donor platelets) and HLA-matched platelets obtained by pheresis.** These come as a single pack and represent the apheresed platelets from 3 to 4 liters of blood from a single donor. One unit of platelets obtained by pheresis is equivalent to 5 to 6 units of platelet concentrate.

(2) **Check platelet count** 10 minutes to 1 hour, and then 24 hours, after platelet transfusion to estimate survival of platelets in the patient. Each unit of platelet concentrate should increase the platelet count by 10,000/µL. The expected 1-hour posttransfusion rise in platelets is 15,000 platelets/µL divided by the patient's body surface area in square meters for each unit of platelet concentrate. (Thus, for a person of 2 m², 6 units should produce a rise of 45,000/µL [6 × 15,000/2]).

(3) **Criteria for transfusing platelets:**

(a) For patients with **reduced platelet production**, criteria for transfusion are shown in Table 29-4.

Table 29-4.   Guidelines for platelet transfusion in patients with reduced platelet production

Platelet count	Recommendation
0–5,000/µL	Transfuse with platelets even if there is no evidence of bleeding
6,000–10,000/µL	Transfuse with platelets if there is: Fresh minor hemorrhage Temperature 38°C or active infection Rapid decline in platelet count (>50% per day) Headache Significant gastrointestinal blood loss Presence of confluent petechiae (as opposed to scattered petechiae) Continuous bleeding from a wound or other sites Planned minor procedure such as a bone marrow biopsy
11,000–20,000/µL	Transfuse with platelets if there is more rapid bleeding or if more complicated procedures are anticipated.
>20,000/µL	If major surgery is planned or when life-threatening bleeding occurs, the platelet count should be increased to at least 50,000/µL For intracranial surgery, transfuse to a platelet count of at least 100,000/µL (bleeding time must be checked before surgery and must be normal). In fully anticoagulated patients, is advisable to keep the platelet count to at least 50,000/mL

(b) **Increased platelet destruction.** Platelet transfusions are of limited benefit in patients with thrombocytopenia due to increased destruction as a result of either antibodies or consumption. If potentially life-threatening bleeding complicates thrombocytopenia due to increased destruction, platelet transfusions may be given; however, small increments in the platelet count usually occur. Intravenous γ-globulin, 1 g/kg i.v. daily × 2 days given before the platelet transfusions, might improve the response.

(c) **Dysfunctional platelets.** One must stop any drugs known to cause platelet dysfunction. Although the use of platelet transfusions should be considered, pharmacologic methods of enhancing platelet function, such as desmopressin, should be used if possible (see Section IV.B.1).

(4) **Refractoriness to platelet transfusions** (platelet rise <5,000/μL after 5 to 6 units of platelet concentrates or 1 unit of platelets obtained by pheresis on two separate occasions) is a common problem in multiply transfused patients. Alloimmunization is the most difficult form to treat and therefore is best prevented (see Section IV.A.3). Apparent refractoriness to platelets may be due to shortened platelet life-span from fever, septicemia, DIC, splenomegaly, drugs, infections, or bleeding.

(a) **Evaluation.** Patients who become refractory to platelet transfusions should have a laboratory evaluation for alloimmunization. They should also be evaluated for infection and DIC as well as have all potentially offending medications stopped.

(b) **Therapy.** The therapeutic modalities for ITP (corticosteroids, intravenous globulin, danazol) are generally ineffective for platelet refractoriness due to alloimmunization. Two therapeutic options exist:

(i) **HLA-matched platelets**
(ii) **Cross-matched platelets.** Because platelets are available at most blood centers, if a blood center performs cross-matching it is often easier to obtain cross-matched platelets because no specific donor requirement is required. This product is as effective as HLA-matched platelets in producing a platelet response in the alloimmunized patient. Either platelet concentrates or apheresed platelets can be cross-matched with the recipient. Nonreactive or, in extenuating circumstances, the least reactive platelets can then be selected for transfusion.

b. **Coagulation factor support**
(1) **Fresh-frozen plasma** contains all clotting factors (but not platelets) and should be used for multiple coagulation factor deficiencies. Fresh-frozen plasma requires 20 to 30 minutes to thaw and must be thawed at 37°C or lower.

(2) **Cryoprecipitated antihemophilic factor (AHF)** is a source of factor VIII–von Willebrand factor (vWF) complex, fibrinogen, and factor XIII. Each bag of cryoprecipitated AHF contains about 50% of the factor VIII–vWF complex and 20% to 40% of the fibrinogen harvested from 1 unit of fresh whole blood. Cryoprecipitated AHF is stored in a frozen state and has the advantage of concentrating the clotting factors in a small volume (10 to 15 mL/U). It is used primarily in deficiencies of fibrinogen. The goal is to keep the fibrinogen level higher than 100 mg/dL. The usual dosage of cryoprecipitated AHF to correct hypofibrinogenemia is 1 bag of cryoprecipitated AHF for every 5 kg of body weight. Because 50% is recovered after transfusion, this may only raise the fibrinogen level by about 50 mg/dL. Larger doses may be needed for severe hypofibrinogene-

mia or "flaming" DIC. The patient is evaluated to determine if the laboratory values have been corrected.

(3) **Factor IX concentrates** are available as factor IX complex concentrates, which contain factors II, VII, IX and X, or as coagulation factor IX concentrates. The latter are highly purified factor IX concentrates with little or no other coagulation factors. Several precautions are worth noting regarding the factor IX concentrates.

(a) This concentrate is made from pooled plasma but is treated with viral attenuation processes, such as dry or vapor heat in the case of factor IX complex concentrates (therefore, the risk of hepatitis is significant) and solvent-detergent or monoclonal antibody in the case of coagulation factor IX concentrates. The dose depends on the preparation to be used. The goal is to bring the factor concentration to no more than 50% of normal.

(b) There is a small risk of DIC resulting from the use of factor IX complex concentrates. Patients with liver dysfunction and newborns are at increased risk. The coagulation factor concentrates are far less thrombogenic and should be used in cases at increased risk for venous thrombosis or DIC.

(1) Factor IX concentrates are stored in the lyophilized state. Do not shake when reconstituting.

3. **Leukocyte reduction.** Patients who have not previously received transfusions and who will need long-term blood product support should receive leukocyte-reduced ($<5 \times 10^6$ leukocytes/bag) blood products. Leukocyte reduction may prevent febrile transfusion reactions, prevent cytomegalovirus (CMV) infections, and delay alloimmunization. Two methods of leukocyte reduction by filtration are currently available: prestorage and bedside.

a. **Bedside filtration** involves leukocyte reduction at the time of transfusion. Disadvantages include plugging of the filter, the presence of leukocyte breakdown products, bag breakage, and lack of consistency of products. Filters are available for RBCs and platelets.

  b. **AS-1 or AS-3 prestorage filtered RBCs** are RBCs that have been leukocyte reduced within 8 to 24 hours of collection. Advantages are fewer leukocyte breakdown products, ease of administration, and consistent quality (guaranteed $<5 \times 10^6$ leukocytes/bag). Cost may be perceived as a disadvantage. However, this is offset by the expense of stocking filters, training of staff in the use of filters, and breakage. The only platelet product currently available as a prestorage leukocyte-reduced product is platelets obtained by pheresis.

  4. **CMV-negative blood.** Only patients known to be anti–CMV-negative with impaired immunity should be considered for the use of CMV negative blood. This group includes children for the most part. The use of CMV-negative blood seriously restricts the potential donor pool for these patients. Leukocyte-reduced blood products ($<5.0 \times 106$/bag) are equivalent to CMV negative screened products.

  WBC depletion filters also remove CMV since CMV resides in the WBCs. Irradiation of blood products does not render them CMV free. Frozen-deglycerolized blood is considered free of CMV contamination.

  5. **Irradiated blood products.** These prevent the development of graft-versus-host disease. Irradiated blood products are expensive and should be limited to patients with one of the following indications:

     Congenital immunodeficiency
     Low-birthweight, premature infants
     Intrauterine and exchange transfusions
     Bone marrow transplantation
     Directed blood donations to blood relatives
     Granulocyte transfusions
     High-dose chemotherapy with growth factor or stem cell rescue
     Hodgkin's disease (relative indication)
     Leukemia and non-Hodgkin's lymphoma (relative indication)

B. **Other forms of therapy**
  1. **Desmopressin.** Desmopressin, 0.3 µg/kg i.v. over 30 minutes every 12 to 24 hours for 2 to 4 days, may be used to elevate factor VIII and vWF levels as well as improve platelet function. Tachyphylaxis may occur if therapy is continued for longer periods. Intranasal desmopressin, 0.25 mL b.i.d. using a solution containing 1.3 mg/mL, has been given for minor bleeding episodes.

2. **Fibrin glue.** This is a topical biologic adhesive. Its effects imitate the final stages of coagulation. The glue consists of a solution of concentrated human fibrinogen, which is activated by the addition of bovine thrombin and calcium chloride. The resulting clot promotes hemostasis and tissue sealing. The clot is completely absorbed during the healing process. The best adhesive and hemostatic effect is obtained by applying the two solutions simultaneously to the open wound surface. Fibrin glue has been used primarily in surgical settings. It has been most effective when used for surface, low-pressure bleeding. There is a small risk of anaphylactic reaction because of the bovine origin of the thrombin.

3. **Antifibrinolytic agents.** Epsilon aminocaproic acid (EACA) and tranexamic acid have been used to control bleeding associated with primary fibrinolysis as seen in patients with prostatic carcinoma and in a small number of patients with refractory thrombocytopenia. Great care must be taken in the use of these agents because of a possible increased risk of thrombosis. EACA may be used topically to control small-area, small-volume bleeding.

4. **Oprelvekin (interleukin-11).** Oprelvekin has recently been approved by the US Food and Drug Administration for the treatment and prevention of chemotherapy-related thrombocytopenia. Oprelvekin is a thrombopoietic growth factor that directly stimulates the proliferation of hematopoietic stem cells and megakaryocyte progenitor cells as well as megakaryocyte maturation, resulting in increased platelet production. It is known to cause fluid retention and should be used with caution in patients who have congestive heart failure (CHF), those with a history of CHF, and those being treated for CHF. One must also be cautious using this agent in patients who are receiving diuretic therapy or ifosfamide because sudden deaths have been reported as a result of severe hypokalemia. Oprelvekin should be used to prevent thrombocytopenia, which would be severe enough to require platelet transfusions. Therapy usually begins 6 to 24 hours after the completion of chemotherapy, and patients should be monitored for any signs or symptoms of allergic reactions or cardiac dysfunction.

SELECTED READINGS

Anand SS, Wells PS, Hunt D, et al. Does this patient have deep vein thrombosis? *JAMA* 1998;279(14):1094–1099.

Baker WF Jr. Thrombosis and hemostasis in cardiology: review of pathophysiology and clinical practice. II. Recommendations for antithrombotic therapy. *Clin Appl Thromb Hemost* 1998;4(2):143–147.

Bauer KA, et al. Tumor necrosis factor infusions have a pro-coagulant effect on the hemostatic mechanism of humans. *Blood* 1989;74:165.

Bern MM, et al. Very low doses of warfarin can prevent thrombosis in central venous catheters: a randomized prospective trial. *Ann Intern Med* 1990;112:423.

Beutler E. Platelet transfusions: the 20,000/μl trigger. *Blood* 1993; 81:1411–1413.

Brennan M. Fibrin glue. *Blood Rev* 1991;5:240.

Dzik S. Leukodepletion blood filters: filter design and mechanisms of leukocyte removal. *Transfusion Med Rev* 1993;7:65

Dzik WH. Leukoreduced blood components, laboratory and clinical aspects. In: Rossi EC, et al., eds. *Principles of transfusion medicine,* 2nd ed. 1996:353–373.

Esparaz B, Kies M, Kwaan H. Thromboembolism in cancer. In: Kwaan HC, Samama MM, eds. *Clinical thrombosis.* Boca Raton: CRC Press, 1989:317–333.

Friedberg RC. Clinical and laboratory factors underlying refractoriness to platelet transfusions. *J Clin Apheresis* 1996;11:143–148.

Gelb AB, Leavitt AD. Crossmatch compatible platelets improve corrected count increments in patients who are refractory to randomly selected patients. *Transfusion* 1997;37(6):624–630.

Gibble JW, Ness PM. Fibrin glue: the perfect operative sealant? *Transfusion* 1990;30:741–747.

Ginsberg JS. Management of venous thromboembolism. *N Engl J Med* 1996;335(24)1816–1828.

Griffin MR, Stanson AW, Brown ML, et al. Deep venous thrombosis and pulmonary embolism: risk of subsequent malignant neoplasms. *Arch Intern Med* 1987;147:1907–1911.

Hillyer CD, Emmens RK, Zago-Novaretti M, Berkman EM. et al. Methods for the reduction of transfusion transmitted cytomegalovirus infection: filtration versus the use of seronegative donor units. *Transfusion* 1994:34:929–934.

Hull RD, Pineo GF. Prophylaxis of deep vein thrombosis and pulmonary embolism: current recommendations. *Clin Appl Thromb Hemost* 1998;4(2):96–104.

Humphries JE. Transfusion therapy in acquired coagulopathies. *Hematol Oncol Clin North* Am 1994;8(6):1181–1201.

Kunkel LA. Acquired circulating anticoagulants in malignancy. *Semin Thromb Hemost* 1992;18:416–423.

Lane TA. Leukocyte reduction of cellular blood component: effectiveness, benefits, quality control and costs. *Arch Pathol Lab Med* 1994;118:392–404.

Legler TJ, Fischer I, Dittman J, et al. Frequency and course of refractoriness in multiply transfused patients. *Ann Hematol* 1997;74(4):185–189.

Mannucci DM. Desmopressin: a non-traditional form of treatment for congenital and acquired bleeding disorders. *Blood* 1988;72:1449–1455.

McCarthy PM. Fibrin glue in cardiothoracic surgery. *Transfus Med Rev* 1993;7(3):173–179.

Murgo A. Thrombotic microangiopathy in the cancer patient including those induced by chemotherapy agents. *Semin Hematol* 1987;24:161–177.

O'Connell, Lee EJ, Schiffer CA. The value of 10 min posttransfusion platelet counts. *Transfusion* 1988;28:66–67.

Pisciotto PT, Benson K, Hume H, et al. Prophylactic versus therapeutic platelet transfusion practices in hematology and/or oncology patients. *Transfusion* 1995;35:498–502.

Poon M. Cryoprecipitate: uses and alternatives. *Transfus Med Rev* 1993;7(3):180–192.

Practice parameter for the use of fresh-frozen plasma, cryoprecipitate, and platelets. *JAMA* 1994;271:777–781.

Przepiorka D, LeParc GF, Stovall MA, Werch J, Lichtiger B. Use of irradiated blood components: practice parameter. *Am J Clin Pathol* 1996;106:6–11.

Przepiorka D, LeParc GF, Werch J, Lichtiger B. Prevention of transfusion associated CMV infection: practice parameter. *Am J Clin Pathol* 1996;106:163–169.

Schafer A. The hypercoagulable state. *Ann Intern Med* 1985;102:814–828.

Slichter SJ. Algorithm for managing the platelet refractory patient. *J Clin Apheresis* 1997;2(1):4–9.

Sorenson HT, Mellemkjaer L, Steffensen FH, Olsen JH, Nielsen GL. The risk of the diagnosis of cancer after primary deep venous thrombosis or pulmonary embolism. *N Engl J Med* 1998;338(17): 1169–1173.

Tefferi A, Silverstein MN, Hoagland HC. Primary thrombocythemia. *Semin Oncol* 1995;22(4):334–340.

Trial to Reduce Alloimmunization to Platelets Study Group. Leukocyte reduction and ultraviolet B irradiation of platelets to prevent alloimmunization and refractoriness to platelet transfusions. *N Engl J Med* 1997;337:1861–1869.

Critical Care Issues in Oncology and Bone Metastasis

Salvatore Veltri

Spinal cord compression, cerebral edema, superior vena cava syndrome (SVCS), anaphylaxis, respiratory failure, tumor lysis syndrome, and bone metastasis can be major causes of morbidity and, in some cases, potential mortality in patients with cancer. Because of the critical nature of these complications of cancer and its treatment, oncologists, oncology nurses, and other oncology health professionals must be prepared to recognize the signs and symptoms of these disorders promptly, so that appropriate therapy can be instituted without delay.

I. **Spinal cord compression**
   A. **Tumors.** The most common tumors resulting in spinal cord compression are breast cancer, lung cancer, prostate cancer, and renal cancer, although it may also occur with sarcoma, multiple myeloma, and lymphoma. Purely intradural or epidural lesions are uncommon because more than three fourths of cases arise from either metastasis to a vertebral body or other bony parts of the vertebra or, less commonly, direct extension from a paravertebral soft tissue mass. Seventy percent of the bone lesions are osteolytic, 10% osteoblastic, and 20% mixed. More than 85% of patients with metastases to the vertebra have lesions that involve more than one vertebral body.
   B. **Symptoms and signs.** The most common early symptoms seen in patients with spinal cord compression are localized vertebral or radicular pain. These are not from the cord compression per se but rather from involvement of the vertebral structures and nerve roots at the level of the compression. Localized tenderness to pressure or percussion over the involved vertebrae is often seen on physical examination. Because pain is seen initially in up to 90% of patients, localized back pain, radicular pain, or spinal tenderness in a patient with cancer should evoke the clinical suspicion of the physician and prompt further evaluation to determine whether the patient has potential or early cord compression. Muscle weakness, evidenced by subjective symptoms or objective physical findings, is present in 75% of patients by the time of diagnosis. The clinician must be aware that progression of this symptom can vary from a gradual increase in weakness over several days to a precipitous loss of function over several hours that may worsen rapidly to the point of paraplegia. If muscle weakness is present, it is incumbent on the physician to act urgently to obtain

consultation with the neurosurgeon and the radio-therapist. It is not appropriate to wait until the next morning! By the time there is muscle weakness, most patients also have sensory deficits below the level of the compression and changes in bladder and bowel sphincter function. When compression is diagnosed late or if treatment is not started emergently, only 25% of patients who are unable to walk when treatment is started regain full ambulation.

C. **Diagnosis.** Magnetic resonance imaging (MRI) is now considered the diagnostic modality of choice, although high-resolution computed tomography (CT) with myelography is an alternative. Plain radiographs and bone scans give evidence of metastases to vertebrae but in and of themselves are not diagnostic of spinal cord involvement.

When there is evidence of bony involvement of the spine on a plain radiograph or bone scan, our approach is to obtain an MRI for those patients who have subjective or objective evidence of weakness, radicular pain, paresthesia, or sphincter dysfunction because these patients are at highest risk of spinal cord compression. Routine MRIs in patients who have completely asymptomatic bony spine metastases (without pain, tenderness, or neurologic findings on a comprehensive clinical examination) are not cost-effective. In patients with only localized pain or tenderness to correspond with the bone scan or radiographic findings, the yield of additional tests is much lower. Thus, the clinical determination of whether to obtain additional invasive or costly diagnostic tests is more difficult and requires a careful assessment of all clinical features of the patient. All patients with spinal metastasis require close follow-up, and they and their families must be urged to report relevant symptoms immediately.

D. **Treatment**

1. **Corticosteroids.** When a radiologic study identifies the level of cord compression or a neurologic deficit is detected on physical examination, dexamethasone may be started to reduce spinal cord edema. A recommended dose is 10 mg i.v. as a loading dose, and then 4 to 6 mg p.o. or i.v. every 6 hours to be continued through the initial weeks of radiation therapy. Thereafter, the dexamethasone therapy may be tapered.

2. **Radiotherapy**

   a. Although the preferences of individual centers vary, we generally recommend the **immediate initiation of radiotherapy** once cord compression is diagnosed. This is based on both randomized and nonrandomized studies showing no significant improvement in outcome for patients treated with surgery plus radiation versus those treated with radiation alone. In addition, metastatic disease to the spine is often not totally resectable, so that follow-up radiation therapy is frequently required. Third, because patients with evidence of spinal metastases frequently have either overt or microscopic evidence of metastases elsewhere that would likely grow during the postoperative recuperation period after surgery, the use of radiotherapy instead allows the initiation of some form of systemic therapy concurrently.

    b. **Radiation therapy** is most frequently given to a total dose of 40 to 45 Gy with daily dose fractions of 200 to 250 cGy. Alternatively, 400 cGy daily may be given initially for the first 3 days of therapy, and then subsequently decreased to standard-dose levels for the completion of the radiation course.

    c. **The clinical response** to radiation is dependent not only on the degree of cord involvement and the duration of symptoms but also on the underlying cell type. In general, patients with severe deficits, such as complete paraplegia or a long duration of neurologic deficit, are unlikely to have return to normal function. This underscores the need to diagnose and treat these patients rapidly. Lymphoma, myeloma, and other hematologic malignancies, along with breast and small cell lung carcinoma, tend to be more responsive than adenocarcinomas of the gastrointestinal tract, renal cancer, and others.

  3. **Surgery.** Surgery (whether decompressive laminectomy for posterior lesions or newer anterior approaches for other lesions) still plays a crucial role in selected patients. Indications for surgery include worsening of neurologic signs or symptoms or the appearance of new neurologic findings during the course of radiation treatment; vertebral collapse at presentation; a question of spinal stability; and disease recurrence within a prior radiation port. In selected patients, the use of surgery to remove disease in the vertebral bodies followed by stabilization can result in dramatic improvement in pain and function.

II. **Cerebral edema**

  A. **Clinical evaluation**

    1. **Neurologic signs and symptoms.** Intracranial metastases are commonly manifested by a variety of neurologic symptoms and signs, including headache, change in mentation, visual disturbances, cranial nerve deficits, focal motor or sensory abnormalities, difficulty with coordination, and seizures. In the more critical condition of brainstem herniation, there may be gradual to rapid loss of consciousness, neck stiffness, unilateral or bilateral pupillary abnormalities, ipsilateral hemiparesis, or respiratory dysfunction; the specific findings depend on whether there is uncal, central, or tonsillar herniation. Any neurologic complaint from a patient with cancer should be viewed with a high index of suspicion by members of the oncology team, especially if metastasis to the brain is commonly associated with the patient's tumor type.

The history and physical examination provide the first clue to the presence of a metastatic lesion or associated cerebral edema. In general, a history of gradual progression of neurologic symptoms before the development of a significant deficit is more consistent with a metastatic lesion, whereas the absence of symptoms followed by the abrupt onset of a severe deficit is suggestive of a cerebrovascular event.

2. **Radiologic studies.** MRI is the imaging modality of choice because it has greater sensitivity than CT in detecting the presence of metastatic lesions and in determining the extent of cerebral edema. CT is substituted for MRI in many institutions because of availability, ease of administration with shorter test time, and less cost. However, although CT is sufficient to detect the presence of cerebral edema in most patients, it is necessary to realize that CT fails to diagnose some lesions and may underestimate cerebral edema. If CT of the brain reveals no definite abnormality in the presence of persistent neurologic findings, MRI is the recommended next step. In general, we do not believe that delaying appropriate imaging studies (either CT or MRI) to examine plain skull radiographs or to obtain radionuclide studies in patients experiencing neurologic difficulties is warranted.

Warning: In a patient with cancer who has focal neurologic signs or symptoms, headache, or alteration in consciousness, a lumbar puncture to evaluate for possible neoplastic meningeal spread should not be done until a CT scan or MRI shows no evidence of mass, midline shift, or increased intracranial pressure. To do the lumbar puncture without this assurance could precipitate brainstem herniation, which is often rapidly fatal.

B. **Treatment**
1. **Symptomatic therapy.** Once the presence of cerebral edema is established, dexamethasone,

10 to 20 mg i.v. to load followed by 6 mg i.v. or p.o. four times daily, should be started. The rationale for the use of steroids centers around the etiology of cerebral edema. It appears that the invasion of malignant cells releases leukotrienes and other soluble mediators responsible for vasodilation, increased capillary permeability, and subsequent edema. Dexamethasone inhibits the conversion of arachidonic acid to leukotrienes, thereby decreasing vascular permeability. Additionally, steroids appear to have a direct stabilizing effect on brain capillaries. There is some evidence to suggest that patients who do not have lessening of cerebral edema with the dexamethasone dose just described may respond to higher doses (50 to 100 mg/day). Because of the risk of gastrointestinal bleeding and other side effects of doses higher than 32 mg/day, higher doses are usually not given for more than 48 to 72 hours.

Patients with severe cerebral edema leading to a life-threatening rise in intracranial pressure or brainstem herniation should also receive mannitol, 50 to 100 g (in a 20% to 25% solution) infused intravenously over about 30 minutes. This may be repeated every 6 hours if needed, although serum electrolytes and urine output must be monitored closely. Patients with severe cerebral edema should be intubated to allow for mechanical hyperventilation to reduce the carbon dioxide pressure to 25 to 30 mm Hg to decrease intracranial pressure.

2. **Therapy of the intracerebral tumor.** Once the patient has been stabilized, appropriate therapy for the cause underlying the cerebral edema should be implemented. Radiation is the usual modality for most metastases, but surgery may be considered for suitable candidates with easily accessible lesions.

3. **Nonmalignant causes of cerebral edema**, such as subdural hematoma in thrombocytopenic patients and brain abscess in immunocompromised patients, must always be considered.

III. **Superior vena cava syndrome.** The superior vena cava is a thin-walled vessel located to the right of the midline just anterior to the right main-stem bronchus. It is ultimately responsible for the venous drainage of the head, neck, and arms. Its location places it near lymph nodes that are commonly involved by malignant cells from lung primary tumors and lymphomas. Lymph node distention or the presence of a mass may compress the adjacent superior vena cava, leading to SVCS. Similarly, the presence of a thrombus due to a hypercoagulable state secondary to underlying malignancy or a thrombus developing around an indwelling central venous catheter may also lead to the development of this syndrome.

A. **Symptoms and signs.** Patients who develop SVCS commonly complain of dyspnea, orthopnea, paroxysmal nocturnal dyspnea, and facial, neck, and upper extremity swelling. Associated symptoms may include cough, hoarseness, and chest and neck pain. Headache and mental status changes also may be seen. A patient's symptoms may be gradual and progressive, with only mild facial swelling being present early in the course of this disorder. These early changes may be so subtle that the patient is unaware of them. Physical examination may reveal a spectrum of findings from facial edema to marked respiratory distress. Neck vein distention, facial edema or cyanosis, and tachypnea are commonly seen. Other potential physical findings include the presence of collateral vessels on the thorax, upper extremity edema, paralysis of the vocal cords, and mental status changes.

B. **Radiologic evaluation.** Patients may often be diagnosed by physical findings plus the presence of a mediastinal mass on chest radiographs. Although previously it was thought that the superior venocavogram was required to establish the diagnosis and delineate the extent of obstruction, current opinion now appears to favor the use of CT instead. CT permits a more detailed examination of surrounding anatomy, including adjacent lymphadenopathy; may differentiate between extrinsic compression and an intrinsic lesion (primary thrombus); poses less risk to the patient; aids in treatment planning for radiation therapy; and allows for possible percutaneous biopsy of a compressing mass.

SVCS may occur in patients with subclavian catheters. The injection of contrast material into these catheters is useful to determine the presence of a thrombus. However, a thrombus forms in the venous vasculature distal to the caval obstruction in most patients with SVCS secondary to external compression. Thus, a clot may be primary or secondary; determination of the cause and the appropriate treatment depends on both the clinical situation and the radiologic findings.

C. **Tissue diagnosis.** Although some patients present with such severe respiratory compromise as to require emergent treatment, most patients are clinically stable and may undergo biopsy for a tissue diagnosis. Tissue may be acquired through multiple methods, including bronchoscopy, CT-guided biopsy, mediastinoscopy, or mediastinotomy. Thoracotomy is the most invasive option and is rarely needed. Because of increased venous pressure and dilated veins distal to the obstruction, extreme care must be taken to ensure adequate hemostasis after any biopsy procedure.

D. **Treatment.** Initially, patients with SVCS may be treated with oxygen for dyspnea; furosemide, 20 to

40 mg i.v., to reduce edema; and dexamethasone, 16 mg i.v. or p.o. daily in divided doses. The benefit of dexamethasone is not clear. In patients with lymphoma, there is probably a lympholytic effect with resultant decrease in tumor mass; in patients with most other tumors, the effect is probably limited to decreasing any local inflammatory reaction from the tumor and from subsequent initial radiotherapy.

1. **Neoplasms.** Therapy for SVCS ultimately involves radiation therapy for most tumors but possibly chemotherapy as a single modality for particularly sensitive tumor types, such as small cell lung cancer, lymphomas, and germ cell cancers. Radiation therapy may be given in relatively high-dose fractions (e.g., 4 Gy) for several days, followed by a reversion to "standard doses" thereafter. We usually continue dexamethasone for about 1 week after the start of radiation treatment.

2. **Thrombi.** SVCS secondary to vascular thrombi may require the use of thrombolytic therapy. Both streptokinase, 250,000 units by i.v. bolus over 30 minutes, and urokinase, 4,400 units/kg by i.v. bolus over 10 minutes, have been used. Although 50% to 75% of patients have resolution of clots with thrombolytic therapy when treated within 7 days of occurrence, thrombi that have been present for longer than 7 days are unlikely to be treated successfully. Avoid thrombolytic therapy in patients with a tumor that might bleed. Anticoagulation with heparin after thrombolytic therapy is recommended; patients whose catheters become patent and functional should receive low-dose warfarin (1 mg/day p.o.) thereafter.

   For patients with thrombi secondary to external superior vena cava pressure, thrombolytics are not usually used, but patients are commonly anticoagulated with heparin and then warfarin to prevent propagation of the clot (see Chap. 29.)

IV. **Anaphylaxis**
   A. **Causes.** Anaphylaxis is one of the most catastrophic, although infrequent, potential side effects of chemotherapy. Anaphylaxis is a hyperimmune reaction mediated by the release of immunoglobulin E. This emergency situation may arise in oncology patients who are exposed to serum products, bacterial products such as L-asparaginase, certain cytotoxic agents (such as paclitaxel [Taxol] or the Cremophor component of paclitaxel), antibiotics such as penicillin, iodine-based contrast material, latex allergy, and monoclonal antibodies (which have murine components). However, virtually any drug can lead to a hyperimmune response resulting in anaphylaxis.

B. **Clinical manifestations.** Patients may display anxiety, dyspnea, and presyncopal symptoms. Urticaria, generalized itching, and evidence of bronchospasm and upper airway angioedema may occur. Peripheral vasodilation may result in significant hypotension and may lead to syncope.

C. **Management.** Prompt recognition and treatment can be invaluable in blunting an adverse response and may prevent a reaction from becoming life-threatening. Patients must be assessed rapidly to ensure that an open airway is present and maintained. Supplemental oxygen should be given for respiratory symptoms. Endotracheal intubation may be necessary. If severe laryngeal edema rather than bronchospasm is the cause of respiratory distress, tracheostomy or cricothyrotomy is necessary.

1. **Epinephrine**, 0.3 to 0.5 mg (0.3 to 0.5 mL of 1:1,000 epinephrine or 3 to 5 mL of a 1:10,000 solution) i.v. is given every 10 minutes for severe reactions with laryngeal stridor, major bronchospasm, or hypotension, for a maximum of three doses (1 mg) or until the episode resolves, whichever occurs first. For milder reactions, a dose of 0.2 to 0.3 mL of 1:1,000 epinephrine may be given subcutaneously and repeated every 15 minutes twice. In the event of life-threatening anaphylaxis, 0.5 mg (5 mL of a 1:10,000 solution) should be given intravenously; this dose may be repeated once in 10 minutes if needed. Because of the cardiovascular stress associated with epinephrine, its use in relatively minor allergic reactions, such as pruritus alone, should be avoided. Alternatively, epinephrine may be administered through the endotracheal tube if intravenous access is unavailable.

2. **Intravenous fluids** (either normal saline or lactated Ringer's solution) may be given for hypotension. Hypotension unresponsive to these measures requires the use of vasopressors, such as dopamine.

3. **Albuterol or metaproterenol aerosol treatments** can be used to treat bronchospasm.

4. **Diphenhydramine**, 25 mg i.v., may be followed by a second dose if necessary. Blood pressure must be monitored because hypotension can result.

5. **Corticosteroids** have a slow onset of action measured in hours. Although their administration may be reasonable for their later effects, they do not have a primary role in the acute management of this emergent condition. Hydrocortisone, 100 to 500 mg i.v., or methylprednisolone, 125 mg i.v., may be given for their later effects.

6. **Cimetidine**, 300 mg i.v., or other H_2-blocker, may be given for urticaria; it has no significant

role in acute, severe episodes, although it has a preventive role in averting reactions from paclitaxel along with dexamethasone (Decadron) and diphenhydramine.

V. Respiratory failure

A. **Causes.** The development of respiratory failure in patients with cancer may occur secondary to many potential causes.

- Bacterial or other pneumonias, especially in patients neutropenic due to therapy
- Sepsis (and other causes of the systemic inflammatory response syndrome)
- Interstitial pulmonary spread of cancer
- Overwhelming parenchymal pulmonary metastases
- Radiation injury
- Lung damage secondary to chemotherapy agents (such as bleomycin, high-dose cyclophosphamide, or methotrexate)
- Pulmonary edema secondary to cardiac damage from cytotoxic agents (like doxorubicin) or biologic agents ("capillary leak syndrome" with interleukin-2 [IL-2])
- Retinoic acid syndrome from tretinoin (all-*trans*-retinoic acid) therapy of acute promyelocytic leukemia
- Pulmonary embolus developing from deep venous thrombosis in a debilitated patient

B. **Management.** The management of severe respiratory failure requires intubation and mechanical ventilation, which is usually managed by pulmonologists or critical care specialists. However, because the prognosis of most patients with advanced solid tumors who develop respiratory failure is poor, careful consideration of a patient's entire medical situation must be made. Relevant factors include the patient's underlying medical illnesses, such as concurrent cardiopulmonary disease, and their particular tumor type and potential for response to antineoplastic therapy. It is prudent—some would say imperative—to ascertain well in advance of the emergency the wishes of patients and their families regarding intensive care unit support and full resuscitative measures.

C. **Prevention.** If possible, progressive steps to prevent or lessen the possibility of the development of respiratory failure should be undertaken. These include the following:

1. **Careful monitoring of granulocyte counts** to be aware of patients at risk for bacterial infection.

2. **Routine lung auscultation of patients receiving agents with potential pulmonary toxicity** followed by appropriate action in the event of pulmonary findings. This may include giving furosemide if indicated and discontinu-

ing offending agents (like bleomycin) before the development of serious symptoms. Reasons for discontinuing bleomycin therapy include unexplained exertional dyspnea, fine bibasilar rales, fine bibasilar reticular shadows on chest radiograph, and significant fall in pulmonary function tests from pretreatment levels.

3. **Ensuring that patients are ambulatory or that antithrombotic precautions are taken for hospitalized patients who are bedridden.**

4. **Consideration of underlying cardiopulmonary disease, prior chest irradiation, and so forth,** before patients are considered to be candidates for systemic therapy is most important. Concurrent illnesses may proscribe the selection of or modify the dosing of cytotoxic agents (such as cisplatin, which requires substantial intravenous hydration) and biologic agents (like IL-2, before which patients' cardiac and pulmonary function should be tested).

VI. **Tumor lysis syndrome.** This syndrome may be seen with any tumor that is undergoing rapid cell turnover as a result of high growth fraction or high cell death due to therapy. In general, acute leukemia, high-grade lymphoma, and less commonly, solid tumors, such as small cell lung cancer and germ cell cancers undergoing therapy, are the most commonly associated tumor types. Tumor lysis syndrome is characterized by the metabolic abnormalities of hyperuricemia, hyperkalemia, and hyperphosphatemia leading to hypocalcemia. Severe clinical situations, including acute renal failure, and serious cardiac dysrhythmia, including ventricular tachycardia and ventricular fibrillation, may develop. It is therefore important for physicians to be aware of which patients might be at risk for this syndrome, attempt to prevent its onset, monitor patient's blood chemistry values carefully, and initiate treatment promptly.

A. **Prevention.** It is useful to start all patients who have tumor types that predispose to this complication on allopurinol, 600 mg/day p.o for 1 or 2 days, at least 24 hours before initiating chemotherapy. Thereafter, patients may receive allopurinol, 300 mg/day p.o.

For patients who must be treated immediately, allopurinol is started at the same dose just described, urine should be alkalinized (pH $\geq$ 7), and i.v. fluid hydration with a "brisk diuresis" of about 100 to 150 mL/h of urine maintained. This can be achieved through the use of intravenous crystalloid, with 1 ampule (44.6 mEq) of sodium bicarbonate in each liter of intravenous solution. If the desired urine output is not reached after adequate hydration, furosemide, 20 mg i.v., may be given to facilitate diuresis. If routine monitoring of urine shows pH < 7.0, an additional ampule of sodium bicarbonate may be added to each liter of infused fluid. Acetazolamide, 250 mg p.o. q.i.d., may also be added to keep urine alkaline.

B. Monitoring. During the course of chemotherapy for patients at risk of tumor lysis syndrome, serum electrolytes, phosphate, calcium, uric acid, and creatinine levels should be checked before therapy and at least daily thereafter. Patients at high risk (e.g., high-grade lymphoma with large bulk) should have these parameters checked every 6 hours for the first 24 to 48 hours. In addition, patients who show any initial or subsequent abnormality in any of these parameters should have appropriate therapy initiated and have measurements of abnormal parameters repeated every 6 to 12 hours until completion of chemotherapy and normalization of laboratory values.

C. Treatment. Patients who have evidence of tumor lysis syndrome must have adequate hydration with half-normal saline solution. Aluminum hydroxide can be used to treat hyperphosphatemia.

Hyperkalemia may be treated in multiple ways. However, the clinician must differentiate between methods that reduce serum potassium by driving this ion intracellularly (as is done with dextrose and insulin or sodium bicarbonate) and methods that lead to actual potassium loss out of the body (as with furosemide through the urine and with sodium polystyrene sulfonate resin [Kayexalate] through the gut). If hyperkalemia or hypocalcemia occurs, an electrocardiogram should be obtained, with continuous monitoring of the cardiac rhythm until these abnormalities are corrected. In addition, because of the potential cardiac arrhythmias secondary to hyperkalemia with hypocalcemia, cardioprotection could be achieved through the use of intravenous calcium.

We recommend the following:

1. For patients with mild elevation of potassium (serum potassium no higher than 5.5 mEq/L), increasing intravenous hydration using normal saline solution with a single dose (20 mg) of intravenous furosemide is often sufficient. An alternative to normal saline is the use of 2 ampules of sodium bicarbonate (89 mEq) in 1 liter of 5% dextrose/water.

2. For patients with serum potassium levels between 5.5 and 6.0 mEq/L, increased intravenous fluids, furosemide, and oral sodium polystyrene sulfonate resin, 30 g, with sorbitol may be used.

3. For patients with serum potassium levels of more than 6.0 mEq/L or evidence of cardiac arrhythmia, several options may be combined. Intravenous calcium gluconate, 10 mL of a 10% solution or 1 ampule, is given first, followed by increased intra-

venous fluids, furosemide, plus 1 ampule of 50% dextrose and 10 units of regular insulin intravenously. Oral sodium polystyrene sulfonate resin with sorbitol also may be used except in patients with a history of congestive heart failure or reduced left ventricular function. Dialysis may be used for refractory hyperkalemia.

VII. Hypercalcemia

A. Causes of tumor hypercalcemia

1. **Associated tumors.** Hypercalcemia is relatively common in patients with malignancy. In one study it was shown that the most common cause of hypercalcemia in hospitalized patients is malignancy. Hypercalcemia of malignancy can be associated with bone metastasis, or it may occur in the absence of any direct bone involvement by the tumor. Based on the findings of study on 433 patients with hypercalcemia of cancer, 86% of the patients had identifiable bone metastasis. More than one half (n = 225) of the cases were accounted for by patients with breast carcinoma, and cancer of the lung and kidneys accounted for a smaller proportion. Patient with hematologic malignancies accounted for approximately 15% of the cases. These patients usually had hypercalcemia in the presence of diffuse tumor involvement of bone, although in a small percentage there was no evidence of bone involvement.

2. **Humoral mediators.** In approximately 10% of the cases of malignancy, hypercalcemia develops in the absence of radiographic or scintigraphic evidence of bone involvement. In this group of patients, the pathogenesis of hypercalcemia appears to be secondary to humoral mediators, including PTH related peptide, and a number of osteoclast activating factors. A number of cytokines with potent bone resorbing activities have been identified. These cytokines may account for the previously designated osteoclast activating factor (OAF). There is evidence indicating that prostaglandins PGs play a role in the hypercalcemia of malignancy. PGs are potent stimulators of bone resorption. There may also be the coexistence of tumor with primary hyperparathyroidism or other cause of hypercalcemia (e.g., Vitamin D intoxication, sarcoidosis).

B. Symptoms, signs, and laboratory findings. Hypercalcemia often produces symptoms in patients with cancer and, in fact, may be the patients major problem. Polyuria and nocturia, resulting from the impaired ability of the kidneys to concentrate the urine, occur early. Anorexia, nausea, constipation,

muscle weakness, and fatigue are common. As the hypercalcemia progresses, severe dehydration, azotemia, mental obtundation, coma, and cardiovascular collapse may appear. In addition to hypercalcemia, the laboratory studies may reveal hypokalemia and increased BUN and creatinine levels. Patients with hypercalcemia of malignancy frequently have hypochloremic metabolic alkalosis, whereas with primary hyperparathyroidism, metabolic acidosis is more common. The concentration of serum phosphorus is variable. PTH levels may be normal, low or high, but marked elevations are rarely seen. Bone involvement is best evaluated by a bone scan, which is often positive in the absence of radiographic evidence of bone involvement.

C.   **Treatment.** The management of hypercalcemia of malignancy has two objectives: (1) reducing elevated levels of serum calcium, and (2) treating the underlying cause. When hypercalcemia is mild to moderate (serum calcium $< 12 - 13$ mg/dl) and the patient is not symptomatic, adequate hydration and measures directed against the tumor (e.g., surgery, chemotherapy, or radiation therapy) may suffice. Severe hypercalcemia, on the other hand, is a life-threatening condition requiring emergency treatment. Therefore, for more severe degrees of hypercalcemia, other measures must be taken, including enhancement of calcium excretion by the kidney in patients with adequate renal function and the use of agents that decrease bone resorption.

The agents used for treatment of hypercalcemia have differences in the time of onset and duration of action as well as in their potency. Therefore, effective treatment of severe hypercalcemia requires the use of more than one modality of therapy.

A suggested approach to the treatment of severe hypercalcemia is:
1.   Rehydration with 0.9% sodium chloride
2.   Calcitonin 4–8 units/kg/i.v. every 6–12 hr for the initial 48–72 hours
3.   Pamidronate (Aredia) 60–90 mg in 1000 ml/0.9% sodium chloride infused over 24 hours
4.   Saline diuresis (0.9% sodium chloride + furosemide)
   1.   **Rehydration**. Rehydration and restoration of intravascular volume is the most important initial step in the therapy of hypercalcemia. Rehydration should be accomplished using 0.9% sodium chloride (normal saline) and often requires the administration of 4–6 liters over the first 24 hours. Rehydration alone causes only a mild decrease of the serum calcium levels ($\approx$10%). However, rehydration improves renal function facilitating urinary calcium excretion.

2. **Saline diuresis.** After adequate restoration of intravascular volume, forced saline diuresis may be used. Sodium competitively inhibits the tubular resorption of calcium. Therefore, the i.v. infusion of saline causes a significant increase in calcium clearance. Because of the large amounts of saline that may be required to correct hypercalcemia, it is advisable to monitor the central venous pressure continuously. The infusion of normal saline (0.9% sodium chloride) at a rate of 250–500 ml/hr, accompanied by the i.v. administration of 20–80 mg of furosemide q/2–4h, results in significant calcium diuresis and mild lowering of the serum calcium in the majority of patients. This type of therapy requires strict monitoring of cardiopulmonary status to avoid fluid overload. Also, it requires ready access to the laboratory to prevent electrolyte imbalance, since the urinary losses of sodium, potassium, magnesium, and water must be replaced to maintain metabolic balance. In some cases the infusion of saline at rates of 125–150 ml/h plus the addition of furosemide 40–80 mg intravenously once or twice a day may reduce the serum calcium until other measures aimed at inhibiting bone resorption take effect.

3. **Calcitonin** (Calcimar) is a peptide hormone that inhibits osteocytic and osteoclastic bone resorption. Salmon calcitonin, when given by infusion, will cause a modest reduction of serum calcium levels, usually by 1–3 mg/dl, which commonly reverses after discontinuation of therapy. To avoid anaphylactic reactions, skin testing should be performed prior to the administration of calcitonin. To avoid inconsistencies in the response, it is recommended that albumin (approximately 5 gm) be added to the infusion to coat the infusion set and prevent absorption of the peptides to the walls of the set. The usual initial dose of calcitonin is 4–8 U/kg, either i.v., SQ or IM q6-12h according to the serum calcium levels. Nausea with or without vomiting has been noted in approximately 10% of the patients treated with calcitonin. It is more common at the beginning of the treatment and usually subsides with continuous administration. Local inflammatory reactions at the site of SC or IM injection have been reported in about 10% of the patients. Skin rashes and flushing occurred occasionally.

4. **Bisphosphonates** (Diphosphonates)

   a. **Mechanism of action.** The diphosphonates are potent inhibitors of normal and abnormal bone resorption and also inhibit bone formation. They bind to the surface of calcium phosphate crystals and inhibit crystal growth and dissolution. In addition, they may directly inhibit osteoclast resorptive activity.

b. **Disodium pamidronate** (Aredia) pamidronate (3-amino-l, hydroxypropylidene-1, 1-bisphosphonic acid) is a very potent inhibitor of bone resorption and the most effective agent for the treatment of hypercalcemia of malignancy. Pamidronate has become the treatment of choice for hypercalcemia of malignancy. The hypocalcemic action of pamidronate is dose related.

(1) **Dosage and administration.** For symptomatic, moderate hypercalcemia (corrected serum calcium 12–13.5 mg/dl) the recommended dose of pamidronate is 60–90 mg given intravenously as a single dose over 24 hours. For severe hypercalcemia (serum calcium >13.5 mg/dl) a single intravenous dose of 90 mg over 24 hours should be given. Pamidronate is available in vials containing 30, 60 or 90 mg of lyophilized powder. Each vial should be reconstituted with 10 ml of sterile water for injection and the desired dose dissolved in 1000 ml of either 0.45%, 0.9% saline or 5% dextrose solution.

(2) **Side effects**. Pamidronate is usually well tolerated and no serious side effects have been reported. Mild fever with temperature elevations of 1°C have been noted in 27% of patients after 24–48 hours of administration. The transient fever is presumed to be due to release of cytokines from osteoclasts. Pain, redness, swelling and induration at the site of infusion occurs in approximately 20% of patients. Hypocalcemia, hypophosphatemia or hypomagnesemia may be seen in 15% of the patients.

c. **Disodium etidronate** (didronel) is no longer commonly used in treatment of hypercalcemia of malignancy.

5. **Gallium nitrate.** Gallium nitrate inhibits bone resorption by reducing the solubility of bone crystals. Gallium nitrate infused at a dose of 200 mg/m² decreases the serum calcium to normal in approximately 75% of patients with hypercalcemia of malignancy. A drawback of

gallium nitrate therapy is the prolonged duration of treatment necessary to normalize the serum calcium (5 days of infusion).

    a. Dosage and administration. The recommended dose of gallium nitrate is 200 mg/m^2 daily for 5 consecutive days. Gallium nitrate is available in vials containing 500 mg/20 ml (25 mg/ml). The daily dose should be diluted in 1000 ml of 0.9% saline of 5% dextrose and infused intravenously over 24 hours. In patients with mild symptomatic hypercalcemia a dosage of 100 mg/m^2/day for 5 days may be used.

    b. Side effects. Nephrotoxicity as demonstrated by rising BUN and creatinine has been seen in approximately 12% of patients treated with gallium nitrate. Simultaneous use of aminoglycosides and other nephrotoxic drugs increases the risk of renal insufficiency.

  6. Plicamycin (Mithracin) is a potent antineoplastic agent that was initially used for the treatment of some malignant tumors of the testes. Plicamycin inhibits bone resorption and causes hypocalcemia. Plicamycin at dosages of 15–25 µg/kg/day infused intravenously usually reverses hypercalcemia within 48 hours in patients with cancer. Plicamycin should be used only for the treatment of hypercalcemia of malignancy that has been refractory to other modalities of therapy.

    a. Dosage and administration. Mithracin is available in vials containing 2,500 µg as a freeze-dried preparation. The vials should be reconstituted with 4.9 ml. Of sterile water. Each ml of the reconstituted solution contains 500 µg (0.5 mg) of plicamycin. The recommended dose is 15 to 25 µg/kg infused intravenously over 4 to 6 hours. The appropriate dose of plicamycin should be diluted in 1000 ml of 0.9% saline or 5% dextrose and infused intravenously over a period of 4–6 hours. The response of the serum calcium and evaluation for signs of toxicity should be done over the ensuing 48h. If hypercalcemia persist, the infusion can be repeated for 3 or 4 days.

    b. Side effects. The most serious form of toxicity associated with plicamycin use is a bleeding diathesis which may begin as an episode of epistaxis and progress to hematemesis and generalized bleeding.

The bleeding diathesis is the result of multiple abnormalities of coagulation and thrombocytopenia.

7. **Glucocorticoids.** Large initial doses of hydrocortisone, 250–500 mg i.v. q8h (or its equivalent), can be effective in the treatment of hypercalcemia associated with lymphoproliferative diseases, such as non-Hodgkin's lymphoma and multiple myeloma, and in patients with breast cancer metastatic to bone. However, it may take several days for Glucocorticoids to lower the serum calcium level. Maintenance therapy should be started with prednisone, 10–30 mg/day PO. The mechanisms by which glucocorticoids lower the serum calcium are multiple and involved.

8. **Oral phosphate supplements** (Neutra-Phos or Fleet Phospho-Soda). Oral phosphate therapy is an adjunct for the chronic treatment of hypercalcemia of malignancy. Oral phosphate decreases the intestinal absorption of calcium and enhances the deposition of insoluble calcium salts in bone and tissue. Oral phosphate supplements at dosages of 1.5–3.0 gm/day of elemental phosphorus can result in mild lowering of the serum calcium levels as well as a reduction in urinary calcium excretion. Diarrhea usually limits the amount of phosphate that can be given. Phosphate supplements should never be given to patients with renal failure or when hyperphosphatemia is present, since soft tissue calcification may occur. Monitoring of the level of calcium and phosphorus as well as the calcium times phosphorus ion product is important to prevent metastatic calcifications.

9. **PG inhibitors.** Nonsteroidal anti-inflammatory agents inhibit cyclo-oxygenase and thereby block PG synthesis. Inhibitors of PG synthesis have been effective in rare cases of metastatic renal cell carcinoma and squamous cell carcinoma of the lung. Indomethacin, 50 mg t.i.d., is the most potent inhibitor of prostaglandin synthesis. Aspirin, 1 gm t.i.d., has also been shown to be effective in selected cases.

VIII. **Bone metastasis.** Metastases to bone occur frequently from many types of tumors and have great potential for morbidity. Bone involvement can be a source of constant pain, limiting a patient's activity and quality of life. The consequences of spinal involvement have been discussed already. The occurrence of a pathologic fracture in a weight-bearing bone has catastrophic implications: Patients who are consequently immobilized or bedridden are predisposed to a variety of complications, including deep venous thrombi, pulmonary emboli, aspiration pneumo-

nia, and decubitus ulcers, as well as psychosocial consequences, including depression.

A. Clinical findings. Bone involvement with metastatic disease can be manifested by a spectrum of clinical presentations. This can vary from constant
aching pain through nocturnal exacerbations of pain
to sharp pains brought on by pressure, weight bearing, other use, or range of motion of the affected site.
Tenderness of an affected bone area may or may not
be present. Tenderness or sharp pain with weight
bearing often implies a greater degree of disruption
of the bony architecture and thus a greater potential
for fracture, particularly in a weight-bearing area.

B. Radiologic findings. These often depend on the
type of malignancy involved as well as the extent of
the metastases. Multiple myeloma is a prime example of a malignancy that leads to pure osteolytic lesions. Consequently, radionuclide bone scans are
rarely useful in the evaluation of patients with this
disease. Rather, a metastatic skeletal survey (plain
radiographs) is preferable. In contrast, prostate cancer most commonly has purely osteoblastic lesions.
Therefore, a radionuclide bone scan would be the diagnostic test of choice. In general, most tumor types
have the potential to yield either type of bone lesion
or both. A radionuclide bone scan may be done to permit a "global view" in these patients.

The presence of "hot spots" in the spine, in weight-
bearing bones such as the femur, or in other major
long bones such as the humerus should lead the clinician to assess the patient further with plain radiographs of these bones. Patients who display significant cortical thinning of long bones or large lytic bone
metastases are at high risk of developing pathologic
fractures with great morbidity. These patients should
be evaluated both by orthopedic surgery for consideration of prophylactic surgery to stabilize the affected
bone and by radiation oncology for treatment of the
tumor to permit regeneration of normal bone.

C. Treatment

1. Surgery. Because rapid return of the patient to
as normal a life as possible is an overriding concern when treating patients with metastatic
disease, surgical stabilization is most often the
initial step in treating pathologic fractures of
long bones. If the fracture is the initial manifestation of tumor relapse, biopsy confirmation
can also be obtained. Whereas fractures at sites
of significant residual bony architecture can be
satisfactorily stabilized with an intramedullary
rod or pin, marked lytic destruction may neces-
sitate additional structural support, such as
methylmethacrylate cement to fill the intramedullary canal and cortical defects. Pathologic fractures of non–weight-bearing bones can

be managed by splinting (ribs) or sling immobilization (humerus or clavicle) while delivering radiotherapy to promote healing. Fixation may also be used in the upper extremities to speed recovery of function, particularly of the humerus. Surgical stabilization of the spine may also be used in selected circumstances (provided the patient has an anticipated survival time of more than 3 months) and can result in significant pain relief and reduction in risk of cord and nerve root compression.

2. **External-beam therapy.** Radiation doses of 15 to 20 Gy in three to five fractions leads to complete relief of pain in about 50% of patients, with an additional 30% of patients having some decrease in pain, whereas 80% to 90% show significant improvement with 30 to 40 Gy. The alleviation of symptoms can be expected within 2 to 3 weeks. For patients who may be expected to have more prolonged survival, higher doses over a larger number of fractions may be used. Most patients receive optimal results from courses of 30 Gy in 10 fractions (2 weeks) or 40 Gy in 15 fractions (3 weeks).

   Radiotherapy fields should include the area of evident bone involvement, as shown on radiograph and bone scan, with a sufficient extension to prevent relapse at the portal margin. It is seldom necessary to treat the entire bone unless the entire bone is involved because encroachment on marrow reserve may compromise any systemic chemotherapy that might also be indicated.

3. **Strontium-89 therapy.** A more recent approach to the therapy of symptomatic bone metastases is through the use of the radioisotopes, including strontium 89, which is given by intravenous injection. This isotope is highly selective for bone, is an emitter of β radiation, and has low penetration into surrounding tissue. Strontium's affinity to metastatic bone disease is reported to be 2 to 25 times greater than its affinity to normal bone. This therapy is especially useful in patients with breast or prostate cancer who have many metastatic bone sites or who have received maximal external-beam irradiation to a specific site. Palliative effects may be seen in other types of tumors as well. Pain relief may occur as early as 1 to 2 weeks after the first injection. Multiple studies indicate that 10% to 20% of patients experience complete pain relief, whereas another 50% to 60% have at least a moderate reduction in symptoms. Responses last 3 to 6 months. Patients who experience some relief of symptoms may receive multiple

doses at 3-month intervals if there has been adequate hematologic recovery.

The toxicity of strontium 89 is primarily hematologic, involving both leukocytes and platelets. About 10% of patients may experience a transient "flare" of their bone pain, similar to what is seen with tamoxifen therapy in breast cancer. This flare reaction often foreshadows a response to treatment. Other new radioisotopes for the palliation of painful bone metastases include samarium 153 and rhenium 186.

4. **Biphosphonates**. Pamidronate and other bisphosphonates (etidronate and clodronate) are specific inhibitors of osteoclastic activity. They are effective for the treatment of hypercalcemia associated with malignancies and can reduce bone pain, especially in multiple myeloma.

SELECTED READINGS

Allen KL, Johnson TW, Hibbs GG. Effective bone radiation as related to various treatment regimens. *Cancer* 1986;37:984.

Arrambide K, Toto RD. Tumor lysis syndrome. *Semin Nephrol* 1993;13(3):273–280.

Bern MM, Lokich JJ, Wallach SR, et al. Very low dose of warfarin can prevent thrombosis in central venous catheters. *Ann Intern Med* 1990;112:423–428.

Ciesielski-Carlucci C, Leong P, Jacobs C. Case report of anaphylaxis from cisplatin/paclitaxel and a review of their hypersensitivity reaction profiles. *Am J Clin Oncol* 1997;20(4):373–375.

Cohan RH, Leder RA, Ellis JH. Treatment of adverse reactions to radiographic contrast media in adults. *Radiol Clin North Am* 1996;34(5):1055–1076.

Coleman RE, Purohit OP. Osteoclast inhibition for the treatment of bone metastases. *Cancer Treat Rev* 1993;19:79–103.

Comis RL. Bleomycin pulmonary toxicity: current status and future directions. *Semin Oncol* 1992;19(2):64–70.

Cooper PR, Errico TJ, Martin R, Crawford B, DiBartolo T. A systematic approach to spinal reconstruction after anterior decompression for neoplastic disease of the thoracic and lumbar spine. *Neurosurgery* 1993;32:1–8.

Escalante CP. Causes and management of superior vena cava syndrome. *Oncology* 1993;7(6):61. (In this same issue are three reviews of this article which lend further perspective to this disorder.)

Fleisch H. Bisphosphonates: a new class of drugs in diseases of bone and calcium metabolism. In: Brunner KW, Fleisch H, Senn H-J, eds. *Recent results in cancer research. Vol. 116: Bisphosphonates and tumor osteolysis.* Berlin-Heidelberg: Springer-Verlag, 1989:1–28.

Garmatis CJ, Chu FC. The effectiveness of radiation therapy in the treatment of bone metastases from breast cancer. *Radiology* 1978;126:235.

Gray BH, Olin JW, Graor RA, et al. Safety and efficacy of thrombolytic therapy for superior vena cava syndrome. *Chest* 1991;99:54–59.

Hauser MJ, Tabak J, Baier H. Survival of patients with cancer in a medical critical care unit. *Arch Intern Med* 1982;142:527.

Johnston FG, Uttley D, Marsh HT. Synchronous vertebral decompression and posterior stabilization in the treatment of spinal malignancy. *Neurosurgery* 1989;25:872.

Jones DP, Mahmoud H, Chesney RW. Tumor lysis syndrome: pathogenesis and management. *Pediatr Nephrol* 1995;9(2):206–212.

Kanis JA, McCloskey EV, Taube T, O'Rourke N. Rationale for the use of bisphosphonates in bone metastases. *Bone* 1991;12[Suppl 1]:S13–S18.

Katin MJ, et al. Hematologic effects of 89-strontium treatment for metastases to bone. *Proc Am Soc Clin Oncol* 1993;3:12.

Lippman M, Rumley W. Medical emergencies. In: Dunagan WC, Ridner ML, eds. *Manual of medical therapeutics.* Boston: Little, Brown, 1989:484–485.

Man Z, Otero AB, Rendo P, Barazzutti L, Sanchez Avalos JC. Use of pamidronate for multiple myeloma osteolytic lesions. *Lancet* 1990;335:663.

McAfee PC, Bohlman HH. One-stage anterior cervical decompression and posterior stabilization with circumferential arthrodesis. *Am J Bone Joint Surg* 1989;71:78.

Porter AT, Davis LP. Systemic radionuclide therapy of bone metastases with strontium-89. *Oncology* 1994;8(2):93.

Robinson RG. Radionuclides for the alleviation of bone pain in advanced malignancy. *Clin Oncol* 1986;5:39.

Samarian-153 lexidronam for painful bone metastases. *Med Lett Drugs Ther* 1997;39(1008):83–84.

Seifert V, Zimmerman M, Stolke D, Wiedemayer H. Spondylectomy, microsurgical decompression and osteosynthesis in the treatment of complex disorders of the cervical spine. *Acta Neurochir* (Wien) 1993;124:104–113.

Soffen EM, Greenberg A, Boumann J, Corn BW. The role of strontium-89 systemic radiotherapy in the management of osseous metastases from prostate cancer. *Techniques Urol* 1997;3(2):76–80.

Thiebaud D, Leyvraz S, von Fliedner V, et al. Treatment of bone metastases from breast cancer and myeloma with pamidronate. *Eur J Cancer* 1991;27:37–41.

Weissman DE. Steroid treatment of CNS metastases. *J Clin Oncol* 1988;6:543–551.

Woods JA, Lambert S, Platts-Mills TA, Drake DB, Edlich RF. Natural rubber latex allergy: spectrum, diagnostic approach, and therapy. *J Emerg Med* 1997;15(1):71–85.

Malignant Pleural, Peritoneal, and Pericardial Effusions and Meningeal Infiltrates

Walter D. Y Quan, Jr.

Malignant pleural, peritoneal, and pericardial effusions and malignant meningeal infiltrates are uncommon early in the course of the malignancy. They occur more frequently with disseminated disease and often herald a poor prognosis. Although pleural and peritoneal effusions may initially have little adverse effect on quality of life, when progressive, they (as well as pericardial effusions and meningeal infiltrates) can result in incapacitating disability and death. It is therefore necessary for the clinician to have a high index of suspicion for these problems and to be prepared to take appropriate action and deliver palliative treatment promptly.

I. **Pleural effusions**
   A. **Causes.** Malignant pleural effusions arise in association with malignant cells lining the pleura, exuded into the pleural space, or blocking veins or lymphatics. The most common malignancy associated with pleural effusions in women is carcinoma of the breast, whereas in men, it is carcinoma of the lung. Other causes of malignant pleural effusions include lymphoma, mesothelioma, and carcinomas of the ovary, gastrointestinal tract, urinary tract, and uterus. Malignancy is not the only cause of effusions, even in patients with known neoplastic disease; therefore, it is important to attempt to exclude other possible causes, such as congestive heart failure, infection, and pulmonary infarction.
   B. **Diagnosis**
      1. **Clinical diagnosis.** Effusions may be asymptomatic or may be suspected because of respiratory symptoms, such as shortness of breath with exertion or at rest, orthopnea, paroxysmal nocturnal dyspnea, or occasionally chest pressure or cough. The patient may feel more comfortable when lying on one side when the effusion is unilateral. On physical examination, dullness to percussion, decreased tactile fremitus, diminished breath sounds, and egophony are typical signs over the area of the effusion.
      2. **A chest radiograph** should be obtained to confirm the clinical impression. If fluid appears to be present, a lateral decubitus film must be obtained to help estimate the volume of the effusion and how free it is within the pleural space.
      3. **Diagnostic thoracentesis** should be performed. Ultrasonographic guidance is helpful if

loculation is present. Fluid should be obtained for bacterial, acid-fast, and fungal cultures, for cytologic examination, and for determining protein concentration (>3 g/dL in most exudates), lactate dehydrogenase (LDH) level, specific gravity, and cell count. The cytologic examination is important because if the results are positive, as in 50% to 70% of patients with malignant effusion, the diagnosis is established. Other parameters of the pleural fluid that may be helpful in establishing that the fluid is an exudate and not a transudate include a specific gravity of more than 1.015, protein concentration that is more than 0.5 times the serum protein concentration, LDH level more than 0.6 times the serum LDH level, and low glucose level. A cytologic examination of fluid from a newly discovered pleural effusion is wise, regardless of whether the patient is known to have malignancy, because for nearly half of all malignant effusions, this finding is the first sign of malignancy. Analyzing pleural fluid for carcinoembryonic antigen (CEA) may be helpful in some patients. Levels higher than 20 ng/mL are suggestive of adenocarcinoma, although they do not substitute for a tissue diagnosis in patients who have no history of malignancy. CEA elevations may be seen in adenocarcinomas from various primary sites, including the breast, lung, and gastrointestinal tract. Elevated levels between 10 and 20 ng/mL may reflect malignancy or benign disorders such as pulmonary infection. The role of assessing other tumor markers on a routine basis has not been established. Likewise, the utility of monoclonal antibodies and gene rearrangement studies in patients with lymphomas to distinguish reactive mesothelial or lymphocytic cells from malignant cells has yet to be determined. The routine use of a "panel of tumor markers" is costly and time-consuming.

4. **Pleural biopsy** may be helpful in establishing the diagnosis in up to 20% of patients for whom the pleural fluid cytology results are negative.

5. **Thoracotomy or pleuroscopy** with direct biopsy may be done in patients who have negative cytology and pleural biopsy results but in whom there is still high suspicion of malignancy.

C. **Treatment.** As malignant pleural effusions are generally a sign of systemic rather than localized disease, the best therapy is treatment that effectively treats the malignancy systemically. Unfortunately, effective systemic treatment is often not possible, particularly when the malignancy is commonly refractory to systemic treatment (e.g., in non–small cell carcinoma of the lung) or in patients who have previously been heavily treated and in whom systemic therapy is no longer effective. In these circumstances, locoregional therapy is required for palliation of the patient's symptoms.

1. **Drainage.** Many malignant pleural effusions recur within 1 to 3 days after simple thoracentesis; about 97% recur within 1 month. Chest tube drainage (closed tube thoracotomy) allows the pleural surfaces to oppose each other and, if maintained for several days, may result in obliteration of the space and improvement in the effusion for several weeks to months. It does not appear to be as effective when used alone as when a cytotoxic or sclerosing agent is added, and therefore, one of these agents is commonly instilled into the space while the chest tube is in place.

2. **Cytotoxic and sclerosing agents.** Historically, the most widely used agent for intra-pleural administration has been the intravenous preparation of tetracycline. However, because the intravenous form is no longer commercially available in the United States, clinicians are required to use alternatives, chiefly bleomycin, doxycycline, and talc. Other agents, including fluorouracil, interferon-α, and methylprednisilone acetate have been less commonly used. Randomized prospective trials comparing sclerosing agents have been hindered by relatively small numbers of patients accrued and are in conflict. In general, there appears to be similar efficacy, but the agents vary in toxicity, ease of administration, and cost. For optimal effectiveness, drainage of pleural fluid as completely as possible is required before instillation.

   a. **Method of administration.** The drug to be used is diluted in 50 to 100 mL of saline and instilled through the thoracostomy tube into the chest cavity after the effusion has been drained for at least 24 hours and the rate of collection is less than 100 mL/24 hours. Throughout the procedure, care must be taken to avoid any air leak. The thoracostomy tube is clamped, and the patient is successively repositioned on his or her front, back, and sides for 15-minute periods during the next 2 to 6 hours. The tube is then reconnected to gravity drainage or suction for at least 18 hours to ensure that the pleural surfaces remain opposed and to prevent the rapid accumulation of any fluid in reaction to the instillation. Some clinicians repeat the instillation daily for a total of 2 to 3 days. For most of the agents listed here, this has no proved benefit. Exceptions include methylprednisolone acetate and doxycycline, which appear to be more effective with additional doses. If the drainage is less than 40 to 50 mL over the previous 12 hours, the tube may be removed and a chest radiograph obtained to be certain that pneumothorax has not occurred during removal of the tube. If the thoracostomy tube continues to drain more than 100 mL/24 hours after the last instillation, it may be necessary to leave it in place for an additional 48 to 72 hours to ensure that a maximum amount of adhesion between the pleural surfaces has taken place. Because the use of sclerotic agents can be painful, it is prudent for the clinician to consider the use of scheduled narcotic analgesia, particularly during the initial 24 hours.

b. **Recommended agents.** One must consider efficacy, side effects, and cost when choosing a sclerosing agent. Bleomycin is probably the most widely used agent and, in one prospective study, was shown to be more effective than tetracycline. It is also more expensive per dose than the other agents. Talc is the least expensive, but this must be balanced against the costs of related procedures, including thoracoscopy and anesthesia. Fluorouracil is relatively inexpensive, but the reported experience with this agent is not great. Minocycline or doxycycline may be reasonable alternatives to tetracycline, but the relative numbers of reported patients treated with these agents are small. Clearly, prospective studies of currently available agents to assess not only response but also cost and morbidity are needed.

(1) **Bleomycin,** 1 mg/kg or 40 mg/m^2, has relatively little myelosuppressive effect and is highly effective.

(2) **Fluorouracil,** 2 to 3 g (total dose) may have a theoretical advantage in sensitive carcinomas, but whether that advantage is significant has not yet been established. Pain is generally minimal. Occasional patients may experience a depressed white blood cell count, especially at the higher dose.

c. **Alternative agents**

(1) **Talc** has been used successfully but requires thoracoscopy and general anesthesia.

(2) **Doxycycline,** 500 mg, may cause pleuritic chest pain. An injection of

10 mL of 1% lidocaine (100 mg) through the chest tube may reduce this symptom.

(3) **Interferon-α**, 50 million units, typically causes influenza-like symptoms. Lower doses appear to be ineffective. Patients treated with interferon should be premedicated with acetaminophen, 650 mg before administration and then repeated in 6 hours. Meperidine, 25 mg i.v. by slow push, may be given for rigors from interferon.

(4) **Methylprednisolone acetate**, 80 to 160 mg, appears to be well tolerated.

d. **Responses.** A combination of chest tube drainage and instillation of one of the agents discussed in Section I.C.2.b or c controls pleural effusions more than 75% of the time. The durations of response are short, with a median between 3 and 6 months unless the patient's systemic disease comes under adequate control. In that circumstance, the effusion may not recur for years or at least until the systemic disease once more emerges.

e. **Side effects** common to most agents include chest pain, fever, and occasional hypotension. These effects are usually not severe and may be controlled by standard symptomatic management. Fever after pleurodesis is usually not due to infection.

3. **Thoracotomy and pleural stripping** may be tried subsequently for effusions refractory to medical treatment.

II. Peritoneal effusions

A. **Causes.** Malignant peritoneal effusions usually occur in association with diffuse seeding of the peritoneal surface with small malignant deposits. The impairment of subphrenic lymphatic or portal venous flow may result in peritoneal effusions. Alternatively, it has been postulated that a "capillary leak" phenomenon mediated by tumor cells or immune effector cells could be a contributing factor. Carcinoma of the ovary is the most commonly associated malignancy in women, whereas in men, gastrointestinal carcinomas are most common. Other neoplasms that may cause peritoneal effusions include lymphoma, mesothelioma, and carcinomas of the uterus and breast. Liver metastasis by itself, unless it is far advanced, is not usually associated with symptomatic peritoneal effusions.

B. **Diagnosis**

1. **Symptoms and signs.** Patients may be completely symptom free or have so much fluid that they have severe abdominal distention, abdom-

inal pain, and respiratory distress. In the presence of peritoneal metastases, there may be abnormal bowel motility that at times resembles a paralytic ileus and may result in loss of appetite, early satiety, nausea, and vomiting. On examination, the lower abdomen and flanks bulge when the patient is supine. Confirmatory signs include shifting dullness, a fluid wave, diminished bowel sounds, or the "puddle sign" (periumbilical dullness when the patient rests on knees and elbows).

2. **Radiographic studies.** Ascites may be suggested on a recumbent film of the abdomen, although radiographs are less sensitive than computed tomography (CT) or ultrasound in detecting fluid. CT is also helpful in defining whether there are enlarged retroperitoneal nodes, tumor masses in the abdomen or pelvis, or liver metastases in association with the ascites.

3. **Paracentesis** is used to distinguish malignancy from other causes of peritoneal effusions, including congestive heart failure, hepatic cirrhosis, and peritonitis. Malignant cells are found in about half of patients in whom the effusion is due to malignancy. Other tests are less reliable, and treatment decisions must often be based on incomplete data. Elevated LDH and protein levels, along with a negative Gram's stain and cultures, are supportive but nonspecific for malignancy. The use of monoclonal antibodies to identify tumor cells is still experimental.

C. **Therapy.** As with malignant pleural effusions, malignant peritoneal effusions as a rule are optimally treated with effective systemic therapy. (The possible exception to this is peritoneal effusions from carcinoma of the ovary. In this circumstance, there may be advantage to intraperitoneal therapy because most systemic disease is on the peritoneal surface.) If the patient is resistant to all further systemic treatment, regional treatment should be tried, but the likelihood of success is less and the complications greater with peritoneal effusions than with pleural effusions. Success probably is less because of the greater likelihood of loculations to areas inaccessible to therapy and the impossibility of obliterating the peritoneal space in the same way that the pleural space can be obliterated. Complications are greater because of the increase in adhesions caused by instillation therapy and the resultant increase in obstructive bowel problems.

1. **Paracentesis** may be helpful in acutely relieving intraabdominal pressure. If the ascites has caused impairment of respiration, paracentesis may give temporary relief. Rapid withdrawal of

large volumes of fluid (>1 liter) can result in hypotension and shock, however, and if frequent paracenteses are performed, severe hypoalbuminemia and electrolyte imbalance may result. Repeated procedures could also subject the patient to increased risk of peritonitis or bowel injury. This procedure thus results in only temporary benefit.

2. **Bed rest and dietary salt restriction,** although helpful in the treatment of various nonmalignant causes of ascites, are of less benefit in malignant ascites.

3. **Diuretics** may be helpful in reducing ascites, but care must be taken not to be too vigorous in attempts at diuresis because of the possibility of dehydration and hypotension. A reasonable choice of diuretic is a combination of hydrochlorthiazide, 50 to 100 mg/day, and spironolactone, 50 to 100 mg/day.

4. **Intracavitary therapy.** Radioisotopes, cytotoxic drugs, and sclerosing agents have been used with some benefit for treating malignant ascites; but, overall, probably fewer than half of patients have a satisfactory response. The utility of these agents has less to do with direct tumor cytotoxicity and more with the induction of a local inflammatory response with subsequent sclerosis. The radioactive isotopes gold 198 and phosphorus 32 should be used only by those with experience and appropriate certification. Cytotoxic agents such as fluorouracil are associated with less risk to the person administering the therapy.

   a. **Method.** The peritoneal fluid should be drained slowly through a Tenckhoff catheter over a 24- to 36-hour period. The potential distribution of the therapeutic agent can be determined by instilling technetium 99m glucoheptonate macroaggregated albumin in 50 mL of saline and obtaining an abdominal scintigram. Two liters of warmed 1.5% peritoneal dialysate solution is instilled, allowed to remain for 2 hours, and then drained. The chemotherapeutic agent is next mixed with 2 liters of fresh 1.5% dialysate solution containing 1,000 units of heparin per liter. After warming, this solution is instilled through the Tenckhoff catheter. For some agents, draining after 4 hours is recommended.

   b. **Agents**
      (1) **Cisplatin**, 50 to 100 mg/m² (especially for carcinoma of the ovary). Drainage is optional. Saline diuresis is recommended. Dosages higher than

100 mg/m² should not be used without protection by intravenous sodium thiosulfate. Cisplatin is repeated every 3 weeks.

(2) **Fluorouracil**, 1,000 mg (total dose) in normal saline with 25 mEq sodium bicarbonate per liter. Drainage is optional. Treatment is given on days 1 to 4 monthly.

(3) **Mitoxantrone**, 10 mg/m². Drainage is optional. This dose has been administered on a weekly basis, although white blood cell counts must be monitored.

(4) **Interferon-α**, 50 million units (for ovarian cancer). Drainage is optional. This dose has been administered weekly for 4 weeks or longer. Patients should be premedicated with acetaminophen before and every 4 hours on the day of therapy.

(5) **FUDR**, 3 g in 1.5 to 2 liters of normal saline given daily for 3 days every 3 to 4 weeks, has been used in colon, gastric, and ovarian cancer.

(6) **Other agents** that have been used intraperitoneally include carboplatin, methotrexate, cytosine arabinoside, etoposide, bleomycin, thiotepa, and doxorubicin. High-dose interleukin-2 (IL-2) with lymphokine-activated killer cells has shown activity in ovarian and colorectal cancer but at the cost of significant toxicity, including peritoneal fibrosis, which in general has prevented the administration of more than one or two cycles. The use of lower IL-2 doses has not been well explored.

5. **Peritoneal–venous shunts** (Denver shunt, LeVeen shunt) may offer palliative relief for refractory ascites because recurrent paracentesis leads to infection and leakage of peritoneal fluid through the paracentesis sites. Potential disadvantages are shunt occlusion, the systemic dissemination of cancer, and disseminated intravascular coagulation.

III. **Pericardial effusions.** Although 5% to 10% of patients dying with disseminated malignancy have cardiac or pericardial metastases, far fewer have symptomatic pericardial effusion. However, although malignant pericardial effusions are not particularly common, they are of great importance because of their potential to cause acute cardiac tamponade and death.

A. **Causes.** The most common neoplasms causing pericardial effusions are carcinomas of the lung and breast, leukemias, lymphomas, and melanoma.

B. **Diagnosis**

1. **Clinical diagnosis.** Patients with developing cardiac tamponade may exhibit a variety of grave symptoms, including extreme anxiety, dyspnea, orthopnea, precordial chest pain, cough, and hoarseness. On examination, they are likely to have engorged neck veins, generalized edema, tachycardia, distant heart tones, lateral displacement of the cardiac apex, a low systolic blood pressure and low pulse pressure, and a paradoxical pulse. They may also have tachypnea and a pericardial friction rub.

2. **Electrocardiogram** (ECG) may show nonspecific low-voltage, T-wave abnormalities, elevation of ST segments, and ventricular alterans or the more specific total electrical alterans. Premature beats and atrial fibrillation also occur.

3. **Chest radiograph** typically shows an enlarged cardiac silhouette, often with a bulging appearance suggestive of an effusion ("water-bottle heart"). There is frequently an associated pleural effusion.

4. **Echocardiography** can confirm the diagnosis and provide important information on the location of the effusion within the pericardium.

5. **Pericardiocentesis** reveals neoplastic cells on cytologic examination in more than 75% of patients.

C. **Treatment**

1. **Volume expansion and vasopressor support** is applied (if necessary) to maintain blood pressure. Adequate oxygenation must be maintained. Diuretics are contraindicated.

2. **Pericardiocentesis** under ECG and blood pressure monitoring should be done in emergent circumstances. If the patient can be stabilized, or in cases of pericardial effusion without tamponade, pericardiocentesis under two-dimensional ECG is preferable because it significantly reduces the incidence of cardiac laceration, arrhythmia, and tension pneumothorax as a complication of the procedure.

3. **Instillation of chemotherapeutic or sclerosing agents.** Because pain may be associated with the intrapericardial therapy, lidocaine (Xylocaine), 100 mg, may be administered intrapericardially as a local anesthetic. (Check with the cardiologist on the safety for each patient.) After the cytotoxic or sclerosing agent is instilled, the pericardial catheter is clamped for 1 to 2 hours and then allowed to drain. One of the following agents may be used:

   a. **Fluorouracil**, 500 to 1,000 mg in aqueous solution as supplied commercially. This dose is generally not repeated.
   b. **Thiotepa**, 25 mg/m^2 in 10 mL of normal saline may be preferred in tumor deemed sensitive to alkylating agents. Myelosuppression may occur. The dose is usually not repeated.
       Complications of intrapericardial therapy include arrhythmias, pain, and fever.
   4. **Radiotherapy** with radioisotopes or 2,000 to 4,000 cGy external-beam therapy may help control effusions.
   5. **Systemic chemotherapy** (with standard regimens) after pericardiocentesis is a possible alternative for newly diagnosed, potentially responsive malignancies such as leukemias and selected lymphomas. Chemotherapy, intrapericardial or systemic, or radiotherapy controls the effusion for at least 30 days in 60% to 70% of patients. If they are ineffective, surgical intervention to create a pericardial window may be necessary and can be effective for several months. It is not recommended, however, unless simpler measures fail.

IV. **Malignant subarachnoid infiltrates**
   A. **Causes.** Leptomeningeal involvement with non–central nervous system cancer is an uncommon complication of most neoplasms, although in children with acute lymphocytic leukemia who have not received prophylactic treatment, the incidence approaches 50%. Of the nonleukemic diseases, breast carcinoma and lymphomas (primarily Burkitt's and T-cell lymphoblastic) account for about 30% each in cases of malignant subarachnoid infiltrates. Carcinoma of the lung and melanoma account for 10% to 12% each.
   B. **Diagnosis**
       1. **Clinical diagnosis.** Patients commonly present with headache, change in mental status, cranial nerve dysfunction, or spinal root–derived pain, paresthesia, or weakness. Any onset of change in neurologic status, particularly of cerebral, cranial nerve, or spinal root origin, should alert the clinician to the possibility of subarachnoid infiltrates.
       2. **Diagnostic studies**
           a. **CT of the head** should be done to look for any intracranial mass. If none is present, a lumbar puncture should be done.
           b. **A lumbar puncture** is done, and the following are evaluated or performed:
               Opening pressure
               Cytology of centrifugal specimen for malignant cells
               Total cell count and differential

Cerebrospinal fluid (CSF) chemistry, including glucose and protein

Microbiologic studies: India ink, Gram's stain, cultures (routine, acid-fast, fungi), and special studies as indicated by the clinical situation

c.   **Magnetic resonance imaging or myelography with CT follow-up** is performed if signs or symptoms of cord compression are present.

C.   **Treatment.** Malignant subarachnoid infiltrates may be treated with radiotherapy, intrathecal chemotherapy, or a combination of the two.

1.   **Radiotherapy.** The radiation field is usually limited to the most involved field (frequently the brain), and intrathecal chemotherapy is used to control the infiltrates elsewhere. This technique is used even though the entire neuraxis is usually involved because total craniospinal irradiation causes severe myelosuppression, which limits the patient's tolerance to concurrent or subsequent cytotoxic chemotherapy.

2.   **Chemotherapy** may be administered by lumbar puncture or preferably into a surgically implanted (Ommaya) reservoir that communicates with the lateral ventricle. The latter has the advantages of being easily accessible in patients who require repeated treatments and of giving a better distribution of drug than can be obtained through lumbar puncture. The disadvantage is that of a foreign object that predisposes to infection and seizures. When the Ommaya reservoir is used, a volume of CSF equal to that to be injected (6 to 10 mL) should be removed through the reservoir with a small-caliber needle. The chemotherapy should then be given as a slow injection. When the chemotherapy is given through lumbar puncture, the volume of injection (usually 7 to 10 mL) should be greater than that of the CSF withdrawn, so as to have a higher closing than opening pressure. This method facilitates distribution of the drug and minimizes post–lumbar puncture headache. The most commonly used drugs are the following:

a.   **Methotrexate**, 12 mg/m^2 (maximum, 15 mg) twice weekly until the CSF clears of malignant cells, then monthly.

b.   **Cytarabine**, 30 mg/m^2 (maximum, 50 mg) twice weekly until the CSF clears of malignant cells, then monthly.

c.   **Thiotepa**, 2 to 10 mg/m^2 twice weekly until the CSF clears of malignant cells, then monthly.

Each of the agents is given in preservative-free saline or, if available, buffered preservative-free diluent similar to Elliot's B solution. Any subsequent flush solution should be of similar composition. Other drugs used to treat effusions (e.g., fluorouracil, mechlorethamine, or radioisotopes) must not be used to treat meningeal disease.

D. Response to treatment. Most patients with meningeal leukemia or lymphoma respond to a combination of radiotherapy and intrathecal chemotherapy. Carcinomas are less likely to improve, but mild to moderate improvement may be seen in up to 50% of patients.

E. Complications. Aseptic meningitis or arachnoiditis, seizures, acute encephalopathy, myelopathy, leukoencephalopathy, and radicular neuropathy may result from intrathecal chemotherapy with or without radiotherapy.

Bone marrow suppression is not usually severe unless the patient undergoes spinal irradiation or systemic chemotherapy as well. Oral leucovorin can be given after the intrathecal methotrexate (10 mg leucovorin p.o. every six hours for six to eight doses, starting either at the same time or 24 hours after the methotrexate) to prevent marrow toxicity. Serious complications are infrequent, however, and in patients with advanced metastatic disease, they usually are not a major problem.

SELECTED READINGS

Pleural Effusions

Andrews CO, Gora W. Pleural effusions: pathophysiology and management. *Ann Pharmacother* 1994;28:894–903.

Bartal AH, Gazitt Y, Zidon G, Vermeulen B, Robinson E. Clinical and flow cytometry characteristics of malignant pleural effusions in patients after intracavitary administration of methylprednisolone acetate. *Cancer* 1991;67:3136.

Bayly TC, Kisner DL, Sybert A, Macdonald JS, Tsou E, Schein PS. Tetracycline and quinacrine in the control of malignant pleural effusions: a randomized trial. *Cancer* 1978;41:1188–1192.

Chernow B, Sahn SA. Carcinomatous involvement of the pleura: an analysis of 96 patients. *Am J Med* 1977;63:695.

Friedman MA, Slater E. Malignant pleural effusions. *Cancer Treat Rep* 1978;5:49.

Fuller DK. Bleomycin versus doxycyclines: a patient-oriented, approach to pleurodesis. *Ann Pharmacother* 1993;27:794.

Gebbia N, Mannino R, DiDino A, et al. Intracavitary treatment of malignant pleural and peritoneal effusions in cancer patients. *Anticancer Res* 1994;14: 739–745.

Goldman CA, Skinnider LF, Maksymiuk AW. Interferon instillation for malignant pleural effusions. *Ann Oncol* 1993;4:141–145.

Hamed H, Fentiman IS, Chaudary MA, Rubens RD. Comparison of intracavitary bleomycin and talc for control of pleural effusions secondary to carcinoma of the breast. *Br J Surg* 1989;76:1266–1267.

Hausheer FH, Yarbro JW. Diagnosis and treatment of malignant pleural effusions. *Cancer Metastasis Rev* 1987;6:23.

Herrington JD. Chemical pleurodesis, with doxycycline 1 g. *Pharmacotherapy* 1996;16:290–295.

Johnson WW. The malignant pleural effusion: a review of cytopathologic diagnoses of 584 specimens from 472 consecutive patients. *Cancer* 1985;56:905.

Kessinger A, Wigton RS. Intracavitary bleomycin and tetracycline in the management of malignant pleural effusions: a randomized study. *J Surg Oncol* 1997;36:91–83.

Kitamura S, et al. Intrapleural doxycycline for control of malignant pleural effusion. *Curr Ther Res* 1981;30:515.

Mansson T. Treatment of malignant pleural effusion with doxycycline. *Scand J Infect Dis* 1988;53:29.

Ostrowski MJ. Intracavitary therapy with bleomycin for the treatment of malignant pleural effusions. *J Surg Oncol* 1989;[Suppl 1]:7.

Ostrowski MJ, Halsall GM. Intracavitary bleomycin in the management of malignant effusions: a multicenter study. *Cancer Treat Rep* 1982;66:1903.

Pavesi F, Lotzniker M, Cremaschi P, et al. Detection of malignant pleural effusions by tumor marker evaluation. *Eur J Cancer Clin Oncol* 1988;24:1005–1011. Published erratum appears in *Eur J Cancer Clin Oncol* 1988;24:1559.

Surland LG, Weisberger AS. Intracavitary 5-fluorouracil in malignant effusions. *Arch Intern Med* 1965;116:431.

Tamura S, Nishigaki T, Moriwaki Y, et al. Tumor markers in pleural effusion diagnosis. *Cancer* 1988;61:298–302.

Van Hoff DD, LiVolsi V. Diagnostic reliability of needle biopsy of the parietal pleura: a review of 272 biopsies. *Am J Clin Pathol* 1975;64:200.

Walker-Renard PB,Vaughan LM, Sahn SA. Chemical pleurodesis for malignant pleural effusions. *Ann Intern Med* 1994;120:56–64.

Weissberg D. Bleomycin and talc for control of pleural effusions. *Br J Surg* 1990;77:955.

Peritoneal Effusions

Baker AR. Treatment of malignant ascites. In: DeVita S, Hellman, Rosenberg SA, eds. *Cancer: principles and practice of oncology,* 3rd ed. Philadelphia: JB Lippincott, 1989:2317.

Berek JS, et al. Intraperitoneal recombinant alpha-interferon for "salvage" immunotherapy in stage III epithelial ovarian cancer. A Gynecologic Oncology Group study. *Semin Oncol* 1986;13(Suppl 2):61.

Bitran JD. Intraperitoneal bleomycin: pharmacokinetics and results of a phase Il trial. *Cancer* 1985;56:2420.

Kelsen DP, Saltz L, Cohen AM, et al. A phase 1 trial of immediate postoperative intraperitoneal floxuridine and leucovorin plus systemic 5-fluorouracil and levamisole after resection of high risk colon cancer. *Cancer* 1994;74:2224–2233.

Lacy JH, Wieman TJ, Shivley EH. Management of malignant ascites. *Surg Gynecol Obstet* 1984;159:397.

Leichman L, Silberman H, Leichman CG, et al. Preoperative systemic chemotherapy followed by adjuvant postoperative intraperitoneal therapy for gastric cancer: a University of Southern California pilot program. *J Clin Oncol* 1992;10:1933–1942.

Markman M, Hakes T, Reichman B, et al. Phase II trial of weekly or biweekly intraperitoneal mitoxantrone in epithelial ovarian cancer. *J Clin Oncol* 1991;9: 978–982.

Muggia FM, Jeffers S, Muderspach L, et al. Phase I/II study of intraperitoneal floxuridine and platinums (cisplatin and/or carboplatin). *Gynecol Oncol* 1997;66: 290–294.

Muggia FM, Liu PY, Alberts DS, et al. Intraperitoneal mitoxantrone or floxuridine: effects on time-to-failure and survival in patients with minimal residual ovarian cancer after second-look laparotomy: a randomized phase II study by the Southwest Oncology Group. *Gynecol Oncol* 1996; 61:395–402.

Nicoletto MO, Fiorentino MW, Viante O, et al. Experience with intraperitoneal alpha2a interferon. *Oncology* 1992;49:467–473.

Papac RJ. Treatment of malignant disease in closed spaces. In: Baker FF, ed. *Cancer: a comprehensive treatise.* Vol. 5. New York: Plenum, 1977.

Reichman B, Markman M, Hakes T, et al. Phase I trial of concurrent intraperitoneal and continuous intravenous infusion of fluorouracil in patients with refractory cancer. *J Clin Oncol* 1988;6:158–162.

Speyer JL, Beller U, Colombo N, et al. Intraperitoneal carboplatin: favorable results in women with minimal residual ovarian cancer after cisplatin therapy. *J Clin Oncol* 1990;8:1335–1341.

Steis RG, Urba WJ, VanderMolen LA, et al. Intraperitoneal lymphokine-activated killer cell and interleukin-2 therapy for malignancies limited to the peritoneal cavity. *J Clin Oncol* 1990;8:1618–1629.

Sugarbaker PH, Gianola FJ, Speyer JC, et al. Prospective, randomized trial of intravenous versus intraperitoneal 5-fluorouracil in patients with advanced primary colon or rectal cancer. *Surgery* 1985;95:414.

Pericardial Effusions

Buzaid AC, Garewal HS, Greenberg BR. Managing malignant pericardial effusion. *West J Med* 1989;150:174–179.

Callahan JA, Seward JB, Nishimura RA, et al. Two-dimensional echocardiographically guided pericardiocentesis: experience in 117 consecutive patients. *Am J Cardiol* 1985;55:476–479.

Helms SR, Carlson MD. Cardiovascular emergencies. *Semin Oncol* 1989;16:463.

Liu G, Crump M, Gross PE, Dancey J, Shepherd FA. Prospective comparison of the sclerosing agents doxycycline and bleomycin for the primary management of malignant pericardial effusion and cardiac tamponade. *J Clin Oncol* 1996; 14:3141–3147.

Maher ER, Buckman R. Intrapericardial installation of bleomycin in malignant pericardial effusion. *Am Heart J* 1986;111:613–614.

Shepherd FA, Ginsberg JS, Evans WK, Scott JG, Oleksiuk F. Tetracycline sclerosis in the management of pericardial effusion. *J Clin Oncol* 1985;3:1678–1682.

Theologides A. Neoplastic cardiac tamponade. *Semin Oncol* 1978;5:181.

Malignant Subarachnoid Infiltrates

Gutin PH, Levi JA, Wiernik PH, Walker MD. Treatment of malignant meningeal disease with intrathecal thiotepa: a phase II study. *Cancer Treat Rep* 1977;61:885–887.

Olson ME, Chernik NL, Posner JB. Infiltration of the leptomeninges by systemic cancer. *Arch Neurol* 1974;30:122–137.

Managing Cancer Pain

Charles S. Cleeland and Eduardo D. Bruera

Patients should not have to suffer needlessly from cancer pain. Most pain from cancer can be adequately controlled with analgesics given by mouth. When this is not possible, a variety of more sophisticated pain management techniques can provide good pain control. It is estimated that about 95% of patients could be free of significant pain with the techniques we have available today, at least until the last week or two of life. Unfortunately, many patients do not benefit from adequate pain control. Estimates based on surveys in the United States indicate that less than half of all patients with cancer obtain optimal pain control. Poorly controlled pain has such catastrophic effects on the patient and his or her family that proper management of pain must have the highest priority for those who take care of patients with cancer. Mood and quality of life deteriorate in the presence of pain, and pain has adverse effects on such measures of disease status as appetite and activity. Severe pain may be a primary reason why both patients and their families stop treatment and why the occasional patient seeks relief through physician-assisted suicide. Improving the practice of anticipating, evaluating, and treating pain will benefit most patients.

I. **Prevalence, severity, and risk for pain.** Most cancer patients with terminal disease need expert pain management; between 60% and 80% of such patients have significant pain. Pain is also a problem for many patients much earlier in the course of their disease. Patients with months or years to live may be compromised by poorly controlled pain. Persistent pain is rarely a problem before metastatic cancer is present. When the cancer has metastasized, however, the percentage of patients with pain increases dramatically. In the United States, even with the availability of a full range of analgesics and other pain treatments, 60% of all outpatients with metastatic disease have cancer-related pain, and one third report pain so severe that it significantly impairs their quality of life. Multicenter studies indicate that about 40% of outpatients with cancer pain do not receive analgesics potent enough to manage their pain. Patients in minority treatment settings, female patients, and older patients are at greater risk for poorly controlled pain due to undermedication.

II. **Etiology of cancer pain**
    A. **Direct tumor involvement** is the most common cause of pain, present in about two thirds of those with pain from metastatic cancer. Tumor invasion of bone is the physical basis of pain in about 50% of these patients. The remaining 50% of these patients experience tumor-related pain that is due to nerve compression or infiltration or involvement of the gastrointestinal tract or soft tissue.

B. **Persistent posttherapy pain,** from long-term effects of surgery, radiotherapy, and chemotherapy, accounts for an additional 20% of all who report pain with metastatic cancer, with a small residual group experiencing pain from non–cancer-related conditions.

C. Most patients with advanced cancer have **pain at multiple sites** caused by multiple mechanisms. A new complaint of pain in a patient with metastatic cancer should first be thought of as disease related, but indirectly related, manageable causes should also be considered.

The sensation of pain is generated either by stimulation of peripheral pain receptors or by damage to afferent nerve fibers. Peripheral pain receptors can be stimulated by pressure, compression, and traction as well as by disease-related chemical changes. Pain due to stimulation of pain receptors is called *nociceptive pain.* Damage to visceral, somatic, or autonomic nerve trunks produces *neurogenic* or *neuropathic pain.* Neuropathic pain is thought to be caused by spontaneous activity in nerves damaged by disease or treatment. Patients with cancer often have nociceptive and neuropathic pain simultaneously. Neuropathic pain is less responsive to opioid analgesics and requires the additional use of other drugs.

III. **Assessment of pain.** Proper pain management requires a clear understanding of the characteristics of the pain and its physical basis. The changing expression of cancer pain demands repeated assessment because new causes of pain can emerge rapidly, and pain severity can increase quickly. In patients with advanced disease, pain from multiple causes is the rule and not the exception. A careful history includes questions concerning the location, severity, and quality of the pain as well as the effect the pain is having on the patient's life.

A. **Pain severity.** Inadequate pain assessment and poor physician–patient communication about pain are major barriers to good pain care. Physicians and nurses tend to underestimate pain intensity, especially when it is severe. Patients whose physicians underestimate their pain are at high risk for poor pain management and compromised function. A small minority of patients with cancer may complain of pain in a dramatic fashion, but many more patients underreport the severity of their pain and the lack of adequate pain relief.

There are several reasons for this reluctance to report pain, including the following:

Not wanting to acknowledge that the disease is progressing

Not wanting to divert the physician's attention from treating the disease

Not wanting to tell the physician that pain treatments are not working

Patients may not want to be put on opioid analgesics because of the following reasons:

Not wanting to become addicted

Fearing the psychoactive components of opioids

Being concerned that using opioids "too early" will endanger pain relief when they have more pain

Fearing that being placed on opioids signals that death is near

Having accepted religious or societal norms or teachings that pain should be endured

Presenting information that addresses these concerns in a straightforward manner will allay most of these fears and should be considered as an essential step in providing pain control. It is important that patients understand that they will function better if their pain is controlled. Patient education materials available from state cancer pain initiatives and from the National Cancer Institute, American Cancer Society, and the Agency for Health Care Policy and Research (AHCPR) can be very useful for both patients and families and should be given to patients when they develop pain.

Communication about pain is greatly aided by having the patient use a scale to rate the severity of their pain. A simple rating scale ranges from 0 to 10, with 0 being "no pain" and 10 being pain "as bad as you can imagine." Used properly, pain severity scales can be invaluable in titrating analgesics and in monitoring for increases in pain with progressive disease. Mild pain is often well tolerated with minimal impact on a patient's activities. However, there is a threshold beyond which pain is especially disruptive. This threshold has been reached when patients rate the severity of their pain at 5 or greater on a 0 to 10 scale. When pain is too great (7 or greater on this scale), it becomes the primary focus of attention and prohibits most activity not directly related to pain. Although it may not be possible to eliminate pain totally, reducing its severity to 4 or less ought to be a minimum standard of pain therapy.

B. **Diagnostic steps.** Those who treat patients with cancer should be familiar with the common pain syndromes associated with the disease:

1. Having the patient show the area of pain on a drawing of a human figure aids identification of the syndrome. This can be particularly helpful in indicating areas of referred pain, common with nerve compression.

2. Careful questioning concerning the characteristics of the pain is essential for physical diagnosis.

3. In addition to severity, these characteristics include the temporal pattern of the pain (constant or episodic) and its quality. Episodic or "incident" pain is much more difficult to control than is continuous pain.

4. Other important characteristics of pain are its relationship to physical activity and what seems to alleviate the pain.

5. The physical examination includes examination of the painful area as well as neurologic and orthopedic assessment.

6. Because bone metastases are a common cause of pain, and pain can occur with changes in bone density not detectable on radiographs, bone scans can be helpful. Magnetic resonance imaging (MRI) is useful in the evaluation of retroperitoneal, paravertebral, and pelvic areas as well as the base of the skull. Myelography may be necessary in determining the cause of pain if MRI cannot be performed.

7. Diagnostic nerve blocks can provide information concerning the pain pathway. Diagnostic blocks can also determine the potential effectiveness of neuroablative procedures that destroy the pain pathway.

C. **The impact of pain on the patient.** When pain is of moderate or greater severity, we can assume that it has a negative impact on the patient's quality of life. That impact, including problems with sleep and depression, must be evaluated. A reduced number of hours of sleep compared with the last pain-free interval, difficulties with sleep onset, frequent interruptions of sleep, or early morning awakening suggest the need for appropriate pharmacologic intervention, often the addition of a low-dose antidepressant at bedtime. Just as patients hesitate to report severe pain, they may hesitate to report depression. Having the patient report depression or tension on a scale of 0 to 10 may help overcome some of this reluctance. Significant depression should be treated through psychiatric or psychologic consultation, especially if it persists in the face of adequate pain relief.

It is important to differentiate between physical pain and psychological stress. A small number of patients in severe psychosocial distress express their concerns as a report of physical pain. Although it is important to recognize severe somatization and to provide psychiatric referral or counseling to these patients, it is equally important to recognize true physical pain. Too often, physicians misdiagnose true pain as depression or anxiety. Accurate pain assessment in patients who are cognitively impaired, particularly those with agitation, may be extremely difficult. These patients present with symptoms that may be attributable to either agitated delirium or pain. As a guide, patients in whom pain was well controlled before the development of delirium are unlikely to be agitated due to uncontrolled pain. Frequent discussions between various health care professionals and the patient's family are required.

D. **The addicted patient.** Some patients with severe alcoholism or drug addiction may request analgesics for their psychological effects. This is unlikely to occur in patients without a clear history of severe addictive behavior. Patients who are recovered alcoholics or drug abusers may be difficult to treat because of their resistance to taking analgesics. In any case, if this diagnosis is suspected, the issue should be discussed openly with the patient and an agreement should be reached about the use of opioids for the management of pain as opposed to mood alterations. With this group of patients, long-acting opioids or continuous infusion are preferable to short-acting opioids or patient-controlled analgesia. Prescriptions by a single physician would make the negotiation process with a patient much simpler. Although their care is more complex, patients with drug or alcohol addiction should never be denied appropriate pain medications.

IV. **Treatment**

A. **General aspects.** All health care professionals who see patients with cancer should be familiar with the AHCPR guidelines, *Management of Cancer Pain*. The prompt relief of pain from cancer frequently involves the use of simultaneously rather than serially administered combinations of drug and nondrug therapies. Identification of a treatable neoplasm as a factor in pain production calls for appropriate radiotherapy (e.g., to bone metastases), chemotherapy, or, in some instances, surgical debulking. Until such treatment can be effective (this may take days to weeks), the patient's pain must be managed with analgesics. In many instances, analgesics are the only pain treatment available because of the patient's condition, the physical basis of the pain, or limited treatment options. The principles of pharmacologic management of pain are evolving through studies of analgesic effectiveness and research on the use of combinations of palliative medications.

There is a growing consensus concerning the types of drugs to use, their routes of administration, and how best to schedule them. The first step is the choice of analgesic drug to be used (nonopioid, opioid, or a combination of both). The second step is the choice of adjuvant drugs, which can increase analgesic effectiveness and can produce other palliative effects to counter the disruptive consequences of pain.

B. **Nonsteroidal antiinflammatory drugs (NSAIDs)**

1. **Mechanism of action and selection of agents.** NSAIDs constitute the majority of nonopioid analgesics. Their effect on the inflammatory process is a key to their analgesic property. Tumor growth produces inflammatory and mechanical effects in adjacent tissues that can trigger the release of prostaglandins, bradykinin, and serotonin, which in turn may precipitate or

exacerbate pain in the surrounding tissues. Prostaglandin-mediated actions on peripheral receptors probably include both direct activation and sensitization to other analgesic substances. Prostaglandins are frequently associated with painful bone metastasis because of their involvement in bone reabsorption. The NSAIDs appear to exert their analgesic, antipyretic, and antiinflammatory actions by blocking the synthesis of prostaglandins. Table 32-1 gives the usual starting doses and dose ranges for several commonly used NSAIDs.

By virtue of their different mechanisms of action and toxicity profiles, the NSAIDs and opioids are often administered together. Enteric-coated aspirin is one of the first-choice drugs for mild to moderate cancer pain. Other NSAIDs, such as ibuprofen, diflunisal, naproxen, and choline magnesium trisalicylate (Trilisate), have established value in the management of clinical pain. These drugs are better tolerated than aspirin but are usually significantly more expensive. Individual differences in response to the various NSAIDs are not yet well understood.

Acetaminophen is a peripherally acting analgesic that does not inhibit peripheral prostaglandin synthesis. Therefore, it does not have antiinflammatory effects or the side effects associated with the use of NSAIDs. Acetaminophen should be considered in patients who have contraindications to the use of NSAIDs.

Commercial preparations containing codeine or oxycodone and acetaminophen or aspirin are among the most widely prescribed scheduled analgesics and are frequently administered to patients with cancer. This is generally appropriate because of the synergistic effects of the

Table 32-1. Starting doses and dose ranges of some nonsteroidal analgesic agents

Drug	Starting dose (mg)	Frequency	Dose range
Aspirin	650	q4–6h	Up to 1,300 mg q6h
Choline magnesium trisalicylate	500	q6h	Up to 1,000 mg q6h
Diflunisal	500	q8–12h	Up to 1,500 mg daily
Ibuprofen	400	q4–6h	Up to 2,400 mg daily
Naproxyn	250	q8–12h	Up to 1,250 mg daily
Piroxicam	10	q12–24h	Up to 20 mg daily
Tolmetin	400	q8h	Up to 1,800 mg daily

combination. Such a combination is reported to be particularly effective for bone pain.

2. **Side effects.** NSAIDs have a number of potentially serious side effects, including gastritis and gastrointestinal hemorrhage, bleeding due to platelet inhibition, and renal failure. Most of these side effects are related to the prostaglandin inhibitory effect of these drugs and are therefore common to all these drugs. Renal failure due to the inhibition of renal medullary prostaglandins can be of particular concern in patients who might also be receiving opioids. Decreased renal elimination of active opioid metabolites might result in somnolence, confusion, hallucinations, or generalized myoclonus. Therefore, kidney function should be monitored in patients receiving a combination of NSAIDs and opioids.

Gastrointestinal complications include gastric pain, nausea, vomiting, hemorrhage, and in extreme cases, perforation. Gastrointestinal damage is mediated by prostaglandin inhibition. The most common form of nephrotoxicity associated with NSAIDs is renal failure, related to prostaglandin inhibition and consequent vasodilation. Hepatic injury has been reported with the use of aspirin, benoxaprofen, and phenylbutazone and, less commonly, with diclofenac, ibuprofen, indomethacin, naproxen, pirprofen, and sulindac. Sulindac, however, appears to be associated with a higher incidence of cholestasis.

NSAID use is also associated with a variety of hypersensitivity reactions involving the skin (rash, eruption, itching), blood vessels (angioneurotic edema, vasomotor disorders), and respiratory system (rhinitis, asthma). In particular, aspirin may cause anaphylactic crisis, a syndrome characterized by dyspnea, sudden weakness, sweating, and collapse. Undesirable hematologic effects of NSAIDs include platelet dysfunction, aplastic anemia, and agranulocytosis. Factors often considered in the empiric selection of an NSAID for a given patient include its relative toxicity, cost, and dosage schedule and the patient's prior experience. The use of certain aspirin analogs (choline magnesium trisalicylate) has been suggested to be associated with a low incidence of gastropathy and platelet dysfunction. The effects of NSAIDs used as single agents in the management of cancer pain are characterized by a ceiling effect, beyond which further increases in dose do not enhance analgesia.

A new generation of cyclooxygenase-2 (COX-2) NSAIDs have entered clinical trials and are expected to be available within the next year. These agents are inhibitors of COX-2, the enzyme expressed in inflamed tissues, and have minimal or no effects on COX-1 (the enzyme expressed normally in the stomach and kidney). Therefore, the safety profile of these agents is expected to increase dramatically, making them much safer for patients with cancer.

C. Opioid analgesics

1. When to start therapy. The choice of an opioid analgesic as opposed to a nonopioid analgesic follows from an assessment of the severity of pain. The decision is relatively easy when pain is mild (choose nonopioid) or severe (choose opioid, usually in combination with a nonopioid). The choice is more difficult when the patient reports moderate pain, especially when there is reason to suspect that the patient may be underreporting pain severity. Several studies have documented that many patients with cancer are inadequately managed because of the physician's reluctance to use opioids in dosages and with schedules known to be sufficient to relieve moderate pain.

Opioid analgesics should be prescribed promptly as soon as there is evidence that pain is not well controlled with nonopioid analgesics. Usually, nonopioid analgesics can be continued as a way of maximizing analgesia because their site of action is different from that of the opioids.

2. Schedule of treatment and selection of dose. Except in a minority of patients whose pain is clearly episodic, analgesics should be given on an around-the-clock basis, with the time interval based on the duration of effectiveness of the drug and the patient's report of the duration of effectiveness. There is evidence that total opioid requirement is lower when opioids are given on a scheduled basis, thereby preventing peaks of pain. Putting patients in the position of having to ask for medication or continually making a judgment about whether their pain is severe enough to take analgesics focuses their attention on pain, reminds them of their need for drugs, and allows pain to reach a severity not readily controlled by the same doses that would be effective with scheduled administration. Nevertheless, there may be large individual differences in the required dose of opioid, depending on such factors as the patient's opioid use history, activity level, and metabolism. The patient's report of pain severity and pain relief is the best guideline for opioid titration.

3. **The so-called weak opioids,** including codeine and oxycodone, usually formulated in combination with acetaminophen or aspirin, can provide active patients with good pain relief for long periods of time. As disease advances, oral administration of the more potent opioids provides most patients with pain relief. Recent data demonstrate that oxycodone as a single entity should be considered a potent opioid. There is considerable agreement that meperidine should not be used on a chronic basis because of its toxic metabolite normeperidine, which is a central nervous system (CNS) stimulant, has a long serum half-life, and has no analgesic properties. Oral administration is preferred, but the physician must remain flexible to changes that are dictated by the patient's ability to use orally administered drugs. This may include the use of opioid and nonopioid suppositories and other alternate routes of administration (transdermal, sublingual, rectal, subcutaneous).

4. **Oral morphine,** either in immediate- or sustained-release preparation, is the analgesic of choice for moderate to severe cancer pain. Long-acting formulations of morphine and other opioids are convenient for both the patient and the health care staff. Immediate-release morphine is much cheaper, however, and is as effective. A typical starting dose for immediate-release oral morphine is 10 to 30 mg every 4 hours in patients not currently receiving opioids. When a patient is switching from another opioid (usually codeine or oxycodone) to morphine, it is important to calculate the equianalgesic morphine dose as a basis for determining what morphine-equivalent doses are the threshold for pain control (Table 32-2). The starting dose may not be sufficient, and relatively rapid upward titration may be needed, especially if pain is severe.

    The upward titration of morphine and other oral opioid analgesics can be done by giving a supplemental "boost" using 50% of the scheduled dose 2 hours after the scheduled dose if there is still significant pain and the patient is not overly sedated or lethargic. The scheduled dose is then set at 150% of the initial scheduled dose. Because of the time it takes to achieve a steady state, there may need to be some readjustment downward if the patient is unduly sleepy or is lethargic at the time of the scheduled dose. The supplemental dose may be given after any scheduled dose (even if there was an increase in the scheduled dose) as long as a sufficient time has passed for the drug to be absorbed from the stomach. An alternative way to

Table 32-2. Opioid dosing equivalence

Drug	Approximate equianalgesic dose	
	Oral	Parenteral
Morphine	30 mg q3–4h*	10 mg q3–4h
Hydromorphone	4–8 mg q3–4h	1.5 mg q3–4h
Codeine[†]	130 mg q3–4h	
Propoxyphene[†]	See comment below[‡]	
Hydrocodone[†]	30 mg q3–4h	
Oxycodone[†]	30 mg q3–4h	
Methadone	5–20 mg q6–8h[§]	5–10 mg q6–8h[§]
Levorphanol	4 mg q6–8h[§]	2 mg q6–8h[§]
Meperidine[‖]	300 mg q2–3h	100 mg q3h
Transdermal fentanyl	25–µg/h patch = 8–22 mg/24 h i.v. or i.m. morphine sulfate = 45–134 mg/24 h p.o. morphine sulfate	

* Slow-release formulations of oral morphine that are available have 8- to 12-h durations of analgesic action.
[†] Codeine, propoxyphene, hydrocodone, and oxycodone are often given as combination products with aspirin, acetaminophen, or both.
[‡] Propoxyphene is a weak analgesic; 65–130 mg is equivalent to about 650 mg of aspirin. It has a duration of action of 3–4 h; however, its duration of action increases with chronic dosing.
[§] The duration of analgesia of methadone and levorphanol may be significantly longer than 6–8 hours in some patients.
[‖] Not recommended for chronic use.
From Weissman DE, et al. *Handbook of cancer pain management.* 4th ed. Madison, WI: The Wisconsin Cancer Pain Initiative, 1993.

titrate is simply to add 50% to the next scheduled dose, but staying with the previously determined schedule (usually every 4 hours). When the doses of opioid are higher (e.g., morphine, 100 mg every 4 hours), some clinicians use less, for example, 20% to 30% (20 to 30 mg) as the boost, but incrementally add to the dose with each scheduled treatment until adequate pain relief has been achieved. Depending on the understanding of the patient and family, it is often best to have the patient check in with a physician or nurse after every other dose increase to be sure the treatment plan is understood, safe, and effective.

5. **Long-acting preparations.** When an effective dose of short-acting morphine has been established, the required 24-hour dose for a long-acting preparation can be calculated. An additional supply of short-acting morphine, given when necessary, will help the patient manage

"breakthrough" pain. Consistent need for this additional short-acting morphine (e.g., three or four doses daily) dictates an upward adjustment of the dose of sustained-release drug. Orders for immediate-release morphine should allow for some upward titration of dose by the patient or by the nurse. Each dose of short-acting morphine for breakthrough pain is usually 15% to 25% of the 24-hour dose of long-acting morphine. If more than this is required, it is usually an indication for increasing the dose of the long-acting preparation.

6. Although the **opioid agonist-antagonist analgesics** have established effectiveness in the control of acute (especially procedurally related) pain, their use in chronic cancer pain is limited by the possibility of precipitous withdrawal in the patient who has been taking morphine-type drugs, by their analgesic ceiling effect (when the drug does not provide more pain relief), and by the lack of an oral form of administration (with the exception of pentazocine, which yields a relatively high proportion of patients reporting disturbing psychomimetic effects).

7. **Alternative potent opioids** may sometimes have less side effects than morphine. Methadone is an agonist opioid analgesic that has the advantage of extremely low cost and lack of known active metabolites. However, because of its long and unpredictable half-life and relatively unknown equianalgesic dose as compared with other opioids, methadone should only be used by pain specialists who are experienced in its use. Other alternatives are levorphanol, which has a longer half-life than morphine, and single-entity oxycodone and hydromorphone, which has a half-life similar to morphine. Equivalent starting doses can be selected from Table 32-2, but if the patient has been on high doses of morphine, care must be taken not to switch cavalierly to proportionally higher doses of the alternative because unexpected side effects may occur.

8. **Alternate routes.** About 70% of patients benefit from the use of an alternate route for opioid administration sometime before death. The duration for which patients need these routes varies between hours and months. Although intermittent injections can be effective for a brief period of time, this method is painful for the patient, time-consuming for the nursing staff, and difficult to manage at home.

   a. **Intravenous infusion.** A number of studies have shown that intravenous infusions of opioids produce stable blood levels of drug and that they are safe and effective for treating both postoperative and cancer pain. Intravenous infusion using a patient-controlled analgesia pump may be very effective in gaining rapid control over pain that has gotten out of hand. It may also be of value when the patient cannot take medications orally and does not wish to take suppositories. The main problem associated with continuous intravenous infusions is the prolonged maintenance of an intravenous line. Patients may need to be subjected to numerous venipunctures when peripheral intravenous lines are used. Totally implantable intravenous catheters represent a major improvement, permitting long-term intravenous access. However, these catheters are expensive and need to be surgically implanted, and their maintenance requires considerable nursing expertise and patient teaching. If such a catheter is already available in a patient with advanced cancer who has pain, it certainly could be used for the administration of opioids. Starting doses of morphine for severe pain are 2 to 3 mg hourly as a continuous infusion, with patient-controlled boosts of 1 mg every 6 to 15 minutes. At the end of 24 hours, 50% of the patient boosts can be added to the total 24-hour dose of the continuous infusion until the patient is requiring less than one boost hourly. At that time, a shift to oral analgesics can be started, if the patient is able to take oral medications. If the doses of intravenous morphine are high, the shifting to appropriate oral doses may take several days. It is usually safe and effective to give a 24-hour dose of long-acting morphine orally that is equal in milligrams to the 24-hour requirement intravenously, and simultaneously to reduce the intravenous dose (continuous infusion rate) by half. Boosts can be given by mouth, but the patient should have the intravenous boost option as reassurance. The next day, the 24-hour intravenous dose required (continuous plus boosts) can be added orally to the previous day's oral dose (long-acting plus short-acting) and the infusion further reduced. The same process is repeated until the patient is getting adequate pain relief with the oral morphine. The infusion can usually be stopped and needed boosts given orally by the third or fourth day.

b. **Subcutaneous route.** This route has been found to be safe and effective for the administration of morphine, hydromorphone, and levorphanol. Subcutaneous opioids can be administered as a continuous infusion using a portable or nonportable pump (use as small a volume as possible, e.g., <5 mL/h) or as an intermittent injection. A butterfly needle can be left under the skin for about 7 days, making both intermittent injections and continuous infusion painless. The needles are frequently inserted in the subclavicular region, anterior chest, or abdominal wall. This allows patients to have free limbs.

c. **Rectal route.** Most of the experience reported in the literature is with the short-term use of rectal opioids for the management of acute pain. Both solid and liquid solutions have been used. Although there is considerable interindividual variation in the bioavailability of rectally administered morphine, there is general consensus that this drug is well absorbed after rectal administration. A number of authors have treated terminally ill patients with cancer with rectal morphine, with good pain control until death. Advantages of the rectal route include the absence of the need for the insertion of needles and the use of portable pumps. However, rectal administration can be uncomfortable or psychologically distressing for some patients; absorption may be decreased by the presence of stool in the rectum, by diarrhea, or simply by normal bowel movements; and progressive titration may be difficult because of the limited availability of different commercial preparations.

d. **Transdermal route.** The recent development of a transdermal preparation of fentanyl citrate has revitalized an interest in this route. Pharmacokinetic data suggest that transdermal fentanyl is well absorbed, although there is considerable delay in reaching steady-state blood levels and a slowly declining plasma concentration after removal of the patch. The 72-hour dosing of the patch makes it convenient to use, and treatment appears to be well tolerated.

e. **Transmucosal route.** Fentanyl citrate can also be formulated in a candied matrix to allow it to be administered orally as a lozenge on a stick. Oral transmucosal fentanyl citrate (OTFC) appears to be rapidly effective for breakthrough pain or for procedures. Dose equivalency studies have suggested that OTFC is about 10 times more potent than parenteral morphine. Starting doses are usually 200 μg, with dosing intervals of 4 to 6 hours. Drug dose requires titrating up as with other agents with single doses of up to 1,600 μg.

f. **Spinal route.** Some patients suffering from localized pain syndromes might benefit from intraspinal administration of opioids. The advantage of this route is the lack of systemic side effects of opioids and the fact that a relatively small dose of drugs is necessary. The disadvantage is the need for the insertion of catheters into the epidural or intrathecal space, the need for expensive infusion pumps, and in many patients, the rapid development of tolerance to the analgesic effect of different opioids. To overcome this rapid development of tolerance, some clinicians have used a combined infusion of opioids and local anesthetic. Because of the complexity associated with this route, it should only be considered in selected patients and after an adequate trial of systemic opioids and adjuvant drugs. The insertion of the catheter and the maintenance of the spinal analgesic regimen should be under the control of a pain specialist.

9. **Adverse effects of opioids.** Fear of the inability to manage side effects is one of the main reasons cited by oncologists that they limit their use of opioids. Yet, most of the agents used in chemotherapy are associated with more potent side effects than the opioids. The analgesic and side effects of opioid agonists are not identical for all patients. Some patients may require a higher equivalent dose of a certain opioid agonist to achieve adequate analgesia. This higher equivalent dose may result in a higher incidence of side effects, such as nausea or sedation. Therefore, when significant toxicity occurs in a patient treated with a certain opioid agonist, such as morphine, it may be appropriate to change to another opioid, such as hydromorphone. In addition, after prolonged treatment, high dosages, or renal failure, patients may experience the accumulation of active metabolites of opioid agonists. Active metabolites have been identified for both morphine and hydromorphone. This accumulation results in CNS side effects, such as sedation, generalized myoclonus, confusion, and in some patients, agitated delirium or grand mal seizures. In these patients, it is also useful to change from one opioid to another.

It is important to understand the side effect liability of these analgesics and be prepared to deal with side effects prophylactically or when they do occur. *Most patients develop tolerance for side effects much more rapidly than they develop tolerance for the analgesic effects of the opioids.*

   a.   **Sedation.** This occurs in most patients during the beginning of opioid treatment or after a major increase in dose. Most patients develop rapid tolerance to this side effect, and while the sedation disappears within 3 to 5 days, the analgesic effect persists. When sedation occurs in patients with cancer receiving a stable dose of opioid, it is necessary to suspect the potential accumulation of active opioid metabolites, such as morphine-6-glucuronide. This occurs more frequently in patients who are receiving high doses of opioids or present with renal failure. It is also important to suspect other non–opioid-related causes, such as hypercalcemia, because these patients are frequently very ill. Opioid-induced sedation can be managed by opioid rotation (some opioids have a higher ratio of analgesic effects to sedation than others) or by the addition of amphetamine derivatives, such as methylphenidate, starting with 5 mg p.o. b.i.d. daily, or dextroamphetamine/amphetamine, 5 mg b.i.d. (last dose no later than 3 PM to avoid insomnia).

   b.   **Nausea and vomiting.** Most patients present with these symptoms after initial administration or a major increase in dose. Some authors propose the use of prophylactic antiemetics on a regular basis during the first days of treatment because in most patients, nausea disappears after that period. The mechanism for the nausea is central. These side effects can be well antagonized by antidopaminergic agents, such as metoclopramide, 10 mg p.o. q.i.d. Dexamethasone, 2 to 4 mg p.o. q.i.d., is also a useful antiemetic that potentiates metoclopramide in these patients but has significant side effects when used for more than 1 or 2 weeks. As with sedation, nausea is a multicausal syndrome in patients with cancer who are receiving opioids: Severe constipation, cancer-induced autonomic failure, gastritis, increased intracranial pressure, and opioid metabolite accumulation are all possible causes of nausea.

c. **Constipation.** This is probably the most common adverse effect of opioids, and it is necessary to anticipate constipation when opioid therapy is started. Opioids act at multiple sites in the gastrointestinal tract and spinal cord. The result is decreased intestinal secretions and peristalsis. Although tolerance to both sedation and nausea develops quickly, it develops very slowly to the smooth muscle effects of opioids, so that constipation persists when these drugs are used for chronic pain. At the same time that the use of opioid analgesics is initiated, provision for a regular bowel regimen, including stimulants and stool softeners, should be instituted to diminish this adverse effect (see Chap. 27).

d. **Respiratory depression.** This is the most serious adverse effect of opioid analgesics. Opioids can cause increasing respiratory depression to the point of apnea. In humans, death due to overdose of opioids is nearly always due to respiratory arrest. At equianalgesic doses, the morphine-like agonists produce an equivalent degree of respiratory depression. When respiratory depression occurs, it is usually in opioid-naïve patients after acute administration of an opioid and is associated with other signs of CNS depression, including sedation and mental clouding. Tolerance quickly develops to this effect with repeated drug administration, allowing the opioid analgesics to be used in the management of chronic cancer pain without significant risk of respiratory depression. If respiratory depression occurs, it can be reversed by the administration of the specific opioid antagonist naloxone. In patients chronically receiving opioids who develop respiratory depression, naloxone in a 1:10 dilution should be titrated carefully to prevent the precipitation of severe withdrawal syndromes while reversing the respiratory depression. Long-acting drugs, such as methadone, fentanyl patches, or slow-release morphine, are likely to cause a higher incidence of respiratory depression. The accumulation of active opioid metabolites and the simultaneous use of other depressants, such as benzodiazepines or alcohol, are risk factors for respiratory depression. Although this is the most feared side effect of opioid analgesics, it occurs seldom in patients receiving chronic opioid therapy for the treatment of cancer pain.

e. **Allergic reactions.** These occur infrequently with opioids. However, it is common that patients are described as "allergic" to a number of opioid analgesics. This commonly results from a misinterpretation by the patient or clinician of some of the common side effects of opioids, such as nausea, sedation, vomiting, or sweating. In most instances, a simple discussion with the patient is enough to clarify this issue.

f. **Urinary retention.** The increase in the tone of smooth muscle of the bladder induced by opioids results in an increase in the sphincter tone leading to urinary retention. This is most common in elderly patients. Attention should be directed to this potential transient side effect, and catheterization may be necessary for management.

g. **"Newer" side effects.** During recent years, as a result of increased education in the assessment and management of cancer pain, patients have been receiving higher doses of opioids for longer periods of time than ever before. This more aggressive use of opioids is associated with additional side effects, usually only seen in patients with late-stage disease receiving high doses of opioids.

   (1) **Cognitive failure.** Patients can experience a transient decrease in concentration and psychomotor coordination after starting opioids or after a sudden increase in the opioid dose. In some patients, the opioid-induced cognitive failure can be permanent. Some of the cognitive effects can be reversed by the administration of amphetamine derivatives, such as methylphenidate. Screening tools, such as the Mini-Mental State questionnaire, are useful in patients receiving high doses of opioids.

   (2) **Other central effects.** Organic hallucinations, myoclonus, grand mal seizures, and even hyperalgesia have been observed in patients receiving high doses of opioids for long periods. These effects are likely due to the accumulation of active opioid metabolites. Improvement is frequently seen after a change in the type of opioid. Hallucinations may improve on low doses of haloperidol, 0.5 to 2 mg b.i.d.

   (3) **Severe sedation and coma.** When coma occurs in patients receiving a

stable dose of opioids for a long period of time, it should be suspected that accumulation of active opioid metabolites has occurred. These patients usually improve quickly after discontinuation of opioids.

    (4) Pulmonary edema. Although noncardiogenic pulmonary edema is a well-recognized complication of opioid overdose in addicts, it had not been recognized until recently as a potential complication of cancer pain treatment. Pulmonary edema usually occurs when patients have undergone rapid increases in dose, usually as a result of severe neuropathic pain. Even though the mortality of the syndrome is very low among patients presenting with acute opioid overdoses, because of the conservative nature of the treatment of terminally ill patients with cancer, the mortality of pulmonary edema is much higher within this population.

    (5) Myoclonus. Myoclonus may occur in patients who are on opioids for long periods, particularly with higher doses and toward the end of life when metabolic problems may also be present. Although it is often not disturbing to the patient, if it does become a clinical problem, it can be treated with clonazepam, 0.5 mg p.o. b.i.d. to start, with titration every 3 days up to a maximum daily dose of 20 mg.

V. Adjuvant drugs. Opioid analgesics are the most important drugs for the treatment of cancer pain. Although these drugs can, in most patients, control severe pain even when they are used appropriately, they may produce new symptoms or exacerbate preexisting symptoms, most notably nausea and somnolence. This aspect of treatment with opioid compounds is particularly problematic in patients with advanced cancer. The combination of severe pain, anorexia, chronic nausea, asthenia, and somnolence is a frequent finding in patients with advanced cancer. The term *adjuvant drug* has been used in a variety of ways, even in the context of cancer pain management. For the purposes of the following paragraphs, an adjuvant drug meets one or more of the following criteria:

- Increases the analgesic effect of opioids (adjuvant analgesia)
- Decreases the toxicity of opioids
- Improves other symptoms associated with terminal cancer

Most symptomatic patients with cancer receive more than one or two adjuvant drugs. Unfortunately, there is still limited consensus on the type and dose of the most appropriate adjuvant drugs.

Claims have been made for the adjuvant analgesic effect of many drugs, but unfortunately, most of the evidence for these effects is anecdotal. Controlled clinical trials are needed to define more clearly the indications and risk-to-benefit ratios. These agents, some of which have the potential to produce significant toxicity, can aggravate the toxicity of opioids.

A. Tricyclic antidepressants. Despite the frequent use of these agents in British hospices and South American and European cancer centers, the use of tricyclics in North American cancer centers has been uncommon. Tricyclic antidepressants have been found to be useful for a variety of neuropathic pain syndromes, especially when pain has a prominent dysesthetic or burning character. Both amitriptyline and desipramine have been found to be effective in the management of postherpetic neuralgia, diabetic neuropathy, and other neurologic conditions. There is, however, only limited evidence for a significant analgesic effect in cancer pain. Clinical experience and expert consensus suggest that tricyclics should be tried for the management of pain of central, deafferentation, or neuropathic origin.

The optimal drug and dosing regimens are unknown. Amitryptyline, 25 mg at bedtime, is a safe starting dose; if it is not overly sedating and the patient does not experience bothersome anticholinergic side effects, the dose may be increased every three days to a maximum total daily dose of 150 mg. The effects of newer antidepressants, such as the selective serotonin uptake inhibitors or specific monoamine oxidase inhibitors, on pain control have not been clearly established. Until further evidence is available, the more traditional tricyclics should be used as adjuvant analgesics. The toxic effects of these drugs are mainly autonomic (dry mouth, postural hypotension) and centrally mediated (somnolence, confusion). Because their use may contribute to symptoms already present in debilitated patients, they should be administered cautiously in those who are very ill.

B. Anticonvulsants. Carbamazepine, phenytoin, valproic acid, and clonazepam, alone or in combination with the tricyclic antidepressants, have been used successfully to treat neuropathic pain. Based on the well-documented efficacy for the treatment of trigeminal neuralgia, considerable experience and expert consensus suggest the use of these agents for neuropathic cancer pain syndromes, including neural invasion by tumor, radiation fibrosis or surgical scarring, herpes zoster, and deafferentation. Based on clinical observations, improvement can be expected in a proportion of patients whose predominant complaint is pain of a shooting, lancinating, burning, or hyperesthetic nature.

1. **Carbamazepine** can be started at 100 mg b.i.d., with the dose escalated to maximum efficacy every several days. If 400 to 600 mg/day is not effective, it is not likely that higher doses will have a substantial therapeutic ratio.

2. **Gabapentin** has been proposed in recent years as an effective and potentially better tolerated agent in these very debilitated patients. The effective dose of gabapentin is generally 900 to 1,800 mg/day. It is given in divided doses, three times a day. Titration to an effective dose can take place rapidly, over a few days, giving 300 mg on day 1; 300 mg twice a day on day 2; and 300 mg three times a day on day 3. To minimize potential side effects, especially somnolence, dizziness, fatigue, and ataxia, the first dose on day 1 may be administered at bedtime. Effective doses in the treatment of neuropathic pain in patients with cancer are not well established.

   Side effects of therapy with this group of agents are potentially serious, particularly in patients with advanced cancer, and can include bone marrow depression, hepatic dysfunction, somnolence, ataxia, diplopia, and lymphadenopathy. Periodic monitoring of complete blood cell count and liver function is recommended.

C. **Corticosteroids.** Controlled studies suggest that the administration of corticosteroids to selected patients with advanced cancer results in decreased pain and improved appetite and activity. Unfortunately, the duration of the effects is probably short-lasting. The mechanism by which corticosteroids appear to produce beneficial symptom effects in patients with terminal cancer is unclear but may involve their euphoriant effects or the inhibition of prostaglandin metabolism. The optimal drug and dosing regimens have not been established. For the treatment of painful conditions, prednisone or dexamethasone is often administered in doses totaling 30 to 60 mg p.o. daily and 8 to 16 mg p.o. daily, respectively. As soon as symptomatic relief is obtained, attempts should be made to decrease the dose progressively to the minimally effective dose. Although long-term side effects are not an important consideration in many patients with advanced cancer, treatment may produce limiting side effects in these patients, particularly immunosuppression (candidiasis occurs in most patients), proximal myopathy, and psychiatric symptoms. The incidence of psychologic disturbances ranges from 3% to 50%, with severe symptoms occurring in about 5% of patients. The spectrum of disturbances ranges from mild to severe affective disorders, psychotic reactions, and global cognitive impairment.

D. **Clonidine.** Clonidine, an α_2-adrenergic agonist, is administered epidurally. It has been shown in one controlled trial to be effective for cancer-related pain, especially neuropathic pain, at epidural doses of 30 µg/h.

E. **Approaches to metastatic bone pain**

   1. **Strontium 89.** Strontium 89 and a number of other isotopes have been found to be useful in the treatment of pain in patients with bony metastases. This agent is more useful in patients with multiple pain locations who might not benefit from radiation therapy. The main limitations of this agent are its high cost and the potential for severe and prolonged hematologic toxicity, mainly thrombocytopenia.

   2. **Bisphosphonates.** These agents have been found to be significantly better than placebo in patients with bone pain due to a variety of primary tumors. Pamidronate and clodronate are the agents that have been most frequently studied. Because of their poor oral bioavailability, these drugs are most useful when given intravenously every 3 to 4 weeks (pamidronate) or intravenously or subcutaneously every 2 to 4 weeks (clodronate). In addition to pain control, these drugs can significantly reduce a number of other complications of osteolysis, such as hypercalcemia, fractures, and need for radiation therapy. A new generation of bisphosphonates with increased oral bioavailability will be available during the next year.

   3. **External-beam radiotherapy.** Radiation therapy can effectively control bone pain in about 70% of patients within 2 to 4 weeks. This treatment is most useful in patients with a single or small number of painful areas. A single administration may be as effective as multiple smaller fractions, reducing the cost and discomfort of transportation back and forth associated with multiple doses.

VI. **Neuroablative procedures.** Evaluation of the physical basis of the pain may indicate that a neuroablative procedure, in which the pain pathway is destroyed, would be of benefit for pain control. As aggressive opioid analgesia becomes more accepted, most patients with cancer do not require these neuroablative interventions. Destruction of the pain pathway can be accomplished surgically or through destructive nerve blocks using an agent such as phenol. The major barrier to the more widespread application of these techniques is the limited number of practitioners expert in their use. The most frequently used neurosurgical procedure is the anterolateral or spinothalamic cordotomy. This is often performed as closed percutaneous cordotomy by stereotactically placing a radiofrequency needle in the anterolateral quadrant of the cervical spinal cord. Unilateral pain control can unmask significant pain on the opposite side of the body. For pain of head and neck cancer, procedures such as percutaneous radiofrequency coagulation of the glossopharyngeal nerve may be used. Nevertheless, performance of such procedures does not eliminate the need to administer and monitor the effectiveness of analgesics. Because of afferent regeneration, destructive procedures have had their greatest application in patients whose expected life-span is only a few months.

Destructive anesthetic block of the celiac plexus has been used for several decades in the management of pain in the abdominal region. This block, which can be preceded by reversible diagnostic block, is a boon to many patients suffering from the severe pain accompanying cancer of the pancreas and may also be helpful for pain from cancers of the liver, gallbladder, or stomach. The effectiveness of the destruction of the celiac plexus for pain relief is supported by at least one randomized clinical trial. If success is achieved with the diagnostic block, lasting disruption of the pain pathway can be achieved using alcohol or phenol. Pain from rib metastases or tumors of the chest wall can be relieved with intercostal nerve blocks. Intrathecal and epidural nerve blocks have provided pain relief, but those procedures carry a risk of sensory and motor deficit.

VII. **Coping or behavioral skill techniques.** Teaching specific skills to manage pain can be of help to many patients, especially those who face pain for months to years. Evaluation and prescription of the specific skills most beneficial to the individual can often be obtained through consultation with a behavioral psychologist, psychiatrist, or nurse pain specialist. Such techniques should never be used as a substitute for appropriate analgesia. The skills include relaxation, self-hypnosis, and other distraction and cognitive control techniques. These measures can affect the sensation of pain by reducing muscle tension on pain-generating lesions as well as by maximizing the patient's ability to cope with the pain and remain as active as the disease permits. All patients need education about the nature of their pain, the methods that can be used to relieve it, and how they can cooperate with their health care providers to achieve good pain control.

SELECTED READINGS

Agency for Health Care Policy and Research. *Management of cancer pain.* Rockville, MD: U.S. Department of Health and Human Services, 1994.

Bruera E, Ripamonti C. Adjuvants to opioid analgesics. In: Patt R, ed. *Cancer pain.* Philadelphia: JB Lippincott, 1992:142–159.

Bruera E, Ripamonti C. Alternate routes of administration of opioids for the management of cancer pain. In: Patt R, ed. *Cancer pain.* Philadelphia: JB Lippincott, 1992:161–184.

Cleeland CS, Gronin R, Hatfield AK. Pain and its treatment in outpatients with metastatic cancer. *N Engl J Med* 1994;330:592–596.

Eisele JH Jr, Grigsby EJ, Dea G. Clonazepam treatment of myoclonic contractions associated with high-dose opioids: a case report. *Pain* 1992;49:231.

World Health Organization (WHO). *Cancer pain relief and palliative care.* Geneva: WHO, 1990.

33

Emotional and Psychiatric Problems in Patients with Cancer

Kathleen S. N. Franco-Bronson
and Kristi S. Williams

I. **General principles.** Clinical psychiatric disorders occur in up to half of patients with cancer at some point during their treatment. Delirium, depression, and anxiety are those most frequently seen and may coexist in the same patient. Careful monitoring for the early symptoms of psychiatric distress is important to the care of these patients. The clinician should inquire regularly about symptoms in the affective and cognitive domains. Symptom clusters help differentiate anxiety, depression, and acute confusional states from other psychiatric disorders. Once an accurate diagnosis is made, appropriate treatment that may include medication can be planned for the target symptoms. More than one psychiatric diagnosis may be present, requiring a hierarchical approach. For example, if both delirium and depression are present, the cause of the delirium should be determined and treated before starting antidepressant therapy (which could worsen the delirium). Once the delirium has improved, treatment for the depression can be considered. When major depression and an anxiety disorder coexist, treatment for the depression is started first and may adequately manage both disorders.

II. **Acute confusional states**

   A. **Precepts.** Psychiatrists are often asked to assist in the care of "agitated" patients. The initial request may be for medication advice, but prescribing psychotropic drugs without understanding the cause of the patient's distress can have serious consequences. Delirium is characterized by fluctuating levels of alertness and consciousness, shortened attention and concentration, rapidly changing moods, irregular sleep–wake cycles, garbled or slurred speech, hypervigilance, and behavior not consistent with good judgment. The delirious patient may also have delusional ideas, hallucinations, or appear depressed. Visual, auditory, tactile, and occasionally olfactory hallucinations can be present. The more sensory modalities that are involved in the hallucinations, the greater is the likelihood that the patient is experiencing an acute confusional state.

   B. **Etiologies**

      1. **Medications** remain the most common reason for acute confusional states. The most frequently identified medications to cause de-

lirium are sedatives, narcotic analgesics, anxiolytics, anticholinergic drugs, and corticosteroids.

2. **Metabolic causes** are often seen in patients with cancer and include hypernatremia and hyponatremia, hyperthyroidism and hypothyroidism, poorly controlled diabetes mellitus, vitamin deficiencies (B_{12}, folate, thiamine), and hypercalcemia.

3. **Infections** of the respiratory, urinary, central nervous, and other systems are common, especially in immunosuppressed patients.

4. **Chemical withdrawal** from benzodiazepines, alcohol, and other drugs can induce delirium.

5. **Medical illness**, such as tumors, cardiac arrhythmias, congestive heart failure, liver disease, trauma, strokes, renal failure, and a variety of other conditions, can cause acute changes in mental status.

C. **Therapeutic approach.** Once an acute confusional state is identified, the primary therapeutic approach is to treat the cause. Antipsychotic medications may be helpful for managing symptoms such as hallucinations, delusions, and extreme agitation, but they do not treat the cause of the delirium.

1. **Orientation** aids in the reduction of confusion.

   a. It is helpful to orient the patient frequently to place, time, and why they are at the hospital, and to give current explanations of procedures. This routine should be done once or more per shift when the delirious patient is awake. Because patients' attention, concentration, and recent memory are frequently impaired, they often do not recall instructions given to them earlier. Leaving a large, legibly written note card with the patient's name, date, hospital name, and so on is beneficial in some instances.

   b. A large calendar, a clock, and family pictures or mementos can assist the patients in feeling less estranged from their environment.

   c. Some patients are reassured by a small night light in their room, which cuts down on illusions or misinterpretations. Patients with compromised vision or hearing are particularly distraught when they are even less able to discern what is happening around them, and they should be provided with their hearing aids and glasses.

2. **Medication** helps to control hallucinations, delusions, and psychotic agitation. The lowest dose to control symptoms is usually preferable.

a. **Haloperidol** (Haldol) (Table 33-1) is a butyrophenone, antipsychotic agent with potent dopamine-blocking action. It is less likely to produce cardiovascular, respiratory, gastrointestinal, and general anticholinergic side effects than many of the other antipsychotic medications. However, moderate doses may cause extrapyramidal symptoms. The starting dose in a patient with an acute confusional state is 0.25 to 2 mg p.o. or i.m., on an as-needed or regular dosing schedule every 4 to 6 hours. A marked advantage of haloperidol is that sedation is minimized while controlling agitation. There are exceptions to the usually preferred low doses of antipsychotic medications. For example, if patients tolerate higher doses with few side effects, they may benefit by having improved pain control. Intravenous haloperidol has not

Table 33-1. Antipsychotic medications: prominent characteristics and dosage for patients with cancer

Agent	Starting Dose (mg)*	Characteristics
Phenothiazines		
Chlorpromazine (Thorazine)	10–25	Significant hypotension risk, lowers seizure threshold, highly sedating, anticholinergic
Thioridazine (Mellaril)	10–25	Similar to chlorpromazine but more likely to alter electrocardiogram; not available i.m.
Perphenazine (Trilafon)	4	Moderate sedation and hypotension
Trifluoperazine (Stelazine)	2	High frequency of extrapyramidal side effects
Others		
Haloperidol (Haldol)	0.5–2.0	Good for acute delirium, high frequency of extrapyramidal side effects, available i.v., i.m., or p.o.
Risperidone (Risperdal)	0.5–1.0	Some α-adrenergic effects, mild extrapyramidal as dose increases, p.o. form only
Olanzapine (Zyprexa)	5	More sedation, orthostasis, weight gain; less extrapyramidal side effects; p.o. form only

* Dose generally can be repeated every 4–6 h (other than risperidone and olanzepine), either on an as-needed or a regular schedule (e.g., b.i.d.).

been approved by the U.S. Food and Drug Administration, although it is commonly used in the seriously agitated patient. Half the oral dosing is prescribed when the medication is given intravenously. Some patients require larger intravenous doses to control symptoms. Avoid very high doses in patients with alcoholic cardiomyopathy, those prone to torsade de pointes or similar arrhythmias, and those with an excessively long QTc interval. Extrapyramidal side effects are minimal with intravenous administration.

b. **Risperidone** (Risperdal) is less likely to produce extrapyramidal side effects but is available only in oral form.

c. **A delirious patient** with vision or hearing impairment is likely to hallucinate during periods of excessive sedation.

d. If the patient demonstrates a **predictable period of confusion,** such as during the early evening ("sun-downing") when there is less environmental activity, a once-a-day dose at that time may be adequate.

e. **When increasing the dose of antipsychotic drugs,** muscle spasms, restlessness, or pseudoparkinsonian symptoms may occur. Adding a small amount of trihexyphenidyl (Artane) 1 to 2 mg b.i.d., benztropine (Cogentin) 1 mg b.i.d., or diphenhydramine (Benadryl) 25 mg b.i.d. can often reduce the side effects. However, increasing the level of anticholinergic activity with these choices may cause an atropinic-like psychosis. Constipation, urinary retention, dry mouth, tachycardia, and increasing confusion are warnings of this potential problem, especially when multiple anticholinergic medications (e.g., antiemetics, analgesics) are being prescribed. Therefore, antiparkinsonian drugs are not prescribed prophylactically but only if clearly indicated. Ondansetron (Zofran) may be substituted for other antiemetics, reducing extrapyramidal symptoms and avoiding the need for an antiparkinsonian medication. Many antiemetics (e.g., droperidol) are also antipsychotics.

f. **Benzodiazepines,** such as lorazepam (Ativan), can be given 0.5 to 2.0 mg every 8 hours. They can be administered in small doses to a patient who needs some sedation without added anticholinergic activity or those whose cardiac status is at risk (i.e., heart block) if the antipsychotic medication is increased. Using both benzodiazepines and antipsychotics is sometimes helpful. One pattern might be 0.5 to 2 mg haloperidol at 4 PM, 1 to 2 mg of lorazepam at 8 PM, and so forth if the patient is agitated.

    g. Increasing delirium. Too much medication may have been given if the patient's level of agitation increases with higher doses.

    h. Hypotension. Avoid adding other antipsychotics, e.g., thorazine, as they predispose to hypotension and shock. If the blood pressure does drop significantly, norepinephrine bitartrate (Levophed) or a similar choice may be necessary because the antipsychotic medications block the action of dopamine. The half-life of the antipsychotic is generally 24 to 48 hours.

III. Depression. Patients with cancer have various emotional responses to their diagnoses. The mourning period for some is brief, does not inhibit their ability to interact with family and friends, and does not hinder participation in their own treatment. Support from others, acceptance of their feelings, and time may be all that is necessary for them to continue the emotional work ahead. However, about one fourth of patients with cancer develop longer, more severe depression. The greatest risk of depression is at the time of first relapse. There are many variables that influence this process, including emotional conflicts with loved ones, disproportionate guilt, previous losses that were never resolved, long-standing debilitating illness, some personality characteristics such as dependency, and inadequate support systems. Any of these factors, along with a family history of depression, are warnings for the physician to heed.

  A. Therapeutic approach

    1. Emotional support at frequent intervals from the physician is generally needed. Some patients explore old emotional conflicts, whereas others just need a safe person to whom they can express their feelings. It is important for patients to be able to hold on to hope. A degree of denial is acceptable, normal, and upheld. Only when this denial makes it impossible for a patient to make informed treatment decisions is it necessary to probe into the denial.

Psychotherapy of a supportive nature is often provided by the primary care physician, oncologist, psychiatrist, clergy, nurse, family, or friend individually or in any combination. For patients who wish to explore ambivalence, a professional psychotherapist trained in psychodynamic or interpersonal therapy is a good option. Cognitive therapy is helpful in letting go of detrimental interpretations while increasing one's ability to deal with emotional pain.

2. **Psychiatric care** may be particularly instrumental when the patient's preexisting personality style is interfering with treatment. Anniversary responses to previous losses, important family events, or past hospitalizations may have a great impact on the presentation of the depression and deserve exploration by a psychotherapist if a pattern is found. If there is a designated psychiatric consultant, this individual must work closely with the rest of the oncology team, communicating in a helpful way to the patient, family, and staff.

   If a patient has felt depressed, distressed, or irritable for some time or describes a loss of pleasure from formerly enjoyable relationships or activities, inquiry about the following symptoms is necessary: insomnia or hypersomnia; alteration in appetite with expected weight change; reduced interest in family, sexuality, work, or hobbies; increased guilt; low energy level; poor concentration; thoughts of death or suicide; frequent crying episodes; and psychomotor hypoactivity or hyperactivity. When the diagnosis of depression in the medically ill patient is being made, the emphasis is placed on psychological features as opposed to physical ones. These include rumination or repetitive negative thoughts, increased tearfulness, withdrawal from family or friends, and anhedonia. These symptoms are characteristic of a major depressive disorder for which antidepressant medications in addition to psychotherapy are recommended. In some studies, group therapy for patients with breast cancer have improved quality of life and may prolong survival.

3. **Medications.** Patients with cancer are often undertreated for major depression that has been mistaken as an "understandable" consequence of their illness or as simple grief. Evidence is beginning to accumulate that psychosocial adjustment and improved life adaptation, in general, occur when patients with cancer and major depression are treated with antidepressant medications.

   a. **Selection of agents and their side effects.** An antidepressant medication should be selected on the basis of its tendency to sedate or activate, cause orthostatic changes, or produce anticholinergic effects. Medication selection should also be tailored to the patient's symptom cluster, such as the need for sedation or weight gain versus the need for activation (Tables 33-2 and 33-3). Route of metabolism and elimination may also figure into a choice,

Table 33-2. Characteristics of commonly used heterocyclic antidepressants

Antidepressant	Sedation*	Anticholinergic actions[†]	Other Characteristics
Amitriptyline (Elavil, Endep)	+4 to +5[‡]	+4 to +5	Also available i.m., orthostasis, quinidine like, good for neuropathic pain
Doxepin (Sinequan, Adapin)	+4	+3 to +4	Highest appetite increase, orthostasis, good for neuropathic pain
Nortriptyline (Pamelor, Aventyl)	+3	+3	Less likely to cause orthostasis than other tricyclic antidepressants

* Associated with histaminergic blockade; appetite increase follows somewhat familiar trends.
[†] Constipation, dry mouth, and urinary retention.
[‡] Scale of 1–5, where 1 is least and 5 is most.
Note: Do not use tricyclic if QTc >450. Tricyclics can also suppress respiratory drive.

as may the medication's tendency to cause seizures.

Highly anticholinergic medications frequently produce dry mouth, blurred vision, tachycardia, and constipation. They can also produce urinary retention, ileus, and acute confusion. The drugs that are also antihistaminergic can increase sedation, appetite, and hypotension. Medications that produce α-adrenergic receptor blockade are associated with increased orthostatic hypotension, dizziness, and reflex tachycardia.

b. **Dosages** (Table 33-4). Weak, debilitated, or elderly patients need protection from many of these side effects. Starting out with small doses and gradually increasing the dose is prudent. Splitting doses may also be helpful for minimizing side effects and maximizing pain relief from these medications.

If a patient has a personal history, family history, or previous response to medication (e.g., steroids) that reflects mania or hypomania, it is necessary to proceed carefully, perhaps with a mood stabilizer such as lithium, or to consult psychiatry. (Table 33-5).

Table 33-3. Characteristics of commonly used nonheterocyclic antidepressants

Anti-depressant	Sedation*	Anticho-linergic actions†	Other Characteristics
Bupropion (Wellbutrin)	+1	+1	Associated with increased seizure risk especially if organic brain pathology or eating disorder is present; more activating; less weight gain
Fluoxetine (Prozac)	+1	+1	May cause restlessness and gastrointestinal upset; more activating; less weight gain; safe in patients with renal disease, but may accumulate in those with liver disease
Sertraline (Zoloft)	+1	+1	Similar to fluoxetine, more diarrhea; short half-life
Paroxetine (Paxil)	+1	+2	Similar to fluoxetine, more anticholinergic
Venlafaxine (Effexor)	+2	+1	Both serotonin and norepinephrine reuptake inhibitor; increases blood pressure at higher doses
Mirtazapine (Remeron)	+4	+2	Weight gain, potential increase in cholesterol, sedation
Nefazodone (Serzone)	+3	+2	Some sedation, less sexual side effects, mild orthostasis

* Associated with histaminergic blockade; appetite increase follows somewhat similar trends.
† Constipation, dry mouth, urinary retention, and so on.
‡ Scale of 1–5, where 1 is least and 5 is most.

    c. Monoamine oxidase inhibitors (MAOIs) may be used to treat major depression or panic disorder but are somewhat inconvenient in that tyramine dietary restrictions and medication interactions require much attention. They are often tried as an alternative when other choices have failed.

IV. Anxiety

    A. Approach to the problem. As grieving is described as normal, so is anxiety in patients with cancer. However, this anxiety varies in its cause, severity, and

Table 33-4. Dosages for antidepressant therapy

Drug	Starting daily dose (mg)	Average daily dose for patient with cancer (mg)
Amitriptyline	10–25	75–150
Bupropion	75–150	300
Doxepin	25	75–150
Fluoxetine	10–20	20
Nefazodone	50	300
Nortriptyline	10–25	50–100
Paroxetine	10–20	20
Sertraline	25–50	100
Venlafaxine	25	75 mg (37.5 mg b.i.d.)

treatment. A detailed history of the onset, characteristics, and length of distress is important. Knowledge of the patient's previous symptoms, current and past physical illness, substance abuse, and medication usage is essential to the evaluation process. Antianxiety agents may be helpful for alleviating patients' distress and helping them to cope with other problems associated with their cancer (Table 33-6).

B. Problems that present as anxiety. The duration of the symptoms is one of the first factors to assess in the anxious patients.

1. **Suspect an adjustment disorder** when maladaptive anxious symptoms have persisted less than 6 months and apparently represent an adjustment to learning the diagnosis or reactions to the treatment. This kind of anxiety may benefit from supportive therapy, relaxation therapy, or benzodiazepines.

2. **Generalized anxiety.** If the anxiety has been present for more than 6 months, continuing no matter what environmental alterations occur, and is accompanied by signs of physical tension or poor attention to conversation or other daily activities, the patient is likely to have generalized anxiety. Supportive therapy, relaxation tapes, biofeedback, buspirone, and benzodiazepines are useful.

3. **Brief, isolated episodes of anxiety** that come and go lead the examiner to consider other diagnoses.

   a. **Panic attacks.** If the patient has repeated "attacks" that have a rapid onset and last 20 minutes to a few hours, and if they are accompanied by tachycardia, palpitations, hyperventilation, sweating, dizziness, and the wish to flee, without a physical or chemical explanation, they are most likely

Table 33-5. Other medications used to treat affective disorders

Drug	Starting dose	Average dose for cancer patients	Disorders	Pretreatment workup	Follow-up studies	Comment
Stimulants* Methylphenidate (Ritalin)	2.5–5.0 mg qam	5–20 mg qam + noon	Medically ill patient with depression	CBC, check vital signs	CBC	
Pemoline (Cylert)	18.75 mg qam	37.5 mg qam + noon	Medically ill patient with depression,	Liver function tests, check vital signs	Liver function tests	Can bite tab and absorb sublingually under tongue
Lithium carbonate (Eskalith, Eskalith CR, Lithobid)	300 mg qhs	300 mg t.i.d.	Depression‡ (may need to add an antidepressant); mania‡ (may need to add clonazepam or an antipsychotic)	ECG, electrolytes, UA, BUN/creat., thyroid T₄, TSH), CBC (esp. WBC & platelets)	Lithium level initially 2 times/wk. Gradually lengthen to q3mo; thyroid studies q6mo or earlier if indicated. UA/BUN/creatinine, CBC if infection	Monitor blood level 12 hr after evening dose. 0.8–1.0 mEq/liter *is* most effective; watch for hypothyroidism diabetes insipidus, nephropathy, dehydration
Anticonvulsants Carbamazepine (Tegretol)	100 mg b.i.d.	200 mg t.i.d.	Depression or mania	CBC, reticulocytes, serum iron, liver function tests, UA, BUN, ECG	CBC, thyroid studies, blood level	Watch for leukopenia, thrombocytopenia, hepatoxicity, decreased effect of Warfarin
Valproic acid (Depakene, Depakote)	15 mg/kg/day	500–750 mg/day (divided into t.i.d. doses)	Mania	Liver function tests, CBC	Liver function tests CBC, blood level	Watch for hepatotoxicity, especially in young children

Table 33-5. *(Continued)*

Drug	Starting dose	Average dose for cancer patients	Disorders	Pretreatment workup	Follow-up studies	Comment
Benzodiazepines Clonazepam (Klonopin)	0.5 mg qhs	2 mg or higher	Mania	CBC, liver function tests	CBC, liver function tests	Do not withdraw rapidly; impaired renal function and respiratory distress require extremely cautious use
Alprazolam (Xanax)	0.5 mg qhs	1 mg t.i.d. or higher	Minor depression	Liver function tests		Do not withdraw rapidly (reduce daily dose by 0.25 mg weekly); use cautiously if respiratory impairment

* Check on weight, pulse, blood pressure. Tolerance may develop, and doses may require adjustment.
† Caution required because of multiple drug interactions.
‡ Natural or corticosteroid induced.
CBC, complete blood cell count; ECG, electrocardiogram; UA, urinalysis; BUN, blood area nitrogen; TSH, thyroid stimulating hormone.

Table 33-6.   Antianxiety agents and nighttime sedatives

Agent	Half-life (Hours)	Onset	Starting Dose (mg)*
Benzodiazepines			
Triazolam (Halcion)	1.5–3.5	Rapid	0.125 (qhs)
Oxazepam (Serax)†	8–20	Moderate	10 (t.i.d.)
Lorazepam (Ativan)†	10–20	Rapid	0.5 (t.i.d.)
Temazepam (Restoril)†	12–24	Rapid	15 (qhs)
Alprazolam (Xanax)	12–24	Moderate	0.25 (t.i.d.)
Chlordiazepoxide (Librium)	12–48	Moderate	10 (b.i.d.)
Clonazepam (Klonopin)	20–30	Rapid	0.5 (b.i.d.)
Diazepam (Valium)	20–90	Rapid	2–5 (b.i.d.)
Clorazepate (Tranxene)	20–100	Rapid	7.5 (b.i.d.)
Flurazepam (Dalmane)	20–100	Rapid	15 (qhs)
Imidazopyrine			
Zolpidem (Ambien)†	1.5–4.5	Rapid	5 (qhs)

Antidepressants (for panic disorder)
   Start at lower doses than for depression; i.e., an imipramine starting dose of 10 mg t.i.d.

β-Blockers (for autonomic symptom control)
   Propranolol (Inderal), 10–20 mg t.i.d.
   Atenolol (Tenormin), 25–50 mg daily

Antipsychotics (for anxiety associated with delirium)

Antihistamines
   May be safer in some cases when respiratory impairment is a complication; also used for insomnia.
   Diphenhydramine (Benadryl), 25 mg; starting doses b.i.d. or t.i.d.
   Hydroxyzine (Vistaril), 50 mg; starting doses t.i.d. or q.i.d.

* If chronic alcohol or benzodiazepine use exists, it is probable that the dose needed is at least double the starting doses listed.
† Preferred in the elderly.
Note: Elderly or extremely debilitated patients should be given lower doses. Caution should be taken when prescribing long-acting sedating medications because they have been associated with a high incidence of falls and hip fracture.

panic attacks that existed before the cancer. They are best treated with benzodiazepines such as clonazepam and alprazolam, antidepressants such as tricyclics, selective serotonin recept inhibitors (SSRIs), or mono animal oxidore inhibitors (MAOIs). β-Blockers to block autonomic symptoms may be tried if performance anxiety around specific activities is identified.
   b. **Organic causes are often responsible for the anxiety.**
      (1) **Hypoxia.** Repeating episodes of anxiety accompanied by alterations in intellectual functioning, poor orientation, reduced judgment, shortened

attention, a rapidly fluctuating mood, and difficulty with memory suggest hypoxia. When anxiety is induced by hypoxia, it is wise to reduce central nervous system (CNS) depressant medications and give small doses of an antipsychotic drug if the anxiety is accompanied by delirium. Antipsychotic medications, however, often produce akathisia, an extrapyramidal restlessness that mimics anxiety. Alternating the antipsychotic drug with small doses of a short half-life benzodiazepine is one option for organically induced anxiety—if respiratory status or arterial blood gas measurements do not worsen.

(2) **Liver disease and other physical disorders.** If anxiety is associated with liver disease, start by reducing CNS depressant medications. When needed, small, infrequent doses of a short-acting benzodiazepine that requires conjugation but not oxidation in the liver are prescribed. These include lorazepam, oxazepam, and temazepam. Many other physical disorders can also produce anxious symptoms, including various brain tumors, pheochromocytoma, carcinoid, hyperthyroidism, cardiac arrhythmias, drug or alcohol withdrawal, and hyperparathyroidism.

(3) **Medications** such as theophylline, corticosteroids, antidepressants, and antipsychotic drugs can produce anxiety. Anxiety is frequently one of multiple symptoms associated with benzodiazepine or narcotic analgesic withdrawal.

c. **Precipitants** can be identified in patients with cancer that initiate the previously discussed adjustment disorder lasting generally no longer than 6 months. Posttraumatic stress disorder, less often seen in patients with cancer, follows a distressing event outside the range of usual human experience. More frequently observed, however, are patients who describe intense fears of needles, radiotherapy rooms, or confined-space scanning devices. Often, the history unfolds to describe previously existing phobias. These patients, like those with anticipatory anxiety about procedures or chemotherapy, may be assisted with relaxation or desensitization techniques, imagery, antianxiety medications, and assurance. If patients begin to experience procedures, treatments, or interpersonal situations as being particularly stressful, anticipatory anxiety intensifies the requirement for larger doses of as-needed medication to attain some relief. Therefore, regular scheduling of antianxiety medication similar to that of pain medication is in order.

V. Insomnia

   A. **Principles.** Difficulty falling asleep may be associated with anxiety, whereas awakening in the middle of the night is generally more closely related to depression. In addition, there are a variety of physical disorders that cause sleeping irregularities. The sleep–wake cycle is almost always disturbed in a delirious patient, no matter what the cause. Pain often awakens a patient with cancer. Medications can awaken some patients directly (e.g., fluoxetine) or indirectly (e.g., diuretics). Aside from sorting out these influences, the physician must take into account the environment. Is the patient too hot or cold? Is the ward too brightly lit or too noisy? Do the patients awaken each time they are checked by the night staff? When any or several of these concerns are corrected, sleeping medication may not be necessary, although the need for sedatives remains in some patients.

   B. **Benzodiazepines** (see Table 33-6). This class of drugs is most often prescribed if a patient needs nighttime sedation. The shorter half-life benzodiazepines (i.e., lorazepam or temazepam) with a rapid onset produce less daytime grogginess than those with a longer half-life. Short-acting agents tend to accumulate less and are safer for patients with liver disease. On the other hand, longer half-life drugs (i.e., diazepam or flurazepam) with a rapid onset produce less unwanted awakening during the very early morning.

   C. **Antihistamines** (see Table 33-6). These medications may be chosen if the physicians are hesitant to prescribe benzodiazepines, such as for patients with respiratory disease. A disadvantage may be the higher anticholinergic potential of these drugs compared with the benzodiazepine family.

   D. **Others.** Chloral hydrate, 500 to 1,000 mg, an old standby hypnotic, can still be used as long as patients are free of gastrointestinal or liver disease. Barbiturates, such as amobarbital sodium, are occasionally used to treat some refractory sleeping disturbances for a short time but are not routinely used because they induce respiratory depression and have addictive potential.

SELECTED READINGS

Bezchlibnyk-Butler KZ, Jeffries JJ, eds. *Clinical handbook of psychotropic drugs.* 6th ed. Seattle: Hogrefe and Huber, 1996.

Breitbart W. Identifying patients at risk for, and treatment of major psychiatric complications of cancer. *Support Care Cancer* 1995; 3:45.

Holland JC, Rowland JH, ed. *Handbook of psycho-oncology.* New York: Oxford University Press, 1989.

Kane FJ, Remmel R, Moody S. Recognizing and treating delirium in patients admitted to general hospitals. *South Med J* 1993;86:985.

Lecrubier Y, Puech A. Neuropharmacology. In: Costa JE, Silva E, Nadelson CC, eds. *International Review of Psychiatry.* Vol. 1. Washington, D.C.: American Psychiatric Press, 1993:441.

Lipowski ZJ. *Delirium: Acute confusional states.* New York: Oxford University Press, 1990.

Marmelstein H, Lesko L, Holland JC. Depression in the cancer patient. *J Psycho-oncol* 1992;1:199.

Massie MJ, Gagnon P, Holland JC. Depression and suicide in patients with cancer. *J Pain Symptom Manage* 1994;9:325.

Massie MJ, Holland JC. Depression and cancer. *J Clin Psychiatr* 1990;51[Suppl]:S12.

McDaniel JS, Musselman DL, Nemeroff CB. Cancer and depression: theory and treatment. *Psychiatr Ann* 1997;27:360.

McDaniel JS, Musselman DL, Porter MR, et al. Depression in patients with cancer: diagnosis, biology and treatment. *Arch Gen Psychiatry* 1995;52:89.

Olin J, Massand P. Psychostimulants for depression in hospitalized cancer patients. *Psychosomatics* 1996;37:57.

Roth AJ, Holland JH. Psychiatric complications in cancer patients. In: Brain MC, Carbone PP, eds. *Current therapy in hematology-oncology.* 5th ed. St. Louis: CV Mosby, 1995:609.

Spiegel D, Bloom JR, Kraemer HC, Gottheil E. Effect of psychosocial treatment of patients with metastatic breast cancer. *Lancet* 1989;2:888–891.

Stiefel FC, Kornblith AB, Holland JC. Changes in the prescription patterns of psychotropic drugs for cancer patients during a 10-year period. *Cancer* 1990;65:1048.

Wise MG, Taylor SE. Anxiety and mood disorders in medially ill patients. *J Clin Psychiatry* 1990;51[suppl 1]:27.

Zonderman DB, Costa PT, McCrae PR. Depression as a risk for cancer morbidity and mortality in a nationally representative sample. *JAMA* 1989;262:1191–1195.

Nomogram for determining body surface of adults from height and mass[a]

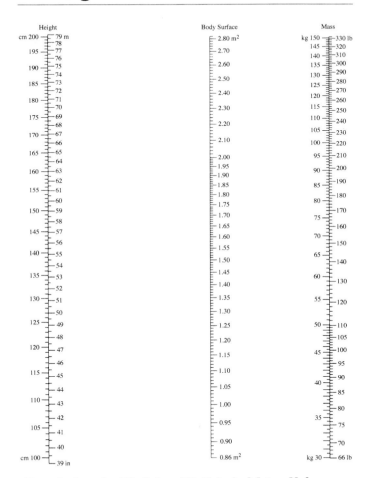

Height	Body Surface	Mass

[a] From the formula of Du Bois and Du Bois. *Arch Intern Med,* 17:863,1916 [$S = M^{0.425} \times H^{0.725} \times 71.84$, or $S = \log M \times 0.425 + \log H \times 0.725 + 1.8564$ (S, body surface in cm²; M, mass in kg; H, height in cm)]. Source: C Lenter (ed.), *Geigy Scientific Tables* (8th edition, vol. 1). Basel, Switzerland: Ciba-Geigy, 1981, p. 227.

Nomogram for determining body surface of children from height and mass[a]

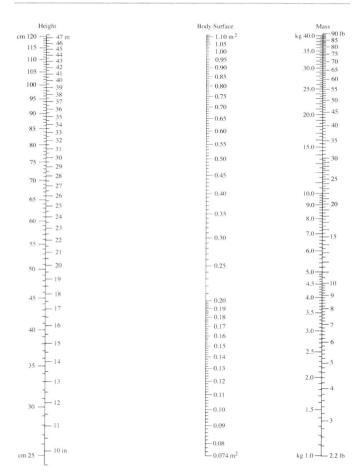

Height	Body Surface	Mass

[a] From the formula of Du Bois and Du Bois. *Arch Intern Med*, 17:863,1916 [$S = M^{0.425} \times H^{0.725} \times 71.84$, or $S = \log M \times 0.425 + \log H \times 0.725 + 1.8564$ (S, body surface in cm^2; M, mass in kg; H, height in cm)]. Source: C Lenter (ed.), *Geigy Scientific Tables* (8th edition, vol. 1). Basel, Switzerland: Ciba-Geigy, 1981, p. 226.

Screening recommendations by the American Cancer Society

| Test or procedure | Population | | Frequency |
	Sex	Age	
Sigmoidoscopy, flexible, or	M & F	50 and over	Every 5 years
Colonoscopy, or			Every 10 years
Double-contrast barium enema			Every 5–10 years
Fecal occult blood test	M & F	50 and over	Every year
Digital rectal examination	M & F	40 and over	Every time sigmoidoscopy, colonoscopy, or double-contrast barium enema is done
Prostate examination[a]	M	50 and over	Every year
Pap test	F	All women who are, or who have been, sexually active or have reached age 18 should have an annual Pap test and pelvic examination. After a woman has had three or more consecutive satisfactory normal annual examinations, the Pap test may be performed less frequently at the direction of her physician.	
Pelvic examination	F	18–40	Every 3 years with Pap test
		Over 40	Every year
Endometrial tissue sample	F	At menopause if at high risk[b]	At menopause and thereafter at the discretion of the physician

continued

Appendix C (*Continued*)

| Test or procedure | Population | | Frequency |
	Sex	Age	
Breast self examination	F	20 and over	Every month
Breast clinical physical examination	F	20–40	Every 3 years
		Over 40	Every year, close to time of mammogram
Mammography	F	40 and over	Every year
Health counseling and cancer checkup[c]	M & F	20–40	Every 3 years
	M & F	Over 40	Every year

[a] Annual digital rectal examination and prostate-specific antigen (PSA) should be performed on men 50 years and older who have at least a 10-year life expectancy, and to younger men who are at high risk. If either is abnormal, further evaluation should be considered.

[b] History of infertility, obesity, failure to ovulate, abnormal uterine bleeding or unopposed estrogen or tamoxifen therapy.

[c] To include health counseling and depending on the person's age, might include examination for cancers of the thyroid, testicle, prostate, ovaries, lymph nodes, oral region, and skin as well as for some non-malignant disease.

From the American Cancer Society. Cancer Facts and Figures. 1998. Atlanta.

Selected Oncology Web Sites

1. American Society of Hematology
   http://www.hematology.org/index.cfm
2. American Cancer Society (ACS statistics, other information, links to states)
   http://www.cancer.org
3. American Society of Clinical Oncology
   http://www.asco.org
4. Agency for Health Care Policy and Research homepage
   http://www.ahcpr.gov
5. Search MEDLINE: PubMed and Internet Grateful Med
   http://www.nlm.nih.gov/databases/freemedl.html
   a. Welcome to PubMed (handy for searching medline and getting abstracts)
      http://www.ncbi.nlm.nih.gov/PubMed
6. Harvard Center for Cancer Prevention
   http://www.hsph.harvard.edu/organizations/ canprevent/index.html
7. Health Services/Technology Assessment Text
   http://text.nlm.nih.gov
8. National Cancer Institute's CancerNet Cancer Information (NCI information, including PDQ, clinical trials information, Journal of National Cancer Institute, statistics)
   http://cancernet.nci.nih.gov
   a. Treatment information for health professionals
      http://cancernet.nci.nih.gov/h_treat.htm
   b. Cancer Therapy Evaluation Program (CTEP) homepage (site for common toxicity criteria)
      http://ctep.info.nih.gov
9. Rxlist, the Internet Drug Index (some cancer drugs as well as other drugs)
   http://www.rxlist.com
10. Newspapers, TV and the weather (to keep some attachment to the real world)
    a. The Weather Channel
       http://www.weather.com (if in case, like me, you have no windows in your office)
    b. CNN Interactive
       http://www.cnn.com
    c. New York Times
       http://www.nytimes.com
    d. Newspapers around the world
       http://excite.com/news/world_newspapers

Subject Index

Page number followed by *t* indicates a table.